KININS V
Part B

ADVANCES IN EXPERIMENTAL MEDICINE AND BIOLOGY

Recent Volumes in this Series

KININS V
Part B

Edited by

Keishi Abe
Tohoku University School of Medicine
Sendai, Miyagi, Japan

Hiroshi Moriya
Science University of Tokyo
Tokyo, Japan

and

Setsuro Fujii
The Osaka Foundation for Promotion of
  Fundamental Medical Research
Otsu, Shiga, Japan

PLENUM PRESS • NEW YORK AND LONDON

Library of Congress Cataloging in Publication Data

International Kinin Congress (5th: 1987: Tokyo, Japan)
(Advances in experimental medicine and biology; v. 247)
"Proceedings of the Fifth International Kinin Congress, held November 29–December 3, 1987, in Tokyo, Japan"—T.p. verso.
Bibliography: p.
Includes index.
1. Kinins—Congresses. 2. Kallikrein—Congresses. I. Abe, Keishi, 1933–   . II. Moriya, Hiroshi. III. Fujii, Setsurō, 1925–   . IV. Series.
QP552.K5I54   1989   89-3935
599′.01924
ISBN-13: 978-1-4615-9548-9   e-ISBN-13: 978-1-4615-9546-5
DOI: 10.1007/978-1-4615-9546-5

Second half of the proceedings of the Fifth International Kinin Congress,
held November 29–December 3, 1987, in Tokyo, Japan

© 1989 Plenum Press, New York
Softcover reprint of the hardcover 1st edition 1989
A Division of Plenum Publishing Corporation
233 Spring Street, New York, N.Y. 10013

PREFACE

The physiological and pathological significance of the kallikrein-kinin system was recently explored extensively, resulting in a rapid accumulation of information regarding their potential importance. This publication provides an integrated picture of the latest information on the kallikrein-kinin system. It contains contributions from morphologists, geneticists, biochemists, pharmacologists, physiologists, and clinicians.

The Fifth International Kinin Congress (Nov. 29-Dec. 3, 1987) provided a forum for the exchange of information and ideas on the kallikrein-kinin system. The participation of more than 350 scientists from 23 countries reflects the widespread interest and international scope of research activity in the physiological and pathological functions of the kallikrein-kinin system. A total of 275 papers including posters were presented, attesting to the unquestioned success of this Congress. These proceedings, in two volumes, contain the collective studies presented, studies of high scientific standard that provoked stimulating and fruitful discussions. Also included in these volumes are the two plenary lectures presented by Dr. H.A. Margolius (USA) and Dr. S. Nakanishi (Japan).

During the last decade our knowledge of the role of the kallikrein-kinin system in health and disease has been greatly advanced by the development of antagonists to bradykinin and the introduction to clinical practice of converting enzyme inhibitors. Symposia on converting enzyme and on recent advances in research on the kallikrein-kinin system are included in the proceedings.

On behalf of the organizing committee, the editors of these volumes express their sincere gratitude for the support of the Ministry of Education, the Scientific Council of Japan, and the following academic societies in the various branches of medical science: the Japanese Biochemical Society, the Japanese Pharmacological Society, the Pharmaceutical Society of Japan, the Japan Hematological Society, Japanese College of Angiology, the Japanese Rheumatism Association, and the Japanese Society of Allergology. We also wish to thank the following sponsors: Uehara Memorial Foundation, the Naito Foundation, the Mochida Memorial Foundation for Medical and Pharmaceutical Research, the Pharmaceutical Manufacturers Association of Tokyo, Osaka Pharmaceutical Manufacturers Association, Bayer Yakuhin Ltd., Sanwa Kagaku Kenkyusho Co., Ltd., CIBA-GEIGY (Japan) Ltd., Nippon Roche K.K., Fujimoto Pharmaceutical Corporation, and many others.

Satellite meetings in Kyoto, Sapporo, and Tokushima provided additional opportunities for interaction and friendship. Our social times together left some unforgettable memories.

We hope these volumes will provide not only an update of current knowledge, but also stimulate further research into the role of the kallikrein-kinin system in health and disease.

We would like to express our sincere thanks to the editors of Plenum Press for their cooperation in publishing these volumes speedily and attractively.

Keishi Abe
Setsuro Fujii
Hiroshi Moriya

KALLIKREIN AND OTHER PROTEASE INHIBITORS

TISSUE KININOGENASES

PLASMA KALLIKREIN-KININ AND RELATED SYSTEMS

KININOGENS, KININS, AND RELATED SUBSTANCES

KININASES

KALLIKREIN-KININ IN HEALTH AND DISEASES

CONTENTS - PART A

KININ RECEPTORS AND ANTAGONISTS

PLASMA KALLIKREIN-KININ AND RELATED SYSTEMS

TISSUE KALLIKREINS

KALLIKREIN-KININ IN HEALTH AND DISEASES

NATRIURESIS AND KALLIKREIN-KININ

HUMAN KALLISTATIN, A NEW TISSUE KALLIKREIN-BINDING PROTEIN:

PURIFICATION AND CHARACTERIZATION

Maoyin Wang, Joseph Day, Lee Chao and Julie Chao

Departments of Pharmacology and Biochemistry
Medical University of South Carolina
Charleston, S.C. 29425, U.S.A.

A new and specific tissue kallikrein-binding protein was identified in mammalian serum and in secreted transformed-cell culture media (Chao et al., Biochem. J. 239: 325-331, 1986). We have designated this kallikrein-binding protein as "kallistatin". Human kallistatin has been purified from serum, using chromatographic steps including DEAE-Sephadex, hydroxylapatite, Cibacron blue-Sepharose, Sephacryl S200, and preparative polyacrylamide gel electrophoresis. The purified kallistatin consists of a single polypeptide chain with an apparent molecular weight of ~ 54 kDa and isoelectric point of ~ 5.0. Kallistatin was eluted as a single peak on reverse-phase HPLC. The purified kallistatin and ^{125}I-labelled human tissue kallikrein form a ~ a 92 kDa SDS- and heat-stable complex. The complex formation is pH dependent and is inhibited by 0.1% (W/V) of deoxycholate or SDS but not by 0.5% (W/V) of Triton X-100, digitonin, Lubrol or CHAPS. A ~ 54 kDa protein was identified in partially purified kallistatin by polyclonal anti-kallistatin antibodies in Western blot analysis and by its binding to ^{125}I-labelled-human tissue kallikrein in ligand blotting. The role of kallistatin in regulating tissue kallikrein activity and metabolism may now be evaluated.

INTRODUCTION

Release of tissue kallikrein into the vasculature of some organs has been demonstrated, and it is clear from several studies that tissue kallikreins circulate systemically (1-3). The enzymatic activity of circulating tissue kallikrein appears to be very low, and the presence of high molecular weight complexes of kallikrein in sera suggests that circulating kallikrein may be bound to inhibitors (3). Specific tissue kallikrein-binding proteins have not yet been identified. We have recently identified a new kallikrein-binding protein in the systemic circulation and in the secreted media of human lung fibroblasts (W-138), rodent neuroblastoma-glioma hybrids (NG-108) (4) and mouse anterior pituitary cells (At T20). Purified and ^{125}I-labelled tissue kallikrein and the binding protein specifically form a ~ 92 kDa SDS- and heat-stable complex. We have also isolated and identified ~ 92 kDa endogenous kallikrein and binding protein complex in human plasma (4), rat urine, and kidney (5,6). The results presented here show the purification and characterization of tissue kallikrein-binding protein from human plasma.

Experimental

Binding Assay of Binding Protein to Tissue Kallikrein

Human urinary kallikrein was purified to homogeneity and labelled with ^{125}I according to the lactoperoxidase method (7). Aliquots of human plasma or eluates from column fractions (desalted with Sephadex G-25 if necessary) were incubated with ^{125}I-human urinary kallikrein and the kallikrein-binding protein complex was separated and identified followacrylamide electrophoresis and densitometric scanning of the autoradiograms (4).

Preparative Gel Electrophoresis

Preparative SDS-PAGE was utilized following DEAE-Sephadex, hydroxylapatite, Cibacron blue-sepharose, and Sephacryl S200 column chromatography. A 7.5-15% linear gradient polyacrylamide slab gel (14 x 16 x 0.15 cm) containing 0.1% SDS was used for preparative electrophoresis. Sample of ~ 1 mg protein was electrophoresed and the gel was immersed into ice-cold 1 M KCl solution for 30 min at 4°C until the precipitated protein bands became visible. Protein bands with electrophoretic mobility from 45,000 to 67,000 daltons were cut; and the gel slices were crushed and eluted into 1.0 ml of 0.01 M sodium phosphate, pH 7.0, on a rocker platform at 4°C for 12 h. The gel fragments were removed and the filtrate was spun in a Microfuge for 10 min. The supernatant after micro desalting with Sephadex G25 were examined for both protein staining and binding activity to kallikrein.

High-Pressure Liquid Chromatography (HPLC)

The HPLC apparatus consisted of a Varian 5060 Chromatograph equipped with a Varian recorder and two wavelength variable UV detectors. A Vydac 214 TP54 protein C_4 column (0.4 x 25 cm) was used for the separation. The elution system consisted of a linear gradient of acetonitrile in the presence of trifluoroacetic acid (TFA). Solvent A consisted of 0.1% TFA in water, and solvent B contained 0.1% TFA in acetonitrile/water (90:10) (V/V). Elution was performed at a flow rate of 1% acetonitrile/ min at room temperature, using the linear gradient specified in the legends of the figure.

Western Blotting and Ligand Blotting

Kallistatin recovered from preparative gels were used to raise antibodies in rabbits as described (8). In Western blot analysis, kallistatin was rendered visible by immunoperoxidase staining as described previously (9). For ligand binding the blots were first saturated with 3% BSA and then soaked at 37°C for 4 h in 0.01 M Tris, pH 7.8, containing ^{125}I-human urinary kallikrein (5 x 10^5 cpm/ml), 1% BSA, 0.05% Tween-20, and 0.02 M NaCl. The blots were washed 3 to 4 times with 0.01 M Tris-HCl, pH 7.8, containing 0.02 M NaCl, 0.05% Tween-20 for 10 min each. The blots were air dried and exposed to X-ray film at -70°C for 24-48 h.

RESULTS

Purification of human tissue kallikrein-binding protein

Kallikrein-binding proteins present in the fractions of various chromatographic steps were assayed by incubating the aliquots with ^{125}I-labelled kallikrein (Mr ~ 38 kDa); and the presence of kallikrein-binding protein was monitored by the detection of a radiolabelled ~ 92 kDa SDS-stable protein complex by PAGE. Purification of kallikrein-binding protein from human plasma was carried out in the following steps:

Step 1: DEAE-Sephadex Chromatography. Human plasma (50 ml) was centrifuged at 10,000 g for 30 min to remove any precipitates. Plasma sample was dialyzed against 0.05 N NaCl, 0.01 M sodium phosphate, pH 7.0, for 24 h at 4°C and then passed through a DEAE-Sephadex column (2.5 x 25 cm), previously equilibrated with the same buffer, until the absorbance of the effluent at 280 nm dropped to below 0.05 unit. The adsorbed proteins were then eluted with a linear NaCl gradient from 0.05 to 0.4 M. Fractions containing kallikrein binding activity were eluted at 0.15-0.25 M NaCl, 0.01 M sodium phosphate, pH 7.0 as indicated in the shaded area (Fig. 1a).

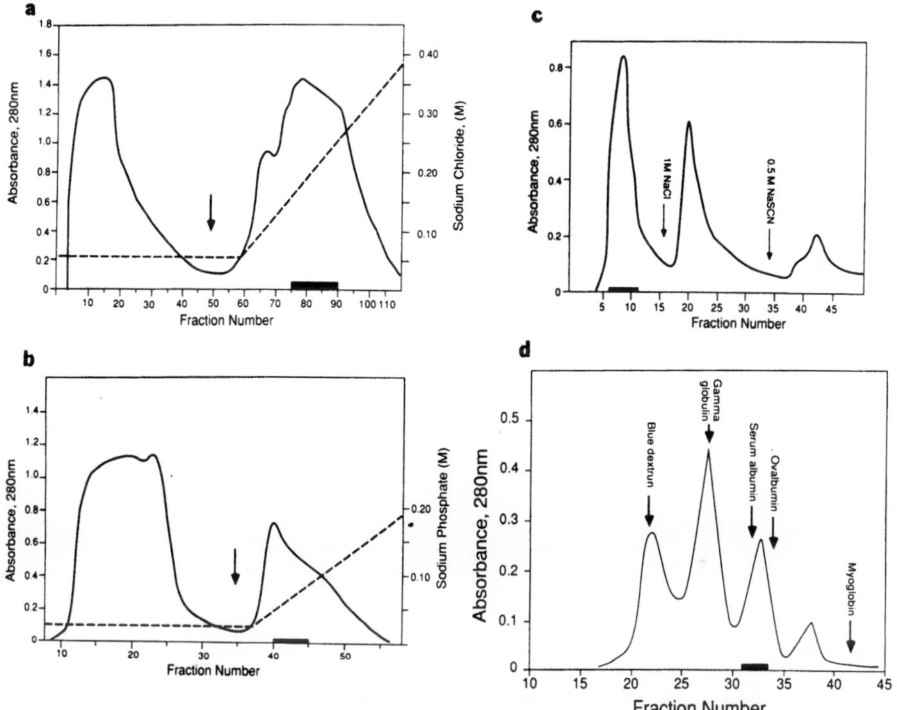

Figure 1. (a) DEAE-Sephadex chromatography of kallikrein-binding protein.
(b) Hydroxylapatite chromatography of kallikrein-binding protein. (c) Cibacron Blue-sepharose chromatography of kallikrein-binding protein. (d) Sephacryl S200 column chromatography of kallikrein-binding protein. The solid bar represents the fractions with kallikrein-binding activity.

Step 2: Hydroxylapatite Chromatography. Fractions containing kallikrein-binding fractions were pooled and dialyzed against 0.01 M sodium phosphate, pH 7.4, and applied to a hydroxylapatite column (3.0 x 25 cm) equilibrated with the same buffer. The column was subsequently washed with the equilibration buffer and the elution was performed with a linear gradient of 0.01 M to 0.2 M sodium phosphate, pH 7.4. Kallikrein-binding protein activity was eluted at 0.04-0.07 M sodium phosphate, pH 7.4, as indicated in the shaded area (Figure 1b).

Step 3: Cibacron Blue-Sepharose Chromatography. The fractions containing kallikrein binding activity were pooled and passed through a Blue-sepharose CL-4B column (2.5 x 20 cm) equilibrated with 0.02 M sodium phosphate, pH 7.0. The adsorbed proteins were eluted with 1 M NaCl in 0.02 M sodium phosphate, pH 7.0, and then followed by 0.5 M sodium thiocyanate. Kallikrein-binding activity appeared only in the flow-through fractions (Fig. 1c).

Step 4: Sephacryl S200 Chromatography. Fractions containing kallikrein-binding activity from the Blue-Sepharose CL-4B column were combined, lyophilized, and dissolved in 0.1 N NaCl, 0.01 M sodium phosphate, pH 7.0. The protein solution was applied and eluted from a Sephacryl S200 column (2.5 x 95 cm) with 0.1 N NaCl, 0.01 M sodium phosphate, pH 7.0 (Fig. 1d).

Step 5: Preparative Polyacrylamide Gel Electrophoresis. Kallikrein-binding protein was purified further by preparative SDS-PAGE.

Characterization of Kallikrein-binding protein

Kallikrein-binding proteins eluted from a preparative gel were assayed for the kallikrein-binding activity and separated on a SDS-PAGE under reducing conditions. Fig. 2A shows protein staining with Coomassie Blue, whereas Fig. 2B shows that kallikrein-binding protein migrates as a single protein band with apparent molecular weight of 54 kDa, which forms a 92 kDa SDS- and heat-stable complex upon binding to ^{125}I-human urinary kallikrein. In two-dimensional gel separation, the purified kallikrein-binding protein appeared in the 1st-dimensional isoelectric focusing with pI of ~ 5.0 and in the 2nd-dimensional SDS-gel with estimated Mr of ~ 54 kDa (data not shown). Gel filtration on a

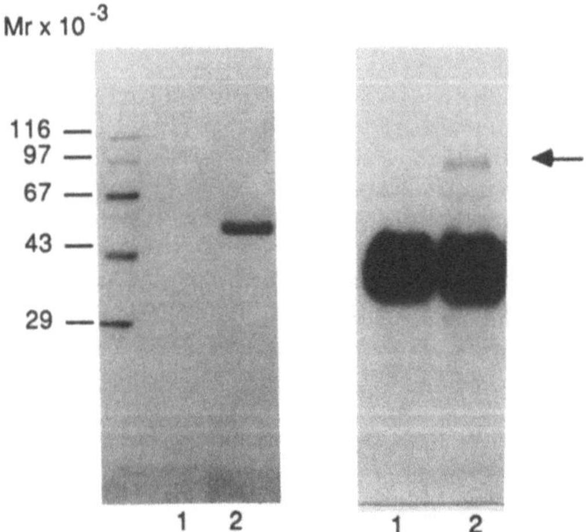

Figure 2. Polyacrylamide gel electrophoresis of human kallikrein-binding protein. Purified human kallistatin (~5 µg) was incubated with ^{125}I-labelled human urinary kallikrein, and electrophoresis was performed in a linear gradient (7.5-15%) polyacrylamide gel. (A) Coomassie blue protein staining. (B) Autoradiograms. ^{125}I-human urinary kallikrein (lane 1), ^{125}I-human urinary kallikreikn incubated with purified human kallistatin (lane 2).

Sephacryl S200 column revealed kallikrein-binding activity in the
fractions between bovine serum albumin and ovalbumin with estimated
molecular weight of ~ 54 kDa (Fig. 1d). Reversed-phase high pressure
liquid chromatography (HPLC) of purified human kallikrein-binding
protein showed a single sharp peak at 56 min with a small shoulder peak
at 67 min, indicating more than 95% homogeneity of the binding protein
(Fig. 3).

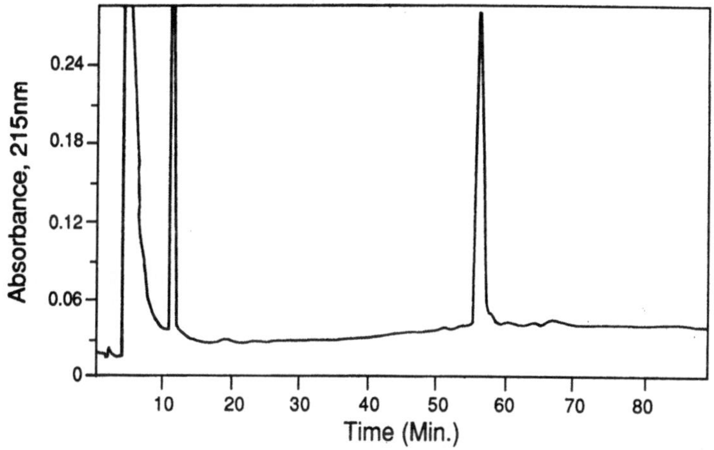

Figure 3. Reversed-phase HPLC of human kallikrein-binding protein. The
         protein (50 µg) injected at time 0 min and eluted with a 3-70%
         acetonitrile gradient in 0.1% trifluoroacetic acid in 70 min.
         The elution peak at 12 min is formic acid, and the peak eluted
         at 56 min is human kallikrein-binding protein.

The complex formation between tissue kallikrein and the binding
protein is pH dependent. When Tris-HCl buffer, pH 7.0-9.0, was used in
the assay buffer, the binding was maximum at pH 8.5. There was no
significant difference of the complex formation when 0.01 M sodium
phosphate, pH 7.0, or phosphate-buffered saline, pH 7.3, was used.
Neutral detergents such as Triton X-100, digitonin, and Lubrol at 0.5%
(W/V) had no effect on the complex formation of kallikrein and kallikrein-binding protein. In contrast, anionic detergents such as deoxycholate or SDS at 0.1% (W/V) completely prevented complex formation
(Fig. 4).

Western Blot and Ligand Blot Analyses of Kallikrein-Binding Protein

Antiserum raised in rabbits against purified human kallikrein-binding protein was subsequently used in immunoblot analysis of partially
purified fractions from human plasma. The nitrocellulose was blocked,
followed by incubation with polyclonal anti-kallikrien-binding protein
antiserum. Western blot analysis on nitrocellulose showed that the
antibody specifically localized a single 54 kDa band (Fig. 5) and that
this band also bound ^{125}I-human urinary kallikrein in ligand blot analysis (Fig. 5). The results from ligand blot analyses confirmed that the
~ 54 kDa protein identified in Western blotting is a kallikrein-binding
protein.

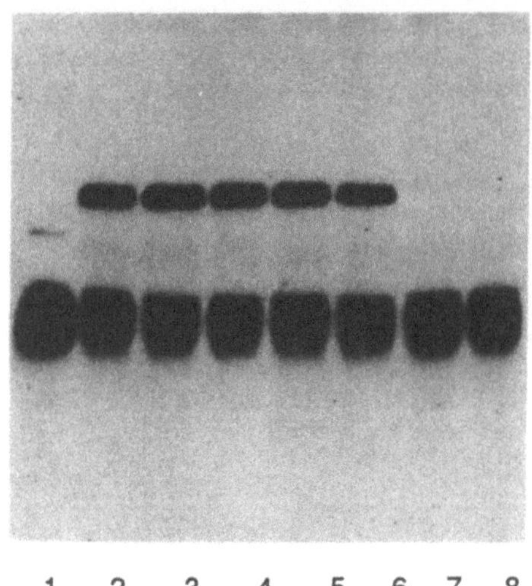

Figure 4. Effect of detergents on kallikrein and binding protein complex formation. Lane 1, ^{125}I-kallikrein alone; lanes 2-8, ^{125}I-kallikrein incubated with human plasma with the addition of detergents. No detergent added (lane 2), 0.5% (W/V) Triton X-100 (lane 3), 0.5% digitonin (lane 4), 0.5% Lubrol (lane 5), 0.5% CHAPS (lane 6), 0.1% sodium deoxycholate (lane 7), 0.1% sodium dodecylsulphate (lane 8).

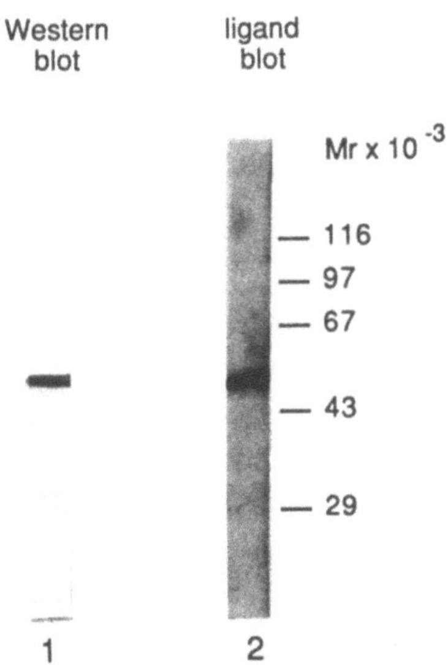

Figure 5. Western blot and ligand blot analyses of human kallikrein-binding protein.

DISCUSSION

In the present report, we describe the purification and characterization of a tissue kallikrein-binding protein from human serum. The purified binding- protein and tissue kallikrein form a 92 kDa SDS- and heat-stable complex. The apparent molecular weight of kallikrein-binding protein is ~ 54 kDa as determined by SDS-PAGE, gel filtration, and ligand blotting. The binding protein is an acidic protein with isoelectric point ~ 5.0. We have designated this kallikrein-binding protein "kallistatin".

The binding of kallikrein to kallistatin is specific, since other serine proteinases such as plasma kallikrein, urokinase, or thrombin cannot compete with the binding. Kallistatin is acid- and heat-labile, while the complex is quite resistant to acid, heat, alkali, or hydroxylamine treatment (4). The complex formation is inhibited completely by anionic detergent but not by neutral detergents. The binding site may involve active site residues (serine or histidine) of tissue kallikrein since active site-blocked kallikrein can no longer form complexes with kallikrein-binding protein (4).

Kallistatin is a specific binding protein for tissue kallikrein. Previously we have shown that kallistatin is distinct from known plasma protease inhibitors (4). In the present study, we have also excluded the possible identity of kallistatin with Protease Nexin I and II (serine protease regulators) from human foreskin fibroblast cell cultures and with plasminogen activator inhibitor from bovine endothelium. Tissue kallikrein cannot form SDS- and heat-stable complexes with purified Protease Nexin I and II under reducing conditions (data not shown). In contrast to Protease Nexins with PI ~ 7.5, kallistatin is an acidic protein.

The biological function of kallistatin is unknown at this time, but it could exert a regulatory effect on kallikrein metabolism. Tissue kallikrein activity may be regulated at the level of biosynthesis, by secretion from producer cells, by the activation of inactive proenzyme forms or by the stimulation or inhibition of the enzyme activity of the activators. Our preliminary studies show that kallistatin cannot form a complex with prokallikrein (latent enzyme) (data not shown). A similar case has been described (10) for urokinase, which is synthesized and secreted as a proenzyme from human foreskin fibroblasts and thus escapes the inhibition from Protease Nexin-like inhibitors secreted from the same cells. Synthesis and secretion of prokallikrein has been identified in rat pancreas, kidney, pituitary, and brain (11-15). These findings suggest that prokallikrein may be protected and that kallistatin may participate in modulating active kallikrein in tissues or in circulation. The biological function of kallistatin and the fate of the kallikrein-kallistatin complex will be further investigated.

REFERENCES

1. W.J. Lawton, D. Proud, M.E. French, J.V. Pierce, H.S. Keizer, and J.J. Pisano, Characterization and origin of immunoreactive glandular kallikrein in rat plasma, Biochem. Pharmacol. 30: 1731-1737 (1981).
2. S.F. Rabito, A.G. Scicli, and O.A. Carretero, Immunoreactive glandular kallikrein in plasma, in "Enzymatic Release of Vasoactive Peptides," F. Gross, and G. Volgel, eds. pp247-258, Raven Press, New York (1980).

3. K. Shimamoto, R.K. Mayfield, H.S. Margolius, J. Chao, W. Stroud, and A.P. Kaplan, The measurement of immunoreactive glandular kallikrein in human serum and its clinical application, <u>J. Lab. Clin. Med</u>. 103: 731-738 (1984).

4. J. Chao, D.M. Tillman, M. Wang, H.S. Margolius and L. Chao, Identification of a new tissue kallikrein-binding protein, <u>Biochem J</u>. 239: 325-331 (1986).

5. C. Woodley, J. Chao, H.S. Margolius, and L. Chao, Specific identification of tissue kallikrein in exocrine tissues and in cell-free translation products with monoclonal antibodies, <u>Biochem. J</u>. 231: 721-728 (1985).

6 . J. Chao and L. Chao, Rat Urinary Kallikrein, <u>in</u> "Methods in Enzymology, Immunochemical Techniques," G. DiSabato, J.J. Langone, and H. Van Vunakis, eds. Academic Press, N.Y., in press (1986).

7 . K. Shimamoto, J. Chao, and H.S. Margolius, The development and application of a direct radioimmunoassay for human urinary kallikrein, <u>J. Clin. Endocrinol. Metab</u>. 51: 840-848 (1980).

8. J. Chao, and H.S. Margolius, Isozymes of rat urinary kallikrein, <u>Biochem. Pharmacol</u>. 28: 2071-2079 (1979).

9. J. Chao, C. Woodley, L. Chao, and H.S. Margolius, Identification of tissue kallikrein in brain and in the cell-free translation product encoded by brain mRNA, <u>J. Biol. Chem</u>. 258: 15173-15178 (1983).

10. D.L. Eaton, R.W. Scott, and J.B. Baker, Purification of human fibroblast urokinase proenzyme and analysis of its regulation by proteases and protease nexin, <u>J. Biol. Chem</u>. 259: 6241-6247 (1984).

11. C. Woodley, J. Chao, and L. Chao, Immunologic analysis of rat pancreatic prokallikrein activation, <u>Biochem. Biophys. Acta</u> 829: 408-414 (1985).

12. R. Matsas, D. Proud, K. Nustad, and G.S. Bailey, Rapid purification of a prekallikrein from rat pancreas, <u>Anal. Biochem</u>. 113: 264-270 (1981).

13. K. Nishimura, H. Shimizu, and T. Kokubu, Existence of prokallikrein in the kidney. Its biochemical properties compared to three active glandular kallikreins from kidney, serum and urine, <u>Hypertension</u> 5: 205-210 (1983).

14. Powers, C.A., Anterior pituitary glandular kallikrein: trypsin activation and estrogen regulation, <u>Mol. Cell. Endocrinol</u>. 46, 163-174 (1986).

15. J. Chao, L. Chao, Identification of latent tissue kallikrein, prolactin and growth hormone secretion in GH_3 pituitary cells using modified radioimmunoassays, <u>Mol. Cell Endocrinol</u>., in press.

THE DESIGN OF SPECIFIC INHIBITORS OF TISSUE KALLIKREIN

AND THEIR EFFECT ON THE BLOOD PRESSURE OF THE RAT

James Burton and Athanassios Benetos*

Evans Department of Clinical Research
University Hospital
Boston, MA USA

*Boston University Medical Center
Boston, MA USA

INTRODUCTION

The role of tissue kallikrein (E.C. 3.4.21.35) in the maintenance of blood pressure is controversial. Administration of kinins, the product of cleavage of kininogen by tissue kallikrein, lowers blood pressure in test animals (Reviewed in Haddy et al., 1970). This is though to occur by several mechanisms including the release of endothelium derived relaxing factors (Toda et al., 1987).

Most experiments aimed at clarifying the role of kinins in the maintenance of normal blood pressure are indirect. Blaine et al. (1985) and Oldham et al. (1986) reported that administration of converting enzyme inhibitors to salt depleted animals lowered blood pressure more than when renin inhibitors were given alone. Precise studies by Iimura et al. (1986) show that in humans the decrease in blood pressure caused by acute administration of converting enzyme inhibitors is better correlated with increases in circulating kinin levels than with decreases in angiotensin II levels. The implication of these experiments is that potentiation of kinin levels contributes to the hypotensive action of converting enzyme inhibitors. Kinins could thus have some role in controlling normal blood pressure.

In direct experiments, Benetos et al. (1986) reported that administration of a kinin receptor blocker raised blood pressure in test animals. While this is consistent with kinins having a role in blood pressure regulation, the pressor action may also have been due to catecholamine release (Mulinari et al., 1988).

Clearly, much circumstantial evidence indicates that kinins may be involved in blood pressure control. Since there are multiple sources of tissue kallikrein in the body, a specific inhibitor, rather than ablation, must be used to clarify the physiologic role of the enzyme.

---

*Present address: Dr. A. Benetos, 109 Agiaf Zonis, Poatia Koliatfou,
          Athens, Greece.

The design of specific inhibitors of tissue kallikrein was initiated to produce experimental drugs which could be used to define the role of kinins in vivo. Since serine proteinases are involved in many diverse physiologic functions such as blood clotting and complement fixation, inhibitors of tissue kallikrein must have high specificity to yield clear results in physiologic experiments.

Previously reported inhibitors such as aprotinin (Fritz et al., 1979) and the chloromethylketones (Kettner, et al., 1980) bind tightly to tissue kallikrein, but are relatively non-specific and cannot be used to clearly show which, if any, role tissue kallikrein plays in vivo.

Examination of the sequences of the naturally occurring substrates of the serine proteases (McRae et al., 1981) indicates that the amino acid residue which occurs at position P_2 usually has a small side chain. The kallikreins are unique among the naturally occurring serine proteases in recognizing a bulky amino acid residue (phenylalanine) at this position.

The impression that the S_2 subsite of tissue kallikrein will accommodate a bulky amino acid residue is supported by a study with tripeptide nitroanilides which have the sequence D-Cha-Xaa-Arg-4NA* (Okunishi et al. 1986). Binding constants (K_I, μM) for a series of tripeptides in which the residue at P_2 (Xaa) was varied were: Cha, 2.1; Phe, 3.7; Leu, 5.9; and Pro, 16.0. The correlation between the size of the side chain at P_2 and the strength of binding to the proteinase indicates that the amino acid residue at this position may, in part, make kininogen a specific substrate for tissue kallikrein. Inhibitors based on the amino acid sequence of kininogen around the cleavage site – "substrate analog approach" (Burton, 1984) – may thus be relatively specific for tissue kallikrein.

Okunishi et al. (1985) showed that the substrate analog KKI-5 which has the sequence Ac-Pro-Phe-Arg-Ser-Val-Gln-NH$_2$ is a relatively specific competitive inhibitor for tissue kallikrein (Table 1). Replacement of the N-terminal acetylproline group with the bulky cyclohexylacetyl group [cHxAc] yielded the competitive inhibitor KKI-7 which has an even better specificity for tissue kallikrein (Table 1). In addition KKI-7 binds to human tissue kallikrein about 40-fold better than KKI-5.

About 30 proteinases and hormone receptors have been evaluated for inhibition by KKI-5 and KKI-7. The subset of these which are thought to play some role in blood pressure control are shown in Table 1. None of the proteinases or receptors is significantly inhibited. KKI-7 thus meets in vitro requirements as an experimental drug for the specific inhibition of tissue kallikrein.

IN VIVO EXPERIMENTS

In vivo tests of the effect of KKI-7 on blood pressure were done with the standard rat model of blood pressure (Benetos et al., 1986; Fig 1). Laboratory rats were fitted with a arterial and venous catheters. After 24 hrs for recovery, the animals were infused into the jugular vein with

---

*Standard IUPAC-IUB nomenclature is used for the amino acids. 1972, J. Biol. Chem., 247:977. Cha, cyclohexylalanine; Xaa, variable amino acid, 4NA, p-nitroanilide.

TABLE 1

Tests for the Specificity of Tissue Kallikrein
K_I (μM)

Protease	Species	KKI-5	KKI-7
Tissue kallikrein	Human	156	4
Tissue kallikrein	Rat	--	30
Tonin	Rat	843	ND
Plasma Kallikrein	Cow	1255	244
Renin	Human	ND	--
Converting Enzyme	Rabbit	400	--
Angiotensin II Receptor	Rat	ND	ND
Kallikrein Receptor	Rat	ND	ND
Vasopressin (V1) Receptor	Rat	ND	ND
α_1 and α_2 Receptor	Chicken	ND	ND
β_1 and β_2 Receptor	Chicken	ND	ND
ANP Receptor	Rat	--	ND

ND, not detectable; --, not done; ANP, atrial natriuretic peptide.

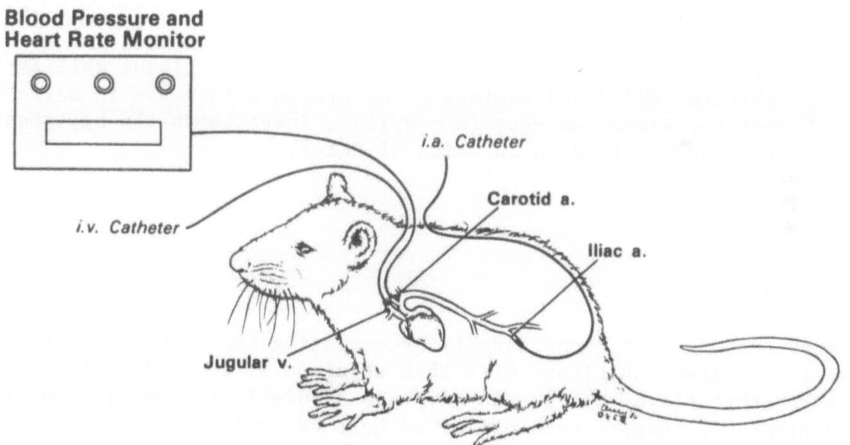

Fig 1 Rat model used to investigate the effect of KKI-7 on rat blood pressure.

various concentrations of KKI-7 dissolved in water:propylene glycol::1:1.
Flow rate was set at 200 μL/min. Maximum concentration of the inhibitor
was 5 mg/mL. The rats were on a normal sodium diet and were restrained,
but conscious during the experiments. Sixteen animals were infused at
each concentration of inhibitor. Eight of the animals (50%) responded to
the infusion and results from these animals averaged (Fig 2).

Blood pressure in the rat rose in response to the inhibitor, but not
the vehicle. The maximum increase (Fig 2) at high doses ($\sim$1.5 mg/kg/min)
is about 30 Torr. ED_{50} for the experiments is 0.8 mg/kg. When infusion
of the inhibitor was terminated, blood pressure of the test animals
returned to normal levels within 3 mins (Fig 2, inset).

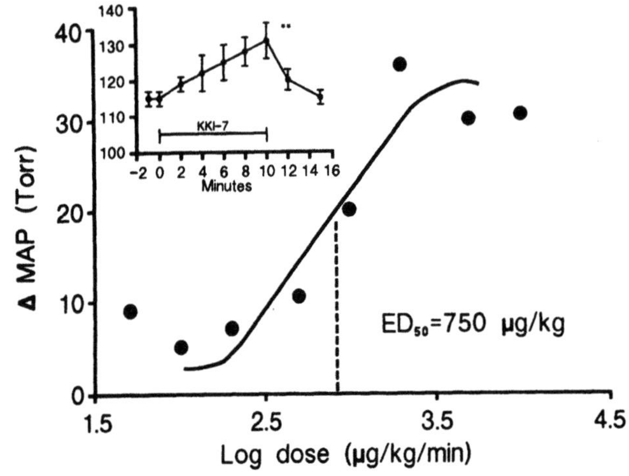

Fig 2   Relationship between the dose of the specific tissue kallikrein
inhibitor KKI-7 and maximum blood pressure increase in salt-
replete, conscious rats (n = 8/16). Inset shows the hypertensive
response obtained on infusion of KKI-7.

DISCUSSION

Previous research, done largely by comparing the hypotensive effect of
converting enzyme inhibitors with that obtained by renin inhibitors,
indicates that tissue kallikrein may have a role in the regulation of
blood pressure. Experiments presented here support this hypothesis by
showing that infusion of an inhibitor which meets _in vitro_ criteria for
specificity raises blood pressure in test animals. While additional
experiments to validate _in vivo_ use of the inhibitor remain to be done,
experiments presented here are the first direct evidence that tissue
kallikrein is involved in the regulation of blood pressure in normal rats.

ACKNOWLEDGMENTS

Support for this research came from the NIH grant HL-38212. We are
grateful for the synthesis, purification, and characterization of KKI-7 by
O. David Carretero.

Benetos, A., Gavras, H., Stewart, J. M. Vavrek, R. J., Hatinoglou, S., Gavras, I., 1986, Vasodepressor role of endogenous bradykinin assessed by a bradykinin antagonist, Hypertension, 8:971.

Blaine, E. H., Nelson, B. J., Seymour, A. A., Schorn, T. W., Sweet, C. S., Slater, E. E., Nussberger, J., Boger, J., 1985, Comparison of renin and converting enzyme inhibition in sodium-deficient dogs, Hypertension, 7:166.

Burton, J., 1984, The design of substrate analog inhibitors of highly specific proteases, in: "Conformationally Directed Drug Design," J. A. Vida, M. Gordon, eds., American Chemical Society, Washington.

Haddy, F. J., Emerson, T. E., Jr., Scott, J. B., Daugherty, R. M., Jr., 1970, The effects of kinins on the cardiovascular system, in: "Handbook of experimental pharmacology, XXV Suppl." E. G. Erdos, ed., Springer Verlag, New York.

Fritz, H., Fink, E., Truscheit, E., 1979, Kallikrein inhibitors, Fed. Proc., 38:2753.

Iimura, O., Shimamoto, K., Tanaka, S., Hosoda, S., Nishitani, T., Ando, T., Masuda, A., 1986, The mechanism of the hypotensive effect of captopril (converting enzyme inhibitor) with special reference to the kallikrein-kinin and renin-angiotensin systems. Jpn. J. Med., 25:34.

Kettner, C., Mirabelli, C., Pierce, J. V., Shaw, E., 1980, Active site mapping of human and rat urinary kallikreins by peptidyl chloromethyl ketones. Arch. Biochem. Biophys., 202:420.

McRae, B. J., Kurachi, K., Heimark, R. L., Fujikawa, K., Davie, E. W., Powers J. C., 1981, Mapping the active sites of bovine thrombin, Factor IX_a, Factor X_a, Factor XI_a, Factor XII_a, plasma kallikrein, and trypsin with amino acid and peptide thioesters: Development of new sensitive substrates, Biochemistry, 20:7196.

Mulinari, R., Benetos, A., Gavras, I., Gavras, H., 1988, Vascular and sympathoadrenal responses to bradykinin and bradykinin analog, Hypertension, In Press.

Okunishi, H., Burton, J., Spragg, J., 1985, Specificity of substrate analogue inhibitors of human urinary kallikrein, Hypertension, 7:I-72.

Okunishi, H., Spragg, J., Burton, J., 1986, The design of substrate analogue tissue kallikrein inhibitors. Hypertension, 8:I-114.

Okunishi, H., Spragg, J., Burton, J., 1987, In vivo assay of specific kallikrein inhibitors, in: Vasodepressor Hormones, Bonner, G., ed., Birkhauser Verlag, Basel.

Oldham, A. A., Arnstein, M. J., Major, J. S., Clough, D. P., 1984, In vivo comparison of the renin inhibitor H77 with the angiotensin-converting enzyme inhibitor captopril, J. Cardiovasc. Pharmacol., 6:672.

Toda, N., Bian, K., Akiba, T., Okamura, T., 1987, Heterogeneity in mechanisms of bradykinin action in canine isolated blood vessels. Eur. J. Pharmacol., 135:321.

SEMISYNTHETIC ARGININE-15-APROTININ, AN IMPROVED

INHIBITOR FOR HUMAN PLASMA KALLIKREIN

H. Tschesche, J. Beckmann, A. Mehlich, A. Feldmann, and
H.R. Wenzel

University Bielefeld, Faculty of Chemistry
D-4800 Bielefeld 1, FRG

C.F. Scott and R.W. Colman

Temple University, Thrombosis Research Center
Philadelphia, PA 19140, USA

Human plasma kallikrein, a product of contact-activated plasma proteolysis, is a serine proteinase with a pronounced preference for arginine residues in the P_1 position of peptide substrates[1]. It is moderately inhibited by aprotinin, the bovine pancreatic trypsin inhibitor (Kunitz)[2] that
has been used as a therapeutic agent in human disease states. Since aprotinin contains a lysine residue at its P_1 reactive-site position 15, we hypothesized that if arginine were substituted for this lysine a more potent
inhibitor for plasma kallikrein might result that could have potential clinical usefulness[3]. Both chemical/enzymatic and recombinant methods have recently become available to synthesize Arg-15-aprotinin and thus to test our
hypothesis. The purpose of this paper is mainly to summarize the semisynthetic approaches[4]; a detailed investigation of the kinetics of inhibition
by Arg-15-aprotinin on human plasma kallikrein, tissue kallikrein, plasmin,
factor XIIa, factor XIa and thrombin was published elsewhere[3].

Fig. 1 outlines our method for the specific cleavage of the reactive-
site peptide bond of aprotinin[5] followed by an 'enzymatic mutation'[6,7] to
yield Arg-15-aprotinin. Both an endo- and an exopeptidase are involved in
hydrolyzing and resynthesizing peptide bonds. It is essential to use kallikrein in the trapping reaction[8] because bovine or porcine trypsin yielded
a product lacking Arg-39[9].

A second semisynthetic method[10] is depicted in Fig. 2. It comprises
carbodiimide-coupling of arginine methyl ester to a suitably protected

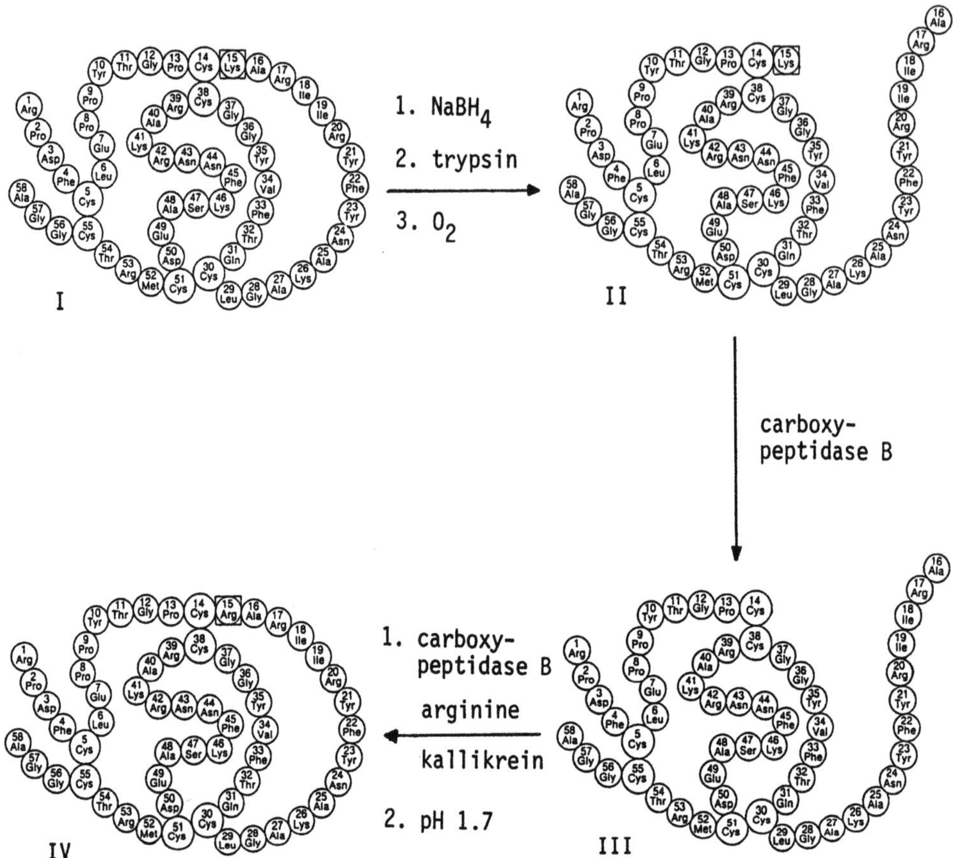

Fig. 1. Semisynthesis of Arg-15-aprotinin by 'enzymatic mutation'. The reaction sequence comprises the following steps: Selective reduction of the Cys-14-Cys-38 disulphide bond of aprotinin (I) with sodium borohydride, tryptic cleavage of the reactive-site peptide bond Lys-15-Ala-16 and re-oxidation of the half-cystine residues to yield 'modified' aprotinin (II). Removal of Lys-15 by carboxypeptidase B providing des-Lys-15 'modified' aprotinin (III). Coupling of arginine to Cys-14 by carboxypeptidase B to yield 'modified' Arg-15-aprotinin in minute amounts which are trapped by complex formation with kallikrein from porcine pancreas thus shifting the carboxypeptidase-catalyzed reaction towards synthesis. Dissociation of the complex at pH 1.7 to yield Arg-15-aprotinin (IV) as the main product.

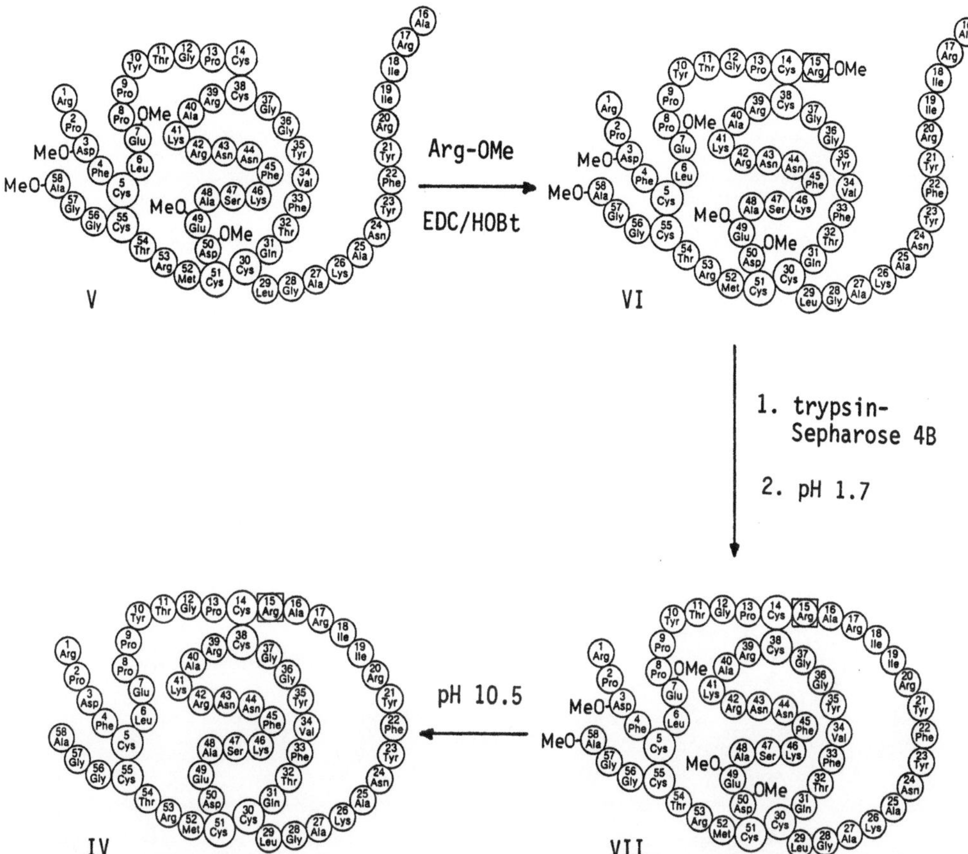

Fig. 2. Semisynthesis of Arg-15-aprotinin using both chemical and enzymatic methods for peptide bond formation. The key intermediate, des-Lys-15 'modified' aprotinin pentamethyl ester (V) is prepared from 'modified' aprotinin (II) as described[4]: Esterification of all six carboxyl groups with acidified methanol. Selective saponification of the Lys-15 methyl ester using endoproteinase Lys-C, from Lysobacter enzymogenes, in dioxane/aqueous citrate-phosphate buffer, 3:2, pH 5.0. Removal of Lys-15 by carboxypeptidase B. Arginine-incorporation then comprises the steps depicted above: Coupling of arginine methyl ester to Cys-14 using N-(3-dimethylaminopropyl)-N'-ethylcarbodiimide/1-hydroxybenzotriazole to yield 'modified' Arg-15-aprotinin hexamethyl ester (VI). Synthesis of the Arg-15-Ala-16 bond and complex formation using trypsin immobilized to Sepharose 4B. Release of Arg-15-pentamethyl ester (VII) from this complex at pH 1.7. Saponification of the methyl ester groups at pH 10.5 to yield Arg-15-aprotinin (IV).

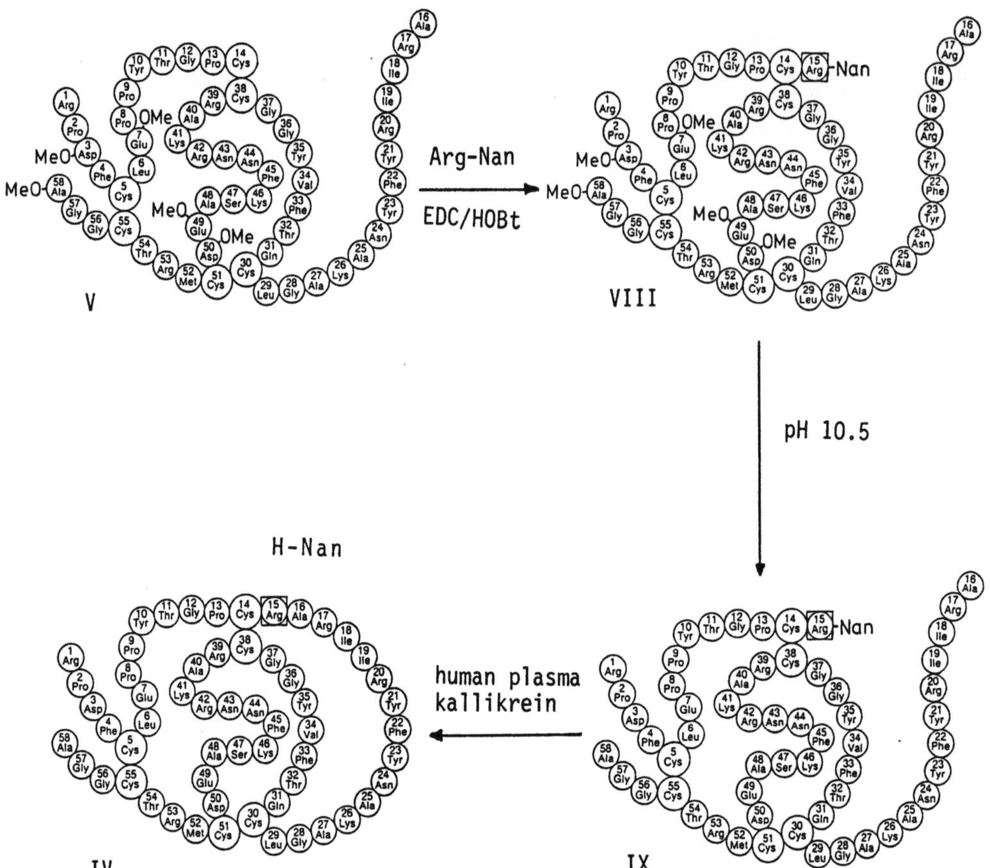

Fig. 3. Semisynthesis and application of an active-site titrant for trypsin-like proteinases. The reactions depicted are: Condensation of arginine
4-nitroanilide to des-Lys-15 'modified' aprotinin pentamethyl ester (V),
see legend to Fig. 2, using N-(3-dimethylaminopropyl)-N'-ethylcarbodiimide/
1-hydroxybenzotriazole. Saponification of the resulting product (VIII) to
yield derivative IX, an Arg-15 'modified' aprotinin with a chromophoric
leaving group, which can be used as active-site titrant for proteinases
with trypsin-like specificity: Upon incubation with human plasma kallikrein
the peptide bond between Arg-15 and Ala-16 is synthesized, and an amount
of 4-nitroaniline which is equimolar to that of the enzyme added is released. The proteinase remains trapped in the complex with Arg-15-aproti-
nin (IV). 4-Nitroaniline can be spectrophotometrically measured at 405 nm.

18

aprotinin derivative[11] followed by trypsin-catalyzed resynthesis of the
reactive-site peptide bond of Arg-15-aprotinin.

Fig. 3 shows a similar reaction sequence which yields a convenient
active-site titrant for human plasma kallikrein and other proteinases with
trypsin-like specificity[12].

The semisynthetic Arg-15-aprotinin was purified by gel filtration and
cation-exchange chromatography. It was characterized by amino acid analysis,
automated Edman degradation, X-ray crystal structure analysis[8], polyacrylamide gel electrophoresis, and high-pressure liquid cation-exchange chromatography[13]. The inhibitor preparation was found to be homogeneous according to all these criteria applied.

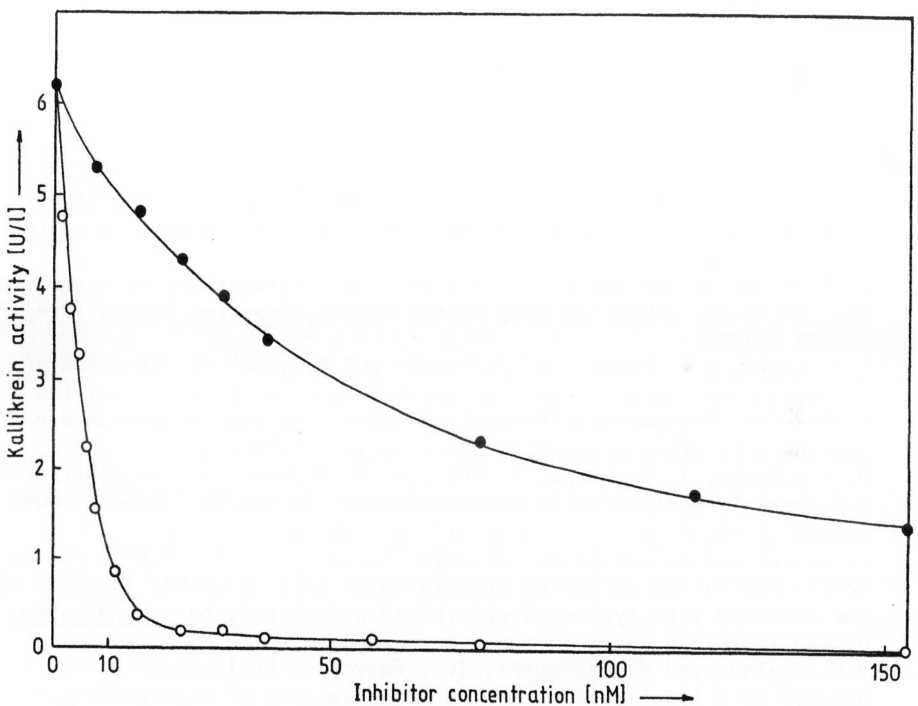

Fig. 4.   Inhibition of human plasma kallikrein by aprotinin
          (●) and semisynthetic Arg-15-aprotinin (o). The
          enzymatic activity was determined using the chromo-
          genic peptide substrate D-prolyl-phenylalanyl-
          arginine-4-nitroanilide[14]. (50 mM Tris/HCl-buffer,
          pH 7.8; 0,4 mM substrate; 25°C).

Fig. 4 shows the titration of human plasma kallikrein with aprotinin and Arg-15-aprotinin respectively. It is evident that the Lys/Arg exchange in the reactive site is accompanied by a considerable increase in affinity of the enzyme for the inhibitor. The complex-dissociation constants estimated from these curves are $4.5 \cdot 10^{-8}$ M for the Lys-15- and $5.9 \cdot 10^{-10}$ M for the Arg-15-aprotinin. Values which are higher by about an order of magnitude have been determined using a different test system[3].

Recently, Arg-15-Glu-52-aprotinin was obtained as recombinant protein from E. coli[15]. The inhibition of various serine proteinases by this homologue closely resembles the inhibition by semisynthetic Arg-15-aprotinin.

Acknowledgement

We thank Bayer AG for supplying us with aprotinin, 'modified' aprotinin and porcine pancreas kallikrein.

Our semisynthetic work has been supported by the Deutsche Forschungsgemeinschaft.

References

1. R.W. Colman, L. Mattler and S. Sherry, Studies on the prekallikrein (kallikreinogen)-kallikrein enzyme system of human plasma, J. Clin. Invest. 48:11 (1969).
2. H. Fritz and G. Wunderer, Biochemistry and applications of aprotinin, the kallikrein inhibitor from bovine organs, Arzneim.-Forsch./Drug Res. 33:479 (1983).
3. C.F. Scott, H.R. Wenzel, H. Tschesche and R.W. Colman, Kinetics of inhibition of human plasma kallikrein by a site-specific modified inhibitor Arg[15]-aprotinin: Evaluation using a microplate system and comparison with other proteases, Blood 69:1431 (1987).
4. H. Tschesche, J. Beckmann, A. Mehlich, E. Schnabel, E. Truscheit and H.R. Wenzel, Semisynthetic engineering of proteinase inhibitor homologues, Biochim. Biophys. Acta 913:97 (1987).
5. H. Jering and H. Tschesche, Preparation and characterization of the active derivative of bovine trypsin-kallikrein inhibitor (Kunitz) with the reactive site lysine-15-alanine-16 hydrolyzed, Eur. J. Biochem. 61:443 (1976).
6. R.W. Sealock and M. Laskowski, Jr., Enzymatic Replacement of the arginyl by a lysyl residue in the reactive site of soybean trypsin inhibitor, Biochemistry 8:3703 (1969).
7. H. Jering and H. Tschesche, Replacement of lysine by arginine, phenylalanine and tryptophan in the reactive site of the bovine trypsin-kallikrein inhibitor (Kunitz) and change of the inhibitory properties, Eur. J. Biochem. 61:453 (1976).
8. W. Bode, J. Walter, R. Huber, H.R. Wenzel and H. Tschesche, The refined 2.2-Å (0.22-nm) X-ray crystal structure of the ternary complex formed by bovine trypsinogen, valine-valine and the Arg[15] analogue of bovine pancreatic trypsin inhibitor, Eur. J. Biochem. 144:185 (1984).
9. R. Richarz, H. Tschesche and K. Wüthrich, Structural characterization by nuclear magnetic resonance of a reactive-site [13]carbon-labelled

basic pancreatic trypsin inhibitor with the peptide bond Arg-39-Ala-40 cleaved and Arg-39 removed, <u>Eur. J. Biochem.</u> 102:563 (1979).

10. J. Beckmann, Semisynthetischer Aminosäureaustausch im reaktiven Zentrum des Trypsin-Kallikrein-Inhibitors, <u>Thesis</u>, Universität Bielefeld (1987).

11. H.R. Wenzel, J. Beckmann, A. Mehlich, E. Schnabel and H. Tschesche, Semisynthetic conversion of the bovine trypsin inhibitor (Kunitz) into an efficient leukocyte-elastase inhibitor by specific valine for lysine substitution in the reactive site, <u>in</u>: "Chemistry of Peptides and Proteins", Vol. 3, W. Voelter, E. Bayer, Y.A. Ovchinnikov and V. T. Ivanov, eds, Walter de Gruyter & Co., Berlin, New York (1986).

12. A. Mehlich, Semisynthetische Untersuchungen zur Struktur-Funktionsbeziehung des Trypsin-Kallikrein-Inhibitors aus Rindermastzellen, <u>Thesis</u>, Universität Bielefeld (1987).

13. H.R. Wenzel, J. Beckmann, A. Mehlich, J. Siekmann, H. Tschesche and H. Schutt, Potentials of high-performance ion-exchange chromatography in protein separations – Synthesis and characterization of aprotinin derivatives and homologues, <u>in</u>: "Modern Methods in Protein Chemistry", Vol. 2, H. Tschesche, ed., Walter de Gruyter & Co., Berlin, New York (1985).

14. G. Claeson, L. Aurell, P. Friberger, S. Gustavsson and G. Karlsson, Designing of peptide substrates. Different approaches exemplified by new chromogenic substrates for kallikreins and urokinase, <u>Haemostasis</u> 7:62 (1978).

15. E. Auerswald, D. Hörlein, G. Reinhardt, E. Schnabel and W. Schröder, Isolation and properties of recombinant Arg-15-Glu-52-aprotinin, <u>Poster</u> at the FEBS Satellite Meeting "Proteinase Inhibitors and Biological Control", Ljubljana/Brdo, Juli 4 – 7 (1987).

IN VIVO INHIBITION OF TISSUE KALLIKREINS BY KININOGEN SEQUENCE ANALOGUE

PEPTIDES

Hideki Okunishi, Jocelyn Spragg*, James Burton [†], and
Noboru Toda

Department of Pharmacology, Shiga University of Medical
Science, Seta, Otsu 520-21 Japan; *Department of Medicine
Harvard Medical School and Department of Rheumatology and
Immunology, Brigham and Women's Hospital, Boston MA 02115
USA; [†]The Evans Memorial Department of Clinical Research
Boston University School of Medicine, Boston MA 02118, USA

SUMMARY

    Kininogen sequence analogs containing amino acid residues around
the Arg-Ser cleavage site of bovine kininogens were prepared with bulky
aliphatic residues in P3 position. KKI-7 (containing a cyclohexylacetyl
group) and KKI-8 (containing an adamantaneacetyl group) both inhibited
human urinary kallikrein (HUK) with K_i of 4 µM. These inhibitors were 40
times more potent than the corresponding peptide containing the
naturally occurring Pro at P3 and were one-seventh as susceptible to
hydrolysis by HUK. Rat submaxillary kallikrein (RSK) and porcine
pancreatic kallikrein (PPK) were also inhibited by these analogs. Both
analogs were poor inhibitors of human plasma kallikrein, while their
capacity to inhibit bovine trypsin was 1/3 and 1/17, respectively, that
to inhibit HUK. In a rat blood flow study, KKI-7 infusion depressed the
response to injected RSK. The response gradually returned toward normal
30 to 60 min after the infusion was terminated. Blood flow increase of
dog jejunal artery in response to infused PPK was blunted by the
simultaneous local infusion of Trasylol, KKI-7, or KKI-8, whereas these
infusions did not alter the response to infused bradykinin. The vehicle
infusion did not attenuate the response either to PPK or bradykinin.
These analogs appear to have greater specificity and stability than
those previously developed and to be appropriate for the _in vivo_
inhibition of glandular kallikreins.

INTRODUCTION

    Glandular kallikreins (EC 3.4.21.35) are serine proteases which
release vasoactive kinins from kininogens. They have been purified from
exocrine glands and their secretions and from kidney and urine. Recent
studies with antisera or polynucleic acids probes suggest that the
glandular kallikreins are also present in other tissues including brain,
pituitary, and pancreatic beta cells. In addition to their action on
kininogens, kallikreins may also cleave other substrates such as
apolipoprotein B-100 of human plasma low density lipoproteins [1],

prorenin and proinsulin (reviewed in [2]). The physiological relevance
of tissue kallilreins is not yet clear, in part because specific
kallikrein inhibitors have not been available. Those reported either are
not highly specific [3] or have some undesirable effects of their
own (reviewed in [2, 4]).

In the course of a program to develop stable, highly specific
inhibitors of glandular kallikreins, it has been found that penta-,
hexa-, and heptapeptides containing the amino acid sequence around the
Arg-Ser cleavage site of bovine kininogens were competitive inhibitors
of human, rat, and pig glandular kallikreins [2, 5]. The inhibitors
showed little inhibition of a number of other highly specific serine
proteases but did inhibit trypsin. Because these inhibitors were rapidly
cleaved by HUK (k_{cat}=190-250/sec), a series of tripeptidyl 4-nitro-
anilide analogs of bradykinin was examined to identify structural
modifications that could yield inhibitors with higher affinity and
stability. The results indicated that substitution of a cyclohexyl-
containing residue for Pro at P3 (nomenclature by Schechter and Berger
[6]) could accomplish these goals [5]. The present study describes the
preparation and initial <u>in vitro</u> and <u>in vivo</u> examination of kininogen
sequence analog inhibitors which incorporate cyclohexylacetic acid or
adamantaneacetic acid in the P3 position.

MATERIALS AND METHODS

<u>Peptide synthesis</u>

Hexapeptide kininogen sequence analogs KKI-7 and KKI-8 were
synthesized as described previously for other kininogen sequence analogs
[5]. Cyclohexylacetic acid or 1-adamantaneacetic acid (both from Aldrich
Chemical Co., Milwaukee WI, USA) were incorporated at the P3 position
using dicyclohexylcarbodiimide (Fluka Chemical Corp., Hauppauge NY,
USA), and [^{3}H]valine (ICN Pharmaceuticals, Irvine CA, USA) was
incorporated in the P2' position. Because both peptides were poorly
soluble in acetic acid, the extraction with 10% acetic acid was followed
by extraction with absolute ethanol in order to increase the yield. For
the same reason, gel filtration on Sephadex was omitted. Instead, the
acetic acid and ethanol extracts were combined, evaporated for ethanol,
lyophilized, dissolved in dimethylsulfoxide(DMSO), and further purified
by isocratic elution from a reverse phase high performance liquid
chromatography(HPLC) preparatory column(Synchropak RP-P, Linden IN,
USA) as described [5]. Both peptides were subjected to HPLC analysis on
Altex Ultrasphere ODS column(Berkeley CA, USA) with an aqueous CH_3CN
(20-70% in 30 min; containing 0.1% trifluoroacetic acid) gradient
elution system and yielded single peaks with absorbance at 220 nm.

<u>In vitro studies</u>

The inhibitor constant(K_i) was determined for highly purified HUK
as reported [5]. The substrate D-Val-Leu-Arg-4-nitroanilide (S-2266, AB
Kabi Diagnostica, Stockholm, Sweden) and HUK were incubated at 37°C in
50 mM tris HCl buffer at pH 9.0. K_i values for RSK (the gift of Dr. N.B.
Oza) and PPK (Bayer AG, Leverkusen-Bayerwerk, FRG) were also determined
in the same assay system. The inhibition of human plasma kallikrein
(Kabi) and bovine pancreatic trypsin (Sigma, St. Louis MO, USA) were
similarly examined with D-Pro-Phe-Arg-4-nitroanilide (S-2302, Kabi) and
<Glu-Gly-Arg-4-nitroanilide (S-2444, Kabi), as respective substrates.
Dixon plots and Cornish-Bowden plots were used to determine K_i values
and type of inhibition [5]. To determine the cleavage of KKI-8 by HUK,
it was incubated with 4 ng of HUK for 30 min at 37°C in 150 µl of 50 mM

tris HCl, pH 9.0. The resultant peptide fragment containing radio-labelled valine was fractionated by HPLC [5] and quantified by liquid scintilation counting.

In vivo studies

The effect of KKI-7 on the blood flow increasing response to RSK was examined in male Sprague-Dawley rats, which were anesthetized with subcutaneous urethane (1.4 g/kg). Polyethylene PE-10 tubings(Clay Adams, Parsippany NJ, USA) were inserted into the right femoral artery and vein for intra-arterial(i.a.) and intravenous (i.v.) injections, respectively. The arterial catheter was inserted so that the tip was located immediately proximal to the aortic bifurcation. A blood flow probe (1.5 mm circumference, Carolina Medical Electronics, King NC, USA) was placed around the left femoral artery and the mean blood flow was monitored with a square-wave electromagnetic flowmeter (Carolina Medical Electronics, model 501). RSK injection (500 ng bolus i.a.) was repeated until a reproducible response was obtained. Then, animals were infused with KKI-7 (206 nmol/22μl/min i.v.) or with DMSO as vehicle (22 μl/min). Control study was also performed to determine whether or not KKI-7 or DMSO affected the blood flow response to bradykinin (2 ng bolus i.a., Bachem, Torrance CA, USA). The magnitude and duration of the response to RSK and bradykinin were compared before, during, and after the i.v. infusion of KKI-7 or the vehicle.

The effect of KKI-8 and KKI-7 on the blood flow increasing response to PPK (Bayer) and bradykinin (Peptide Institute, Inc., Minoh, Osaka, Japan) was examined in dog mesentery in situ. The animals were anesthetized with Nembutal, and respiration was artificially assisted. The abdominal wall was opened by a midline incision, and an flow probe (1 mm diameter, Nihon Kohden, Tokyo, Japan) was placed around one of the jejunal arteries, and the mean blood flow was monitored by an electromagnetic flowmeter (Nihon Kohden, model MFV-2100). An arterial branch, which was located distal to the probe, was cannulated with PE-10 tubing and ligated for the infusion of Trasylol (Bayer), KKI-7, KKI-8, or DMSO vehicle. A neighboring branch, located distal to the above one, was also cannulated for the infusion of PPK (0.68U/68μl/min for 2 min) or bradykinin (68 ng/68 μl/min for 2min). The blood flow increase elicited with PPK and bradykinin was integrated with an IBAS image analysis system (Kontron Messgerate GmbH, Munich, FRG). These responses to PPK and bradykinin were compared before, during and after the infusion of Trasylol, KKI peptides and DMSO vehicle.

RESULTS

Hexapeptide kininogen sequence analogs were synthesized incorporating into the P3 position cyclohexylacetic acid (KKI-7) or adamantaneacetic acid (KKI-8). Each analog was examined for its capacity to inhibit the cleavage of chromogenic substrates by HUK and related enzymes; the data are summarized in Table 1. The graphical analyses indicated that the inhibition was competitive. KKI-8 was cleaved by HUK, but only at 15% the rate at which the hexapeptide containing Pro in the P3 position (KKI-5) was cleaved [5].

In rat models, the injection of 500 ng of RSK over a period of 10 sec elicited a flow increase that usually lasted for 1.5 to 2 min. The systemic infusion of KKI-7 reduced the response to 6 and 26% of the control in two rats. Repeated injections of RSK, after the termination of KKI-7 infusion, indicated that the inhibitory effect of KKI-7 lasted 30 min or longer. In contrast, the response to bradykinin was not

Table 1. Specificity of KKI-7 and KKI-8 on kallikreins
         and trypsin.

ENZYME	K_i (µM)	
	KKI-7	KKI-8
Human Urinary Kallikrein	4.0	4.2
Porcine Pancreatic Kallikrein	45.3	72.7
Rat Submaxillary Kallikrein	29.7	109.3
Human Plasma Kallikrein	244.0	358.0
Bovine Trypsin	12.3	71.8

KKI-7, cyclohexylacetyl-Phe-Arg-Ser-Val-Gln-NH$_2$

KKI-8, adamantaneacetyl-Phe-Arg-Ser-Val-Gln-NH$_2$

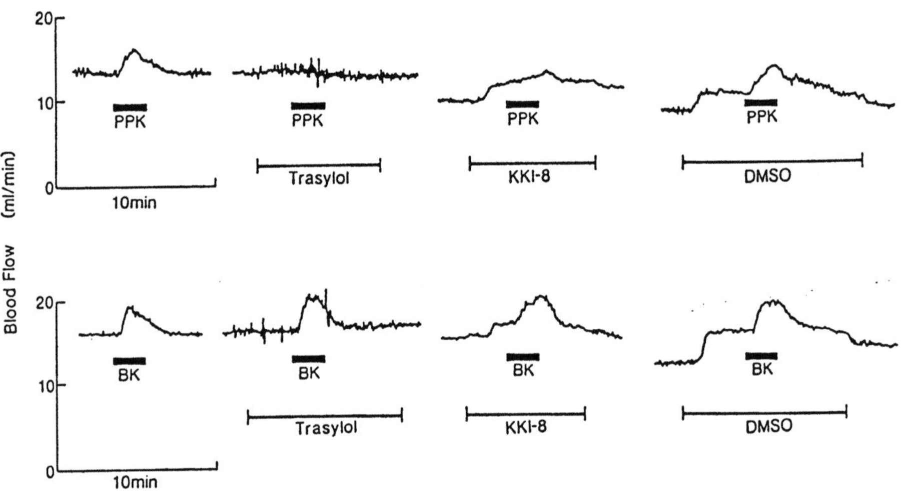

Fig. 1. Effect of Trasylol(5000U/min), KKI-8(227 nmol/32.4 µl/min)
        and DMSO vehicle(32.4 µl/min) on the dog jejunal blood
        flow increase in response to porcine pancreatic kallikrein
        (PPK, 0.68U/68 µl/min) and bradykinin (BK, 68ng/68 µl/
        min). PPK and BK were infused for 2 min as indicated by
        bold bars. Infusion periods of inhibitors and vehicle are
        indicated by horizontal lines. The leftmost recordings are
        the control responses to PPK (upper) and BK (lower),
        respectively. A moderate and reversible increase in the
        basal blood flow caused by the infusion of KKI-8 did not
        differ from that of DMSO vehicle.

influenced by KKI-7. Infusion of the DMSO vehicle itself, at the same rate at which KKI-7 was infused, did not alter the response to RSK or bradykinin.

In dog mesentery, the 2 min-infusion of PPK elicited a jejunal blood flow increase which lasted for 4 to 5 min (Fig. 1). The total flow increase was integrated as 4.12±0.78 ml (n=6). Infusion of KKI-8 itself did increase the basal blood flow, but this effect was not different from that of DMSO vehicle. KKI-8 infused at the rate 227 nmol/32.4 µl/min and 151 nmol/21.5 µl/min reduced the response to PPK to 23.6±12.2% (n=4) and 63.0±4.1% (n=4) of the control, respectively. In two dogs, KKI-8 infused at 378 nmol/54 µl/min reduced the response to 0 and 6.2% of the control. Trasylol infused at 5000 U/min and 2060 U/min also reduced the PPK response to 24.4±8.0% (n=3) and 35.8% (n=2), respectively. KKI-7 infused at 378 nmol/54 µl/min attenuated the PPK response in two dogs to 0 and 4.3% of the control. Vehicle infusion did not attenuate but rather potentiated the PPK response to 124.1±19.0 % (n=5) at the rate of 32.4µl/min, and to 152.5%(n=2) at the rate of 54.0 µl/min as compared to the control. Infusion of bradykinin for 2 min elicited a blood flow increase integrated as 4.54±0.62 ml (n=3), which was comparable to that evoked by PPK (Fig. 1). However, the response to bradykinin was not affected by the infusion of either Trasylol, KKI-8, or DMSO. The PPK response recovered within 5 min after the infusion of KKI-7, KKI-8 or Trasylol was stopped.

DISCUSSION

As expected from the results of a study of tripeptidyl 4-nitro-anilide analogs of bradykinin [5], substitution of the bulky aliphatic residues in the P3 position of kininogen sequence analogs containing the amino acid residues around the Arg-Ser cleavage site leads to increased inhibition of tissue kallikreins. Both KKI-7 and KKI-8 are 40 times more potent as HUK inhibitors than is KKI-5, the hexapeptide containing the naturally occurring Pro at the P3 position. Human plasma kallikrein is relatively little inhibited by either KKI-7 or KKI-8 (Table 1), suggesting that this enzyme has more stringent requirements for the homologous sequence on the C-terminal side of the cleavage site (P1'-P3'). It is noteworthy that KKI-8 is 17 times more potent an inhibitor of HUK than trypsin, while KKI-7 is only 3 times potent. These results suggest that trypsin does not have an S3 subsite that can accept a group as bulky as the adamantane residue and provide a basis for the design of kallikrein inhibitors which more strictly distinguish HUK from trypsin. KKI-8 was hydrolyzed by HUK one-seventh as fast as KKI-5, the hexapeptide containing the native Pro at P3 [5], indicating that this substitution not only leads to increased specificity but also to increased stability.

Because substrate analogs as well as highly purified glandular kallikreins are presently available in limited supply, initial studies to examine the in vivo activity of these compounds necessarily employed small animals or local circulation whose basal blood flow averaged 10 ml/min or less. KKI-7 and KKI-8 proved to be effective inhibitors of glandular kallikreins in vivo and had no effect on the response to bradykinin, indicating that these analogs were neither kinin-receptor agonists nor antagonists, nor had kinin-potentiating activity. The infusion of KKI-7 and KKI-8 in the DMSO vehicle as well as vehicle itself led to a moderate, reversible increase in basal blood flow. No specific adverse effects of the analogs were appreciated during the experimental period. More than 30 min were required until the total recovery of RSK response following the cessation of KKI-7 infusion, suggesting the _in vivo_ stability of KKI-7. In dogs, however, PPK response recovered to the control in 5 min after infusion of either KKI-8, KKI-7 or Trasylol was stopped. This may be attributed to the rapid diffusion of locally infused inhibitors into systemic circulation.

The data presented indicate that substitution of bulky aliphatic residues in the P3 position of kininogen sequence analog inhibitors improves the inhibitory potency and specificity of the peptides and leads to increased resistance to hydrolysis by HUK. The data obtained from _in vivo_ studies may provide a basis for the development of potent and specific tissue kallikrein inhibitors.

ACKNOWLEDGEMENTS

We are grateful to Dr. Peter Gaudron, Drs. Mark and Janice Pfeffer, Dr. Norman Levinsky, Dr. Wilfred Lieberthal, and Dr. Mizuo Miyazaki for advice and facilities used in the _in vivo_ studies, and to Dr. Narendra Oza for providing rat submaxillary kallikrein. We appreciate the excellent technical assistance of Marilyn Pontone, Robert Wolff and Stephen Wood. This work was supported in part by Grants HL-35949, AI-10356, and AM-05577 from the National Institutes of Health. Support from the trustees of the Evans Memorial Foundation, Inc. is gratefully acknowledged.

REFERENCES

1. A. D. Cardin, K. R. Witt, J. Chao, H. S. Margolius, V. H. Donaldson, and R. L. Jackson. Degradation of apolipoprotein B-100 of human plasma low density lipoproteins by tissue and plasma kallikreins. _J. Biol. Chem._ 259:8522-8528 (1984).
2. H. Okunishi, J. Burton, and J. Spragg. Specificity of substrate analogue inhibitors of human urinary kallikrein. _Hypertension_ 7 [Suppl I]:I-72 - I-75 (1985).
3. C. Kettner, C. Mirabelli, J. V. Pierce, and E. Shaw. Active site mapping of human and rat urinary kallikreins by peptidyl chloromethyl ketones. _Arch. Biochem. Biophys._ 202:420-430 (1980).
4. R. Vogel. Kallikrein inhibitors. _in_: Handb. Exp. Pharmacol. vol 25 (Suppl), E. G. Erdos, ed., Springer Verlag, New York (1979).
5. H. Okunishi, J. Spragg, and J. Burton. The design of substrate analogue tissue kallikrein inhibitors. _Hypertension_ 8 [Suppl I]: I-114 - I-118 (1986).
6. I. Schechter and A. Berger. On the size of the active site in proteases. I. Papain. _Biochem. Biophys. Res. Commun._ 27:157-162 (1967).

HIGHLY SELECTIVE SYNTHETIC INHIBITORS WITH REGARD

TO PLASMA-KALLIKREIN ACTIVITIES

S.Okamoto[1], U.Okamoto[2], K.Wanaka[1], A. Hijikata-Okunomiya[3],
M. Bohgaki[1], T. Naito[4], N. Horie[2] and Y. Okada[5]

1) Kobe Research Projects on Thrombosis and Haemostasis
   Saiseikai-Hospital, Kobe 651, Japan
2) Faculty of Nutrition, Kobe-Gakuin University, Kobe 673
3) Kobe University School of Allied Medical Sciences, Kobe 654
4) Showa Denko K.K., Life Science Research Lab., Tokyo 140
5) Faculty of Pharmaceutical Sciences, Kobe-Gakuin University
   Kobe 673

SUMMARY

The synthetic inhibitors of plasma kallikrein (PK) were found, which
are called PKSI-1007, PKSI-0180 and PKSI-0527 in our laboratories. (1) The
inhibitors inhibited PK competitively with D-Pro-Phe-Arg-pNA and the Ki
values obtained were considerably small, 10^{-6} M-10^{-7} M. However, the Ki
values for glandular kallikrein (GK), plasmin (PL), thrombin (TH) and
factor Xa (FXa) were larger. In particular, a selectivity of PKSI-0527
towards PK was very high and the toxicity was weak (i.v. LD_{50} for mice is
over 100 mg/kg). (2) The inhibitors were effective (a) to prevent the
bradykinin formation in the kaolin-activated human plasma and the acid-
treated ascites taken from the mice bearing Sarcoma 180, (b) to prolong
the coagulation time by contact activation, and (c) to inhibit the enhancement of ADP-platelet aggregation by PK. The results indicated that
the some PKSI-inhibitors will be much useful for the basic studies, furthermore they deem to be even promising towards the clinical application.

INTRODUCTION

Most of the proteinases in the coagulation-fibrinolysis system assume
high ability to select its specific substrate, which is enough compared
with the antigen-antibody reaction. Borrowing the terminology of information theory, you may explain that the each substrate bears the "code",
while the corresponding proteinase is equipped with the "decoding machine". However, some chemically modified code, most of them bearing the
nature to simulating the peptide-code, can be the "noise" which is synthetic inhibitor having high selectivity. Our studies have been conducted
along this assumption and fortunately we were able to obtained several
series of synthetic inhibitors of the proteinases.[1, 2, 3] Results obtained
are now to be reported, focusing the problem of the synthetic selective
inhibitors of PK. It should be recalled that the action of aprotinin has
been characterized by its selective inhibition toward GK and PL[4]: Highly
selective synthetic inhibitor of PK has not been reported however.

MATERIALS AND METHODS

Enzyme assay system: Enzyme activities were measured using the chromogenic peptide substrates obtained from Kabi Vitrum. Human PK from Kabi Vitrum, porcine GK from Sigma Chemical Co., human PL from Kabi Vitrum, bovine TH from Mochida Pharmaceutical Co. and bovine FXa from Diagnostic Reagents Ltd. were employed. The hydrolysis of synthetic peptide substrates was estimated principally according to the methods outlined in the data sheet given by Kabi. PKSI-inhibitors used were synthesized by the authors and their colleagues.

BK assay in the plasma: The blood obtained from healthy donors was taken in a plastic tube with 3.8% sodium citrate solution (9:1), which was immediately centrifuged at 3,000 r.p.m. for 10 minutes at 4°C to obtain the intact plasma. Kaolin suspension (0.4 mg/ml) was added to the mixture of 160 µl of the intact human plasma, 20 µl of o-phenanthroline (60 mM) and 20 µl of inhibitor or borate saline buffer (pH 7.4) and incubated for 2 minutes at 37°C and then 80 µl of trichloroacetic acid (TCA, 20%) was added.   The mixture was centrifuged for 10 minutes (3000 r.p.m.) at 4°C. The supernate was assayed according to assay method of MARKIT-A-Bradykinin kit (Dainippon Pharmaceutical Co.).

BK assay in the ascites: The ascites taken from mice bearing Sarcoma 180 adjusted to pH 2 with 1N HCl were incubated for 15 minutes at 37°C and adjusted pH 7.0-7.6 with 1N NaOH. Acid-treated ascites was mixed with one tenth volume of the inhibitor solution or borate saline buffer and incubated at 37°C for 0, 10, 20 and 30 minutes, then one fifth volume of TCA was added prior to bradykinin assay.

PTT: PTT was measured with PTT reagent obtained from Behring institute.

The platelet aggregation: The citrated blood was centrifuged at 1000 r.p.m. for 10 minutes at room temperature to obtain platelet rich plasma (PRP). The platelet count was adjusted to 300,000 platelets/µl. Platelet poor plasma (PPP) was centrifuged at 3,000 r.p.m. for 10 minutes at room temperature. 50 µl of PK (0.06u/ml, 0.12 u/ml) and 50 µl of ADP (20 µM, Sigma) were added to the mixture of 350 µl of PRP, 50 µl of Chrono-Lume (Chrono-Log Co.) and 25 µl of 0.05 M Tris-HCl buffer (pH 7.4). Platelet aggregation and ATP release were monitored with Lumi Aggligometer (Chrono-Log). Inhibitory effect on enhancement of platelet aggregation by PK was examined by the same manner with substituting inhibitor solution for buffer.

RESULTS

(A) <u>Chemical Structure of PKSI-1007</u>

The PKSI-1007 assumed a tripod structure, the basic skeleton of which was L-arginine. This structure showed trans-4-aminomethylcyclohexyl-carbonyl to be at the N-terminal of the arginine molecule and 4-ethoxy-carbonylanilide to be at the C-terminal position (Fig. 1).

(B) <u>Inhibitory Effect of PKSI-Inhibitors</u>

1) <u>Mode of action.</u> The study of the inhibition was made by the plots according to Lineweaver and Burk, indicating that the PK inhibition of PKSI-inhibitors were competitive as shown in Fig. 2 taking PKSI-0527 as a representative. They showed also the competitive inhibition on the different enzymes examined.

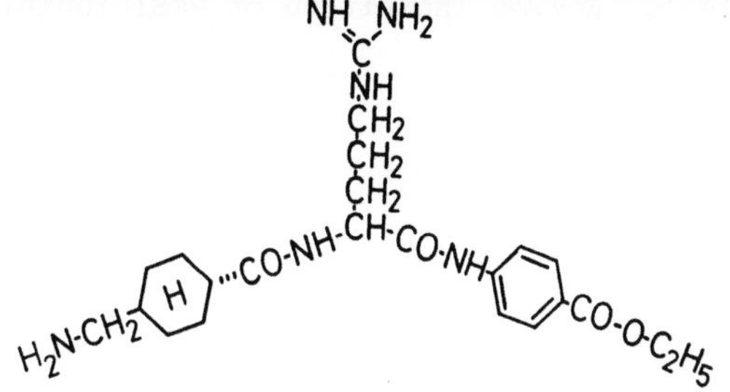

Fig. 1. Chemical structure of PKSI-1007.

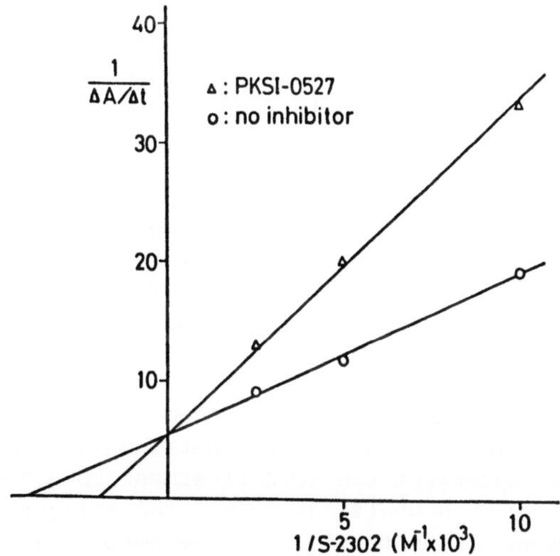

Fig. 2. Mode of action of PKSI-0527.
substrate: D-Pro-Phe-Arg-pNA,
enzyme: human PK.

2) <u>Selectivity.</u> Inhbitory effects of PKSI-inhibitors on the enzymes were measured using the synthetic chromogenic substrates, S-series by Kabi. (a) PKSI-1007 showed Ki value of 8.0 μM for PK. By contrast, Ki of 120 μM for GK, 270 μM for PL and more than 500 μM for TH as well as FXa were obtained. (b) PKSI-0180 was a more potent inhibitor than PKSI-1007, the Ki value for PK being 0.47 μM. (c) PKSI-0527 showed that the Ki value of PK was 0.81 μM, while the Ki values of PL, GK, TH, and FXa were 390 μM, >500 μM, >500 μM and >500 μM respectively. High selectivity towards PK was remarkably demonstrated as seen in Table 1, so far as the enzymes examined concerned. In particular, Ki values of PKSI-0527 for GK, PL, TH, and FXa were hundreds times larger than that for PK, as indicated by the figures in parenthesis. In addition, it can be noted that i.v. LD_{50}/kg in mice was over 100 mg in our preliminary toxicity test, which encourages us to extend the studies towards the in vivo applications.

(C) <u>Effect of PKSI-Inhibitors on Contact Activation</u>

1) <u>BK formation in plasma.</u> The inhibitory effect of PKSI-0180 on the bradykinin formation by kaolin were examined in the intact human plasma. As shown in Fig. 3, the amount of bradykinin formed in the kaolin-activated human plasma decreased by increasing gradually the concentration of PKSI-0180.

Table 1. Enzyme Inhibition of PKSI-inhibitors.

Table 1. Enzyme Inhibition of PKSI-inhibitors.

	P.Kallikrein Ki (µM)	G.Kallikrein Ki (µM)	Plasmin Ki (µM)	Thrombin Ki (µM)	FXa Ki (µM)
PKSI 1007 (Index)	8.0 (1)	120 (15)	270 (34)	>500 (>63)	>500 (>63)
PKSI 0180 (Index)	0.47 (1)	53 (113)	20 (43)	>500 (>1064)	330 (702)
PKSI 0527 (Index)	0.81 (1)	>500 (>617)	390 (481)	>500 (>617)	>500 (>617)

Substrate: S-2302 for P.kallikrein, S-2266 for G.kallikrein, S-2251 for plasmin, S-2238 for thrombin and S-2222 for factor Xa.

2) <u>Coagulation time (PTT).</u> Fig. 3 also shows that PKSI-0180 is able to prolong PTT; the right ordinate indicates the ratio of PTT with different concentration of PKSI-0180 to PTT without inhibitor, while the abscissa is the concentration of PKSI-0180. The results would be reasonably explained by assuming that PK inhibitor is able to prolong PTT by inhibiting PK of the contact system.

3) <u>BK formation in ascites.</u> The Sarcoma 180 was inoculated into the abdominal cavity of mice and the ascites obtained on 8th day was used. The ascites collected underwent the acid-treatment to get rid of kininase. Then the samples were incubated at 37°C, the aliquots taken out were measured of the amount of BK formed. In the control aliquots, the amounts of BK showed remarkable increase with the time course of incubation. While the addition of PKSI-0527 of the final concentrations of 10 µM and 100 µM in the ascites showed the significant decrease of the amount of BK, showing clearly the dose-dependancy of the concentration of PKSI-0527 (Fig. 4). The PKSI-0180 showed also similar effect on suppressing the BK formation in the ascites.

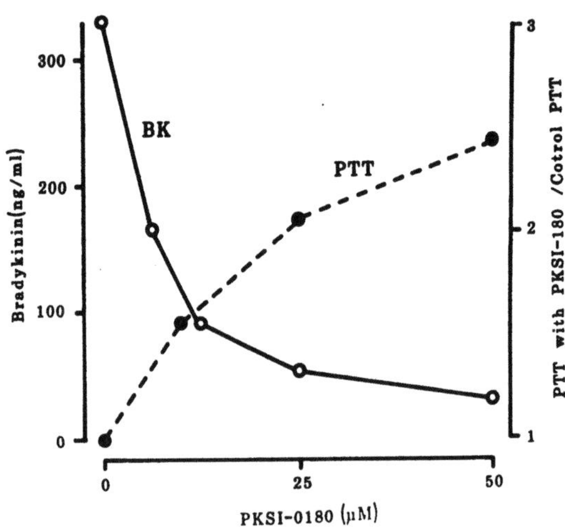

Fig. 3. Inhibitory effect of PKSI-0180 on BK formation by kaolin and PTT.

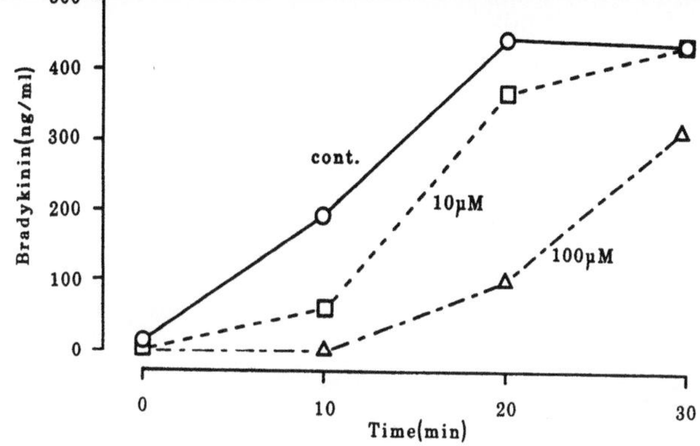

Fig. 4. Inhibitory effect of PKSI-0527 on BK formation
in acid-treated ascites of Sarcoma 180.

D) <u>Effect of PKSI-Inhibitor on Enhancement of Platelet Aggregatin by PK</u>

Fig. 5 shows the enhancing effect of human PK on platelet aggregation induced by ADP. In the upper part of Fig. 5, the aggregation is shown, and in the lower part, the ATP release which was measured by detecting the luminescence from the luciferace-luciferin system. Fig. 5 also indicates that human PK enhanced the platelet aggregation induced by ADP and the second phase as well.

Fig. 6 shows the inhibitory effect of PKSI-0180 on the enhancement of the ADP-platelet aggregation by PK. Results suggest that PK exerts some action to ADP aggregated platelet but the detailed mechanism has not been cleared up yet.

DISCUSSION

Generally speaking, most of the synthetic inhibitors do not exert highly specific or selective inhibition onto a target coagulation proteinase. In particular, this may be the case of the synthetic inhibitors of

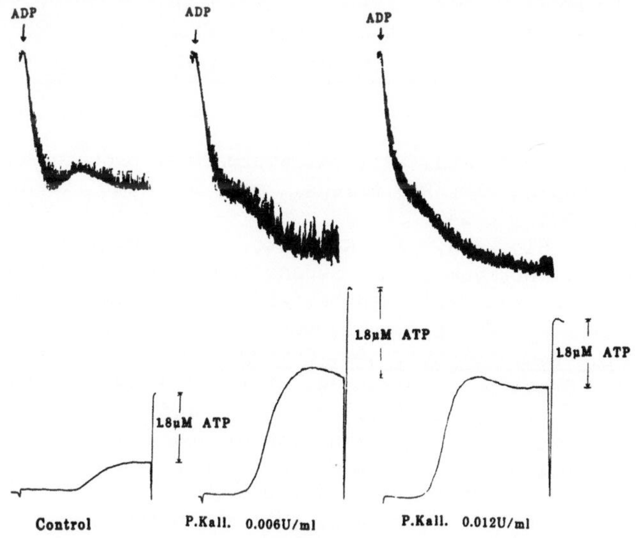

Fig. 5. Enhancing effect of P.kallikrein on
platelet aggregation induced by ADP.

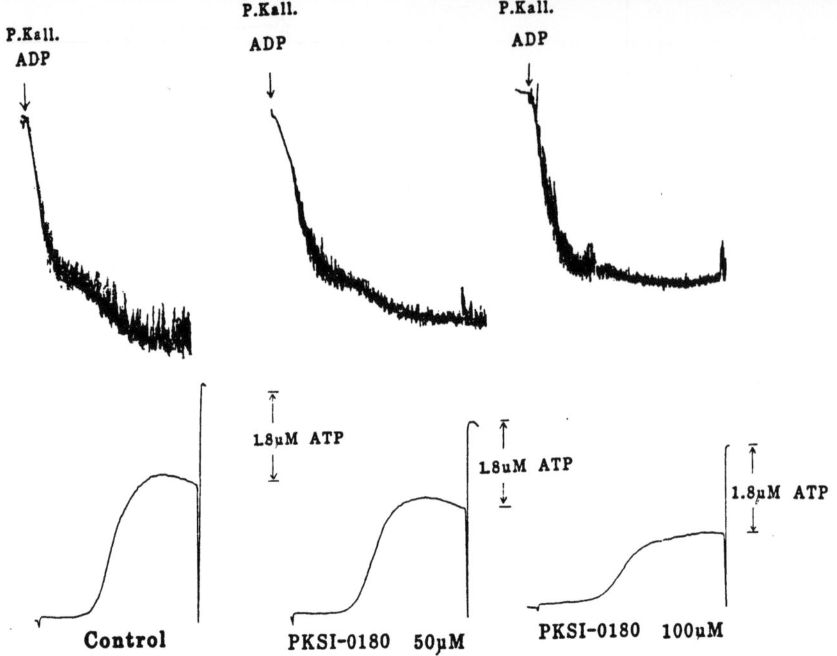

Fig. 6. Inhibitory effect of PKSI-0180 on enhancement
of ADP-platelet aggregation by PK.

PK. In recent several years, approximately 900 kinds of synthetic compounds have been designed so possible as rationally and synthesized by step-wise chemical modification of the weak inhibitors. Thus PKSI-1007, 0180 and 0527 were obtained as the highly selective inhibitors. However, possible role of PK concerning with the contact system should involve the complicated problems in health and desease. The present paper may present some tool for these studies; correlation between coagulation, bradykinin formation, fibrinolysis (and possibly platelet aggregation) in the contact system would be extremely complicated; even so, we do expect that results obtained by using PKSI-inhibitors cast light on a promising prospectiveness to us. Needless to say, further studies are urgenlty required. We should add that they are now under investigation in our laboratories.

REFERENCES

1. S. Okamoto and A. Hijikata, Rational approach to proteinases inhibitors, in: "Drug Design VI", E.J.Ariens, ed., Academic Press, INC., San Francisco (1975), p 143.
2. S. Okamoto, A. Hijikata, R. Kikumoto, S. Tonomura, H. Hara, K. Ninomiya, A. Murayama, M. Sugano and Y. Tamao, Potent inhibition of thrombin by the newly synthesized arginine derivative no. 805. The importance of stereostructure of its hydrophobic carboxamide portion, Biochem. Biophys. Res. Commun., 101:440, (1981).
3. S. Okamoto, U. Okamoto, Y. Okada, A. Hijikata-Okunimiya, K. Wanaka, N. Horie and T. Naito, Coding, decoding and noise of proteinase: a rational approach to plasmin inhibitors, in: "Fundamental and clinical fibrinolysis", Castellino et al. eds., Elsevier Science Publishers B.V., Amsterdam (1987), p 67.
4. H. Fritz, E. Fink and E. Truscheit, Kallikrein inhibitors, Fed. Proc., 38:2753 (1979).

APROTININ CONCENTRATIONS EFFECTIVE FOR THE INHIBITION OF

TISSUE KALLIKREIN AND PLASMA KALLIKREIN IN VITRO AND IN VIVO

Hans Hoffmann[1], Matthias Siebeck[2], Olaf Thetter[2],
Marianne Jochum[1], and Hans Fritz[1]

[1]Abteilung für Klinische Chemie und Klinische Biochemie in der
Chirurgischen Klinik Innenstadt
[2]Chirurgische Klinik Innenstadt und Chirurgische Poliklinik
University of Munich, Munich, FRG

INTRODUCTION

The basic proteinase inhibitor aprotinin (Trasylol[R]) from bovine organs
has been used for the treatment of acute pancreatitis, hyperfibrinolysis,
and traumatic shock for more than 30 years. However, uncertainty has existed
as to the appropriate dosage of aprotinin until recently, when more precise
assays to monitor plasma aprotinin levels were developed (Jochum et al.,
1984; Mueller-Esterl et al., 1984). These assays have been utilized to
monitor aprotinin plasma concentrations in several clinical trials (Jochum
et al., 1987; Clasen et al., 1987).

Plasma concentrations of aprotinin sufficient to inhibit the different
target enzymes were calculated from enzyme kinetics and substrate availability (Philipp, 1978; Fritz, 1978, 1985). To experimentally assess these
theoretical considerations we studied the plasma concentrations of aprotinin
preventing the proteinase action of plasma kallikrein and tissue kallikrein
on their natural target substrates, the high molecular weight (HMW) and low
molecular weight (LMW) kininogen as follows: (i) in in vitro systems the
purified components were applied (tissue kallikrein or plasma kallikrein and
LMW or HMW kininogen); (ii) in experimental animal models either the
purified proteinase (tissue kallikrein) was administered by infusion or the
proteinase (plasma kallikrein) was liberated from its precursor by the induction of contact phase activation.

MATERIALS AND METHODS

Reagents: Aprotinin (Trasylol[R]) was purchased as a sterile isotonic
solution for intravenous administration (vials of 500,000 KIU/50 ml, pH 5,
specific activity 7150 $\pm$ 200 KIU/mg from Bayer AG, Leverkusen, FRG). Human
high molecular weight kininogen (HMWK), low molecular weight kininogen
(LMWK) and plasma kallikrein (HPK) were isolated from freshly drawn plasma
from healthy donors by the method of Mueller-Esterl et al., 1983. Tissue
kallikrein from porcine pancreas (PZ 744997) was kindly donated by Bayer AG,
Leverkusen, FRG. Dextran sulphate (DS) (M_r 500,000) was obtained from Pharmacia Fine Chemicals, Uppsala, Sweden.

units and assays. The kallikrein inactivator unit (KIU) is used to measure the activity of aprotinin. One KIU is defined as the amount of aprotinin which decreases the activity of 2 biological kallikrein units by 50 %. Multiplication of the KIU values by a factor of 0.14 transforms these figures into the corresponding microgram quantities of aprotinin. Aprotinin levels in plasma were measured by a competitive enzyme-linked immunosorbent assay (ELISA) for aprotinin (Mueller-Esterl et al., 1984). Plasma prokallikrein (PPK) levels were measured by a chromogenic substrate assay (S-2302, Kabi Vitrum). Kininogen (HMWK + LMWK) plasma levels were measured by a bradykinin radioimmunoassay after cleavage with trypsin (Uchida and Katori, 1979). Coagulation times were determined by routine methods using diagnostic kits obtained from Behring, FRG. Data are presented as mean $\pm$ SEM.

<u>In vitro studies</u>. All in vitro experiments using purified components were performed in phosphate buffered saline with 1 % bovine serum albumin (pH 7.2, 37^{0}C). By incubating increasing amounts of the inhibitor with a constant amount of the proteinase and kininogen the inhibition stoichiometry of human plasma kallikrein and porcine tissue kallikrein with aprotinin was determined. After a 180 min incubation time the reaction was stopped by acidification and the kinin released was measured by kinin RIA. The concentrations of HMWK (0.8×10^{-6} mol/l) and LMWK (1.8×10^{-6} mol/l) used in vitro were similar to the corresponding physiological plasma levels.

<u>Animal experiments</u>. Weaned piglets weighing 17-23 kg were used. The animals were purchased from the Versuchsgut Oberschleissheim, Veterinary School, University of Munich, FRG. Acepromacine maleate 50 mg (Vetranquil^{R}) was administered intramuscularly for premedication. Anesthesia was induced with 15 mg/kg pentobarbital (Narcoren^{R}) and maintained with repeated injections of 4 mg/kg. One arterial and two venous catheters were inserted via the left femoral vessels for hemodynamic monitoring and blood sampling. After a 1-h baseline period the animals were randomly assigned to different experimental protocols (Table 1). Mean arterial blood pressure (MAP) was monitored with a Bentley Trantec Model 800 transducer and a Sirecust 404 monitor (Siemens AG, Munich, FRG). Blood samples were taken before and at 15 min intervals during the experiment. Platelets were counted manually in EDTA anticoagulated samples (Neubauer chamber). Blood samples were anticoagulated with 3.8 % citrate (1:10) for PPK, aprotinin, Quick, or aPTT determinations, or heparin (5 U/ml) for kininogen measurements, and centrifuged at 20^{0}C with 3000 rpm for 20 min. The supernatant was aliquoted and stored at -80^{0}C until measurement. After the observation period of 2 hours (DS groups, Table 1) and 5 hours (TK groups, Table 1), the animals were sacrificed.

Table 1. Experimental protocols: Animals were given either tissue
kallikrein (TK) or dextran sulphate (DS) simultaneously
with either saline or different doses of aprotinin.

Contact activation [DS 2 mg/kg]	+ saline		(n= 5)	group DS_0
	+ aprotinin	50,000 KIU/kg	(n= 4)	group DS_1
	+ aprotinin	200,000 KIU/kg	(n= 4)	group DS_2
	+ aprotinin	400,000 KIU/kg	(n= 2)	group DS_3
Tissue Kallikrein [TK 50 µg/(kg x h)]	+ saline		(n= 7)	group TK_0
	+ aprotinin	694 KIU/(kg x h)	(n= 6)	group TK_1
	+ aprotinin	1389 KIU/(kg x h)	(n= 6)	group TK_2

In animals assigned to DS groups (see Table 1) activation of the coagulation, fibrinolytic and plasma kallikrein systems was induced by continuous
intravenous infusion of dextran sulphate (DS), 2 mg/kg over 60 min. In
addition, five animals (group DS_0) were given saline; ten animals received
aprotinin in a total dose ranging between 51,000 and 415,000 KIU/kg (groups
DS_{1-3}) intravenously in two equivalent doses, one as a bolus injection
before starting the DS infusion and the other dose was coadministered with
DS over a 60 min period.

Tissue kallikrein (TK) was infused in 19 animals (see Table 1) at a
constant rate of 50 µg/(kg x h) over 3 hours (groups TK_{0-2}). The control
animals (group TK_0) received TK and saline. In the remaining animals TK was
given simultaneously with a 4 hr infusion of aprotinin. The infusion of
aprotinin was started 1 h before TK administration.

RESULTS

Inhibition of tissue kallikrein

Incubation of porcine tissue kallikrein with human LMW and HMW kininogen in vitro resulted in kinin release at tissue kallikrein concentrations
greater than 10^{-10} mol/l. The kinin release from LMWK was effectively
blocked by aprotinin levels greater than 10^{-7} mol/l (4 KIU/ml) (Fig. 1).
This was also demonstrated for HMW kininogen (data not shown).

After tissue kallikrein infusion, mean arterial pressure (MAP) decreased over a 30 min period from 86.5 ± 10.3 mmHg to 76 ± 12.5 mmHg in
group TK_0. After 1 h MAP was restored to baseline level. A similar
transient decrease in MAP (from 100.3 ± 13.2 to 83.7 ± 24.7 mmHg) was
observed in group TK_1, whereas in group TK_2 MAP decreased only slightly
(from 92.6 ± 16.2 mmHg to 86.2 ± 5.1 mmHg).

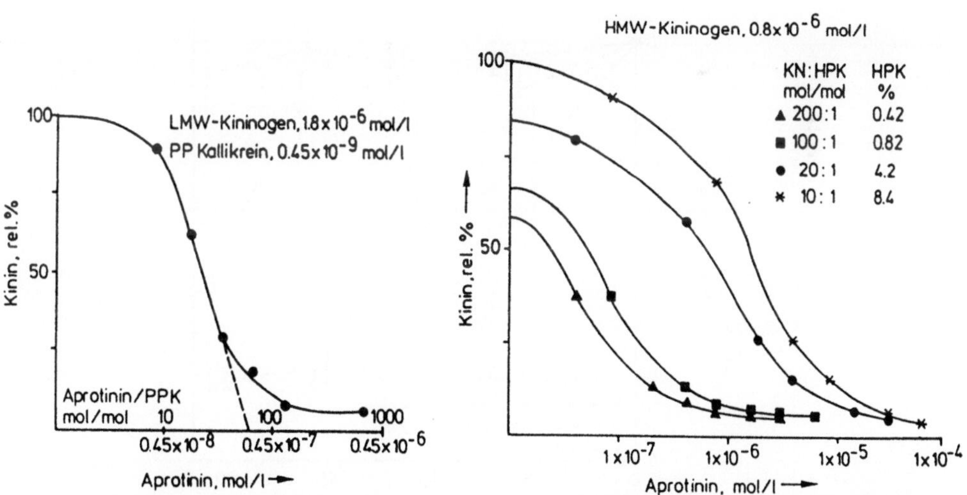

Fig. 1. Dose-response curves of aprotinin on the inhibition of kinin release
from (left) human low molecular weight (LMW) kininogen by porcine
pancreatic (=tissue) kallikrein (PPK) and (right) human high
molecular weight (HMW) kininogen by human plasma kallikrein (HPK) in
the in vitro system. The percent values given correspond to the
degree of plasma prokallikrein activation in relation to the mean
total amount of prokallikrein present in human plasma.

Kininogen concentrations in plasma decreased to 42 ± 17.5 % of the
starting value (100 %) in group TK_0. Aprotinin administration at doses of
694 KIU/(kg x h) in group TK_1, and 1389 KIU/(kg x h) in group TK_2 limited
this fall to 63 ± 6.5 %, and 85 ± 7.6 %, respectively (Fig. 2). In these
experiments the plasma levels of aprotinin ranged from 0.6 to 1.4 KIU/ml in
group TK_1, and from 4 to 7 KIU/ml in group TK_2.

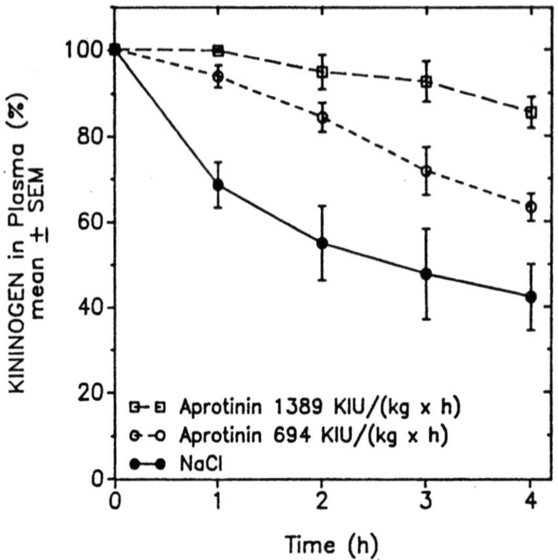

Fig. 2. Plasma kininogen concentrations in animals during an infusion
of tissue kallikrein [50 µg/(kg x h)]. Aprotinin plasma levels
ranged from 0.6 to 1.4 KIU/ml and from 4 to 7 KIU/ml during a
continuous infusion of 694 KIU/(kg x h) and 1389 KIU/(kg x h),
respectively.

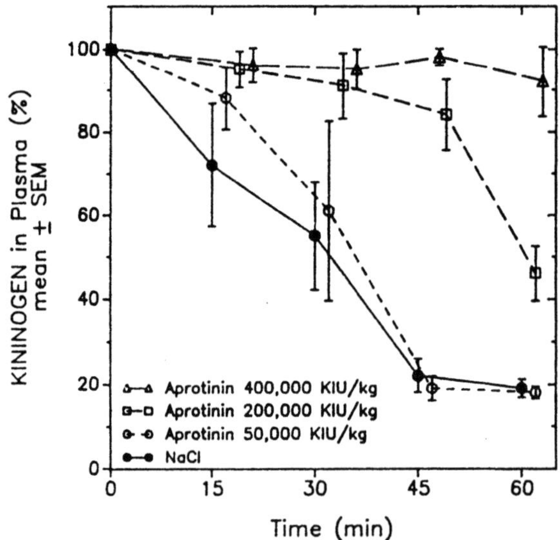

Fig. 3. Plasma kininogen concentrations in animals during activation
of the intrinsic coagulation cascade by continuous infusion of
dextran sulphate (DS), 2 mg/kg over 1 h. Aprotinin plasma
levels ranged from 100 to 150 KIU/ml at a total dose of 50,000
KIU/kg, from 200 to 300 KIU/ml (dose: 200,000 KIU/kg), and from
400 to 500 KIU/ml at a total dose of 400,000 KIU/kg.

<u>Inhibition of plasma kallikrein</u>

When human plasma kallikrein (HPK) was incubated with human kininogen in the in vitro system, HPK concentrations greater than 10^{-9} mol/l were associated with substantial kinin release from HMW kininogen. HPK released kinin not only from HMWK but also from LMWK. At HPK concentrations of 10^{-8} mol/l, 40 % of total HMWK and 20 % of total LMWK was cleaved within 180 min. Aprotinin levels greater than 10^{-5} mol/l (400 KIU/ml) effectively blocked the action of HPK on HMWK (Fig.1) and on LMWK (data not shown). The actual concentrations of aprotinin necessary for complete inhibition of kinin release depended clearly on the amount of plasma kallikrein present. Thus, the inhibitory effectiveness of a certain aprotinin concentration in vivo would depend on the percentage of plasma prokallikrein activated under the given conditions.

Induction of contact activation in animal experiments by continuous infusion of dextran sulphate (DS) over 60 min led to a transient drop in MAP (-66 ± 14 mmHg) and a decrease in plasma prokallikrein (-77 ± 2 %) and kininogen levels (-81 ± 5 %). Administration of aprotinin delayed the onset of MAP reduction and the consumption of kininogen in a dose-dependent manner (administered dose vs. onset of MAP decrease: Pearson $r^2=0.86$; n=8). No MAP reduction at all and only a slight consumption of kininogen (-8 ± 12 %) was observed at plasma aprotinin levels of 400 - 500 KIU/ml in group DS_3 (Fig. 3). Plasma levels of aprotinin in group DS_1 ranged from 100 - 150 KIU/ml and in group DS_2 from 200 - 300 KIU/ml. Platelet count dropped below 200,000 $1/mm^3$ in 4 out of the 5 animals in group DS_0. In the aprotinin treated animals thrombocytopenia developed in 1 of the 4 animals in group DS_2 and in none of two animals in group DS_3.

DISCUSSION

The primary target enzymes of the basic proteinase inhibitor aprotinin (Trasylol[R]) from bovine tissue cells, are serine proteases such as trypsin, plasmin, as well as tissue and plasma kallikrein (Fritz and Wunderer, 1983). In this study aprotinin was assayed for its ability to inhibit the action of tissue kallikrein and plasma kallikrein on their natural substrates, HMW and LMW kininogen, both in vitro and in vivo. The results demonstrate that effective inhibition of tissue kallikrein and plasma kallikrein may be achieved, in vitro and in vivo under concentration conditions known to occur clinically. Human tissue kallikrein and human plasma kallikrein have affinities to aprotinin comparable to those of the corresponding enzymes of porcine origin (Fritz and Wunderer, 1983). Our in vitro studies using purified human compounds, and the in vivo studies using pigs, yielded comparable results. Therefore the inhibitory plasma levels determined may be equally valid in humans. Plasma levels of aprotinin were measured by a recently developed competitive enzyme-linked immunosorbent assay (Mueller-Esterl et al., 1984). This assay has been shown to provide a versatile means to monitor rapidly and precisely aprotinin levels in plasma and body fluids from patients treated with aprotinin (Jochum and Mueller-Esterl, 1985; Clasen et al., 1987).

The activation and release of pancreatic proteases such as trypsin or tissue kallikrein into peritoneal exudates and into the circulation, concomitant with the consumption of endogenous inhibitors and the turnover of kininogen, has been demonstrated in both experimental pancreatitis (Kortmann et al., 1983; Borgstrom and Ohlsson, 1978) as well as clinically in man (Balldin and Ohlsson, 1979). Using continuous tissue kallikrein infusion as a model for kallikrein liberation, e.g. during acute pancreatitis, we studied the inhibition of tissue kallikrein with aprotinin in animal experiments. The dose of kallikrein infused was calculated from the kallikrein

amount present in the porcine pancreas (Frey et al., 1968). The results
obtained revealed that even the maximal continuously liberated dose of
kallikrein, as can be predicted in vivo, may be sufficiently blocked at
aprotinin plasma levels of 4 - 10 KIU/ml (10^{-7} mol/l). This was assessed by
kininogen consumption and measurements of arterial pressure. Keeping in mind
that trypsin is even more sensitive to aprotinin inhibition, concentrations
of 10^{-7} mol/l should also suffice to completely inactivate trypsin released
from the pancreas under inflammatory conditions (Fritz, 1985).

Unlike tissue kallikrein and trypsin, plasma kallikrein (HPK) is much
less efficiently inhibited by aprotinin (Fritz, 1978). HPK plays a major
role in the activation of the coagulation and fibrinolytic cascades. (i) It
triggers the endogenous pathway of blood coagulation via F XII activation,
(ii) it liberates kinin from kininogen, and (iii) it may stimulate polymorphonuclear granulocytes and thus induce the release of lysosomal enzymes
(Mueller-Esterl and Fritz, 1984; Schapira et al., 1983). A pronounced and
rapid activation of HPK has been demonstrated in traumatized and septic
patients, and during cardiopulmonary bypass (McConn et al., 1983; Aasen,
1985; Heller et al., 1987). Activation of HPK occurs on negatively charged
surfaces, e.g. exposed subendothelial structures. Also the cell wall
fractions of bacteria may activate HPK (Kalter et al., 1983). Thus, after
trauma and sepsis, in a short time period, high amounts of active HPK may be
generated from its precursor plasma prokallikrein despite high concentrations of endogenous HPK inhibitors present in plasma.

We used the intravenous infusion of dextran sulphate (DS) as a model
for the induction of in vivo contact activation. In this model about 80 % of
the plasma prokallikrein is activated within 60 minutes. This activation is
paralleled by a transient fall in arterial pressure, a rapid turnover of the
kininogens, a fall in platelet count, and a prolonged coagulation time.
Aprotinin was able to attenuate this response to DS in a clear dose depen-
dend manner. Marginal inhibition was observed at plasma levels of 100
KIU/ml, weak inhibition with 200 KIU/ml, while plasma levels greater than
400 KIU/ml abolished the effect completely. This was confirmed in the in
vitro studies: When physiological concentrations of HMWK were incubated with
small amounts of HPK (corresponding to 1 % of the total HPK pool activatable
in vivo) kinin release was inhibited at aprotinin concentrations of 40
KIU/ml, whereas when higher amounts of HPK were applied (corresponding to
10-20 % of the total HPK pool), only aprotinin concentrations as 400 KIU/ml
properly inhibited the action of HPK on kininogen. These results are in
agreement with theoretical considerations based on enzyme kinetics and
substrate availability which predicted that only aprotinin concentrations of
200-400 KIU/ml would suffice to effectively inhibit plasma kallikrein
(Fritz, 1978; Philipp, 1978).

At exceedingly high aprotinin plasma levels the inhibitory function of
aprotinin may be explained in part by alternative mechanisms. At pH 7.4
aprotinin is a highly positive charged molecule and may avidly bind to
negatively charged surfaces (Fritz and Wunderer, 1983). In our model,
aprotinin may directly bind to DS and thus saturate the negatively charged
activating surface. In addition, it is known from ACD blood that aprotinin
(at concentrations of 400 KIU/ml) may bind to negatively charged molecules
of the platelet membrane surface and thus inhibit platelet aggregation
(Harke et al., 1982). This effect of aprotinin, based on ionic interactions
may be responsible for the absence of thrombocytopenia in the high dose
aprotinin group. However, this non specific effect of aprotinin, in addition
to its role as an enzyme inhibitor may be significant in certain clinical
situations such as after trauma or during cardiopulmonary bypass.

The question arises as to the feasibility of obtaining these plasma
concentrations of aprotinin in clinical situations. Recent studies have been

shown that this is indeed feasible (Clasen et al., 1987). However, due to
the short plasma half life time of the inhibitor a continuous infusion is
necessary to maintain plasma levels within the desired range (Fritz et al.,
1969, Clasen et al., 1987). Very high doses of aprotinin are apparently
tolerated well. Coagulatory or microcirculatory disturbances have not been
observed after administration of 17.5 millon KIU aprotinin within 24 hours
in traumatized patients (Clasen et al., 1987). The dosage regimen used in
this study resulted in initial peak plasma levels of about 400 KIU/ml which
returned to 100-200 KIU/ml during subsequent continuous infusion of 1
million KIU/h over 12 hours. In our study, in two aprotinin-control animals
showing peak plasma levels of 800 KIU/ml after a bolus injection and 400 to
500 KIU/ml during subsequent continuous infusion of aprotinin, apart from a
slight prolongation of the coagulation time, no physiologic change was
noted.

In conclusion, the present study demonstrated that effective inhibition
of tissue kallikrein and plasma kallikrein in vivo is achieved at aprotinin
plasma levels of 4 - 10 KIU/ml (10^{-7} mol/l) and 400 KIU/ml (10^{-5} mol/l),
respectively. In conjunction with the newly developed assays for aprotinin
this data may help to improve the efficacy of proteinase inhibitor therapy.

REFERENCES

Aasen, A.O., 1985, The proenzyme functional inhibition index. A new parame-
    ter for the evaluation of the severely injured and septic patient, Acta
    Chir Scand, suppl. 522:211.
Balldin, G., Ohlsson, K., 1979, Demonstration of pancreatic protease-
    antiprotease complexes in the peritoneal fluid of patients with acute
    pancreatitis, Surgery, 80:451.
Borgstrom, A., Ohlsson, K., 1978, Immunoreactive trypsin in serum and
    peritoneal fluid in acute pancreatitis, Hoppe Seylers Z Physiol Chem,
    359:677.
Clasen, C., Jochum, M., Mueller-Esterl, W., 1987, Feasibility study of very
    high aprotinin dosage in polytrauma patients, Prog Clin Biol Res,
    236A:175.
Frey, E.K., Kraut, H., Werle, E., 1968, "Das Kallikrein-Kinin-System und
    seine Inhibitoren," Enke-Verlag, Stuttgart.
Fritz, H., Oppitz, K.-H., Meckl, D., Kemkes, B., Haendle, H., Schult, H.,
    Werle, E., 1969, Verteilung und Ausscheidung von natuerlich vorkommen-
    den und chemisch modifizierten Proteaseinhibitoren nach intravenoeser
    Injektion bei Ratte, Hund (und Mensch), Hoppe Seylers Z Physiol Chem,
    350:1541.
Fritz, H., 1978, Inhibition of plasmin and plasma kallikrein by the basic
    trypsin-kallikrein inhibitor from bovine organs (Trasylol) and similar
    protease inhibitors: Theoretical considerations, in: "Progress in
    chemical fibrinolysis and thrombolysis, Vol.3," Davidson, J.F., Rowan,
    R.M., Samama, M.M., Desnoyers, P.C., eds., Raven Press, New York.
Fritz, H., Wunderer, G., 1983, Biochemistry and applications of aprotinin,
    the kallikrein inhibitor from bovine organs, Drug Res, 33,4:479.
Fritz, H., 1985, The target enzymes of aprotinin in vitro and in vivo, in:
    "Proteolyse und Proteinaseninhibitoren in der Herz- und Gefaesschirur-
    gie," Dudziak, R., Reuter, H.D., Kirchhoff, P.G., Schumann, F., eds.,
    Schattauer Verlag, Stuttgart.
Harke, H., Stienen, G., Rahman, S., Flohr, H., 1982, Aprotinin-ACD-Blut, II.
    Der Einfluss von Aprotinin auf die Freisetzung zellulaerer Mediatoren
    und Enzyme im Konservenblut, Anaesthesist, 31:165.
Heller, W., Fuhrer, G., Hoffmeister, H.-E., Gallimore, M.J., 1987, Studies
    on shock during extracorporal circulation during aorto-coronary bypass
    operations, Prog Clin Biol Res, 236A:87.
Jochum, M., Jonakova, V., Dittmer, H., Fritz, H., 1984, An enzymatic assay

convenient for the control of aprotinin levels during proteinase inhibitor therapy, <u>Fresenius Z Anal Chem</u>, 317:719.

Jochum, M., Mueller-Esterl, W., 1985, Bestimmung von Aprotinin-Plasmakonzentrationen nach therapeutischer Anwendung von Trasylol, <u>in</u>: "Proteolyse und Proteinaseninhibitoren in der Herz- und Gefaesschirurgie," Dudziak, R., Reuter, H.D., Kirchhoff, P.G., Schumann, F., eds., Schattauer Verlag, Stuttgart.

Jochum, M., Dittmer, H., Fritz, H., 1987, Der Effekt des Proteinaseninhibitors Aprotinin auf die Freisetzung granulozytaerer Proteinasen und Plasmaproteinveraenderungen im traumatisch-haemorrhagischen Schock, <u>Lab med</u>, 11:235.

Kalter, E.S., Van Dijk, W.C., Timmermann, A., Verhoef, J., Bouma, B.N., 1983, Activation of purified human plasma prekallikrein triggered by cell wall fractions of Escherichia coli and Staphylococcus aureus, <u>J Infect Dis</u>, 148:682.

Kortmann, H., Ernst, C., Hoffmann, H., Boenner, G., 1983, Der Einfluss endogen freigesetzter Kinine auf den Verlauf der experimentellen akuten haemorrhagischen Pankreatitis, <u>Langenbecks Arch Chir</u>, Suppl:35.

McConn, R., Wassermann, F., Haberland, G., 1983, The kallikrein-kinin system in the acutely ill: (A) Changes in plasma kininogen in acutely ill patients. (B) The efficacy of pulmonary clearence of bradykinin, <u>Adv Exp Med Biol</u>, 156B:1019

Mueller-Esterl, W., Rauth, G., Fritz, H., Lottspeich, F., Henschen, A., 1983, Human Kininogens, <u>in</u>: "Kininogenases/Kallikrein VI," Haberland, G.L., Rohen, J.W., Fritz, H., Huber, P., eds., Schattauer Verlag, Stuttgart.

Mueller-Esterl, W., Fritz, H., 1984, Human Kininogenases and their function in the kallikrein-kinin system, in: "Proteases: Potential role in health and disease," Hoerl, W.H., Haidland, A., eds., Plenum Publishing Corp., New York.

Mueller-Esterl, W., Oettl, A., Truscheit, E., Fritz, H., 1984, Monitoring of aprotinin plasma levels by an enzyme-linked immunosorbent assay (ELISA), <u>Fresenius Z Anal Chem</u>, 317:718.

Philipp, E., 1978, Calculations and hypothetical considerations on the inhibition of plasmin and plasma kallikrein by trasylol, <u>in</u>: "Progress in chemical fibrinolysis and thrombolysis, Vol.3," Davidson, J.F., Rowan, R.M., Samama, M.M., Desnoyers, P.C., eds., Raven Press, New York.

Schapira, M., Scott, C.F., Boxer, L.A., Colman, R.W., 1983, Activation of human polymorphonuclear leucocytes by purified human plasma kallikrein, <u>Adv Exp Med Biol</u>, 156B:747.

Uchida, Y., Katori, M., 1979, Differential assay method for high molecular weight and low molecular weight kininogens, <u>Thromb Res</u>, 15:127.

ACKNOWLEDGEMENT

The authors whish to acknowledge the kininogen measurements by Prof. Dr. E. Fink, aprotinin measurements by Prof. Dr. W. Mueller-Esterl, and the excellent technical assistance by Mrs. G. Godez, Mrs. A. Oettl, Mrs. E. Schaller, and Mrs. S. Sokal.

CHANGES IN THE KALLIKREIN-KININ-SYSTEM AFTER DIFFERENT DOSE REGIMEN OF APROTININ DURING CARDIOPULMONARY BYPASS OPERATION

W. Heller, G. Fuhrer, M.J. Gallimore,
J. Michel, and H.-E. Hoffmeister

Department of Cardiovascular Surgery, University
of Tübingen, 7400 Tübingen, FRG

Introduction

It has been reported by our group that shortly after the onset of cardiopulmonary bypass an increase in kallikrein like activity and a decrease in prekallikrein and kallikrein inhibition can be detected (9). Furthermore, kallikrein like activities seemed to be somewhat lower and prekallikrein levels were slightly higher in a few patients treated with higher doses of aprotinin. Therefore, we performed another series of studies to investigate the effect of high and low doses of aprotinin. After anaesthesia 5000 KIU/kg body weight (group 1) or 15000 KIU/kg body weight (group 2) of aprotinin were administered. Another dose was given to the prime volume of the heart-lung machine, further infusions of this antiprotease in the same dose were performed 30 minutes after the onset of cardiopulmonary bypass and at the end of extracorporeal circulation.

Material and methods

All patients suffered from coronary artery disease and underwent aorto-coronary venous bypass grafting (n=30). Group 1: 14 patients were treated with the 5000 KIU aprotinin/kg body weight dosage regimen. Group 2: 16 patients received 15000 KIU aprotinin/kg body weight dosage regimen. The administration was performed according to the following schedule:
1) After anaesthesia 2) To the prime volume of the heart-lung machine 3) 30 minutes after the onset of cardiopulmonary bypass 4) At the end of extracorporeal circulation.
For the determination of kallikrein like activity, kallikrein inhibition, prekallikrein, ß-fXIIa-inhibition, factor XII and antithrombin III, blood was taken:
1) Before anaesthesia 2) after thoracotomy 3) immediately after the onset of extracorporeal circulation (ECC). 4) 15 minutes after the onset of ECC 5) 30 minutes after beginning ECC 6) 45 minutes after starting ECC 7) at the end of ECC 8) after operation 9) First post operative day 10) third post operative day 11) seventh post operative day.

Kallikrein like activity, prekallikrein and kallikrein inhibition levels were determined by means of chromogenic substrate assays (Deutsche KabiVitrum GmbH, Munich, FRG) according to the methods of Gallimore and Friberger (1). ß-fXIIa inhibition was measured using ß-fXIIa (Channel Diagnostics, Walmer Deal, Kent, U.K.) and S-2222 (Deutsche KabiVitrum, Munich, FRG).
Factor XII levels were analysed according to a method from Gallimore et al.(2).
For the determination of antithrombin III a commercially available test kit (Deutsche KabiVitrum GmbH, Munich, FRG) was used.
All levels were corrected for hematocrit. Heparin was antagonized in all plasma samples in the ratio 1:1.

Results

Group 1

Patients in this group had high normal prekallikrein levels before operation (123 ± 35%). After thoracotomy no significant changes occurred (120 ± 43%). The onset of cardiopulmonary bypass was associated with a slight fall of this protein (109 ± 43%). A further reduction during ECC could be observed and levels of 100 ± 31% were determined after cardiopulmonary bypass. The levels increased from the end of the operation to the first post operative day (from 106 ± 35% to 118 ± 40%). Prekallikrein levels fell to 101 ± 32% on the third post operative day but increased on day 7 to 111 ± 27% (fig. 1). Factor XII levels were found to be 85 ± 28% before operation and were not significantly changed after thoracotomy (88 ± 36%). During extracorporeal circulation levels were lowered (79 ± 35% 45 minutes after the beginning of ECC) but afterwards the levels reached prebypass values (86 ± 38%). On the first post operative day the levels rose to 101 ± 46%, but a continuous fall to the seventh post operative day could be observed (87 ± 27%).
Kallikrein like activities increased after the onset of cardiopulmonary bypass (from 29 ± 9 U/l to 48 ± 19 U/l). During extracorporeal circulation the levels fell continuously to 35 ± 7U/l. In the post operative period no significant changes were observed (First day 29 ± 7 U/l, seventh day 31 ± 17 U/l, fig. 2).
ß-fXIIa inhibition levels were 109 ± 29% and were not altered during thoracotomy, levels increased slightly after the beginning of ECC, but declined to 117± 67% after cardiopulmonary bypass. A significant increase could be detected in the post operative period and levels of 208 ± 88% were found on day 7. Kallikrein inhibition capacity was 128 ± 35% of normal before operation and was slightly elevated after the administration of the first dose of aprotinin (136 ± 32%). The inhibition rose to 210± 61% when cardiopulmonary bypass was started. 15 minutes later the levels decreased slightly (190 ± 70%), but inhibition capacity increased due to the next infusion of aprotinin 30 minutes after the beginning of ECC (227 ± 73%). During the course of the operation, levels declined to 186 ± 52%. From the first to the seventh post operative day a continuous increase occurred (from 152 ± 75% to 170 ± 60%, fig. 3).
Preoperative antithrombin III activities were in the normal range (95 ± 12%). During operation a slight fall could be

seen and the lowest levels were determined 45 minutes after
the onset of ECC (89 ± 17%). After operation the levels rose
and were above initial values on the seventh post operative
day (111 ± 41%).

<u>Group 2</u>

In patients with higher doses of aprotinin preoperative prekallikrein levels were somewhat lower than in patients from
group 1 (99 ± 20%). Immediately after the onset of cardiopulmonary bypass levels decreased to 90 ± 36%. A further reduction was seen 15 minutes later (86 ± 34%). When aprotinin was
given, a slight fall could be observed in the plasma taken 30
minutes after the beginning of extracorporeal circulation (84
± 36%). At the end of the bypass, levels increased to 94 ±
38%, but were found to be reduced to 89 ± 31% after operation. On the first post operative day prekallikrein levels
rose to 92 ± 27%, but declined again to 82 ± 25% on day 3.
Determination of prekallikrein on the seventh post operative
day showed an increase (105 ± 52%, fig. 1). Before operation
levels of fXII were comparable to those from group 1 (83 ±
18%). The levels increased after thoracotomy but fell to
intial values after the onset of cardiopulmonary bypass
(from 100 ± 44% to 84 ± 37%). During extracorporeal
circulation levels did not change significantly. Levels of 87
± 46% were found after bypass and 95 ± 45% after operation.
The levels increased continuously in the post operative
period (day 1 99 ± 31%, day 3 101 ± 37%, day 7 111 ± 65%).
Kallikrein like activities were elevated after starting the
ECC (sample 1 29 ± 6 U/l, sample 3 45 ± 23% U/l). During the
operation this activity decreased and was found to be 39 ±
15 U/l after surgical treatment. No significant changes
occurred during the post operative period (fig. 2).
ß-fXIIa inhibition capacity increased from 83 + 18% to 112 +
50% when samples taken preoperatively were compared with
those after starting ECC. No significant changes occurred
during the bypass time, but levels decreased to 98 ± 43%
after operation. From the first to the seventh post operative day ß-fXIIa inhibition capacity was significantly elevated.
Preoperative kallikrein inhibition was in the normal range
(104 ± 28%), but rose to 177 ± 78%) after the infusion of
aprotinin. A further increase could be observed when the
prime volume of the heart-lung machine (containing another
dose of aprotinin) was mixed with the blood of the patients
(260 ± 103%). In the following sample (15 minutes later)
levels were slightly reduced (237 ± 104%) but increased again
after the addition of aprotinin (277 ± 134%). The highest
levels were detected after bypass (310 ± 171%). In the post
operative period an acute-phase reaction was seen (from 155 ±
66% on day 1 to 191 ± 104% on day 7, fig. 3).
Patients in this group showed low normal antithrombin III
levels before operation (80 ± 13%). After thoracotomy a
slight increase was observed (98 ± 36%). These activities
were reduced during ECC and mean values of 89 ± 28% were
determined after operation. The levels on day 7 after operation were higher than preoperative values (112 ± 46%).

<u>Discussion</u>

In patients during cardiopulmonary bypass an activation of

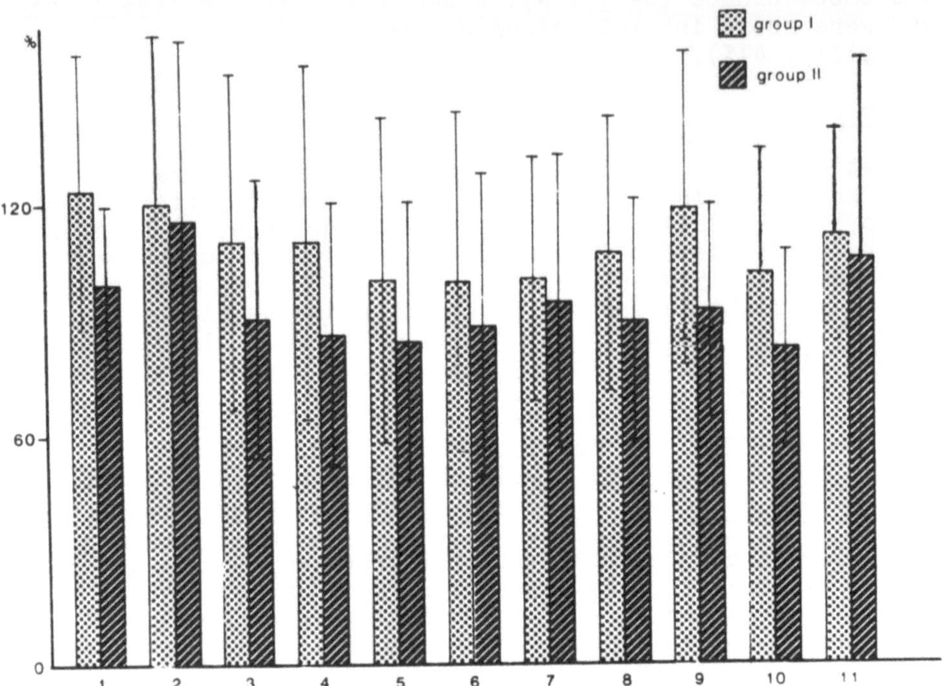

Fig. 1   Prekallikrein levels in patients with two
different doses of aprotinin

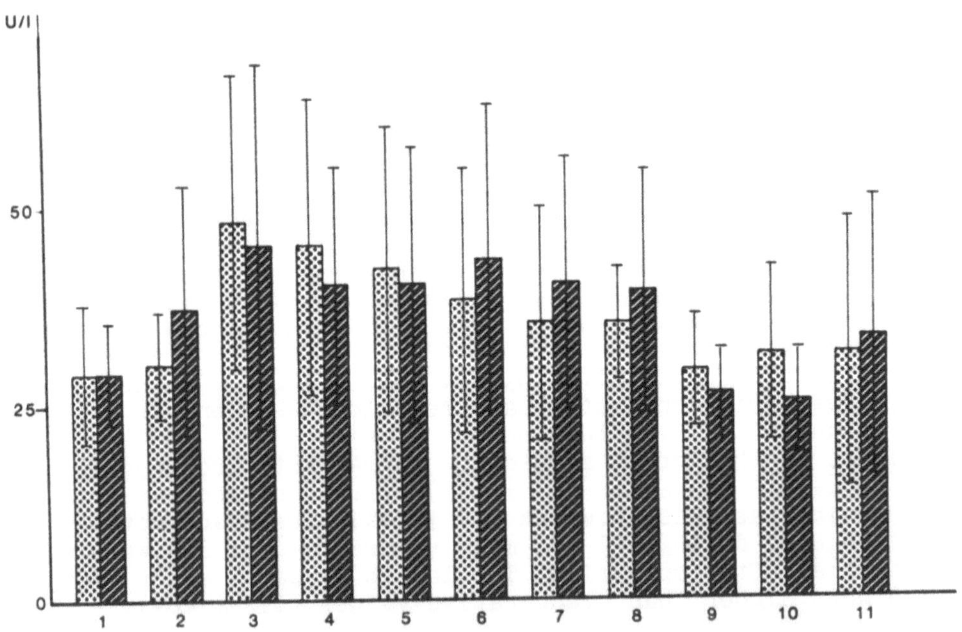

Fig. 2   Changes in kallikrein-like activities
in patients treated with two different
doses of aprotinin

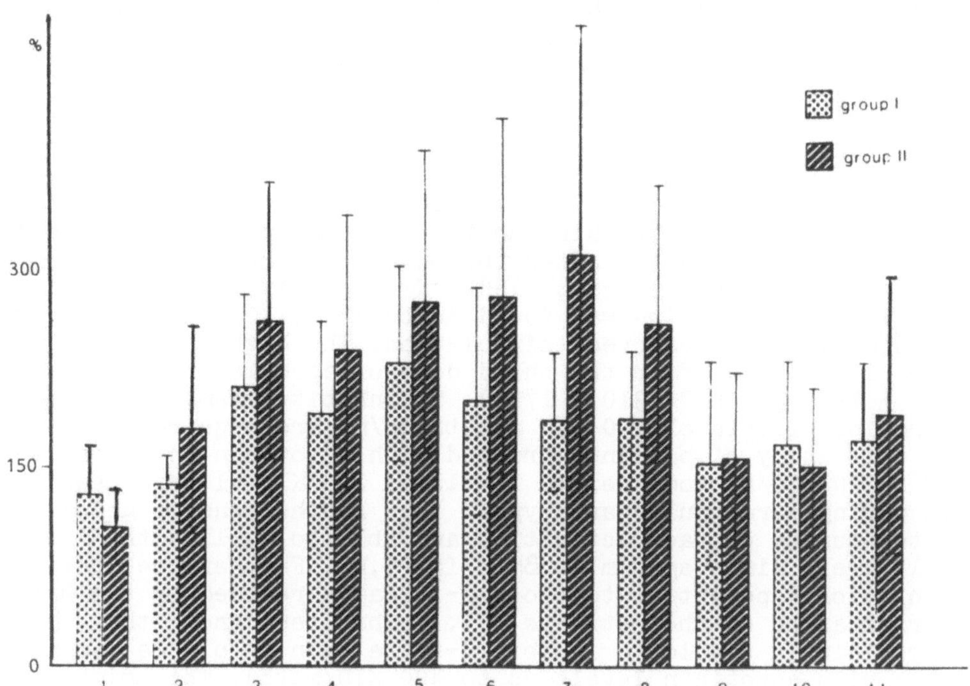

Fig. 3   Levels of kallikrein-inhibition
in patients using two different
dose regimens of aprotinin

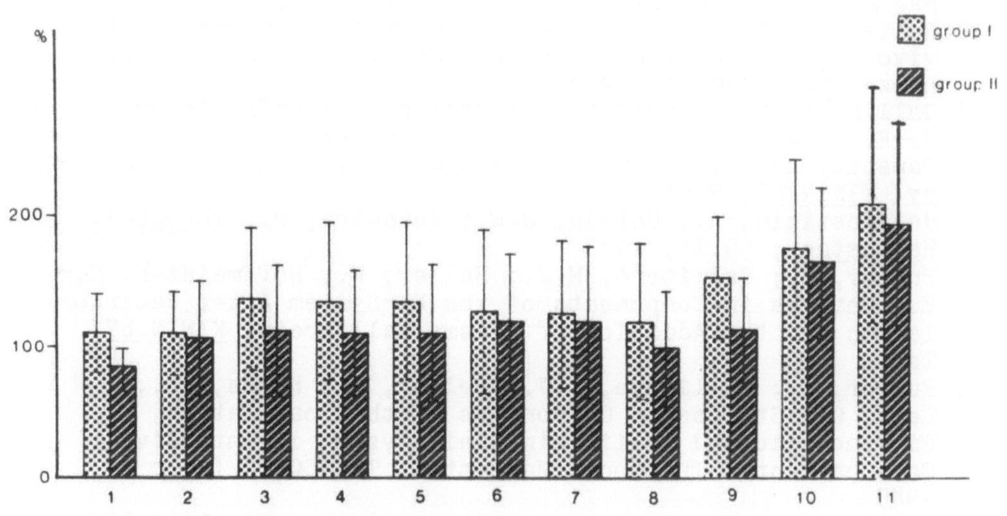

Fig. 4   Inhibition of ß-FXIIa after the
addition of aprotinin
(Group 1: 5000 KIU aprotinin/kg per dose
Group 2:15000 KIU aprotinin/kg per dose)

the contact phase system occurs. This can be shown by an increase in kallikrein like activities and a reduction in prekallikrein, factor XII and ß-fXIIa inhibition when prebypass levels are compared with those after the commencement of extracorporeal circulation. Antithrombin III levels decreased slightly during cardiopulmonary bypass. By the adminstration of aprotinin the kallikrein inhibition capacity was markedly elevated. In patients with 5000 KIU aprotinin/kg body weight levels of this inhibition capacity were 210 ± 61% of normal, immediately after the onset of cardiopulmonary bypass. In the other group (15000 KIU aprotinin a dose) kallikrein inhibition was found to be 260 ± 103% at the beginning of extracorporeal circulation. The highest levels were determined after the third dose of aprotinin (group 1 : 227 ± 73%, group 2: 310 ± 171%). To inhibit plasma kallikrein aprotinin levels of 200 KIU aprotinin/ml are required (3). In this study of patients treated with aprotinin in a dose of 15000 KIU/kg body weight levels of 200 KIU/ml were reached during cardiopulmonary bypass (4). Another enzyme generated during contact activation and able to amplify the kallikrein kinin system is ß-fXIIa (5,6). Furthermore, the inhibitoric potential to block ß-fXIIa is reduced by the heparinization of the patients (7). It has been shown that aprotinin is unable to inhibit ß-fXIIa even in plasma samples with aprotinin levels up to 400 KIU/ml(8). This might be responsible for the changes in both groups. Further studies to reveal the beneficial effects of combined inhibitor therapy are underway in our laboratory.

References

1) Gallimore, M.J.; Friberger, P.. Simple Chromogenic Peptide Substrate Assays for Determining Prekallikrein, Kallikrein Inhibition and Kallikrein Like Activity in Human Plasma. Thromb. Res. 25, p 293, 1982
2) Gallimore, M.J.; Rees, W.A.; Fuhrer, G.; Heller, W.. A Direct Chromogenic Peptide Substrate Assay for Hageman Factor (FXII). Fibrinolysis, 1, pp 123-127, 1987
3) Fritz, H.. Die Zielenzyme des Aprotinin in vitro und in vivo. In: Proteolyse und Proteinaseninhibitoren in der Herz- und Gefäßchirurgie, 1985
4) Gallimore, M.J.; Fuhrer, G.; Heller, W.; Hoffmeister, H.-E.. Augmentation of Kallikrein and Plasmin Inhibition Capacity by Aprotinin Using a New Assay to Monitor Therapy, KININ 87, Tokio
5) de Agostinin, A.; Colman, R.W.; Schapira, M.. Thrombos. Haemostas., 50:11, 1983
6) Fuhrer, G.; Gallimore, M.J.; Heller, W.; Hoffmeister, H.-E.. Changes in Components of the KK-System After Recirculation and the Addition of Plasma Kallikrein. KININ 87, Tokio
7) Fuhrer, G.; Gallimore, M.J.; Heller, W.; Klöss, Th.; Lenz, G.. Studies on Components of the Coagulation, Fibrinolytic and Kallikrein Kinin System in Intensive Care patients. Thrombos. Haemostas. THHADQ 54 (1) p 253, 1985
8) Gallimore, M.J.; Rees, W.A.. Personal communication 1985
9) Fuhrer, G.; Gallimore, M.J.; Heller, W.; Hoffmeister, H.-E.. Studies on Components of the Plasma Kallikrein-Kinin System in Patients Undergoing Cardiopulmonary Bypass. KININ 84

CENTRAL EFFECT OF APROTININ, A SERINE PROTEASE INHIBITOR, ON BLOOD

PRESSURE IN SPONTANEOUSLY HYPERTENSIVE AND WISTAR-KYOTO RATS

Shinji Seto, Masazumi Akahoshi, Shigeru Kusano, Shin-ichi
Kitamura and Kunitake Hashiba

The Third Department of Internal Medicine, Nagasaki
University School of Medicine, Nagasaki, Japan

SUMMARY

We examined the effect of centrally administered aprotinin, a serine
protease inhibitor, on blood pressure (BP) in conscious spontaneously
hypertensive rats (SHR) and Wistar-Kyoto rats (WKY). Twenty-two gauge
needles and polyethylene catheters were implanted into lateral
cerebroventricle and femoral artery, respectively, at 48 hours before the
experiments. In Group 1 (8 SHR, 6 WKY), rats received a bolus intracerebroventricular injection (i.c.v.) of aprotinin (1,000 KIU/kg/10 μl).
A prompt increase of BP was observed in SHR after aprotinin and this
elevation of BP was persisted for over 30 minutes (mean BP : 158.8 ± 2.9
mmHg at control to 168.7 ± 3.2 at 15 min., p<0.01; to 168.3 ± 3.4 at 30
min., p<0.01). On the other hand, BP of WKY decreased gradually after
aprotinin (mean BP : 143.0 ± 3.3 at control to 136.8 ± 2.7 at 15 min.,
n.s.; to 134.2 ± 5.1 at 30 min., p<0.05). The intravenous injection
(i.v.) of aprotinin (Group 2 : 7 SHR, 5 WKY) and the i.c.v. of artificial
cerebrospinal fluid (CSF) (Group 3 : 5 SHR, 6 WKY) did not affect BP in
both SHR and WKY except for the minor transient increas of BP in WKY
immediately after artificial CSF i.c.v.. We performed additional
experiments to study the contributions of sympathetic nervous system and
vasopressin to these changes in BP. Either hexamethonium (Hx : 25 mg/kg
i.v. ; Group 4 : 7 SHR, 5 WKY) or d(CH2)5 arginine vasopressin (AVP-
antagonist : 30 μg/kg i.v. ; Group 5 : 5 SHR, 4 WKY) were given at 60
minutes before aprotinin i.c.v.. In SHR, the pretreatment with Hx
abolished the pressor response to aprotinin, although the pretreatment of
AVP-antagonist did not affect the pressor response. Pretreatments with
both Hx and AVP-antagonist cancelled the depressor response to aprotinin
in WKY. We concluded that the central administration of aprotinin exerted
dual effects ; the pressor effect due to increase of sympathetic nervous
activity in SHR, which may not be related to the inhibition of kinin-
generating activity by aprotinin and the depressor effect due to decrease
of sympathetic nervous activity and vasopressin in WKY, which may be
related to the inhibition of kinin-generating activity of serine protease.

INTRODUCTION

It has been proposed a physiological role of some serine protease(s),
such as kallikrein, in central nervous system on the regulation of BP

through its kinin-generating activity[1]. Recent studies demonstrated that all components necessary for the formation and the metabolism of kinins are present in brain[1] and, further, central administration of kinins increases BP in conscious rats[2,3]. Moreover, it has been reported that the increase in endogenous CSF kinins during ventriculocisternal perfusion with melittin, an activator of membrane-bound kallikrein, was associated with an increase in BP[4]. In addition, it has been demonstrated that the concentration of kinins in CSF of SHR was lower than that of WKY[5] suggesting the existence of the disparity of the central serine proteases activity between hypertensive and normotensive rats. However, the effects of the inhibition of central serine protease activity or a decrease in endogenous CSF kinins on BP has not been fully investigated.

Aprotinin, a reversible inhibitor of kallikrein and other serine proteases, has been used as a tool to study the possible action of the kallikrein-kinin system[6]. Although aprotinin has been reported to have unrecognized properties due to its highly cationic nature besides inhibition of serine proteases[7,8], we elected aprotinin i.c.v. to inhibit the kinin-generating activity of the central serine proteases. This study was designed to determine whether centrally administered aprotinin would decrease BP of SHR and WKY while the rats were conscious resting state, and further, to clarify the role of central serine proteases on BP regulation in hypertensive and normotensive rats. We also studied the contributions of sympathetic nervous system and vasopressin to the responses of BP induced by aprotinin i.c.v.

MATERIALS AND METHODS

Effect of Aprotinin i.c.v. on BP

Male SHR and male WKY were anesthetized by pentbarbital (50 mg/kg intraperitonial), a 22-gauge stainless steel cannula was stereotaxically implanted into lateral ventricle ; 1.0 mm posterior to bregma, 1.5 mm lateral from the midline and 4.5 mm deep from the dura. Cannula was anchored to the skull by jewelers' screws embedded in dental acrylic cement. Each animal was also inserted polyethylene catheters filled with heparinized saline into femoral artery and vein. The catheters were passed subcutaneously and brought through the skin at the scapular region, as previously described[8]. The experiments were performed 48 hours after cannula implantation. Conscious rats were kept semi-restrained in plastic restrainer, and direct mean BP was recorded. In Group 1 (8 SHR : 286.8 ± 10.1 g, 6 WKY : 323.3 ± 5.8 g), after 60 minutes of stabilization period and BP had stabilized, each rat received an bolus dose of 1,000 KIU/kg/10 µl of aprotinin i.c.v. and mean BP was continuously monitored another 30 minutes. As controls, we also conducted 1,000 KIU/kg/10µl of aprotinin i.v. in Group 2 (7 SHR : 266.3 ± 9.6 g, 5 WKY : 296.4 ± 8.6 g) and 10 µl of artificial CSF (Elliot's B solution) i.c.v. in Group 3 (5 SHR : 299.2 ± 13.6 g, 6 WKY : 291.3 ± 7.6 g) after 60 minutes of stabilization period.

Contributions of Sympathetic Nervous System and Vasopressin to the Effect of Aprotinin i.c.v.

In Group 4 (7 SHR : 292.6 ± 7.9 g, 5 WKY : 345.2 ± 20.1 g), hexamethonium (Hx), a ganglion blockade, 25 mg/kg i.v. was administered to block sympathetic nervous activity. Sixty minutes after Hx i.v., they received aprotinin i.c.v. and direct BPs were continuously monitored as in Group 1. Pretreatment with d(CH2)5 arginine vasopressin (AVP-antagonist) 30 µg/kg i.v. was given to block the action of vasopressin in Group 5 (5 SHR : 317.6 ± 2.6 g, 4 WKY : 325.0 ± 25.2 g) at 60 minutes before aprotinin i.c.v.. Direct BPs were continuously monitored as in Group 5.

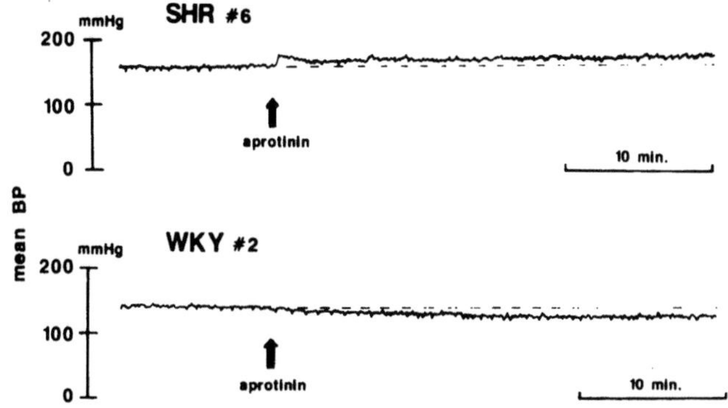

Figure 1. Actual mean BP recordings in SHR(#6), upper panel,
and in WKY(2), lower panel.

RESULTS

Effect of Aprotinin i.c.v. on BP

Figure 1 shows the actual mean BP recordings of SHR and of WKY. In
SHR, aprotinin i.c.v. caused a prompt increase in BP and this elevation of
BP was persisted for over 30 minutes. On the other hand, BP of WKY
decreased gradually after aprotinin i.c.v.. The effects of aprotinin
i.c.v. on mean BP in Group 1 were summarized in Figure 2. Mean BP of SHR
significantly increased after aprotinin i.c.v. for over 30 minutes, and
WKY showed the significant decrease in mean BP by about 6 % at 30 minutes
after aprotinin injection.

Aprotinin i.v. did not affect the mean BP both in SHR and WKY (Group
2, Figure 3). No significant changes in mean BP except for the early
transient increase of mean BP in WKY was observed by artificial CSF
(Elliot's B solution) i.c.v. in Group 3 (Figure 3).

Contributions of Sympathetic Nervous System and Vasopressin to the Effect of Aprotinin i.c.v.

Comparisons of the changes in mean BP (delta mean BP) elicited by
aprotinin alone (Group 1) with those BP changes in groups pretreated with
either Hx (Group 4) or AVP-antagonist (Group 5) were shown in Figure 4.
In SHR, the pretreatment with Hx abolished the pressor response to
aprotinin i.c.v., although the pretreatment with AVP-antsgonist did not
affect this pressor response. In WKY, pretreatments with both Hx and AVP-
antagonist cancelled the depressor response to aprotinin.

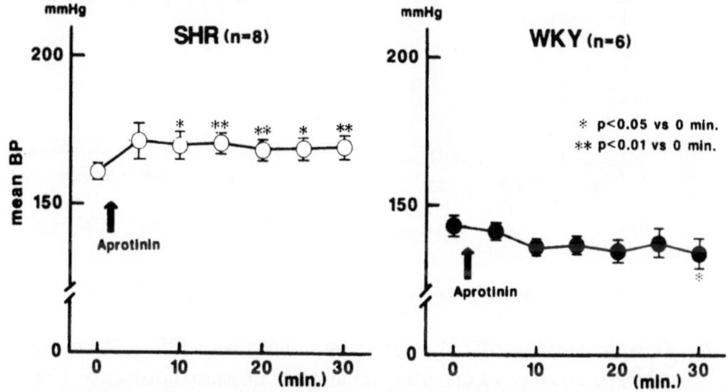

Figure 2. Effect of aprotinin i.c.v. on BP in SHR, left side
of the panel and in WKY, right side of the panel.

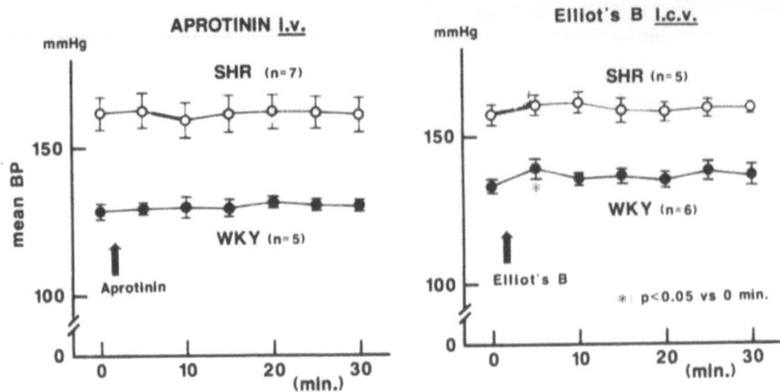

Figure 3. Effect of aprotinin i.v. and articial CSF (Elliot's B) i.c.v. on mean BP. Aprotinin i.v. on left side and Elliot's B i.c.v. on right side of the panel.

DISCUSSION

Serine protease inhibitor, aprotinin, i.c.v. significantly increased BP for over 30 minutes in SHR. Since this elevation of BP was abolished by the pretreatment with Hx, but was not prevented by the pretreatment with AVP-antagonist, aprotinin may selectively exert an effect on sympathetic nervous system and increased sympathetic nervous activity in SHR. On the other hand, BP of WKY decreased gradually by aprotinin i.c.v. and this decrease of BP may be due to the decrease in sympathetic nervous activity and vasopressin, because this depressor effect was cancelled by the pretreatments with both Hx and AVP-antagonist.

The observed pressor effect of aprotinin i.c.v. in SHR may not be due to its inhibitory effect on kininogenase activity of central serine proteases. Since kinins i.c.v. and the increased endogenous CSF kinins were associated with increase in BP[2,4], the inhibition of central serine proteases and resultant decrease in CSF kinins could decrease BP. Moreover, the prompt increase of BP after aprotinin i.c.v. suggests that factor(s) other than inhibition of kinin-generating activity by aprotinin is related to this pressor response. Aprotinion's unrecognized properties due to its highly cationic nature[7] might be related to this pressor effect in SHR. On the other hand, the gradual decrease of BP after aprotinin

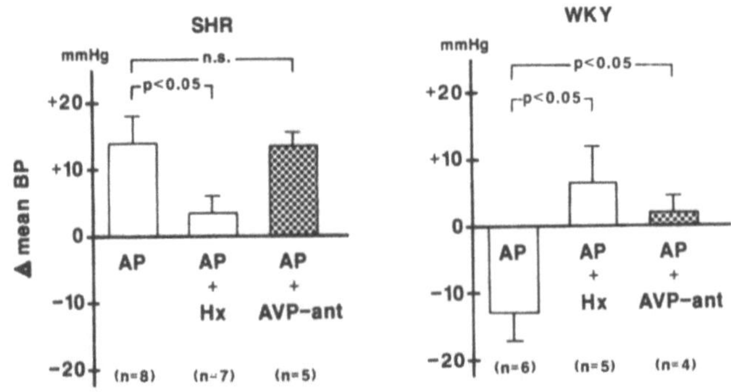

Figure 4. Comparisons of the changes in mean BP after aprotinin (AP) i.c.v. with and without hexamethonium (Hx) or AVP-antagonist (AVP-ant). SHR on the left side and WKY on the right side.

i.c.v. in WKY could be due to aprotinin's inhibitory effect on
kininogenase activity. The abolition of this depressor action by Hx and
AVP-antagonist suggests that aprotinin itself or its inhibitory effect on
kininogenase activity decreases sympathetic nervous activity and
vasopressin. The central vasopressor action of kinins have been reported
to be at least partially mediated by the central alpha-adrenergic[9],
prostaglandin[10] and vasopressin system[11]. Therefore, this depressor
effect could be explained by the decrease of CSF kinins due to aprotinin
i.c.v., in other words, endogenous CSF kinins may involve in the
regulation of BP in WKY. However, Brooks et al. reported that the
increase in vasopressin release induced by kinins i.c.v. did not
contribute to the pressor response to kinins[12].

The difference of the responses of BP between SHR and WKY after
aprotinin i.c.v. may be due to the difference of intrinsic activity of
serine proteases in central nervous system participating in central kinins
formation. In fact, exaggerated sympathetic responses to central
administration of bradykinin[13,14] and reduced endogenous CSF kinins
concentration[5] had been reported in SHR when compared with WKY suggesting
that the intrinsic activity of central serine protease is low or is a
minor compoment of central regulation of BP in SHR. Furthermore, it is
possible that aprotinin i.c.v. unmasked the abnormality, other than
central serine protease, of the central regulation of BP in SHR. Bunag et
al. demonstrated that alpha-adrenergic vasodepressor mechanisms in
supramedullary brain area no longer function normally in SHR by the method
of intracarotid injection of bradykinin into cross-perfused head
preparations[14].

In conclusion, aprotinin i.c.v. appears to exert dual effects;
first, the pressor effect due to the increase of sympathetic nervous
activity observed in SHR, and second, the depressor effect due to the
decrease of sympathetic nervous activity and vasopressin observed in WKY.
Although the pressor effect of aprotinin i.c.v. in SHR may not be related
with the inhibition of kinin-generating activity by aprotinin, the
depressor effect of aprotinin i.c.v. observed in WKY may be due to the
decrease in CSF kinins concentration by aprotinin suggesting that
endogenous CSF kinins may involve in the regulation of BP in WKY.

REFERENCES

1. D. I. Diz, Bradykinin and related peptides in central control of the
   cardiovascular system, Peptides, 6(Suppl 2):57-64 (1985).
2. L. Pearson, G. A. Lambert and W. J. Lang, Centrally mediated
   cardiovascular and EEG responses to bradykinin and eledoisin, Eur.
   J. Pharmacol., 8:153-158 (1969).
3. F. M. A. Correa and F. G. Graeff, Central mechanisms of the
   hypertensive action of intraventricular bradykinin in the
   unanesthetized rat, Neuropharmacology, 13:65-75 (1974).
4. G. R. Thomas, H. Thibodeaux, H. S. Margolius and P. J. Privitera,
   Cerebrospinal fluid kinins and cardiovascular functioin. Effect of
   cerebroventricular melittin, Hypertension, 6(Suppl I):I46-I50
   (1984).
5. K. Hermann, G. Schaechtelin and M. Marin-Grez, Kinins in cerebrospinal
   fluid: Reduced concentration in spontaneously hypertensive rats,
   Experientia, 42:1238-1239 (1986).
6. O. A. Carretero and A. G. Scicli, Possible role of kinins in
   circulatory homeostasis. State of the art review, Hypertension,
   3(suppl I):I4-I12 (1981).

7. R. Vogel and E. Werle E, Kallikrein inhibitors, in: "Handbook of Experimental Pharmacology," vol 25, E. G. Erdos, ed., Springer, New York, pp 213-249 (1970).

8. S. Seto, V. Kher, A. G. Scicli, W. H. Beierwaltes and O. A. Carretero, The effect of aprotinin (a serine protease inhibitor) on renal function and renin release, Hypertension, 5:893-899 (1983).

9. H. Takahashi and R. D. Bunag, Centrally induced cardiovascular and sympathetic nerve response to bradykinin in rats, J. Pharmacol. Exp. Ther., 216:192-197 (1981).

10. K. Kariya, A. Yamauchi and Y. Chatani, Relationship between central actions of bradykinin and prostaglandins in the conscious rat, Neuropharmacology, 21:267-272 (1982).

11. W. E. Hoffman and P. G. Schmid, Separation of pressor and antidiuretic effects of intraventricular bradykinin, Neuropharmacology, 17:999-1002 (1978).

12. D. P. Brooks, L. Share, J. T. Crofton and A. Nasjletti, Interrelationship between central bradykinin and vasopressin in conscious rats, Brain Research, 371:42-48 (1986).

13. T. Unger, R. W. Rockhold, T. Yukimura, R. Rettig, W. Rascher and D. Ganten, Role of kinins and substance P in the central blood pressure regulation of normotensive and spontaneously hypertensive rats, in: "Central Nervous System Mechanisms in Hypertension," J. P. Buckley and C. M. Ferrario, ed., Raven Press, New York, pp115 -127 (1981).

14. R. D. Bunag and H. Takahashi, Exaggerated sympathetic responses to bradykinin in spontaneously hypertensive rats, Hypertension, 3:433 -440 (1981).

AUGMENTATION OF KALLIKREIN AND PLASMIN INHIBITION CAPACITY

BY APROTININ USING A NEW ASSAY TO MONITOR THERAPY

M.J. Gallimore, G. Fuhrer, W. Heller, and
H.-E. Hoffmeister

Dept. of Cardiovascular Surgery, University of
Tuebingen, D-7400 Tuebingen, FRG

Introduction

The broad spectrum proteinase inhibitor aprotinin is widely
used therapeutically in shock, pancreatitis, cardiopulmonary
bypass and other clinical states with hyperfibrinolysis. Until recently aprotinin levels in plasma samples were not
measured routinely, possibly because simple assays were not
available.
We developed a simple assay using plasma kallikrein and a
kallikrein substrate (S-2302) to monitor aprotinin levels in
patients during cardiopulmonary bypass. Aprotinin was infused in a dose of 5000 KIU aprotinin or 15000 KIU aprotinin
per kilogram body weight. Since aprotinin administration
leads to an increase in kallikrein inhibition capacity, we
determined both, total kallikrein inhibition and kallikrein
inhibition due to aprotinin.

Material and methods

For all determinations citrate plasma (9+1) was used. Since
during cardiopulmonary bypass patients were treated with heparin, and some methods for components of the kallikrein-
kinin systems interfere with this drug (1), the anti-Xa levels were analysed and antagonized by the addition of protamine chloride. Total kallikrein inhibition levels were measured by means of plasma kallikrein (Channel Diagnostics,
Walmer, Deal, Kent, UK) and the chromogenic substrate S-2302
(Deutsche KabiVitrum GmbH, Munich) according to the method
of Gallimore et al. (2). Aprotinin was delivered by Bayer AG,
Leverkusen, FRG. Plasma was taken according to the following
schedule:
1) preoperative 2) after thoracotomy 3) immediately after
onset of cardiopulmonary bypass (CPB) 4) 15 minutes after
CPB 5) 30 minutes after CPB 6) 45 minutes after CPB 7) 60
minutes after CPB 8) after commencement of CPB 9) immediately after operation. Aprotinin was given in a dose of 5000
KIU per kg bodyweight (group 1) or 15000 KIU per kg bodyweight (group 2) after anaesthesia (after sample 1), in the
prime volume of the heart lung machine (sample 3), 30 minutes after onset of CPB and after sample 8.

Aprotinin method

Buffer: 6.1 g Tris, 21.1 g NaCl, 3.36 g EDTA, 20 mg polybrene, 0.15 M methylamine, 0.2 % albumin, 3 ml corn inhibitor, pH 7.8

100 µl acetone was mixed with 300 µl plasma in siliconized
glass tubes (30 minutes, temperature +4°C).
300 µl of this mixture was added to 1700 µl buffer.

Diluted plasma or standard   200 µl
Plasma kallikrein   200 µl
Mix and incubate for exactly 5 minutes
S-2302 (1 mmol/l)   200 µl
Mix and incubate for exactly 4 minutes
Acetic acid (50 %)   200 µl

The absorbance is read at 4o5 nm against its blanks which are
prepared by adding the reagents in reverse order without
incubation.

Results

Addition of various amounts of aprotinin to pooled plasma
and testing these samples for the inhibition of kallikrein
results in a straight line (logarithmic) or curve from 0 to
200 KIU aprotinin/ml (Fig. 1).
Total kallikrein inhibition was found to be 115 ± 31 % in
group 1 and 126 ± 44 % in group 2. After the infusion of
aprotinin kallikrein inhibition capacity rose to 126 ± 23%
in group 1. These changes were more pronounced in group 2
(144 ± 77%). Onset of cardiopulmonary bypass (sample 3) was
followed by another augmentation of this inhibition due to
the administration of aprotinin to the prime volume (group
1: 141 ± 28 %; group 2: 173 ± 28 %). According to the
half-life time of aprotinin, levels of kallikrein inhibition fell to 118 ± 24 % in group 1 and 165 ± 30 % in
group 2. 30 minutes after onset of cardiopulmonary bypass
levels of total kallikrein inhibition increased significantly. A continous fall from sample 6 to sample 8 could be observed. At the end of the operation and the antagonization of
heparin combined with another dose of aprotinin total kallikrein inhibition was 131 ± 25 % in group 1 and 184 ± 40 % in
group 2 (fig. 4).
Aprotinin levels increased to 24 KIU/ml in group 1 and were
78 KIU/ml in group 2 in plasma sample 2. A further increase
was seen after the onset of CPB due to priming the heart-
lung machine with another dose of aprotinin. These concentrations fell to 36 ± 5 KIU/ml in group 1 and were 98 ± 14
KIU/ml (sample 4).
Highest levels were detected after the third infusion of
aprotinin (Group 1: 66 ± 9 KIU/ml,group 2 : 210 ± 50 KIU/ml)
In group 2 aprotintin concentration decreased from 210 KIU/
ml to 116 ± 30 KIU/ml and were lowered from 60 KIU/ml to 43
± 19 KIU/ml. After operation aprotinin administration led to
a slight increase of this inhibitor (fig. 2 and 3).

Discussion

Since its introduction as a therapeutic antiprotease very

few studies have been performed to monitor levels of aprotinin in patients receiving this inhibitor. It has been suggested that this has contributed to the difficulty in demonstrating therapeutic effectiveness of aprotinin (3). This led to the development of immunochemical (4,5) and a functional (3) assay for this protein. The latter method utilizes porcine pancreatic kallikrein together with a chromogenic substrate for this enzyme and has been shown to work well with clinical material. We have utilized plasma kallikrein and a plasma kallikrein substrate to develop a simple assay for aprotinin which can be performed manually or on automated clinical chemistry analysers. In this assay acetone was used to destroy natural inhibitors and methylamine was added to block the binding site of alpha-2-macroglobulin. Corn inhibitor was mixed with the buffer to inhibit any factor XII activity which might be generated after the addition of kallikrein. A standard curve for the assay can either be plotted as log E_{405} versus aprotinin in KIU/ml whereby a straight line is obtained (Fig. 1) linear between 0 and 200 KIU/ml aprotinin, or as E_{405} versus aprotinin in KIU/ml whereby a curve results.
The precision of the assay was good and should be better when performed using automated equipment.
Plasma samples from patients treated with aprotinin showed a dose dependant increase in levels of plasma kallikrein inhibition. We called this assay a test for total kallikrein inhibition because natural inhibitors (C1-Inhibitor and alpha-2-makroglobulin) and aprotinin were measured.
Preoperatively levels in this assay were found to be 115 ± 31 % in group 1 and 126 ± 44 % in group 2 with the range from 77 % to 197 %. Administration of the first dose of aprotinin led to a marked elevation of total kallikrein inhibition with higher levels in group 2. In two patients levels were below 100 % which might indicate some consumption during thoracotomy. After onset of cardiopulmonary bypass kallikrein inhibition levels rose in both groups due to another dose of aprotinin in the prime volume of the heart lung machine. 15 minutes later the inhibition capacity fell to 118 ± 24 % in group 1 und 165 ± 30 % in group 2. This reflects the half-life time of aprotinin but could also be caused by activation of plasma defense systems and formation of inhibitor-enzyme complexes.
After having started the infusion of the next aprotinin dose the level rose to 146 ± 28 % (group 1) and 200 ± 18 % (group 2) respectively. Until the commencement of cardiopulmonary bypass kallikrein inhibition capacity decreased slightly (group 1) or was not significantly changed (group 2). Since no further aprotinin administration was performed during this period of time, the course of these levels could be caused by infusion of blood products, e.g. whole blood or fresh frozen plasma. After operation a slight increase was observed (group 1) or levels were almost stable (group 2).
One day after operation the natural inhibitiors (no aprotinin was given postoperatively) caused a kallikrein inhibition capacity of 99 ± 32 % in group 1 and 132 ± 42 % in group 2, respectively.
Using the method for aprotinin 24 ± 21 KIU/ml were detected in group 1 and 78 ± 11 KIU/ml in group 2 after the first dose of aprotinin. A further elevation could be shown after onset of cardiopulmonary bypass due to the addition of apro-

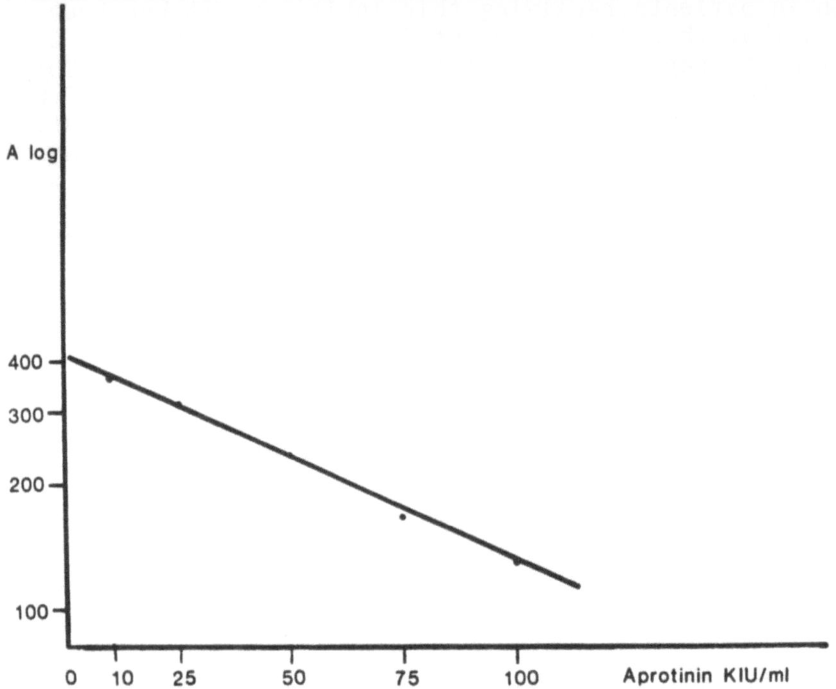

Fig. 1   Standard curve of aprotinin (logarithmic)

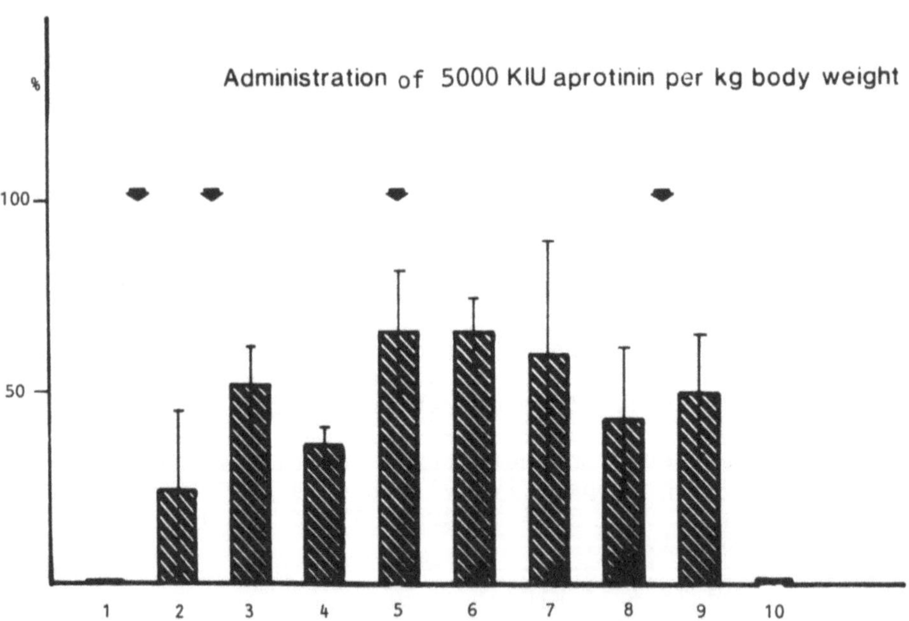

Fig. 2   Levels of aprotinin in patients with low
         dose treatment

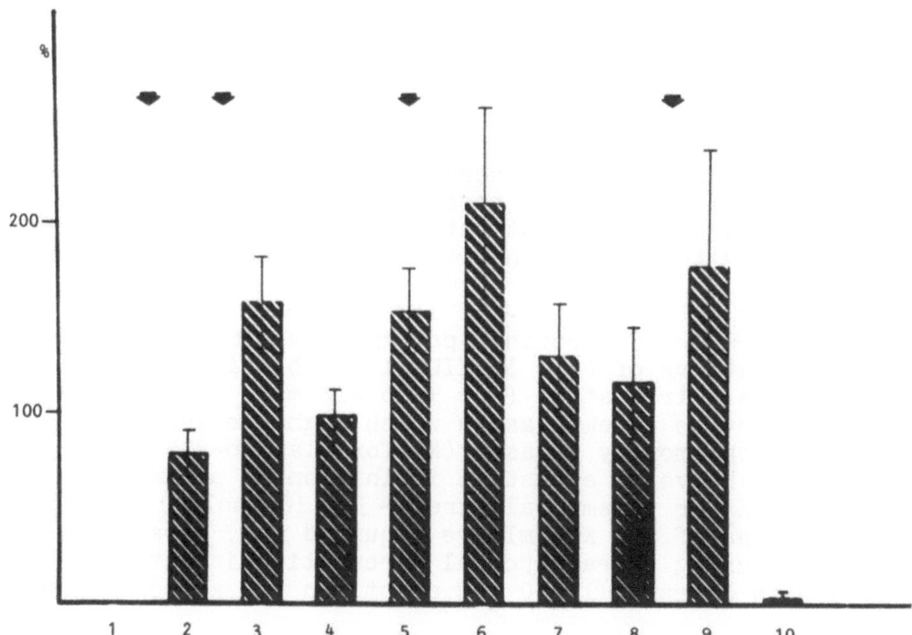

Fig. 3   Aprotinin levels in patients with the
         administration of 15.ooo KIU aprotinin/Kg
         b.w. a dose

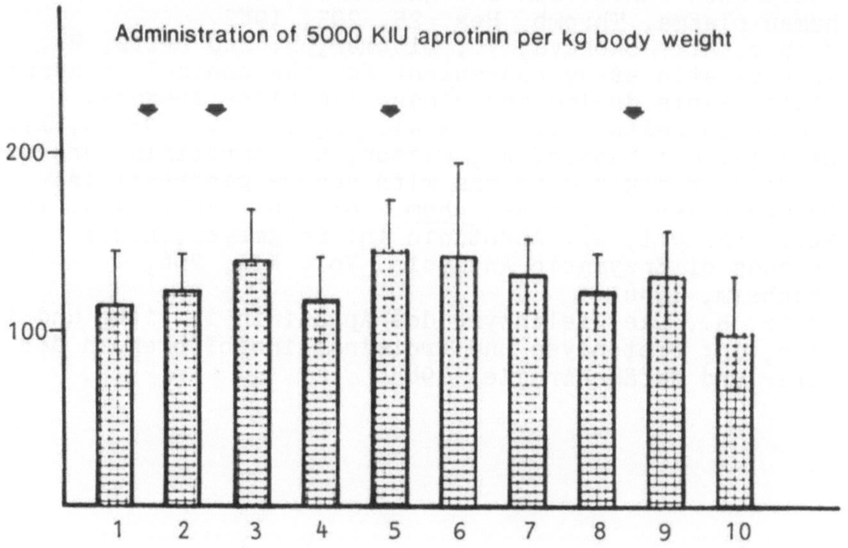

Fig. 4   Kallikrein inhibition levels in patients
         treated with low doses of aprotinin

tinin to the prime volume of the heart-lung machine. In both
groups highest aprotinin concentrations were found after the
third dose of this antiprotease. Due to the half-life time
of aprotinin or complex formation with proteases, levels declined to 43 ± 19 KIU/ml (group 1) and 116 ± 30 KIU/ml
(group 2) at the end of extracorporeal circulation (fig. 2
and 3). Our results show that the simple assays for aprotinin
we have described will be very valuable in monitoring plasma
levels of aprotinin during therapy. Together with the total
kallikrein inhibition assay these enable us to follow the
inhibitory status of the patient and even to differentiate
inhibition due to plasma inhibitors or plasma inhibitors plus
aprotinin.
In this study patients with the lower dose of aprotinin
(four times 5000 KIU aprotinin per kg body weight) had highest concentrations of 66 ± 16 KIU/ml of this inhibitor during
extracorporeal circulation (66 ± 16 KIU/ml). These levels
are sufficient to block plasmin which might be generated
during cardiopulmonary bypass. (K_i for plasmin~2,3 x 10^{-10}
mol/l). To achieve an effective inhibition of plasma
kallikrein (K_i for plasma kallikrein~3 x 10^{-8}mol/l) aprotinin
concentrations of 200 KIU/ml are required (6). These levels
were found during extracorporeal circulation in patients
treated with doses of 15000 KIU aprotinin per kg body weight.

References

1) Fuhrer, G., Heller, W., Hoffmeister, H.-E. (1984)
   Effect of high and low molecular weight heparin preparation on chromogenic substrate assay for components of
   the kallikrein-kinin system. Kinin 84, Savannah
2) Gallimore, M.J. and Friberger, P.. Simple chromogenic
   peptide substrate assays for determining prekallikrein,
   kallikrein inhibition and kallikrein like activity in
   human plasma. Thromb. Res. 25, 293, 1982
3) Jochum, M.; Jonokova, V.; Dittmer, H. and Fritz, H..
   An enzymatic assay convenient for the control of aprotinin levels during proteinase inhibitor therapy.
   Fresenius Zeitschrift 7. Anal. Chem. 317, 719-720, 1984
4) Balldin, G.; Lasson, A.; Olsson, K.. Aprotinin turn-over
   studies in dog and in man with severe pancreatitis.
   Hoppe-Seylers. Z. phys. chem. Vol. 365, 1417-1423, 1984
5) Müller-Esterl, W.. Aprotinin in: Bergmeyer, H.U.:
   Methods of Enzymatic Analysis. Vol. XII, 256,
   Weinheim, 1986
6) Fritz, H.. Die Zielenzyme des Aprotinin in vitro und in
   vivo, in: Proteolyse und Proteinaseinhibitoren in der
   Herz- und Gefäßchirugie, 1985

STUDIES ON THE INHIBITION OF PLASMA KALLIKREIN, C1-ESTERASE

AND ß-FXIIa IN THE PRESENCE AND THE ABSENCE OF HEPARINS

G. Fuhrer, M.J. Gallimore, W. Heller, and
H.-E. Hoffmeister

Department of Cardiovascular Surgery, University
of Tübingen, 7400 Tübingen, FRG

Introduction

We previously reported that the inhibition of plasma kallikrein was elevated and of ß-FXIIa was reduced in platelet
rich compared to platelet poor plasma (5).In the present
study we investigated the effect of added unfractionated
heparin and a low molecular heparin preparation (Fragmin,
KabiVitrum GmbH , Munich, FRG) on the plasma inhibition
of kallikrein, ß-FXIIa and C1-esterase.

Material and methods

For the in vitro studies a plasma pool from 20 healthy
donors was used.
ß-FXIIa- inhibition was analysed by means of ß-FXIIa (Channel Diagnostics, Walmer, Deal, U.K.) and the chromogenic
substrate S-2222 (Deutsche KabiVitrum, Munich, FRG) according to the method described elsewhere (1).
Kallikrein inhibition was assayed using plasma kallikrein
(Channel Diagnostics, Walmer, Deal, U.K.) and S-2302 (Deutsche KabiVitrum, Munich, FRG). The method was published by
Gallimore et al.(2). For C1-esterase inhibition a test kit
from Immuno AG, Vienna, Austria was used. Human C1-inhibitor
was a generous gift from Dr. A. Philapitsch, Immuno AG,
Vienna, Austria. For the heparinization of the plasma a high
molecular weight heparin (Medac, Hamburg, FRG) or a low
molecular weight heparin preparation (Fragmin, Deutsche KabiVitrum , Munich, FRG) was added.

Results

High molecular heparin

After the addition of 0,5 U heparin/ml ß-FXIIa inhibition
decreased from 103% to 82%. Further falls could be detected
using a heparin concentrations of 1,0 or 1,5 U heparin/ml
(77% and 63%) inhibition declined to 57% and 47% respectively when 2 and 3 U heparin/ml were added. These effects diminished after the antagonization of heparin by protamine

chloride in the ratio 1:1 (fig. 1). No significant changes
occurred in heparinized plasmas with levels from 0-3 U hepa-
rin/ml in the kallikrein inhibition assay (without heparin:
99 %, 3 U heparin/ml: 96 %) Cl-esterase inhibition was not
affected by the addition of heparin in concentrations from
0-3 U heparin/ml.
With purified Cl-inhibitor levels of ß-FXIIa-inhibition
decreased to 72% (from 107% to 72%) after the addition of 3U
heparin/ml. Heparin produced no changes in kallikrein and
Cl-esterase inhibition (fig. 2).
To exclude direct effects of heparin on the reaction between
ß-FXIIa and the chromogenic substrate, heparin in various
concentrations was added to buffer and then tested in the ß-
FXIIa inhibition assay (fig. 3). No effects were seen.

Low molecular weight heparin

The addition of a low molecular weight heparin preparation in
various concentrations led to a significant reduction in
ß-FXIIa inhibition. Using 0.5 anti-Xa/ml,levels of ß- FXIIa
inhibition decreased from 91% to 86% and were found to be 80%
in a concentration of 1 anti-Xa low-molecular weight (LMW)
heparin/ml. Inhibition fell to 65% when 1.5 anti-Xa/ml was
added, to 55% with heparin levels of 2.0 anti-Xa/ml and to
35% with 3.0 anti-Xa/ml. The addition of protamine chloride
prior to determination abolished these effects (fig. 4).
No significant changes occurred in kallikrein and Cl-esterase inhibition in the plasma samples in the presence of the
low molecular weight heparin preparation. By testing
purified Cl-inhibitor and various amounts of LMW-heparin in
the assay for ß-FXIIa, Cl- esterase and kallikrein
inhibition,the same pattern could be observed as with plasma, ß-FXIIa inhibition decreased. From 114 to 109% after the
additiion of 0.5 anti-Xa/ml. Further reduction were seen in
samples with levels of 1.0 and 1.5 anti-Xa/ml (98% and 91%).
A level of 82% in the ß-FXIIa inhibition was measured with
2.0 anti-Xa/ml and this inhibition capacity declined to 72%
after the addition of 3.0 anti-Xa/ml (fig.5).

Discussion

Inhibition of plasma kallikrein is higher in platelet rich
than platelet poor plasma, whilst inhibition of ß-FXIIa is
reduced (fig.6). Both unfractionated and fractionated heparins reduce the plasma inhibition of ß-FXIIa, but kallikrein
inhibition and Cl-esterase inhibition are not altered. The
major inhibitor for ß-FXIIa is Cl-inhibitor (7). We
ascertained that the binding properties of ß-FXIIa to
Cl-inhibitor are changed by adding purified Cl-inhibitor to
the buffer containing heparin and ß-FXIIa. A direct effect of
heparin preparations on the reaction between ß-FXIIa and the
chromogenic substrate was excluded by showing an unaltered
pNA-release from S-2222 after the addition of various amounts
of heparin.
ß-FXIIa is generated during contact activation and released
into the bloodstream and activates kallikrein and fibrinolytic systems.
In patients treated with high doses of heparin the inhibition capacity of ß-FXIIa may be reduced to such an extent
that both the activation of fibrinolysis and the kallikrein-
kinin system occur even in the presence of normal Cl-inhibi-

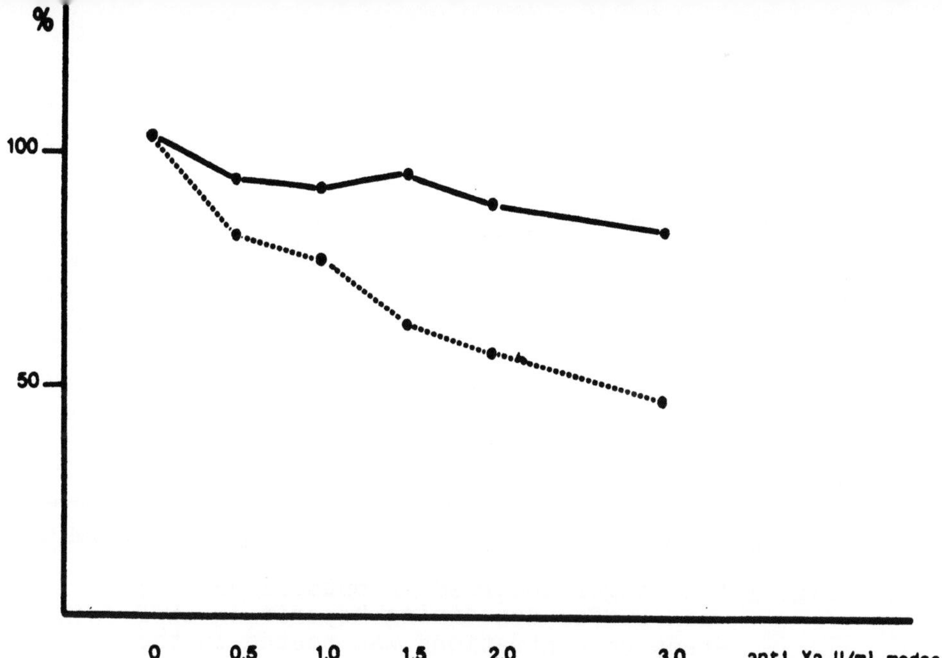

Fig. 1 Beta-FXIIa inhibition in heparinized (---)
plasma samples (unfractionated heparin).
Addition of protamine chloride abolished
these effects (——).

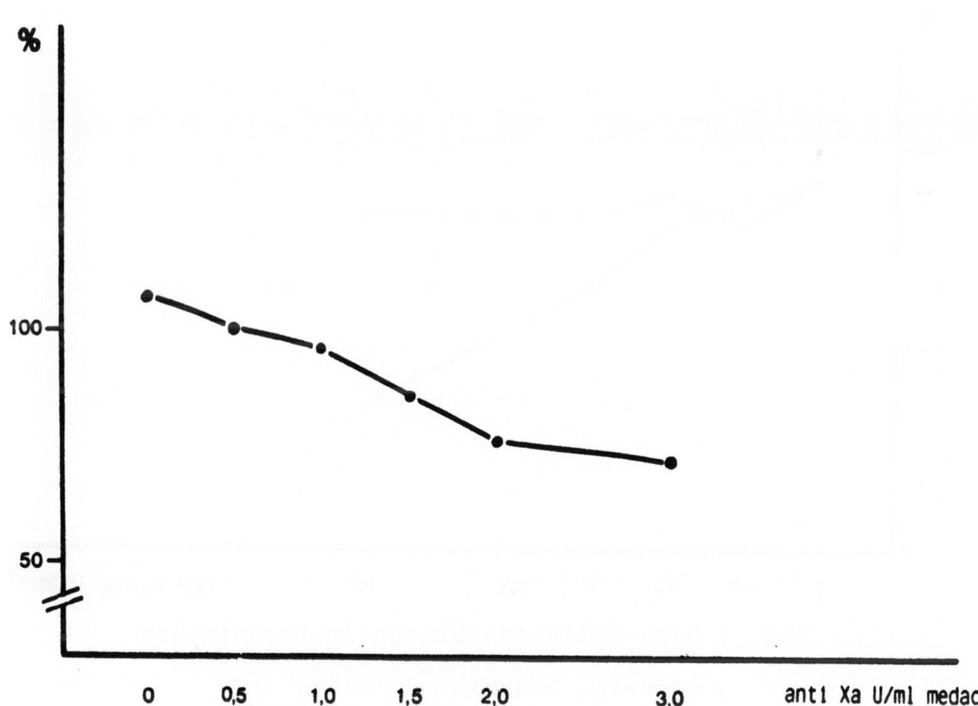

Fig. 2 Beta-FXIIa inhibition in buffer containing
C1-inhibitor and heparin in different
concentrations.

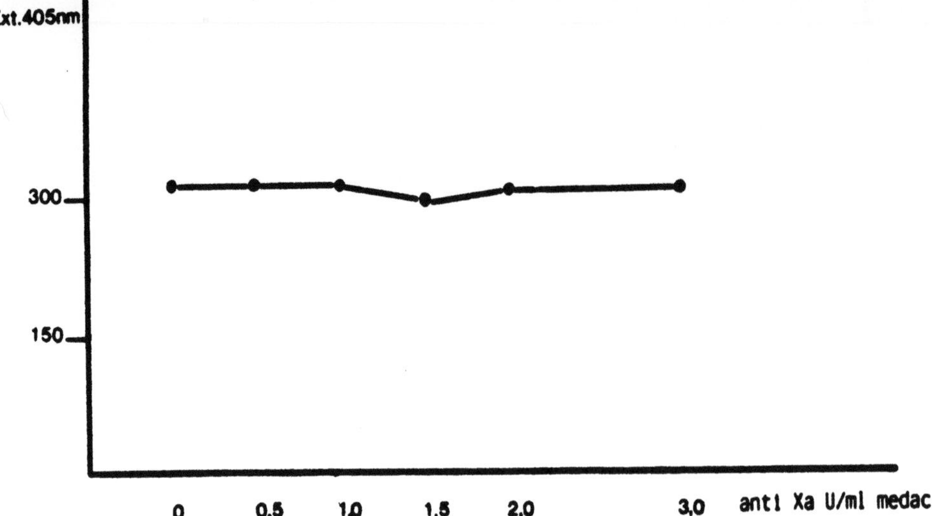

Fig. 3 No changes occurred in optical density
when buffer containing heparin in different concentrations was tested in the
beta-FXIIa inhibition assay.

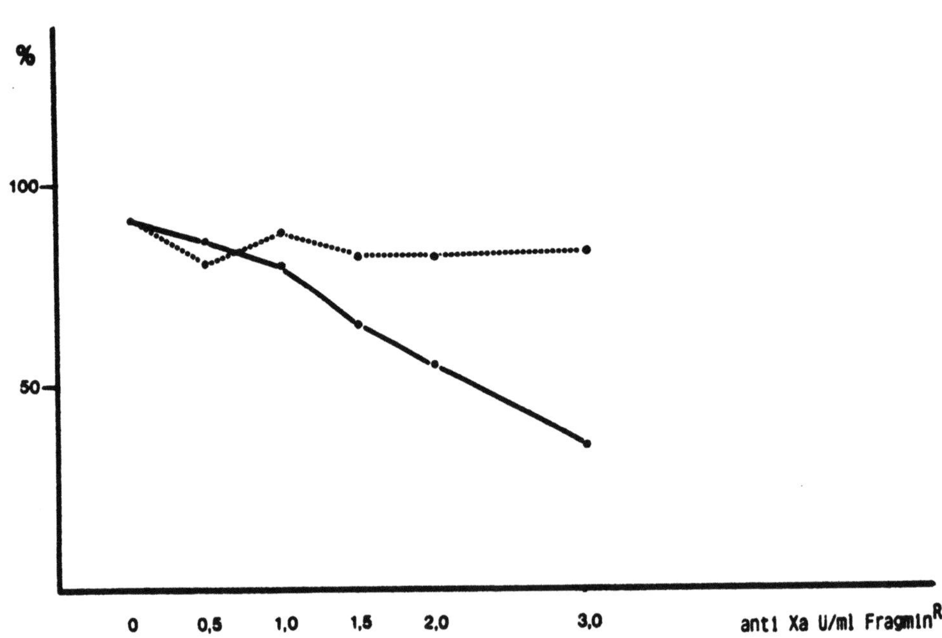

Fig. 4 Beta-FXIIa inhibition in heparinized
(———) plasma samples (fractionated
heparin, Fragmin).
Addition of protamine chloride
abolished these effects (---).

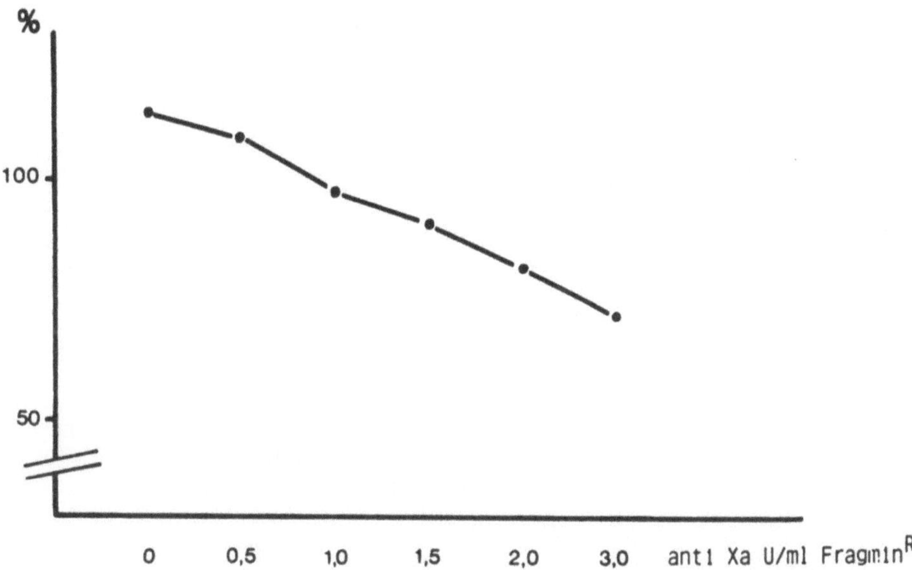

Fig. 5 Effect of fractionated heparin on C1-
esterase inhibition of beta-FXIIa

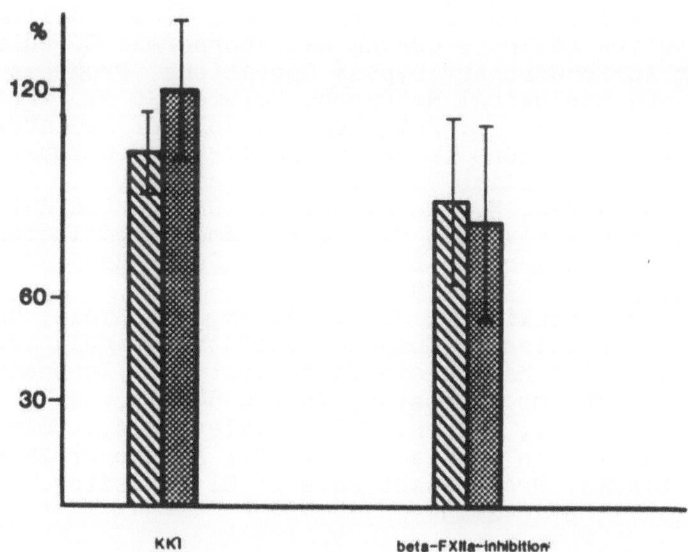

Fig. 6 Effect of platelet rich and platelet poor plasma on inhibition of
plasma kallikrein and beta-FXIIa

tor levels. This pathological situation is present in patients during cardiopulmonary bypass, where immediately after onset of bypass an increase in kallikrein like activity, a reduction in ß-FXIIa inhibition, kallikrein inhibition and prekallikrein levels can be detected (3). Furthermore, hyperfibrinolysis is associated with open heart surgery in most cases (4). Since the action of antithrombin III is accelerated in the presence of heparin, clotting is prevented and disseminated intravascular coagulation does not occur in most of the patients following open heart surgery. In clinical situations associated with thrombocytosis the inhibition of ß-FXIIa could also be reduced. This might lead to marked changes in the above mentioned systems. One can also speculate that this phenomenon plays a role in the local activation of cascades involving the release of platelet enzymes. Therefore in our opinion it is important to ensure a sufficient inhibitoric potential in patients with thrombocytosis or in clinical situations where heparin treatment is required. From the results of this study combined with other findings it seems to be essential to infuse C1-inhibitor concentrates in these patients.

References

1) Fuhrer, G.; Gallimore, M.J.; Heller, W.; Hoffmeister, H.-E.. Reduced ß-FXIIa-Inhibition Capacity in Heparinized Plasma Samples. Thromb.Haemostas.THHADQ 58 (1), p 138, 1987
2) Gallimore, M.J.; Friberger, P.. Simple Chromogenic Peptide Substrate Assays for Determining Prekallikrein, Kallikrein Inhibition and Kallikrein Like Activity in Human Plasma. Thromb. Res. 25, p 293, 1982
3) Heller, W.; Fuhrer, G.; Hoffmeister, H.-E.; Gallimore, M. J.. Studies on Shock during Extracorporeal Circulation during Aorto-Coronary Bypass Operations. Progress in Clinical and Biological Research, Volume 236 A. First Vienna Shock Forum, Part A: Pathological Role of Mediators and Mediator Inhibitors in Shock, pp 87-94, New York, 1987
4) Aasen, A.O.; Gallimore., M.J.; Lilleaasen, P.; Lyngaas, K.; Larsbraaten, M.; Amundsen, E.. Changes in Antiplasmin and Plasmin Activities during Extreme Hemodilution and Open Heart Surgery in Dogs. Europ. Surg. Res., Vol. 11. No. 3, pp 145-153, 1979
5) Fuhrer, G.; Gallimore, M.J.; Heller, W.; Klöss, Th.; Lenz, G.. Studies on Components of the Coagulation, Fibrinolytic and Kallikrein Kinin System in Intensive Care Patients. Thromb.Haemostas. THHADQ 54 (1),p 253, 1985
6) de Agostini, A.; Lijnen, H.R.; Paxlev, R.A., Colman, A.W. Schapira, M.. In Activation of FXII Active Fragment in NormalPlasma. Predominant Role of C1-Inhibitor. J. Clin. Invest. 73, p 1542-1549

THE MAJOR PLASMA KALLIKREIN INHIBITOR IN GUINEA PIG PLASMA WITH

CONTRAPSIN-LIKE NATURE

Takahisa Imamura and Takeshi Kambara

Department of Allergy, Institute for Medical Immunology
Kumamoto University Medical School, Kumamoto 860, Japan

SUMMARY

Kallikrein inhibitor in plasma(KIP) was purified, and the share in
the kallikrein inhibitory capacity of guinea pig plasma was estimated by
depletion of the inhibitory activity of KIP with anti-KIP IgG. And KIP
was characterized the inhibitory activity using various proteases.

The purified KIP exhibited a single band on SDS-gel electrophoresis
and the molecular weight was 64,000. KIP inhibited plasma kallikrein
dose-dependently and time-dependently, forming a complex with kallikrein
with the molecular weight of 137,000.

Since the kallikrein inhibitory capacity of guinea pig plasma was
completely depleted by anti-KIP IgG that inactivated kallikrein
inhibitory activity of KIP, KIP was likely to be the major kallikrein
inhibitor in guinea pig plasma.

KIP inhibited trypsin and elastase, but not chymotrypsin. The
Inhibitory spectrum of KIP was different from the spectrum of each
protease inhibitor in human plasma, but was similar to the spectrum of
contrapsin in mouse plasma.

These results indicated that guinea pig plasma had a different
mechanism for kallikrein inhibition, compared with human plasma.

INTRODUCTION

Guinea pig plasma kallikrein enhances vascular permeability when
injected into the guinea pig skin. The ability of the kallikrein depends
on the kinin generation in the skin through the enzymatic activity of
kallikrein and the blocking of the enzymatic activity of kallikrein by
soybean trypsin inhibitor results in the inhibition of vascular permeability enhancement activity[1]. The observation that the vascular
permeability enhancement induced by kallikrein is short-lasting, indicates the presence of inhibitory mechanisms in the skin for vascular
permeability enhancement caused by kallikrein. Among the mechanisms,
endogenous kallikrein inhibitors are thought to important. $Alpha_2$-

macroglobulin increases more than 10-fold in the skin sites where vascular permeability is enhanced by activated Hageman factor (coagulation factor XII) and inhibits vascular permeability enhancing activity of Hageman factor[2]. It is likely that kallikrein inhibitors discharged into the skin by vascular permeability enhancement have significant roles in terminating the vascular reaction.

Human plasma contains several inhibitors for plasma kallikrein. Cl-inactivator is dominant inhibitor, and α_2-macroglobulin and antithrombin III follow in this order[3]. In guinea pig, however, what kind of protease inhibitor inhibits kallikrein and what inhibitor predominates are unknown. Among trypsin inhibitors in plasma, α_1-protease inhibitor ranks first in human, but in mouse, contrapsin is the major inhibitor[4]. Accordingly, it is probable that major kallikrein inhibitor in guinea pig plasma is different from the inhibitor that corresponds to Cl-inactivator in human.

In the present study, a kallikrein inhibitor in guinea pig plasma was purified and characterized. And the results indicated the inhibitor has contrapsin-like nature and was the major kallikrein inhibitor in guinea pig plasma.

METHODS

Preparation of kallikrein inhibitor in plasma(KIP) and anti-KIP IgG

Kallikrein inhibitor was purified from guinea pig plasma with procedures as follows : DEAE-Sephadex column chromatography(pH 8.0), DEAE-cellulose column chromatography(pH 5.5), CM-Sephadex column chromatography(pH 5.5), and Sephadex G-150 column chromatography. Antiserum to KIP was raised in rabbits by intradermal multiple-site injections of the purified KIP solution emulsified with complete Freund's adjuvant. The IgG fraction was prepared from the antiserum using ammonium sulfate fractionation, CM-Sephadex column chromatography, and DEAE-cellulose column chromatography.

Preparation of guinea pig plasma kallikrein

Guinea pig plasma kallikrein was purified from guinea pig plasma by the method described previously[1].

Measurement of Protease Inhibitory Activity

The inhibitory activity for proteases was measure by the inhibition of amidolytic activity for the protease specific fluorogenic substrate. Fifty microliter of a protease, 50 µl of sample and 390 µl of 20 mM Tris-HCl buffer, pH 8.0, containing 150 mM NaCl and bovine serum albumin (0.1 mg/ml), were incubated in a plastic tube at 37°C for 30 minutes. Then 10 µl of the protease specific MCA(4-methylcoumaryl-7-amide) substrate(5mM) was added and incubated 5 minutes. The enzymatic activity of the protease was stopped by addition of 500 µl of 30 % acetic acid. The amount of 7-amino-4-methyl coumarin released was fluorometrically measured with a fluorescene spectrophotometer with excitation at 380 nm and emission at 440 nm.

Depletion of kallikrein inhibitory activity of guinea pig plasma by anti-KIP IgG

The buffer used for the dilution of guinea pig plasma and anti-KIP IgG and for the incubation was 20 mM Tris-HCl, pH 8.0, containing 150 mM

NaCl, bovine serum albumin(0.1 mg/ml), polybrene(0.1 mg/ml) and 5 mM
EDTA. Fifty microliter of 30-fold normal guinea pig plasma was treated
with 100 µl of anti-KIP IgG in a plastic tube at 37°C for 30 minutes.
Then 50 µl of kallikrein(10^{-8}M) and 290 µl of the buffer were added,
and incubated at 37°C for 30 minutes. Residual kallikrein inhibitory
activity was measured as described above. The effect of anti-KIP IgG on
the kallikrein inhibitory capacity of plasma was expressed with percent
depletion of the capacity. As a control, normal rabbit IgG was used.

Oxidation of KIP

To investigate the effect of oxidation of KIP on protease inhibitory
activity of KIP, KIP was oxidized with N-chlorosuccinimide(NCS) according
to the method of Johnson and Travis[5]. The oxidation of KIP was performed in 50 mM Tris-HCl, 50 mM NaCl, pH 8.0, at room temperature for 15
seconds and residual inhibitory activity for bovine pancreatic trypsin
(10^{-8}M, Sigma) was measured. As a control, human α_1-protease inhibi-
tor(Sigma) was used.

Sodium dodecyl sulfate(SDS)-polyacrylamide slab gel electrophoresis

The interaction of KIP and kallikrein was analyzed by SDS-slab gel
electrophoresis with 10 % gel according to the method of Laemmli[6].
Gel was stained for protein with Coomasie brilliant blue R-250.

RESULTS AND DISCUSSION

Purity of KIP

The purified KIP exhibited a single band at between albumin and
α_1-region on gel electrophoresis at alkaline pH[1]. On SDS-gel
electrophoresis, KIP also exhibited a single band under reduced and
nonreduced conditions and the molecular weight was 64,000.

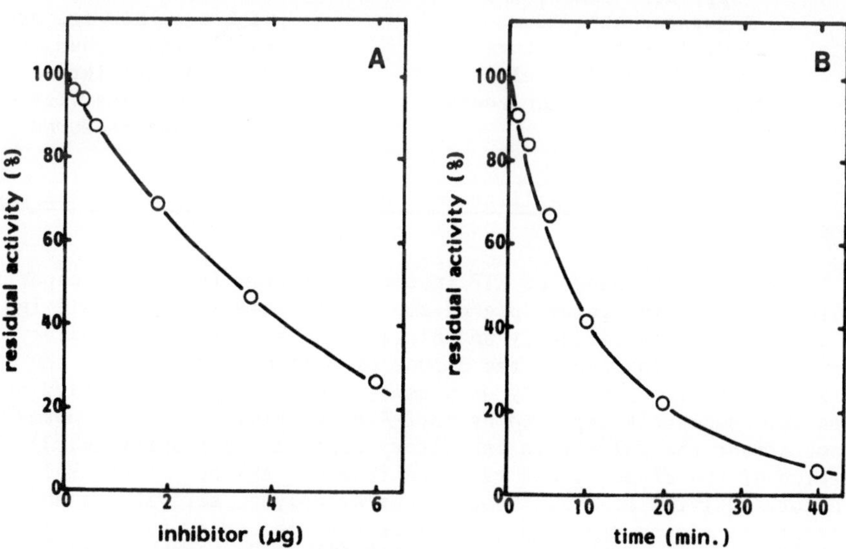

Figure 1.   Inhibition of amidolytic activity of kallikrein by KIP.
A. Kallikrein(10^{-8}M) was incubated with KIP for 30 min..
B. Kallikrein(3×10^{-9}M) was incubated with KIP(3×10^{-7}M).
Z-Phe-Arg-MCA was used as a substrate.

<u>Inhibition of guinea pig kallikrein by KIP</u>

As shown in Fig. 1A, guinea pig plasma kallikrein was inhibited by KIP. Increasing the amount of KIP decreased linearly the amidolytic activity of kallikrein at least up to 80 % inhibition. Decrease of kallikrein activity was linear until 10 minutes, and then levelled off (Fig. 1B). The analysis of interaction of KIP and kallikrein on SDS-polyacrylamide slab gel electrophoresis demonstrated that KIP formed a complex time-dependently(Fig. 2), and the molecular weight of the complex was 137,000. Kinetical properties of KIP for kallikrein is similar to those of contrapsin[7]. Vascular permeability enhancing activity of kallikrein was also blocked by KIP completely[1].

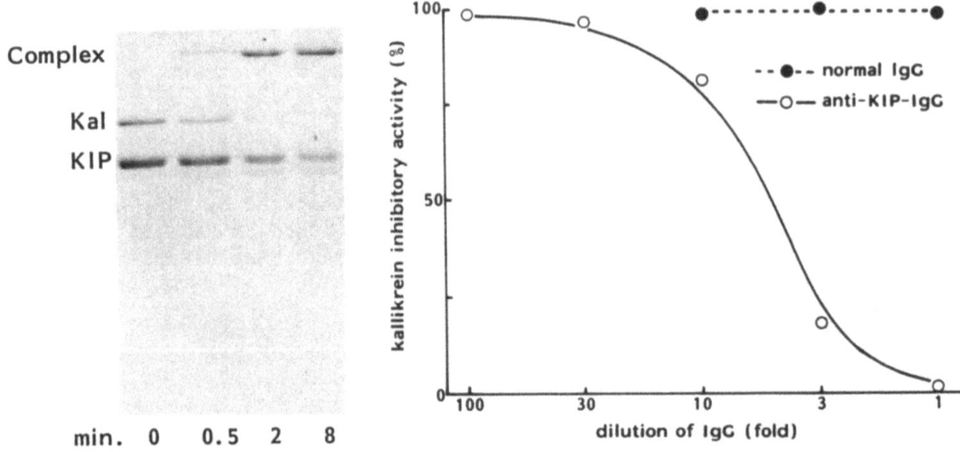

<table>
<tr><td>

Figure 2. SDS-gel electrophoretic analysis of interaction of kallikrein and KIP. Kallikrein(2µg) and KIP (3µg) were mixed, and incubated at 37°C at pH 7.0. Then the mixture was subjected to electrophoresis under nonreduced conditions.

</td><td>

Figure 3. Effect of anti-KIP IgG on kallikrein inhibitory capacity of guinea pig plasma. Plasma diluted 30 fold was incubated with anti-KIP IgG at 37°C for 30 min.. Then, the residual kallikrein inhibitory activity of plasma was measured.

</td></tr>
</table>

<u>Effect of anti-KIP IgG on kallikrein inhibitory capacity of guinea pig plasma</u>

To estimate the share of KIP in the kallikrein inhibitory capacity of guinea pig plasma, guinea pig plasma was treated with anti-KIP IgG that bound to KIP specifically and blocked the kallikrein inhibitory activity of KIP. Increasing the amount of anti-KIP IgG reduced the kallikrein inhibitory capacity of plasma, and finally the capacity of plasma was completely depleted by anti-KIP IgG(Fig. 3). Since normal IgG did not affect the kallikrein inhibitory capacity of plasma(Fig. 3), the depletion of the capacity was resulted from the absence of the kallikrein inhibitory activity of KIP. Most of the amidolytic activity of added kallikrein in plasma depleted the kallikrein inhibitory capacity was inhibited by soybean trypsin inhibitor(10^{-5}M), and the observation indicated that kallikrein was not trapped by α_2-macroglobulin and suggested that α_2-macroglobulin did not compensate for the loss of kallikrein inhibitory activity in plasma after the treatment with anti-KIP IgG. These results demonstrated that KIP was the major kallikrein inhibitor in guinea pig plasma.

70

<u>Inhibition profile of KIP for proteases</u>

The protease inhibitory activity of KIP was characterized using various proteases and the character was compared with that of the protease inhibitor in human plasma. As shown in Table 1, KIP inhibited trypsin and elastase, and for trypsin, KIP inhibited strongly. Since KIP did not inhibit chymotrypsin, KIP was quite different from human plasma protease inhibitors including α_1-protease inhibitor, antithrombinIII, α_1-antichymotrypsin, α_2-antiplasmin, and inter-α-trypsin inhibitor7

Takahara and Sinohara reported a novel trypsin inhibitor in mouse plasma, named contrapsin[4,7]. Table 1 showed the similarity of inhibition profile between KIP and contrapsin, although contrapsin did not inhibit elastase.

Table 1. Inhibition profiles of KIP and contrapsin for proteases

protease	substrate	KIP	Contrapsin[4,7]
plasma kallikrein	Z-Phe-Arg-MCA	+	+
trypsin	Boc-Phe-Ser-Arg-MCA	++	++
chymotrypsin	Suc-Ala-Ala-Pro-Phe-MCA	−	−
elastase	Suc-Ala-Pro-Ala-MCA	+	−
α-thrombin	Boc-Val-Pro-Arg-MCA	±	−

<u>Effect of oxidation on kallikrein inhibitory activity of KIP</u>

Human α_1-protease inhibitor has a methionine residue at the reactive center and the oxidation of the methionine residue at the reactive center resulted in the inactivation of the inhibitory activity of human α_1-protease inhibitor for trypsin[5]. To investigate whether KIP has human α_1-protease inhibitor-like nature, KIP was oxidized and the residual trypsin inhibitory activity was measured. The trypsin inhibitory activity of human α_1-protease inhibitor was inactivated to 50 % by oxidation with 20 fold NCS to the inhibitor molarity, but the trypsin inhibitory activity of KIP was not reduced, even by the oxidation with 40 fold NCS. The result suggested that KIP did not have a methionine residue at the reactive center region and was not identical to α_1-protease inhibitor in human plasma. In fact, we isolated α_1-protease inhibitor-like protease inhibitor that was sensitive to the oxidation, in guinea pig plasma.

According to the study of KIP, it is clear that the inhibition mechanism of guinea pig plasma was different from the mechanism of human plasma. The fact that KIP monopolizes the kallikrein inhibitory activity of plasma may suggest that plasma level of KIP is high as well as that of contrapsin[4], and the large inhibitory capacity of KIP for kallikrein in guinea pig plasma might be relevant to block Hageman factor initiated proteolytic cascade, because the concentration of Hageman factor in guinea pig plasma is four times greater than the concentration of Hageman factor in human plasma and guinea pig Hageman factor has 10 times greater capacity to correct the clotting time of Hageman factor-deficient plasma, compared with the capacity of normal human Hageman factor[9].

ACKNOWLEDGMENT

This work was supported in part by grants from the Japanese Ministry of Education.

REFERENCES

1. T. Imamura, T. Yamamoto, and T. Kambara, Guinea pig plasma kallikrein as a vascular permeability enhancement factor. Its dependence on kinin generation and regulation mechanisms $\underline{\text{in vivo}}$, Am. J. Pathol., 115:92–101 (1984).
2. T. Ishimatsu, T. Yamamoto, K. Kozono, and T. Kambara, Guinea pig macroalbumin. A major inhibitor of activated Hageman factor in plasma with an α_2-macroglobulin-like nature, Am. J. Pathol., 115:57–69 (1984).
3. F. van der Graaf, J. A. Koedam, and B. N. Bouma, Inactivation of kallikrein in human plasma, J. Clin. Invest., 71:149–158 (1983).
4. H. Takahara, and H. Sinohara, Mouse plasma trypsin inhibitors. Isolation and characterization of α-1-antitrypsin and contrapsin, a novel trypsin inhibitor, J. Biol. Chem., 257:2438–2446 (1982).
5. D. Johnson, and J. Travis, The oxidative inactivation of human α-1-protease inhibitor. Further evidence for methionine at the reactive center, J. Biol. Chem. 254:4022–4026 (1979).
6. U. K. Laemmli, Cleavage of structual proteins during the assembly of the head of bacteriophage T4, Nature, 227:680–685 (1970).
7. H. Takahara, and H. Sinohara, Mouse plasma trypsin inhibitors: Inhibitory spectum of contrapsin and alpha-1-antitrypsin, Thromb. Res., 27: 45–50 (1983).
8. J. Travis, and G. S. Salvesen, Human plasma proteinase inhibitors, Ann. Rev. Biochem., 52:655–709 (1983).
9. T. Yamamoto, and C. G. Cochrane, Guinea pig Hageman factor as a vascular permeability enhancement factor, Am. J. Pathol., 105:164–175 (1981).

COMPARATIVE STUDIES ON FAST ACTING PA-INHIBITORS

FROM PIG AND HUMAN PERIPHERAL LEUCOCYTES

Marija Kopitar, Marina Drobnič-Košorok, Vladimir
Cotič, Dušica Gabrijelčič, Roman Jerala and Vito Turk

Department of Biochemistry
J. Stefan Institute
Ljubljana, Yugoslavia

INTRODUCTION

The fibrinolytic system is a multicomponent enyzme system composed of
plasminogen, plasminogen activators and inhibitors. The plasminogen activators catalyze the conversion of plasminogen to plasmin. The regulation of
plasmin activity appears to be accomplished by many processes such as :
activation of plasminogen activators or inhibition of plasminogen activators
and plasmin. The studies of recent years have indicated two types of immunologically and biochemically distinct specific inhibitors of plasminogen
activators : PAI-1 - endothelial cell type PAI[1] and PAI-2- placental type
PAI[2]. The former inhibits tissue type PA (t-PA) as well as urokinase type
(u-PA) whereas PAI-2 is primarily an u-PA inhibitor.

In our laboratory we have studied the proteinase inhibitors from pig
and human leucocytes for a longer period. In the case of leucocyte plasminogen activator inhibitors isolated from pig[3] and human[4] we reported that
these two inhibitors differ in many biochemical characteristics. On the basis
of biochemical and immunological characteristics it was found that human
leucocytic PAI[4] is identical with the placental type PAI-2. We report herein the further characterization of pig leucocytic PAI and its N-terminal
amino part comparison with PAI-1, PAI-2, some serpins, chicken ovalbumin as
well as with rat and human serum albumin.

MATERIALS AND METHODS

Abbreviations : S-2444 = pyro-Glu-Gly-Arg-p-nitroanilide; S-2251 =
H-D-Val-Leu-Lys-p-nitroanilide; pI = isoelectric point; PAGE = polyacrylamide gel electrophoresis; SDS = sodium dodecyl sulphate; Fbg = fibrinogen;
UK = urokinase; PA = plasminogen activator; u-PA = urokinase-type plasminogen activator; t-PA = tissue-type plasminogen activator; PAI = plasminogen
activator inhibitor; p-NPGB = nitrophenilguanidinobenzoate.

Sephadex G-100, low Mr calibration kit, Pharmalyte (pH 3-10), broad pI
calibration kit were supplied by Pharmacia, Sweden. DEAE-cellulose - DE 32
was from Whatman, England. S-2444, S-2251 and human plasmin were purchased
from Kabi, Molndal, Sweden. UK was from Leo Pharmaceutical, Denmark. Fbg
(plasminogen reach) and agar were from Behringwerke, FRG.

Pig and human leucocyte PAI-s were isolated from peripheral blood as reported in 3, 4.

SDS-PAGE

It was carried out in polyacrylamide gel slabs according to Laemmli [5]. Before the experiment samples were either reduced with 0.1 M 2-mercapto-ethanol or with 20 mM dithioerithritol in sample buffer or run unreduced in the sample buffer.

Molecular mass estimation. The Mr of the inhibitors was determined by SDS-PAGE with reduction or without reduction using the molecular weight standards.

Enzyme activity and inhibition assay were performed by the procedures reported in 3, 4 with Fbg and S-2444 as substrates.

The protein was determined by the method of Lowry et al.[6]

Amino acid analysis

The amino acid analysis of the purified inhibitor was determined with Beckmann 118 CD amino acid analyser. Samples were evaporated to dryness in a vacuum concentrator and then hydrolyzed in 6 M HCl or in methan sulphonic acid, 4 M.

Determination of N-terminal amino acid of inhibitor molecule

Amino acid sequencing was performed with automatical Edman degradation on an Applied Biosystems Instruments 470 A, automatical gass sequenator as described in [7] .

For homologous sequences we searched through the Protein Identification Resource (PIR) protein sequence data base, release 10.0, using programs SEARCH and ALIGN.

Immunozation procedures and isolation of polyclonal antibodies

Polyclonal antibodies against purified pig PAI were prepared by injection of antigen into the popliteal lymph nodes of rabbits. In our experiments we used 60 ug of PAI for lymph nodes injections and 30 ug for booster injections into intradermal sites on the back. The titer of the anti-inhibitor serum was determined by Ouchterlony double immunodiffusion analysis.

IgG was purified on a column with protein A Sepharose 4 B according to the Pharmacia pamphlet. IgG was bound at pH 8.0 in 0.1 M Na phosphate buffer and eluted step-wise with 0.1 M, pH 6.0 and pH 4.0, Na citrate- citric acid buffers. The IgG eluted at pH 4.0 was dialyzed against PBS buffer and concentrated by liophylization.

Western blot

In Western blot analysis the pig PAI were electrophoretically transferred onto nitrocellulose filters (Schleicher and Schüll BA 85) by the procedure of Towbin et al. [8] . The immunological detection was obtained on nitrocellulose by polyclonal rabbit antibodies in concentration 10 ug/ml. After the reaction with peroxydase had conjugated antibodies (goat antirabbit), the bound conjugate was immunostained.

RESULTS AND DISCUSSION

The differences and some biochemical characteristics on the pig and human PAI have already been reported. These two inhibitory proteins differ in molecular weight and pI. The human PAI has an Mr of 47 kDa, whereas the pig inhibitor has 65 kDa. pI of human PAI is 5.5-5.7 and 4.4.-4.5 of pig PAI. These two inhibitors also differ in succeptibility to inactivation by cathepsin D. PAI of pig origin could be inactivated by cathepsin D whereas cathepsin D has no effect on the activity of human PAI [3,4]. These two inhibitors showed the same inhibition ability. They specifically inhibit only PA-s but not plasmin, trypsin or thrombin [1,2,3,4,9].

The apparent dissociation constant K_i determined by Henderson[10] for pig and human PAI with HMr u-PA (titrated with pMBG) were found to be 8×10^{-8} M and 1.5×10^{-8} M, respectively.

The second order rate constant $-K_1-$ of the reaction of PAI was determined using HMr u-PA. The molar concentration of the active enzyme was determined by titration with p-NPGB. The value $7.5 \times 10^6 M^{-1}s^{-1}$ was obtained for pig and $2.5 \times 10^6 M^{-1}s^{-1}$ for human PAI.

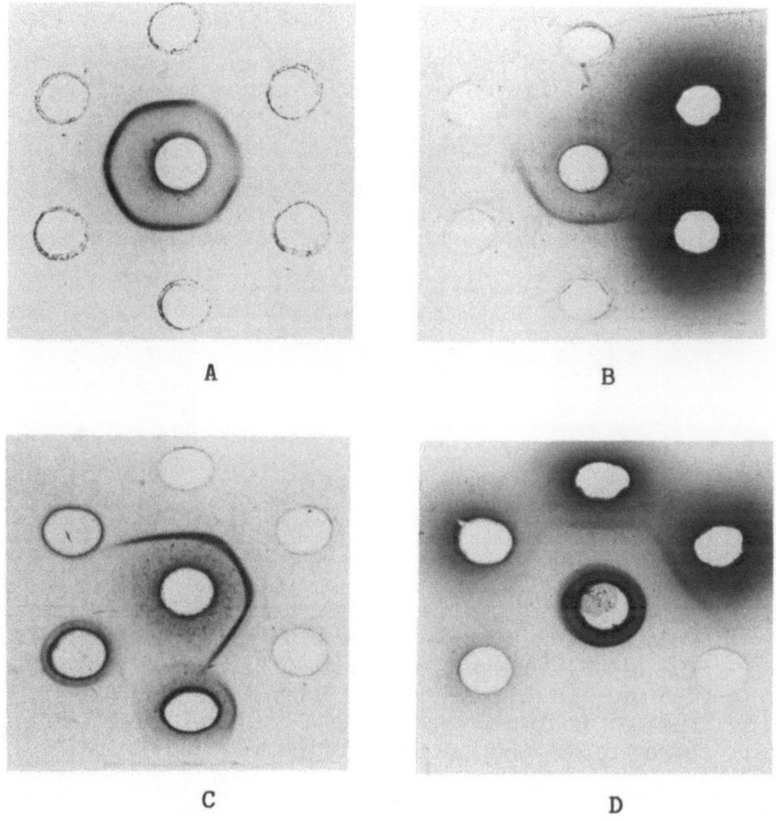

Fig. 1. Double immunodiffusion. A- Well 1 rabbit antiserum against purified pig PAI, wells 2-7 purified pig PAI. B- Well 1 rabbit antiserum against pig PAI, wells 2-3 purified pig PAI, 4-5 normal pig serum. C- Well 1 rabbit antiserum against purified pig PAI, wells 2-4 purified pig PAI, 5-7 purified human PAI. D- Well 1 purified human leucocytic PAI, wells 2-4 rabbit antiserum against purified pig PAI.

The K_i of human PAI with HMr u-PA is the same as those reported by Kruithof [9] for the PAI-2 isolated from Histiocytic Lymphoma cell line U-937. Lecander and coworkers [11] and lately Kruithof have studied the inhibition of LNPI-2 with two chain TPA and single chain TPA and found that PAI-2 much better inhibited the double chain TPA.

The immunological identity of placental PAI with PAI from other sources was first established with our PAI isolated from human peripheral leucocytes [4] . In the present work we reexamined in more detail the immunological properties of pig and human leucocytic PAI. The purified pig PAI was analyzed by double immunodiffusion as shown in Fig.1. Polyclonal antibodies against pig leucocytic PAI crossreacted with pig leucocytic PAI, and they showed a weaker crossreactivity also with human PAI (Fig. 1 C,D) but did not crossreact with pig serum, indicating that this inhibitor protein is not present in normal pig serum.

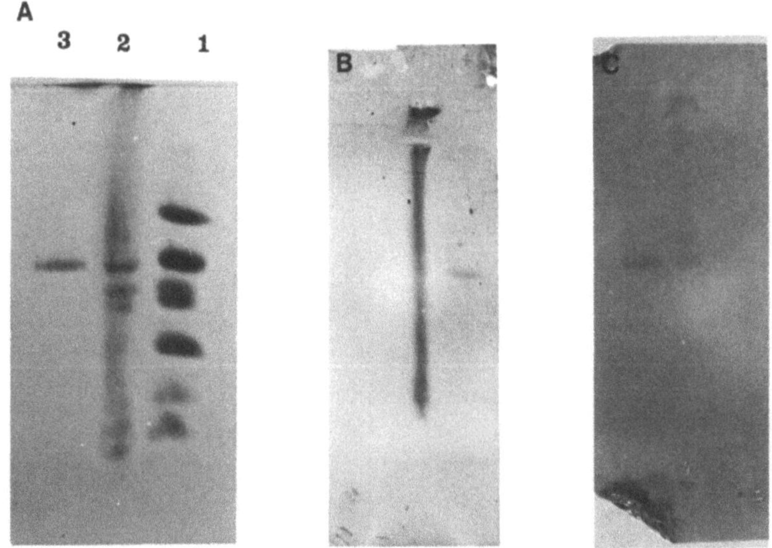

Fig. 2. Western immunoblots of SDS-PAGE gels of pig PAI samples
transferred to nitrocellulose with rabbit antipig PAI
IgG. A- SDS-PAGE gel, standards (1), cytosol (2), purified pig PAI (3); B- cytosol (1) and purified PAI (2)
transferred to nitrocellulose; C- cytosol and PAI transferred to nitrocellulose and stained immunologically.

By immunoblotting of proteins transferred to nitrocellulose from SDS gels (Fig. 2) it was established that purified pig PAI and the starting material- cytosol (alkaline activated) reacted with antibodies and that the inhibitor is present in cytosol only in one molecular form.

Table 1. Amino acid composition of pig PAI, placental PAI-2,
endothelial PAI-1

	residues/mol		
	experimental	theoretical[1]	theoretical[2]
Lysine	58	28	19
Histidine	17	7	13
Arginine	23	15	18
Aspartic acid	55	19	20
Asparagine	–	19	13
Threonine	35	21	20
Serine	26	33	27
Glutamic acid	74	33	15
Glutamine	–	17	23
Proline	28	18	21
Glycine	19	27	21
Alanine	47	31	26
Cysteine	10	6	–
Valine	35	23	33
Methionine	8	18	16
Isoleucine	20	18	15
Leucine	64	39	37
Tyrozine	20	14	9
Phenilalanine	27	25	24
Tryptophan	8	4	9

The experimental values were obtained by amino acid analysis
of the purified inhibitor as described in the experimental
procedures. 1 - the theoretical number of residues/mol of
PAI-2 was deduced from cDNA sequence of placenta inhibitor[2]
and 2- of PAI-1 by the same way from [1].

The amino acid compositions of pig PAI and of placental PAI-2 and of
endothelial PAI-1 are shown in Table 1. It is clearly evident that pig
inhibitor differs in amino acid composition from both known amino acid
compositions of PAI-s.

The amino terminus of the natural PAI from pig leucocyte is alanine. The
amino acid sequencing of the pig PAI resulted in a homogenous sequence for
the first 30 amino acid residues. Comparison of these N-terminal parts of
pig inhibitor to placental PAI-2 and to endothelial PAI-1, antithrombin III
showed only a little similarity as well as to ovalbumin. While pig PAI is
in its N-terminal part of the molecule especially similar to rat albumin or
to human albumin. Thus, 23 identities out of 30 possible matches between
residues. From the data presented, it is evident that pig and human PAI
showed some similarities. They showed immunological identities, shared the
same inhibition spectrum, and both inhibitors contain cysteines in their
molecular structures, whereas the endothelial inhibitor contained no cysteine.

From the known data [1, 2, 3, 4, 9, 10, 11] and from the results presented it is evident that there exist at least three different types of plasminogen activator inhibitors. PAI-1 and PAI-2 do not crossreact with each
other [1, 2], but human leucocytic PAI (identical to placental PAI-2) cross-
reacted with pig leucocytic PAI which differs structurally and in biochemical characteristics from PAI-2. Similarly also a PAI of Mr of about 65 kDa,
which appeared in plasma of pregnant women [11, 2], crossreacted with
PAI-2 (47 kDa). Thus, some immunological identity between PAI-2 and PAIs of
about 65 kDa does exist.

Table 2. Comparison of the amino acid sequence of the N-terminal part of
the pig PAI with the N-terminal part of PAI-2, PAI-1, antithrombin
III (AT III), ovalbumin (OVAL), human serum albumin (HSA) and rat
serum albumin (RSA).

PAI	A E H K S E I A H R F K D E G E R H F K G X V W I X F S Q Y
PAI-2	M E D L C V A N T L F A L N L F K H L A K A S P T G N L F L
PAI-1	P S Y V A H L A S D F G V R V F Q Q V A Q A S K D R N V V F
AT III	V W E L S K A N S R F A T T F Y Q H L A D S K N D N D N
OVAL	m G S I G A A S M E F C F D V F K E L K V H H A N E N I F Y
HSA	S A H K S E V A H R F K D L G E E N F K A L V L I A F A Q Y
RSA	E A H K S E I A H R F K D L G E Q H F K G L V L I A F S Q Y

The data for PAI-2, PAI-1, AT III and OVAL were taken from R.D.Ye and co-workers [2] whereas the data for HSA and RSA were ours as reported in the Methods section.

REFERENCES

1. T. Ny, M. Sawdey, D. Lawrence, J.L. Millau and D.J. Loskutoff, Cloning
    and sequence of a cDNA coding for the human beta-migrating endothelial-
    cell-type plasminogen activator inhibitor, Proc. Natl. Acad. Sci. USA 83:
    6776 (1986).
2. R.D. Ye, T.C. Wun and J.E. Sadler, cDNA cloning and expression in esche-
    richia coli of a plasminogen activator inhibitor from human placenta,
    J. Biol. Chem. 262 : 3718 (1987).
3. M. Kopitar, Isolation and some characteristics of urokinase inhibitors
    isolated from pig leucocytes, Haemostasis 10: 215 (1981).
4. M. Kopitar, B. Rozman, J. Babnik, V. Turk, D.E. Mullins and T.C. Wun,
    Human leucocyte urokinase inhibitors- Purification, characterization
    and comparative studies against different plasminogen activators,
    Thrombosis and Haemostasis 54: 750 (1985).
5. U.K. Laemmli, Cleavage of structural proteins during the assemby of the
    head of the bacteriophage T4, Nature 27: 680 (1970).
6. O.H. Lowry, N.J. Rosebrough, A.L. Farr and R.J. Randall, Protein measu-
    rement with Folin phenol reagent, J. Biol. Chem. 193: 265 (1051).
7. P. Edman and A. Henscher, Sequence determination, in: "Protein Sequence
    Determination," S.B. Needleman, ed., Springer Verlag, Berlin (1975).
8. H. Towbin, T. Stalhelin and J.Gordon, Electrophoretic transfer of pro-
    teins for polyacrylamide gels to nitrocellulose sheets : Procedure and
    applications, Proc. Natl. Acad. Sci. USA 76: 4350 (1979).
9. E.K. Kruithof , J.D. Vassalli, W.D. Schleuning, R.J. Mattaliano and
    F. Bachmann, Purification and characterization of a plasminogen acti-
    vator inhibitor from the Histiocytic Lymphoma cell line U-937, J. Biol.
    Chem. 261: 11207 (1986).
10. P.J.F. Henderson, A linear equation that described the steady-state ki-
    netics of enzymes and subcellular particles interacting with tightly
    bound inhibitors, Biochem. J. 127: 321 (1972).
11. J. Lecander, R.Roblin and B. Astedt, Differential inhibition of two
    molecular forms of melanoma cell plasminogen activator by a placental
    inhibitor, Br. J. Haematol. 57: 407 (1984).

Acknowledgement. The excellent technical assistance of Mrs. Majda Božič
is gratefully acknowledged. Supported by a research grant from The Research
Council of Slovenia.

IN VIVO FUNCTION OF C1-INHIBITOR AND PATHOPHYSIOLOGY OF EDEMA

ATTACK IN PATIENTS WITH HEREDITARY ANGIONEUROTIC EDEMA

J. Kodama*, K. Uchida**, T. Sakata** and F. Funakoshi**

* Institute for Medical Care and Health Maintenance, SANYO
  Electric Group, Health Insurance Association, Osaka, Japan
** National Cardiovascular Center, Osaka, Japan

INTRODUCTION

The autosomal dominant defect of C1-inhibitor(C1-INH) is responsible
for the pathophysiology of hereditary angioneurotic edema(HANE). As documented mainly in vitro, C1-INH inhibits enzyme activity of multiple plasma
proteinases, such as C1r, C1s, activated Hageman factor (αHFa), Hageman
factor fragment(βHFa),activated Factor XI, plasmin and kallikrein(Landerman et al 1962, Donaldson and Evans 1963, Ratnoff et al 1969, Forbes et al
1970, Schreiber et al 1973). Hence, other than the early acting components
of complement system, positive feedback reactions, linked to the contact
phase of intrinsic coagulation cascade, appear as possible direct pathoge-
netic mechanism for the edema attack(Curd et al 1980, Schapira et al 1983,
Witzke et al 1983, Kodama et al 1984, 1986). On the other hand, the prominent clinical symptom of the disease, bouts of localized edema formation
with haemoconcentration and leukocytosis(Kodama et al 1984), is well known
to be elicited by several exogenous triggering stimuli(Osler 1888, Donaldson
and Evans 1963, Frank et al 1976). Those are exposure to cold, emotional
and physical stress, infection, trauma, contusion, compression and usage of
drugs, such as amphetamine and estrogen preparation. Hence, to our opinion,
the hereditary defect of C1-INH represents itself as a condition of prepared-
ness for the edema attack. In addition to this hereditary defect, the action
of the exogenous stimuli upon individual kindreds with the disposition could
initiate a relevant activation process of the responsible plasma proteinase
system.
To challenge such possibilities, we have tried to analyze the pathobiochemistry of the edema attack of HANE by follow up experiments with or without substitution of the Pasteurized C1-INH concentrate(Fuhge et al 1986)
on patients under our control.

METHODS

Table I shows the methods used in our clinical investigation. In the
earlier experiments the parameters were assessed mainly on manual methods
(Kodama et al 1984), and their principles are depicted in the parentheses.
To perform such determinations in the routine laboratory test, we have developed relevant automated assay methods on COBAS BIO centrifugal analyzer(Duncan et al 1985, Uchida et al in press). As reported elsewhere, the within
run and day to day reproducibility for the determination of the inhibitory
activity of C1-INH using Berichrom C1-Inaktivator were n=10, $\bar{X}$=93.0%, SD=3.2

Table I. Methods

Immunological antigen of C$\overline{1}$-INH	(SRID)	Activated partial thromboplastin time	
Inhibitory activity of C$\overline{1}$-INH	(4 step haemolytic titration)	Prothrombin time	
Hageman factor	(aPTT, deficient human plasma)	Antithrombin-III	Automated assay on
Factor XI		α-2-Plasmin inhibitor	COBAS BIO
Factor VII	(PT, deficient human plasma)	Plasminogen	
Antithrombin-III	(SRID)	Prekallikrein	
α-2-Plasmin inhibitor		Inhibitory activity of C$\overline{1}$-INH	
Plasminogen	(affinity chromatography, fibrin agar plate)	Complement components	Haemolytic titration
Plasmin		Thrombelastgram	Standard method on Hellige's apparatus
Antiplasmin			
Fibrin degradation products	(latex agglutination)	Estrone	Ethylether extraction,
Prekallikrein	(amidolytic activity)	Estradiol	fractionation on HPLC, RIA
Kininogens	(differential bioassay)		
Testosterone	n-Hexan-ethylether extraction, RIA	Androstenedione	Petroleumether extraction RIA (Δ^4A. dione-kit)

% and CV=3.4% as well as n=7, $\overline{X}$=90.4%, SD=4.5% and CV=4.9%, respectively.
Immunological antigen amount of C$\overline{1}$-INH was 27.0±10.0 mg/dl.

RESULTS

I : Follow up studies without substitution of C$\overline{1}$-INH concentrate

Results were summarized as follows: 1) In the course of long term observation, the haemolytic activity of C1s, C4 and C2, amidolytic activity of prekallikrein and the blood level of HMW-kininogen decreased progressively. 2) Even in the period of remission, the coagulation activity of Hageman factor and Factor XI was augumented and the free plasmin activity was detectable. Decrease in proteins of antithrombin-III and α-2-plasmin inhibitor occurred concomitantly. 3) During edema attack, moderate haemoconcentration, neutrophile leukocytosis, augumented coagulation activity of Hageman factor, Factors XI and VII, shortening of r+k in the thrombelastgram and the free plasmin activity with a decrease to the undetectable level of α-2-plasmin inhibitor were demonstrated. 4) Following attacks of edema, an elevated blood level of fibrin degradation products and a refractory period for the new attack were noted(Kodama et al 1984,1986).

II : Follow up studies with substitution of C$\overline{1}$-INH concentrate

Figure 1 shows changes of plasma proteinase systems following treatment with 1,500 unit C$\overline{1}$-INH concentrate for facial edema attack of a female HANE

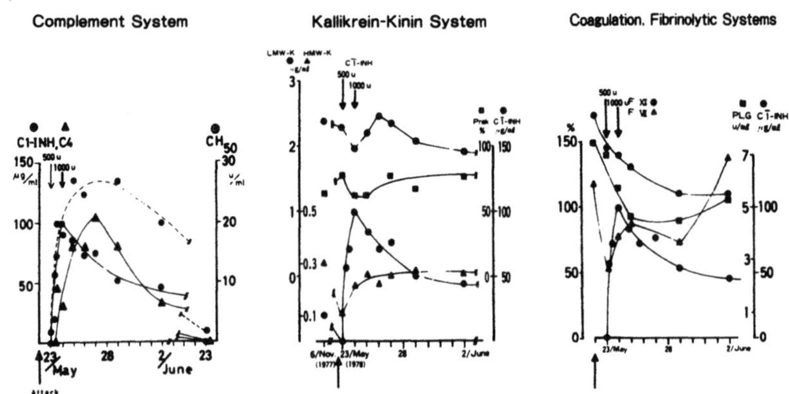

Fig. 1. Course of Complement, Kallikrein-Kinin and Coagulation
Systems following Administration of C$\overline{1}$-INH Concentrate
in a Female Patient in Attack

patient. Details were reported elsewhere(Kodama et al 1984). Hence, changes
only in the kallikrein-kinin system are described here again. The amidolytic
activity of prekallikrein decreased for 48 hrs after substitution. The blood
level of HMW-kininogen increased in parallel to the clinical improvement to
a maximum in 24 hrs and maintained nearly on the same level for 10 days. It
decreased to a very low level at the next occasion of edema attack. LMW-kininogen decreased until 24 hrs and then reached a maximum on day 3.

Table II . Backgrounds of Patients

Case No.	Age (years)	Sex	Body weight (kg)	C1̄-INH* Activity (%)	C1̄-INH* Antigen (mg/dℓ)	Dose (u)	HANE attack
1	56	F	70	33.7	13.4	1500	remission
2	52	F	52	10.7	9.2	1000	remission
3	54	F	58	0.0	5.4	1000	acute (face)
4	53	F	51	0.0	5.3	1000	remission
5	64	F	50	9.4	7.0	1500	remission
6	20	F	68	8.3	trace	1500+1000	acute (hands)
Mean ±SD	49.8 ±15.2	—	58.2 ±8.9	10.4 ±12.3	6.7 ±4.5	—	—

Table II shows backgrounds of patients undergone to our additional substitution experiment. Six female patients from 6 HANE families, 2 in an acute
attack and 4 in remission, were selected. Cases 1, 3 and 5 correspond to the
propositi of the 1st, 3rd and 4th family of the previous report. Case 4 is
the older sister of case 2. Cases 1, 5 and 6 are maintained with Danazol 100
mag daily. The control male patient for the blood level of female sex steroid
hormone, aged 34 in remission, is the propositus of the 7th family. Doses of
C1-INH concentrate were 1,000-2,500 unit as shown in the Table.

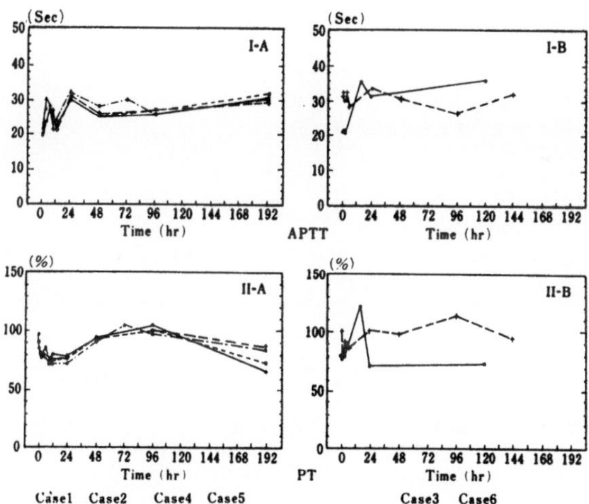

Fig. 2. Course of aPTT and PT of Patients in Remission and in Attack

Figure 2 shows time course of aPTT(in second) and PT(in % value) of
patients in remission(Group A) and in attack(Group B). In Group A and in
case 3, who was not on Danazol maintenance, aPTT was shortened to a level of
20 sec before substitution. Until 24 hrs after substitution, it elongated to
a level of 30 sec, showing an initial biphasic alteration. On day 8, it recovered to the normal level of over 30 sec. PT was decreased until 24 hrs,
like a reflected image of aPTT, reached 100% level on day 4 and then it decreased to 80% level on day 8. In case 3, PT increased to a level of over
100% until 24 hrs after substitution and then it began to decrease.

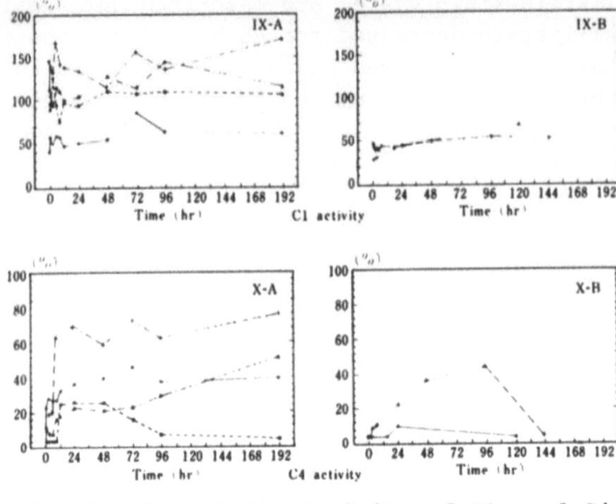

Fig. 3.   Haemolytic Activity of C1s and C4

Figure 3 shows time course of the haemolytic activity of C1s and C4. No uniform tendency was found in the haemolytic activity of C1s, but C4 increased in 5 out of 6 cases. The haemolytic activity of C3 showed no uniform tendency but C2 paralleled to that of C4.

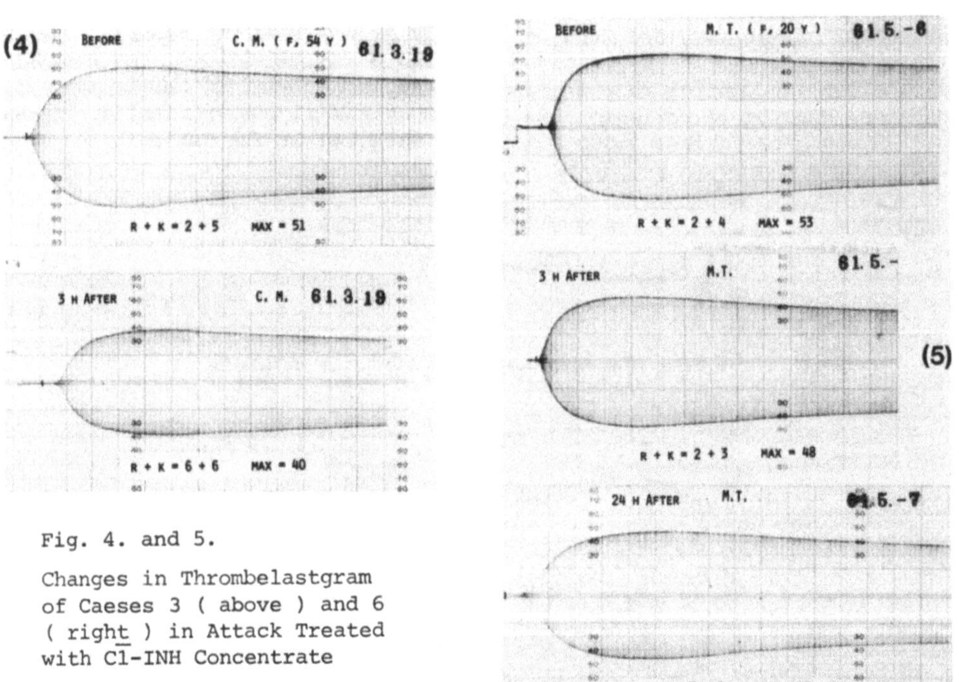

Fig. 4. and 5.

Changes in Thrombelastgram of Caeses 3 (above) and 6 (right) in Attack Treated with C1-INH Concentrate

Figures 4 and 5 show changes of the thrombelastgram of cases 3 and 6 with edema attacks. Case 3, aged 54, was treated with 1,000 unit C1-INH for facial edema. Case 6 had been maintained with Danazol 100 mg daily and had had edema of the both forearms, which was treated with 1,500 unit C1-INH.The edema in case 3 disappeared completely in 3 hrs when the inhibitory activity of C1-INH was 47.9%(Table III). In case 6, the edema did not improve in 3 hrs when the inhibitory activity of C1-INH was 44.4%. Hence, 1,000 unit was additionally substituted and the edema disappeared in 24 hrs. The thrombelast-

Table III . Inhibitory Activity and Protein Amount of $\overline{C1}$-INH
and Blood Levels of Sex Steroids

HANE patient		Case 3 (female, 54)		Case 6 (female, 20)		Control (male, 34)
		before	3 h after	before	3 h after	
$\overline{C1}$-INH						
inhibitory activity	(%)	0	47.9	8.3	44.4	0
antigen amount	(μg/mℓ)	54	145.	0	145	60
Sex steroids						
estrone	(pg/mℓ)	18		140		86.1
estradiol	(pg/mℓ)	<10		104		12.4
androstenedione	(ng/mℓ)	1.5		2.6		3.2
testosterone	(ng/mℓ)	—		—		4.61

gram parameters r+k and maximal amplitude were normalized in parallel to the
clinical improvement. In case 6, the parameters showed again a hypercoagulable changes on day 6 (r+k=2+3, max=55), when the inhibitory activity of
C1-INH became undetectable, although she remained in remission. As shown in
Table III, the blood level of estrone and estradiol in case 6 was much higher
than in case 3. The control male patient in remission showed also much higher
estrogen levels than in case 3.

COMMENTS

Results of our follow up experiements on patients with HANE have revealed the followings: 1) Even in the remission period, the classical pathway of complement system, coagulation cascade and fibrinolytic system are
activated. 2) During attack of edema, not only complement but also coagulation, fibrinolytic and kallikrein-kinin systems are concomitantly activated.
3) C1-INH inhibits in vivo the enzyme activity of kallikrein to generate
bradykinin in the first place. 4) C1-INH functions in vivo as a regulatory
protein molecule for the contact phase of the coagulation cascade.
On the basis of these findings, the interaction between exogenous triggering stimuli and activation of the plasma proteinase systems could be elucidated as follows: 1) Bacterial inflammation and trauma evoke activation of
the coagulation cascade and fibrinolytic system directly or through the protein C mediated reactions(Comp et al 1982). 2) Exposure to cold, emotional
and physical stress and administration of amphetamine are accompanied by the
stimulation of the adrenal-sympathetic-nerve system(Kopin et al 1978),
which evokes concomitant response of the hypothalamico-neurohypophyseal axis
(Mills and Wang 1964). Hence, release of catecholamines and/or "plasminogen
activator releasing hormone"(Mannucci 1974, Cash 1978) can liberate activating enzymes from the endothelial cells of vessels(Loskutoff and Edgington
1977, Wiggins et al 1980), resulting in the activation of enzymes linked to
the contact phase of the coagulation cascade. 3) Comression or contusion
upon soft parts of the body, that are not accompanied by the impairment of
the blood vessels, result in the blood flow entangled in the area, where the
blood supply is maintained by the microcirculation. As a result of electro-
stimulation of the microcirculation, haemorheological changes, activation of
platelets and leukocytes and enhanced vascular permeability can take place
(Tsuchiya et al 1986). The metabolic bursts of leukocytes can be evoked by
substances that are readily generated in the microcirculation of patients
with HANE, such as αHFa, kallikrein, C3a, C5a and leukotriene B_4(Goldman
and Goetzl 1982, Jochum et al 1986, Wachtfogel et al 1986). Activated leukocytes release elastase and superoxyd radicals, resulting in the alteration of
plasma proteinase systems and in the impairment of endothelial cells of
microcirculation. In turn, the Hageman factor homologue is activated, resulting in the enhanced vascular permeability.
Those reactions are modified by several intrinsic and extrinsic factors
as follows: 1) Specific and unspecific inhibitors for individual plasma proteinases, such as α-2-plasmin inhibitor, antithrombin-III, α-2-macroglobulin
and α-1-antitrypsin. The rate of biosynthesis of HMW-kininogen is very slow
(Oh-ishi et al 1979). Hence, the blood level of HMW-kininogen can control

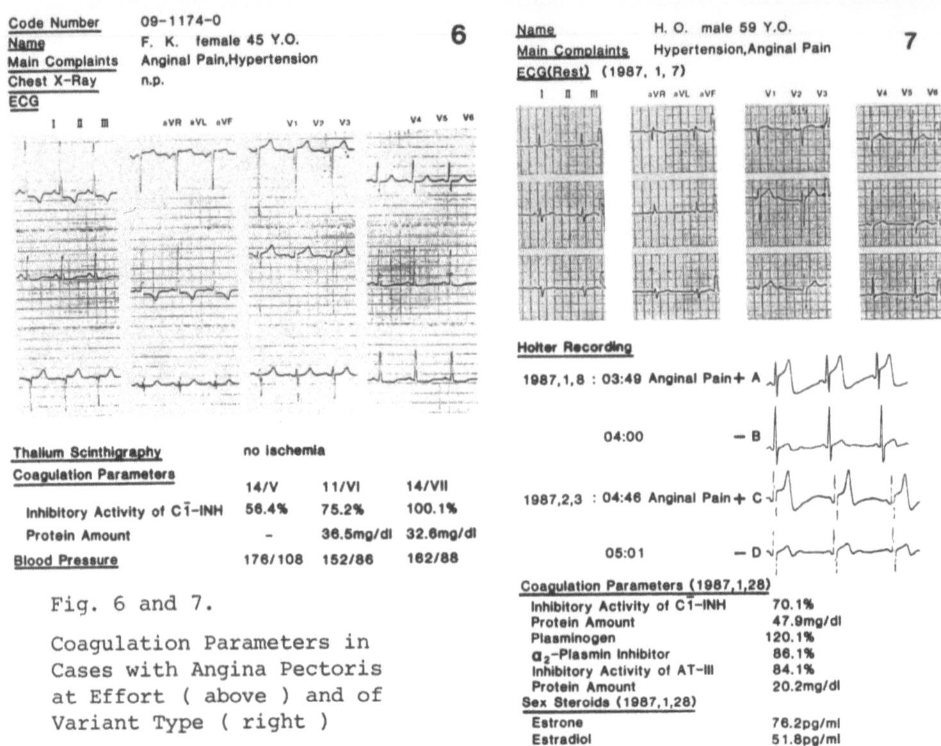

Coagulation Parameters	14/V	11/VI	14/VII
Inhibitory Activity of C$\bar{1}$-INH	56.4%	75.2%	100.1%
Protein Amount	–	36.5mg/dl	32.6mg/dl
Blood Pressure	176/108	152/86	162/88

Fig. 6 and 7.

Coagulation Parameters in
Cases with Angina Pectoris
at Effort (above) and of
Variant Type (right)

Coagulation Parameters (1987,1,28)	
Inhibitory Activity of C$\bar{1}$-INH	70.1%
Protein Amount	47.9mg/dl
Plasminogen	120.1%
α_2-Plasmin Inhibitor	86.1%
Inhibitory Activity of AT-III	84.1%
Protein Amount	20.2mg/dl

Sex Steroids (1987,1,28)	
Estrone	76.2pg/ml
Estradiol	51.8pg/ml

the occurrence of edema attack. 2) Extrinsic factors, such as responsiveness
to the adrenal-sympathetic-nerve stimuli of individual kindreds with the disposition and the blood level of female sex steroids(Williams et al 1977, Altura and Altura 1977).In a male HANE patient sustained control with methyl-
testosterone resulted in a development of gynaecomastia(Ohela 1977). Hence,
in male patient with the disposition the activity of aromatase(Höffken et al
1985) appears responsible for the occurrence of edema attack.

We have found thus an analogy in the exogenous triggering stimuli and
extrinsic modifying factors between HANE attack and thromboembolic diseases,
such as acute myocardial infarct and angina pectoris(Phillips 1978, Enterican et al 1978, Luria et al 1982). Preliminary analyses in cases with angina
pectoris at effort and of variant type are shown in Figures 6 and 7. It is
empasized that there are cases with angina pectoris in which inhibitory activity of C$\bar{1}$-INH decreased and a discrepancy between inhibitory activity and
protein amount of C$\bar{1}$-INH with protein excess has been clearly demonstrated.

REFERENCES

Altura, E. M. and Altura, B. T., 1977, Influence of sex hormones, oral con-
    traceptives and pregnancy on vascular muscle and its reactivity, in:
    "Factors influencing vascular reactivity", O.Carrier and S. Shibata,
    eds., Igaku-Shoin, Tokyo. New York
Cash, J. D., 1978, Control mechanisms of activator release, in: "Progress in
    chemical fibrinolysis and thrombolysis. Vol 3", J. F. Davidson, R. M.
    Rowan, M. M. Samama, P. C. Desnoyers, eds., Raven Press, New York
Comp, P. C., Jacock, R. M., Ferrell, G. L. and Esmon, C. T., 1982, Activation
    of protein C in vivo, J. Clin. Invest., 70: 127-134
Curd, J. G., Prograis, L. J. and Cochrane, C. G., 1980, Detection of active
    kallikrein in induced blister fluid of hereditary angioedema patient,
    J. Ex. Med., 152: 742-747

Donaldson, J. H. and Evans, R. R., 1963, A biochemical abnormality in hereditary angioneurotic edema: Absence of serum inhibitor of C'1-esterase, Amer. J. Med., 35: 37-44

Duncan, A., Bowie, E. J. W., Owen, Jr., C. A. and Fass, D. N., 1985, A clinical evaluation of automated chromogenic tests as substitutes for conventional prothrombin time and activated partial thromboplastin time tests, Clin. Chem., 31: 853-855

Enterican, J. H., Beach, C., Carroll, D., Kenmure, A. C. F., Klopper, A., Mackie, M. and Douglas, A. F., 1978, Raised plasma oestradiol and oestrone levels in young survivors of myocardial infarction, Lancet, 2: 487-490

Forbes, C. D., Pensky, J. and Ratnoff, O. D., 1970, Inhibition of activated Hageman factor and activated plasma thromboplastin antecedent by purified serum C'1 inactivator, J. Lab. Clin. Med., 76: 809-815

Frank, M. M., Gelfand, J. A. and Atkinson, J. P., 1976 Hereditary angioedema: The clinical syndrome and its management, Annals Int. Med., 84: 580-583

Fuhge, P., Gratz, P. and Geiger, H., 1986, Moderne Methode zur Herstellung von Gerinnungstherapeutika, Behring Inst. Mitt., 79: 164-176

Goldman, D.W. and Goetzl, E. J., 1982, Specific binding of leukotriene B_4 to receptors on human polymorphnuclear leukocytes, J. Immunol., 129: 1600-1604

Höffken, K., Miller, A. A., Miller, B., Becher, R. and Schmidt, C. G., 1985, Neue Aspekte in der Hormontherapie des metastasierten Mammakarzinoms, D. M. W., 110: 1799-1802

Jochum, M., Witte, J., Duswald, K. H., Inthorn, D., Welter, H. and Fritz, H., 1986, Pathobiochemistry of sepsis: Role of proteinases, proteinase inhibitors and oxidizing agents, Behring Inst. Mitt., 79: 121-130

Kodama, J., Uchida, K., Yoshimura, S., Katayama, Y., Kushiro, H., Yutani, C., Funahashi, S., Takamiya, O., Matsumoto, Y., Ando, Y., Hashimoto, T., Nagaki, K., Katori, M., Uchida, T., Oh-ishi, S. and Inai, S., 1984, Studies of four Japanese families with hereditary angioneurotic edema: Simultaneous activation of plasma protease systems and exogenous triggering stimuli, Blut 49: 405-418

Kodama, J., Uchida, K., Yutani, CH. and Funahashi, S., 1986, Hereditäres angioneurotisches Ödem: Pathophysiologie und Therapie, Behring Inst. Mitt., 79: 231-240

Kopin, I. J., Lake, C. R. and Ziegler, M., 1978, Plasma level of norepinephrin, Ann. Int. Med., 88: 671-680

Landerman, N. S., Webster, M. E., Becker, E. L. and Ratcliffe, H. E., 1962, Hereditary angioneurotic edema. II. Deficiency of inhibitor for serum-globulin permeability factor and/or plasma kallikrein, J. Allergy, 74: 330-341

Loskutoff, D. J. and Edgington, T. S., 1977, Synthesis of a fibrinolytic activator and inhibitor by endothelial cells, Proc. Nat. Acad. Sci., 74: 3903-3907

Luria, M. H., Johnson, M. W., Pego, R., Seuc, C. A., Manubens, S. J., Wieland, M. R. and Wieland, R. G., 1982, Relationship between sex hormones, myocardial infarction, and occulsive coronary disease, Arch. Int. Med., 142: 42-44

Mannucci, P. M., 1974, Enhancement of plasminogen activator release by vasopressin and adrenaline: A role of cyclic AMP?, Thrombos. Res., 4: 539-549

Mills, E. and Wang, S. C., 1964, Liberation of antidiuretic hormone: Pharmacologic blockade of ascending pathways, Amer. J. Physiol., 207: 1405-1410

Ohela, K., Räsänen, J. A. and Wager, O., 1973, Hereditary angioneurotic edema, Genealogical and immunological studies, Annals of Clinical Res., 5: 174-180

Oh-ishi, S., Uchida, A., Ueno, A. and Katori, M., 1979, Bromelein, a thioprotease from pineapple stem, depletes high molecular weight kininogen by activation of Hageman factor(Factor XII), <u>Thrombos. Res.</u>, 14: 665-672

Osler, W., 1888, Hereditary angioneurotic oedema, <u>Amer. J. Med. Sci.</u>, 95: 362-267

Phillips, G. B., 1978, Sex hormones, risk factors and cardiovascular diseases, <u>Amer. J. Med.</u>, 65: 7-11

Ratnoff, O. D., Pensky, J., Ogston, D. and Naff, G. B., 1969, The inhibition of plasmin, plasma kallikrein, plasma-permeability factor and the C1r subcomponent of the first component of complement by serum C'1 esterase inhibitor, <u>J. Exp. Med.</u>, 129: 315-331

Schapira, M., Silver, L. D., Scott, C. F., Scheier, A. H., Prograis, L. J., Curd, J. G. and Colman, R. W., 1983, Prekallikrein activation and high molecular weight kininogen consumption in hereditary angioedema, <u>New Eng. J. Med.</u>, 308: 1050-1053

Schreiber, A. D., Kaplan, A. P. and Austen, K. F., 1973, Inhibition by C1-INH of Hageman factor fragment activation of coagulation, fibrinolysis and kinin generation, <u>J. Clin. Invest.</u>, 52: 1402-1409

Tsuchiya, M., Suematsu, M., Miura, S. and Nagata, H., 1985, Microcirculatory disturbance in stress condition- a new concept of disseminated intravascular coagulation(DIC) (in Japanese), <u>Seitai no Kagaku</u>, 36: 211-216

Uchida, K., Sakata, T., Funakoshi, F., Koh, H., Kuramochi, M. and Kodama, J., in press, C1-inhibitor and thromboembolic diseases, <u>Jikei Kai Med. J.</u>

Wachtfogel, Y. T., Pixley, R. A., Kucich, U., Abram, W., Weinbaum, G., Schapira, M. and Colman, R. W., 1986, Purified plasma Factor XIIa aggregates human neutrophils and causes degranulation, <u>Blood</u>, 67: 1731-1737

Wiggins, R. C., Loskutoff, D. J., Cochrane, C. G., Griffin, J. H. and Edgington, T. S., 1980, Activation of rabbit Hageman factor by homogenates of cultured rabbit endothelial cells, <u>J. Clin. Invest.</u>, 65: 197-206

Williams, L. T. and Lefkowitz, R. J., 1977, Regulation of rabbit myometrial alpha adrenergic receptors by estrogen and progesterone, <u>J. Clin. Invest.</u>, 60: 815-818

Witzke, G., Bork, K., Benes, P. and Böckers, M., 1983, Hereditary angioneurotic edema and blood coagulation: Interaction between C1-esterase-inhibitor and the activation factors of the proteolytic enzyme system, <u>Klin. Wochenschr.</u>, 61: 1131-1135

EFFECT OF THYROIDECTOMY ON RAT PLASMA T-KININOGEN CONCENTRATION AS DEMONSTRATED BY A NEW AND DIRECT T-KININOGEN RADIOIMMUNOASSAY

Jacob Bouhnik, Françoise Savoie, François Alhenc-Gelas, Thierry Baussant, Francis Gauthier* and Pierre Corvol

INSERM U36, 17, rue du Fer-à-Moulin 75005 Paris, France
* Université F. Rabelais, Lab. Biochimie des Protéines Plasmatiques, 2 bis Bld Tonnelé 37032 Tours Cedex, France

T-kininogen, the third kininogen species has been found up to now only in the rat. Contrary to the two other kininogens, the LMW and the HMW kininogens, it is not a substrate for blood or tissue kallikreins but is for trypsin or cathepsin D which released in vitro Ile-Ser-bradykinin (1). Moreover, its plasma concentration sharply increased after inflammation experimentally induced by different agents, whereas the two other kininogens were unchanged (1, 2).

Previous work has shown that thyroid hormones potentiate and thyroidectomy decreases the inflammatory response of certain connective tissues of the rat to irritating substances (3, 4). Therefore, studies were undertaken to establish the effect of thyroidectomy on the regulation of T-kininogen concentration in the rat.

Male rats of 90 g were surgically thyroparathyroidectomized and given 0.3 % $CaCl_2$ in drinking water throughout the experiments. Blood was collected from the eye with a capillary tube in the presence of sodium citrate. This technique of blood collection is easy and has the advantage of not provoking inflammation and therefore of not interfering with the T-kininogen level contrary to other techniques.

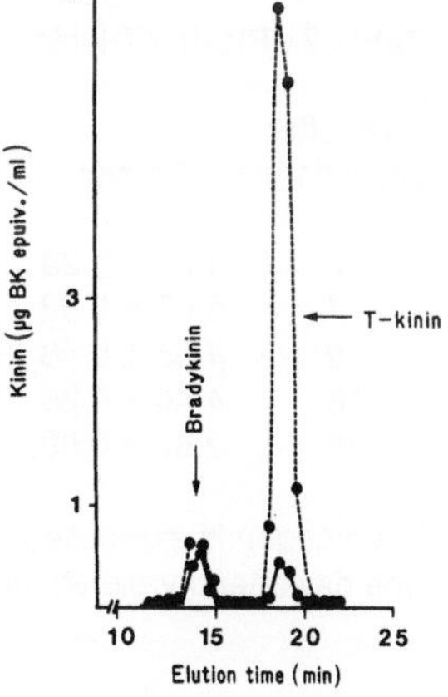

Fig 1 - Reverse phase HPLC of immunoreactive kinins released by trypsin from plasma of normal and turpentine-treated rats. Kinins were measured by RIA using bradykinin as a standard
(●——●) normal plasma (●--●) turpentine treated rat.

T-kininogen was measured by a direct radioimmunoassay that we have developed (2). A good correspondence was obtained between this direct RIA and the T-kinin generating assay. Thus, by direct assay it was found that T-kininogen is increased about 10 fold in rats subcutaneously injected with turpentine, data confirmed by HPLC analysis of the plasma kinins released by trypsin, demonstrating that only T-kinin was increased, bradykinin being unchanged (Fig. 1).

<u>Influence of thyroidectomy on plasma T-kininogen concentration</u>

Two phases were observed after thyroidectomy or sham-operation (Table 1). The first common to thyroidectomized and sham-operated animals was characterized by a significant increase of pasma T-kininogen concentration, about five fold the initial level. Thus, it was not a consequence of the absence of thyroid hormones but an inflammatory reaction due to the surgical operation, that is thyroid ablation or sham-operation. The second phase for the sham-operated animals consisted of a significant decrease of T-kininogen concentration and a return to the normal value from the 16th day to the end of the experiment.

As regards the thyroidectomized rats, the concentration of plasma T-kininogen partially decreased, but from the 9th day to the end, it remained elevated. A simple injection of T3 (10 µg/100 g BW) to thyroidectomized rats decreased significantly T-kininogen concentration from 1.7 nmole/ml plasma to 0.9 nmole.

Table 1 . Effect of thyroidectomy on plasma T-kininogen concentration of the rat

Days after oparation	Control	Sham-operated	Thyroidectomized
0	4.38 ± 0.44	4.38 ± 0.44	4.38 ± 0.44
2	6.25 ± 0.86	20.12 ± 1.93	23.33 ± 1.62
9	3.59 ± 0.34	7.52 ± 1.18	12.02 ± 0.95
16	4.50 ± 0.30	4.80 ± 0.34	11.66 ± 1.61
23	3.54 ± 0.50	4.20 ± 0.32	10.83 ± 0.62
37	4.32 ± 0.50	4.48 ± 0.30	11.96 ± 0.71
51	4.0 ± 0.34	4.95 ± 0.54	16.79 ± 1.16

T-kininogen is expressed in nmole/ml plasma. The values are the mean ± SEM of 7 control, 7 sham-operated and 14 thyroidectomized rats.

When thyroidectomized rats received one day after thyroid ablation a chronic treatment with T3 0.5 µg/100 g BW daily, it was found that from the 9th day after the disappearance of inflammation caused by the operation, T-kininogen concentration was not significantly different from that of the sham-operated animals (Table 2).

Table 2 . Plasma T-kininogen concentration of thyroidectomized rats chronically treated with T3.

Days after oparation	Control	Sham-operated	Thyroidectomized	Thyroidectomized + T3
0	4.21 ± 0.29	4.21 ± 0.29	4.21 ± 0.29	4.21 ± 0.29
1	5.05 ± 0.32	15.66 ± 0.93	18.11 ± 1.54	18.77 ± 0.66
9	4.55 ± 0.48	4.61 ± 0.23	17.32 ± 2.20	5.86 ± 0.62
18	4.46 ± 0.25	4.46 ± 0.41	16.75 ± 1.62	6.38 ± 0.43
26	2.82 ± 0.09	2.95 ± 0.20	13.57 ± 1.20	4.62 ± 0.95

T-kininogen is expressed in nmole/ml plasma. T3, 0.5 µg/100 g BW was administered daily from one day after thyroid ablation. Seven animals were used in each group.

<u>Influence of a laparotomy on plasma T-kininogen concentration in thyroidectomized rats</u>

A single laparotomy in the normal rat caused a significant increase of T-kininogen concentration 4.3 fold the initial level one day after the operation and 5.2 fold at the 6th day (Table 3). In rats thyroidectomized from 7 weeks, T-kininogen concentration increased one day after laparotomy 2.6 fold and 8.2 fold by the 6th day ; this corresponds to a concentration about 25 fold the concentration of non-operated normal control rats (Table 3).

Similar results were observed when the thyroidectomized rats were partially hepatectomized (70%) instead of laparotomized.

Table 3 . Influence of a laparotomy on plasma T-kininogen concentration in normal and thyroidectomized rats.

Days after laparotomy	Control	Control laparotomized	Thyroidectomized laparotomized
0	6.86 ± 0.96	5.68 ± 0.50	17.07 ± 1.18
1	4.46 ± 1.03	24.66 ± 4.18	45.50 ± 6.18
3	5.62 ± 0.75	25.50 ± 2.46	68.93 ± 4.70
6	9.39 ± 0.96	29.50 ± 2.41	140.00 ± 10.75
9	9.21 ± 1.62	20.27 ± 1.55	116.14 ± 12.39
13	5.62 ± 0.45	10.05 ± 1.55	53.29 ± 8.73

T-kininogen is expressed in nmole/ml plasma. The values are the mean ± SEM of 4 controls, 7 control laparotomized and 5 thyroidectomized laparotomized rats.

Influence of thyroidectomy on T-kininogen synthesis by liver slices

Liver slices from normal and thyroidectomized rats were incubated with krebs-Ringer bicarbonate in an atmosphere of 95% O_2, 5% CO_2. It was found that all were increased by thyroidectomy. The release of T-kinininogen in the medium during the two preincubations 2.8 fold, the synthesis of T-kininogen during the 2 h incubation, about 80 % and also the T-kininogen content of the liver homogenate, 3.5 fold (Table 4).

Table 4 . Liver content and biosynthesis of T-kininogen by rat liver slices

	Liver homogenate pmole/g tissue		Incubation medium release p mol/g tissue		
	before incubation	after incubation	R_1	R_2	I
Control	66.7 ± 9.6	68.8 ± 12.0	25.0 ± 2.8	13.3 ± 1.6	47.5 ± 5.4
Thyroidectomized	238.4 ± 55.0	185.0 ± 33.8	64.5 ± 11.3	32.0 ± 11.3	85.3 ± 12.3

Liver slices were preincubated (R_1 and R_2) twice for 15 min. each time and then incubated for 2 h (I). The data are presented as mean ± SEM. Seven animals were used in each group.

Effect of thyroidectomy on the clearance of T-kininogen

T-kininogen was iodinated in the presence of chloramine T with ^{125}I and injected in the jugular vein of normal and thyroidectomized rats. Blood was collected at different times from 5 min. to 24 h after administration of the labeled protein. Clearance data were fitted to a two compartment model. Compartment 1 represented the initial rapid phase from 5 to 60 min. and compartment 2, the second slower phase of clearance for 1 h to 24 h. It appeared that during the first h, corresponding to the repartition of the labeled T-kininogen in the organism, no significant difference was observed between normal and thyroidectomized animals. In the 2nd compartment, between 1 and 24 h, the clearance of T-kininogen was slowed 20 % by thyroidectomy (Table 5).

Table 5 . Clearance of ^{125}I-T-kininogen in normal and thyroidectomized rats.

	Plasma half-life (min ± SEM)	
	Normal	Thyroidectomized
Compartment 1	75 ± 12	80 ± 5
Compartment 2	299 ± 9	356 ± 7

CONCLUSION

Thyroidectomy decreases slightly the turnover rate of T-kininogen. This is in good agreement with the well known effect of thyroid hormones on the catabolism of proteins (5). The increase of the T-kininogen synthesis after thyroidectomy is not a usual effect. However it is not a unique case. A similar effect was reported upon fibrinogen (6). T-kininogen and fibrinogen belong to a particular class of proteins, the acute phase proteins. However, T-kininogen being a cysteine proteinase inhibitor (7), its increase after thyroidectomy can explain previous work indicating that thyroidectomy decreases the inflammatory response (3,4). It is also possible that at the same time, the increase of T-kininogen would supply more T-kinin which would act, as bradykinin, at the level of peripheral vessels facilitating the migration into tissues of phagocytes, for the repair of damaged tissues.

REFERENCES

1 - H. Okamoto and L.M. Greenbaum. Kininogen substrates for trypsin and cathepsin D in human, rabbit and rat plasmas. Life Sci. 32: 2007 (1983).

2 - J. Bouhnik, T. Baussant, F. Savoie, F. Alhenc-Gelas, F. Gauthier and F. Esnard. Direct radioimmunoassay for rat T-kininogen. Biochem. Biophys. Res. Commun. 144: 1090 (1987).

3 - P. Spencer abd G.B. West. Further observations on the relationship between the thyroid gland and the anaphylactoid reaction in rats. Int. Arch. Allergy Appl. Immunol. 20: 321 (1962).

4 - B. Steinetz and G. Di Pasquale. Anti-granuloma and anti-edema properties of corticosterone in hyper and hypothyroid rats. Proc. Soc. Exp. Biol. Med. 125: 673 (1967).

5 - F.L. Hoch. Metabolic effect of thyroid hormones in Handbook of Physiology. Greer MA and Solomon D.H. (eds) American Physiol. Soc. 3: 391 (1974).

6 - C.D. Legrèle, J.M. Felix and R. Jacquot. Effect of thyroid hormones on post natal fibrinogen levels in the rat. Biol. Neonate 46: 61 (1984).

7 - F.Esnard and F. Gauthier. Rat α_1-cysteine proteinase inhibitor. An acute phase reactant identical with α_1 acute phase globulin. J. Biol. Chem. 258: 12443 (1983).

THE PECULIAR T-KININASE ACTIVITY OF RAT MAST CELL CHYMASE

F. Gauthier, T. Moreau, N. Gutman, D. Faucher*, T. Baussant**,
and F. Alhenc-Gelas**

Université François Rabelais,Laboratoire de Biochimie
Faculté de Médecine, F 37032 Tours. * Rhone-Poulenc Santé
F-37260 Monts. ** INSERM U 36, 17, rue du Fer à Moulin
F-75005 Paris

INTRODUCTION

Among the potential functions of kininogens are those of kinin
precursor, lysosomal cysteine proteinase inhibitor, calpain inhibitor
and coagulation initiator (1, 2). With the noteworthy exception of rat T
kininogen which is a typical acute phase reactant all other kininogen
species of low (L) or high (H) Mr reported so far do not respond to an
inflammatory challenge by changing their rate of synthesis.

Possibly related to this behaviour during inflammation, potential
functions of T genes products seem to differ significantly from those of
L and H kininogen so that the major if not unique physiological function
of T kininogen could be that of lysosomal cysteine proteinase inhibitor
(3). A possible kininogenic function for rat T kininogen is still
debated however (4 - 6), though no enzyme working in catalytic amount
has been described so far to be able to specifically release T kinin
from its precursor as would do plasma or tissue kallikreins from L or H
kininogens. The poor involvment of T kininogen as a kinin precursor has
been also demonstrated by Damas et al.(7) and Oh-Ishi et al.(8)
working on L and H kininogen deficient rats .It remains however that
local production of T kinin during the response to specific but still
not well defined stimuli cannot be excluded.

Human mast cells have been reported to release a kininogenase
activity upon degranulation during the allergic response to an IgE
mediated stimulus which in turns allows the local production of vasoactive kinins (9). On the other hand recent experiments in the rat have
shown that mast cell chymase is involved at an early step in the process
of degranulation (10).

The fate of chymase after degranulation is not yet well understood.
Its potent proteolytic activity allows the liberation from IgG$_1$ of
peptides with chemotactic activity emphasizing its function as a
mediator of inflammation (11). Besides, preliminary experiments in our
laboratory have shown that mast cell chymase was able to induce rapid
fragmentation of T kininogen with a possible modification of its
properties in a place and at a time it may be supposed to act in vivo.

The nature of this fragmentation and its consequences on the potential
function of T kininogen have been analysed in this study which reinforce
the hypothesis that the kinin precursor function of this kininogen is of
negligible physiological importance.

MATERIAL AND METHODS

- T kininogen and H kininogen were purified as described previously
(12, 13)
- Mast cell chymase was purified mostly as reported by Kido et al.
(14) using rat peritoneal cells as starting material. Aliquots of crude
supernatant and precipitate obtained after the 27,000 g centrifugation
step were saved to control their proteolytic activity and their
kininogenase activity on purified T kininogen. Purified chymase was
stored at $-70°C$ in 80 mM potassium phosphate buffer pH 8.0, 5 % (w/v)
ammonium sulfate.
- Chymase titration was made mixing constant amounts of protease with
increasing (0.78 to 3.9 µM final) amounts of chymostatin in 80 mM
potassium phosphate buffer pH 8.0 and using 2.5 µM Suc-Leu-Leu-Val-Tyr-
NMec as a substrate. The method was as described elsewhere (15).
- Kinin liberation from T and H kininogens was measured by radioimmunoassay (16) using either chymase, tissue kallikrein or trypsin as well
as crude fractions from the chymase purification procedure as potential
kininogenases and experimental conditions were as described before (15).
- Proteolytic activity of chymase on T kininogen was followed by SDS
polyacrylamide gel electrophoresis under reducing conditions. Chymase/T
kininogen molar ratio varied between 0.015 and 0.6 and incubation was
made for 10 min at 37°C in the chymase conservation buffer before adding
the reduction buffer.
- Proteolytic peptides issuing from partial chymase hydrolysis were
purified by FPLC on Superose 12 then by HPLC on an Aquapore butyl
reverse phase column eluted at 1 ml/min for 30 min with a linear
gradient of 0 - 60% (v/v) acetonitrile in 0.07 % (v/v) trifluoroacetic
acid. Eluted samples (about 500 pmol) were used for sequence analysis on
an Applied Biosystems 477A protein sequencer and identification of PTH
derivatives was performed using an on line associated Model 120A
analyzer. Alternatively , N terminal sequences were determined from
samples electro blotted onto activated glass fiber paper after SDS
p.a.g.e. according to the method of Aebersold et al. (17).

RESULTS AND DISCUSSION

In previous attempts to study the kinin precursor function of rat T
kininogen we have investigated the properties of trypsin (18) and rat
submaxillary gland endopeptidase k (15); both of them are able to
release T kinin but only when reacted in stoichiometric amounts with T
kininogen. Such conditions induced at the same time a large proteolysis
of the precursor which gives rise in any case to potent inhibitory
peptides towards lysosomal cysteine proteinases. These peptides are
released much more easily than immunoreactive kinins and could be of
greater biological significance. However the peculiar feature of T
kininogen as an acute phase reactant could also result in a limited
expression of its potential kinin precursor function particularly at
inflammatory sites where it was shown to accumulate in response to acute
phase conditions (not published results).

Mast cells are involved in the response to inflammatory stimuli
(11) and their activation depend on the activity of chymase which is the
major protease in these cells. The interaction of T kininogen with mast

cell chymase, which could be a phenomenon of biological relevance
during inflammation, was studied as a prerequisite to a search for a
specific T kininogenase activity in these cells.

After purification on octyl-Sepharose and titration by chymostatin,
chymase was incubated with T kininogen as reported under Methods and
samples were analysed by electrophoresis on SDS gels after reduction to
follow proteolysis, and on the other hand, were assayed for their kinin
content. As shown on fig. 1 catalytic amounts of chymase are able to
cleave T kininogen giving rise first to a 62 kD fragment which is
further split into two main fragments of 43 kD and 20 kD when the amount
of chymase is slightly increased. Under these conditions and even after
stoichiometric amounts of chymase were incubated with T kininogen, no
liberation of immunoreactive kinin was observed confirming that chymase
is not a kininogenase. Parallel experiments carried out with crude
extracts of freeze-thawed peritoneal cells after centrifugation revealed
an almost identical electrophoretic pattern and showed that no kinin was
released whatever the experimental conditions used and the sample
tested.

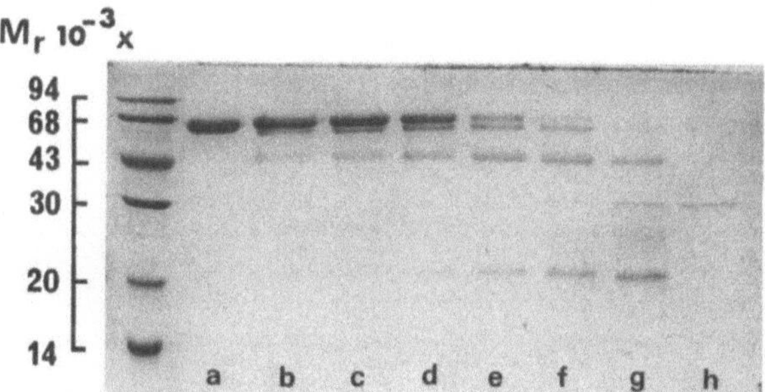

Fig. 1. Proteolysis of the kininogen by mast cell chymase. T kininogen
        (20 µM final) was incubated for 10 min at 37°C with increasing
        amounts of chymase to obtain enzyme/T kininogen molar ratio of
        (a) 0, (b) 0.015, (c) 0.030, (d) 0.06, (e) 0.15, (f) 0.3, (g)
        0.6. Reaction was stopped by heating in reducing buffer and
        samples were analysed by SDS mini gel electrophoresis. Each
        sample contains about 1 µg of T kininogen. Purified chymase
        appears in (h) as a single band of 30,000 kD. Mr markers were
        from Pharmacia.

More surprising was the fact that after chymasetreatment, trypsin
was no more able to release any immunoreactive kinin from T kininogen
though this protease is well known to release T kinin from its precursor
when added in sufficient amount (18).

Hypothesis was therefore put forward that chymase was able to cleave
a peptide bond in the kinin sequence destroying its immunoreactivity.
Control experiments were carried out under the same experimental conditions and using either trypsin treated T kininogen which has released T
kinin or purified bradykinin and T kinin as substrates. Curiously
enough, no significant loss of the immunoreactivity of these peptides
was obtained suggesting that they were resistant to chymase hydrolysis.
This agrees with the results reported by Le Trong et al. (19) who
mentioned the high resistance of bradykinin to chymase hydrolysis.

Bradykinin hydrolysis by chymase may be obtained however after
prolonged time of incubation (20). Further experiments were then carried
out using rat high Mr kininogen treated by chymase under the same conditions as above then by tissue kallikrein which releases bradykinin from
this kininogen. Chymase was still unable to release bradykinin but
complete liberation was obtained in the presence of the kininogenase.
The specificity of chymase as a kininase appeared therefore to depend on
the way the kinin is included and exposed in its precursor.

Cleavage sites of T kininogen by chymase were therefore identified by
determining N terminal amino acid sequences of proteolytic fragments
obtained at different times of incubation or at different enzyme concentrations. Results are shown on fig. 2 which indicate that the initial
cleavage site of T kininogen is located in the bradykinin sequence
involving residue Phe 367 of the precursor. This site of cleavage is
identical with that of kininase I reacting with free kinin (21) which
leads to a loss of the C terminal amino acid of T kinin destroying
almost completely its immunoreactivity (16) as well as the biological
function normally devoted to kinins once liberated from the precursor
(21).

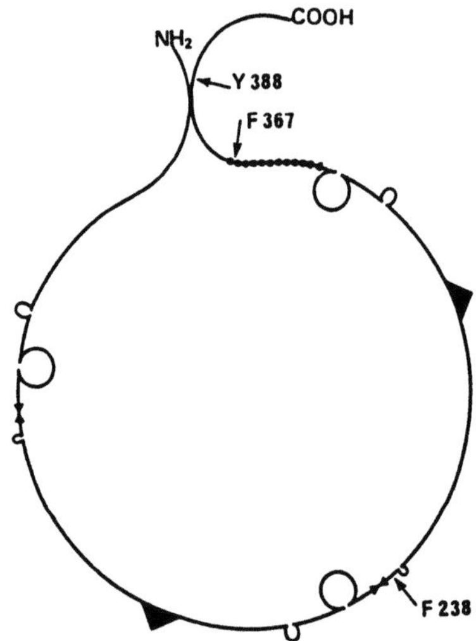

Fig. 2. Representation of the preferential cleavage sites of T kininogen
        by mast cell chymase. Initial cleavages occur at Phe 367 and Tyr
        388 which results in the inactivation of T kinin prior to its
        eventual liberation from the precursor. Cleavage at Phe 238
        allows the liberation of two peptides which retain strong
        inhibitory activity towards cathepsin L.↘corresponds to the
        bradykinin sequence, ▲ indicates the QVVAG sequence which is
        supposed to be involved in the inhibitory site and circles
        represent the putative disulfide loops. The three cystatin like
        domains of the heavy chain are delineated by arrows.

Cleavage at residue Tyr 388 of the light chain also occurs very
rapidly as soon as catalytic amount of chymase are reacted with T
kininogen which explains that no fragment of 6 kD is observed together
with the 62 kD fragment after SDS page analysis as shown on fig. 1.

The third very susceptible peptidic bond which is hydrolysed by
chymase though not so easily as the two former is located after Phe 238
i.e. close to the junction between cystatin like domains two and three.

From this hydrolysis two fragments are liberated corresponding to cystatin like domains 1 + 2 and domain 3 which means that both include one canonical QVVAG sequence which is a part of the inhibitory site. In complete agreement with this result, we found that these two peptides retain strong inhibitory activity towards rat lysosomal cathepsin L and papain (not shown).

From these results it appears that rat mast cell chymase possesses a kininase activity exerting preferentially on T kininogen since neither free kinins nor H kininogen seem to be susceptible to this hydrolysis. In case a T kininogenase is liberated at an inflammatory site, this peculiar kinase activity would provide an additional mean of regulation of the kinin system avoiding large amounts of T kinin to be liberated from T kininogen which is by far the most important kinin reservoir in the rat especially during the acute phase response, without affecting the activity of free kinins and the function of other kinin delivering systems.

ACKNOWLEDGEMENTS : This work was supported by a grant from INSERM (CRE n° 865006). Thanks are due to B. Cérélis for secretarial assistance.

REFERENCES

1. Müller-Esterl, W., Iwanaga, S. and Nakanishi, S., Kininogens revisited, Trends Biochem. Sci., 11, 336-339, (1986).
2. Sasaki, M., Taniguchi, K., Suzuki, K. and Imahori, K., Human plasma α_1- and α_2-thiol proteinase inhibitors strongly inhibit Ca activated neutral protease from muscle, Biochem. Biophys. Res. Commun. 110, 256-261, (1983).
3. Gauthier, F., Gutman, N., Moreau, T. and El Moujahed, A. Possible relationship between the restricted biological function of rat T kininogen (thiostatin) and its behaviour as an acute phase reactant, Biol. Chem. Hoppe Seyler (1987), in press.
4. Barlas, A., Sugio, K. and Greenbaum, L.M., Release of T-kinin and bradykinin in carrageenin induced inflammation in the rat. FEBS Lett., 190, 268-270, (1985).
5. Barlas, A., Gao, X. and Greenbaum, L.M., Isolation of a thiol-activated T-kininogenase from the rat submandibular gland. FEBS Lett., 218, 266-270, (1987).
6. Sakamoto, W., Satoh, F., Gotoh, K. and Uehara, S., Ile-Ser-bradykinin (T-kinin) and Met-Ile-Ser-bradykinin (Met-T-kinin) are released from T-kininogen by an acid proteinase of granulomatous tissues in rats. FEBS Lett., 219, 437-440, (1987).
7. Damas, J., Remacle-Volon, G. and Adam, A.,Inflammation in the rat paw due to urate crystals. Involvement of the kinin system. Naunyn-Schmiedberg's Arch. Pharmacol., 325, 76-79, (1984).
8. Oh-Ishi, S., Hayashi, I., Hayashi, M., Yamakisu, A., Nakano, T. Utsunomiya, Nagashima, Y., Evidence for a role of the plasma kallikrein-kinin system in acute inflammation : reduced exudation during carrageenin-and kaolin-pleurisies in kininogen-deficient rats. Agents Actions, 18, 450-454, (1986).
9. Proud, D., Macglashan, D.W., Newball, H.H., Schulman, E.S. and Lichtenstein, L.M., Immunoglobulin E-mediated release of a kininogenase from purified human lung mast cells. Am. Rev. Respir. Dis., 132, 405-408, (1985).
10. Kido, H., Fukusen, N. and Katunuma, N., Antibody and inhibitor of chymase inhibitit histamine release in immunoglobulin E-activated mast cells. Biochem. Intern., 10, 863-871, (1985).

11. Katunuma, N., Fukusen, N. and Kido, H., Biological functions of serine proteases in the granules of rat mast cells. <u>Adv. Enzyme Regul.</u>, 25, 241-255, (1986).

12. Gauthier, F., Moreau, T. and Esnard, F., Rat T kininogen : an acute phase reactant and a potent inhibitor of cysteine proteinases which could be a kinin precursor. <u>Ciênc. Biol.(Portugal</u>), 11, 93-99, (1986).

13. Reis, M.L., Alhenc-Gelas, F., Alhenc-Gelas, M., Allegrini, J., Kerbiriou-Nabias, D., Corvol, P. and Menard, J., Rat high-molecular-weight kininogen : purification, production of antibodies and demonstration of lack of immunoreactive kininogen in a strain of Brown Norways rats. <u>Biochim. Biophys. Acta</u>, 831, 106-113, (1985).

14. Kido, H., Fukusen, N. and Katunuma, N., A simple method for purification of chymase from rat tongue and rat peritoneal cells. <u>Anal. Biochem.</u>, 137, 449-453, (1984).

15. Gutman, N., Moreau, T., Alhenc-Gelas, F., Baussant, T., El Moujahed, A., Akpona, S. and Gauthier, F., T kinin release from T kininogen by rat submaxillary gland endopeptidase k. <u>Eur. J. Biochem.</u>, (1987) in press.

16. Alhenc-Gelas, F., Marchetti, J., Allegrini, J., Corvol, P. and Menard, J., Measurement of urinary kallikrein activity species differences in kinin production. <u>Biochim. Biophys. Acta</u>, 677, 477-488, (1981).

17. Aebersold, R.H., Tylow, D.B., Hood, L.E. and Kent, S.B.H., Electroblotting onto activated glass. <u>J. Biol. Chem.</u>, 261, 4229-4238, (1986).

18. Moreau, T., Gutman, N., El Moujahed, A., Esnard, F. and Gauthier, F., Relationship between the cysteine proteinase-inhibitory function of rat T kininogen and the release of immunoreactive kinin upon trypsin treatment. <u>Eur. J. Biochem.</u>, 159, 341-346, (1986).

19. Le Trong, H., Neurath, H. and Woodbury, R.G., Substrate specificity of the chymotrypsin-like protease in secretory granules isolated from rat mast cells. <u>Proc. Natl. Acad. Sci. USA</u>, 84, 364-367, (1987).

20. Reilly, C.F., Schechter, N.B. and Travis, J., Inactivation of bradykinin and kallidin by cathepsin G and mast cell chymase. <u>Biochem. Biophys. Res. Commun.</u>, 127, 443-449, (1985).

21. Marceau, F., Lussier, A., Regoli, D. and Giroud, J.P., Pharmacology of kinins : their relevance to tissue injury and inflammation. <u>Gen. Pharmac.</u>, 14, 209-229, (1983).

KININ FORMATION FROM T-KININOGEN

BY SPLEEN ACID KININOGENASES

Keiko Yamafuji and Yoshiko Matsuki

Department of Food and Nutrition
Nakamura Gakuen College
Fukuoka, Japan

INTRODUCTION

We have reported the formation of kinins from rat plasma by spleen acid kininogenases[1] and showed that the acid kininogenases were also found in the lymphocyte derived from rat thymus[2]. In this paper, we will inform the findings that the T-kininogen[3,4] is the major precursor of the kinins formed by the actions of spleen enzymes and that the kinin forming reactions were highly potentiated by the coexistence of thiol compound.

MATERIALS AND METHODS

HMW-kininogen and T-kininogen were the generous gift by Dr.Hisao Kato and Mr.Kei-ichi Enjyoji of National Cardiovascular Center,Research Institute. Synthetic kinins and peptidylMCA were the products of Protein Research Foundation, Osaka. DEAE-Sephadex A-50 and Sephadex G-100 were obtained from Pharmacia Fine Chemicals. The reagents used in SDS-PAGE were purchased from Bio-Rad Laboratories. The other Chemicals used were of the highest grade available.

Preparation of the Enzymes

108g(from 160 rats)of frozen spleen was homogenized in 216ml of ice cold 1mM EDTA. The homogenate was then stirred for 6hrs bringing pH to 3.6 with occasional addition of diluted sulfuric acid. The clear acid extract obtained by centrifugation of homogenate was subjected to ammonium sulfate fractionation. The protein precipitated by the addition of ammonium sulfate to make 70% saturation from the supernatant of 40% saturation was centrifuged and taken up into small amount of water and dialyzed against the elution buffer of gel filtration with three changes in an ice box. Resulting protein (230mg) solution was applied on Sephadex G-100 column(3x90cm) and eluted with 0.9% NaCl containing 1mM EDTA. Kinin forming activity and peptidylMCA hydrolyzing activity were assayed as described in next paragraph. The fractions which showed the kinin formation were divided into two groups; A: partially SH dependent, B: totally SH dependent. The protein were precipitated from each combined fraction by addition of ammonium sulfate.

Abbreviations; MCA:4-methyl-coumaryl-7-amide, U:A_{280}xVolume(ml),2-ME:2-mercaptoethanol,DTT:dithiothreitol, GSH:glutathione.

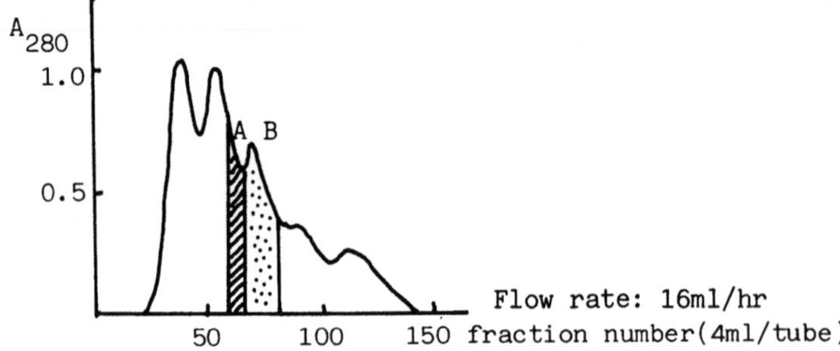

Fig. 1. Gel filtration of rat spleen 40~70 SAS fraction
on Sephadex G-100

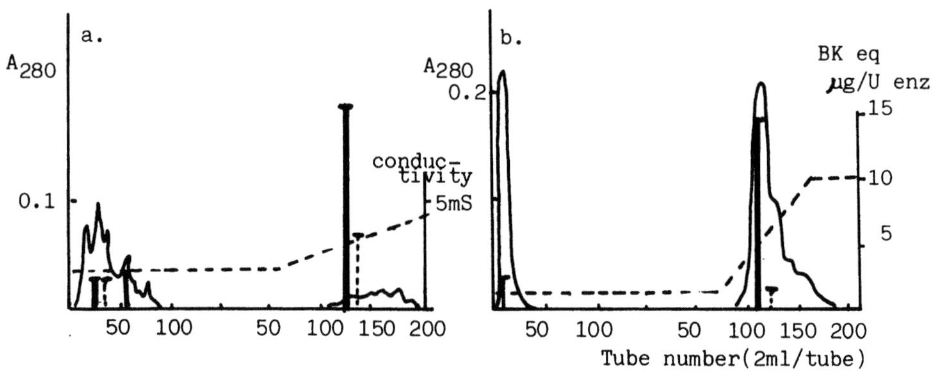

Fig. 2. DEAE-Sephadex A-50 column chromatography of kininogenase fraction
a;Sample A, flow rate 5ml/hr, b; Sample B, flow rate 4ml/hr

The precipitate was then centrifuged,dissolved and dialyzed against the
starting buffer of next chromatography. Thus obtained solution of A(16.6mg)
and B(16.0mg) were applied successively on DEAE-Sephadex A-50 (2x40cm) column
equilibrated with 0.01M phosphate buffer(pH6.0) containing 0.1M or 0.02M
NaCl. Isocratic elution was performed with equilibrium buffer followed by
the linear gradient elution from equilibrium buffer to the same buffer
containing 0.5M NaCl. Purity and the molecular weight of each fraction were
checked by SDS-PAGE using MINIPROTEAN apparatus provided by Bio-Rad Lab.

Enzyme Assay

In general, for the detection of kinin formed, enzyme preparation(0.01U
to 0.02U) was incubated with kininogen(0.1U to 0.2U) in the presence of 40mM
2-ME in 0.1M acetate buffer(pH 4.0) for 2 hours at 37°C. Neutralized, boiled
and centrifuged supernatant was assayed on isolated rat uterus. The effect
on blood pressure was measured by injecting the samples intravenously to male
Wister rat weighing 250g. The hydrolysis of peptidylMCA was measured as the
emission intensity of fluorescence(exitation 380nm,emission 460nm) due to the
formation of 7-amino-4-methylcoumarin according to the method described for
cathepsin B[5] with slight modification of replacing cysteine by DTT. The
reaction products of T-kininogen with the enzymes were analyzed by means of
reverse phase HPLC in use of Waters 600 system equipped with TSK 120A column
Isocratic elution was performed with the phosphate buffer composed of 17%
acetonitrile, 0.25M Na_2SO_4, 0.01M KH_2PO_4 and 0.2% phosphoric acid[6] at the
flow rate of 1ml/min.

Table 1. Kinin formation and substrate hydrolysis by the fractions from
DEAE-Sephadex A-50 Chromatography

Tube number		BK eq from T-KNG		BK eq from HMW-KNG		AMC nmole/U enz	
		ng/200μl	μg/U enz	ng/200μl	μg/U enz	ZPheArgMCA	BzArgMCA
A-I- 21∼30	-SH	5.7	1.6	ND	ND	ND	ND
	+SH	24.0	6.9	1.9	0.6	249	4
A-I- 31∼35	-SH	18.6	4.4	ND	ND	ND	ND
	+SH	46.2	10.9	ND	ND	249	4
A-I- 36∼40	-SH	16.8	6.0	ND	ND	ND	ND
	+SH	21.6	7.7	ND	ND	557	ND
A-G-126∼138	-SH	22.3	15.9	ND	ND	ND	ND
	+SH	66.0	47.1	ND	ND	242	ND
B-I- 6∼10	-SH						
	+SH	40.0	3.8	ND	ND	25	22.7
B-I- 9	-SH	5.7	0.6	ND	ND		
	+SH	56.4	5.1	ND	ND		
B-G- 96∼118	-SH						
	+SH	560	29.5			410	0.6
B-G- 116	-SH	18.5	1.8	ND	ND		
	+SH	144	13.8	10.5	1.0		
B-G-119∼142	-SH						
	+SH	800	42.7			576	0.8

+SH means 40mM of 2-ME for kinin formation and 2mM of DTT for MCA release.

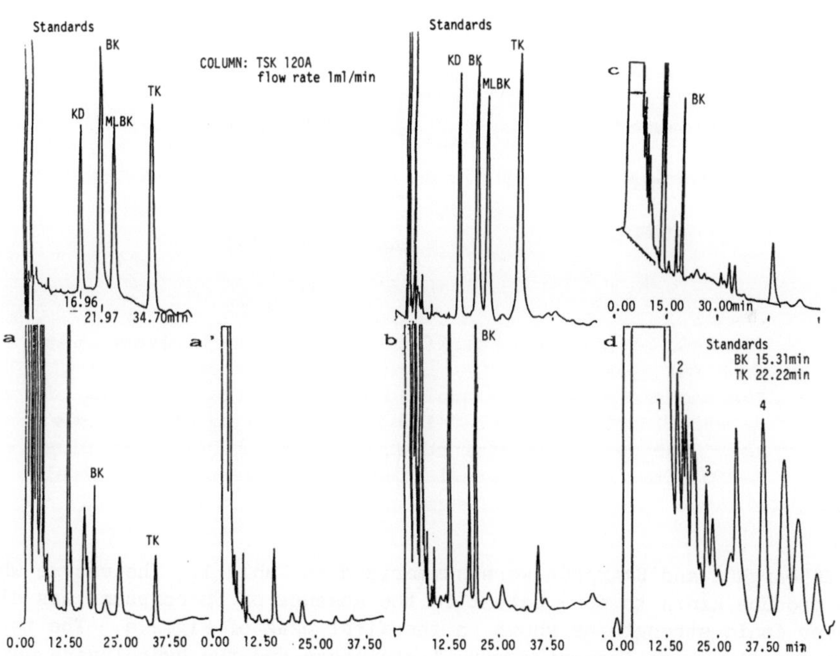

Fig. 3. HPLC of T-kininogen hydrolysate. The enzymes used are a: A-I-126∼
138 with SH, a':without SH, b: B-I-9 with SH, c: B-I-116 with SH
and d: B-96∼118 with SH.

RESULTS AND DISCUSSION

The kinin forming activity was found in the fractions A and B patterned
in the chromatogram of Sephadex G-100 as can be seen in Fig.1. The chromato-
grams of DEAE-Sephadex A-50 of these A and B were shown in Fig.2. a. and b.
respectively. The amounts of kinin formed and the amounts of AMC released

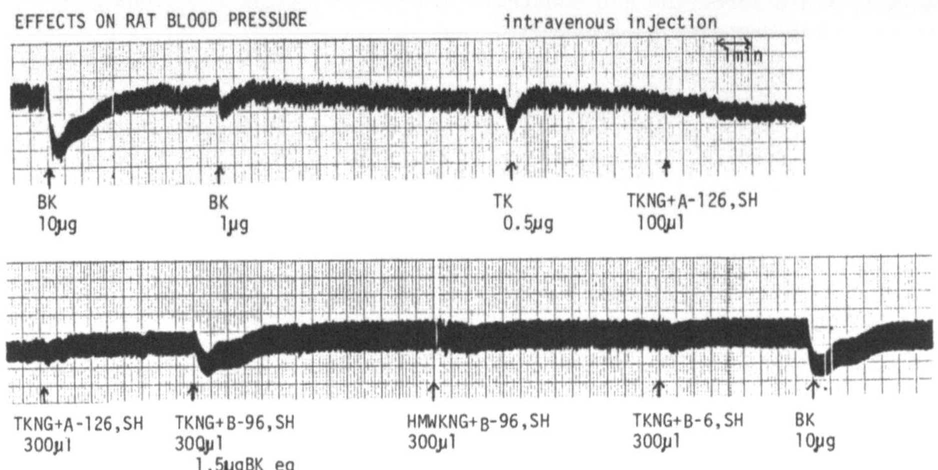

Fig. 4. Effect of T-kininogen hydrolysate on rat blood pressure

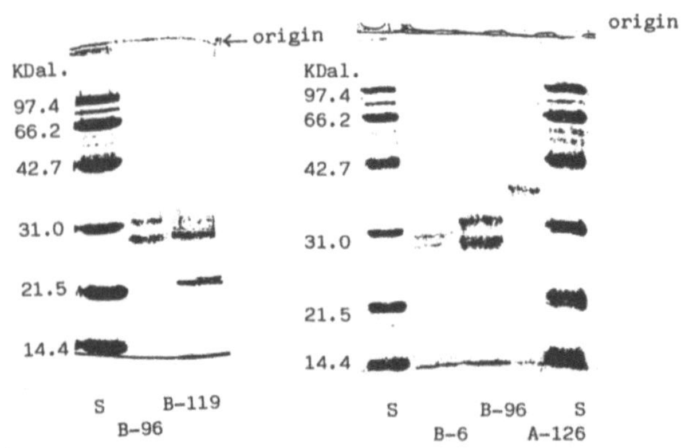

Fig. 5. SDS-PAGE of partially purified SH dependent kininogenases
from rat spleen
The amounts of samples applied were as follows; 2.9 μg of
B-G-96~118, 2.9 μg of B-G-119~142 and 1.2 μg of A-G-126~
138. The gels were stained with Coomassie Brilliant Blue
R-250 after electrophoresis for two hours with 12.5mA/gel.

from ZPheArgMCA and BzArgMCA were summarized in Table 1. The enzyme which
could produce kinin to some extent in the absence of SH compound was eluted
at lower ionic strength as shown in the first peak of Fig.2.a. The three
single fraction were incubated with T-kininogen and the hydrolysate were
examined by HPLC as shown in Fig.3.a,b.and c. The formation of T-kinin was
shown in a and b, though small the amount was. While,T-kinin could not be
identified in c. When the fractions from the peak including No.116 of c.
were combined, concentrated and incubated in the same way except the enzyme
unit used(twice much), the HPLC of the hydrolysate showed far more complicated pattern as shown in d. Among the peaks appeared in d, marked four
peaks(numbered 1 to 4) were detected to have uterus contracting activity.
The active peak 2 seemed to correspond to bradykinin and peak 3 to T-kinin
leaving peak 1 and 4 to be identified. The chromatogram c showed that the
single fraction 116 produced peak 2(BK) and peak 4. Peak 4 may provably be
attributed to MetIleSer-Bradykinin considering the sequence of T-kininogen[7]
and the retention time[8]. The DEAE-Sephadex A-50 fractions following B-118

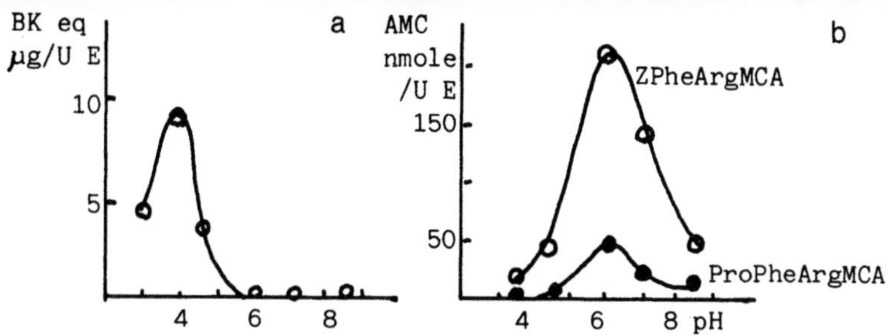

Fig. 6. pH activity curve:
    a. For kinin formation; 50ml of heated plasma was incubated
       with 0.025U of enzyme at the existence of 40mM 2-ME.
    b. For the hydrolysis of peptidylMCA; 10µU of enzyme was
       added to 1ml of 5µM substrate containing 2mM DTT.

Table 2. Hydrolysis of peptidylMCA by B-G-96~118

Substrate	AMC released nmole/U enz/10min	Substrate	AMC released nmole/U enz/10min
ZPheArgMCA	410	SucGluProLeuGluProMCA	2
BocValLeuLysMCA	218	BocLeuSerThrArgMCA	2
ProPheArgMCA	56	GltGlyArgMCA	2
BocIleGluGlyArgMCA	21	BocGluLysLysMCA	1
BocPheSerArgMCA	9	SucAlaAlaProPheMCA	1
BocValProArgMCA	5	BzArgMCA	1
BocLeuGlyArgMCA	3	LeuMCA	0
SucAlaProAlaMCA	2		

0.005U of enzyme was used in 1ml of reaction mixture. Concentration of
substrate was 5µM in 0.1M phosphate(pH6.0) containing 2mM of DTT.

Table 3. The effects of SH compounds on the reaction catalyzed by B-G-96~118

SH compound	Kinin formation from plasma (µg BK eq/U enz)		AMC release from peptidylMCA (nmole AMC/U enz)	
	pH 3.0	pH 4.0	ZPheArgMCA	ProPheArgMCA
2-Mercaptoethanol	4.5	3.2	6	9
Dithiothreitol	17.2	9.6	411	73
Cysteine	ND	8.1	191	47
Glutathione	3.0	9.6	11	7
none	ND	2.0	ND	ND

The concentrations of the SH compounds were as follows; 2-ME, Cys and GSH
were 40mM and DTT was 20 mM for kinin forming reaction, and all were 2mM
for the hydrolysis of synthetic substrates.

were also combined and incubated with T-kininogen. Hydrolysate of this
reaction showed even more production of kinin as listed at the bottom of
Table 1(B-G-119~142). When the HPLC analysis was performed, the same set
of four active peptides as Fig.3.d. were detected but in different hight of
peaks. In Fig. 5, SDS-PAGE showed that B-G-96~118 consists of two proteins
of 28K and 32K dalton, while B-G-119~142 consist of 28K and 22K proteins.
From the results described , it is provable to conclude that 28K protein is
the enzyme which is responsible to the release of kinins. As for
the contribution of 32K or 22K enzyme in the formation of T-kinin, we can

not deduce any firm conclusion yet. As can be seen in Fig.5, A-G-126~138
are fairly pure revealing only on band of 38K. Although this protein which
is pure and T-kinin forming attracts the attention, we will stay with the
dominant and most active protein: B-G-96~118, in this paper. When B-96~118
(0.038U) was incubated with 0.25U of T-kininogne, the amount of kinin formed
was calculated to be 0.94µg in total incubation mixture (300µl) from uterus
assay. The same sample mounted to 1.5µg when estimated from blood pressure
assay as was shown in Fig.4. This observation coincide with the fact that
the peptides longer than bradykinin were released into the hydrolysate.

To look into the substrate specificity of this potent protein, we
examined the reactions on several peptidylMCAs. The results were listed in
Table 2. The most susceptible peptide among those tested was ZPheArgMCA,the
typical substrate of plasma kallikrein[9] and the second place was BocValLeu-
LysMCA, the substrate of plasmin[10]. Considering the persistence of other
plasmin substrates such as BocGluLysLysMCA, it is eventually suggested that
hydrophobic amino acid at P_2 and P_3 site are essential for the attack by 28K
enzyme.

The effects of pH on the kinin forming reaction or on the hydrolysis
of peptidylMCA were investigated. Fig.6 shows the optimum pH of 4.0 and
6.0 for kinin formation and substrate hydrolysis, respectively.

In examining the mode of activation by SH compounds, DTT was recognized
to be the most effective activator as can be seen in Table 3. However, it
seems more important that cysteine or glutathione could positively activate
kinin forming reaction at pH 4.5, since this fact will make it acceptable
to consider the regulation of kinin level by circulating SH compounds in
physiological and pathological conditions.

The separation of the enzymes are now at the last stage. The differen-
tiation or identification of acid kininogenases from or with SH dependent
cathepsins are the urgent problems to be solved.

ACKNOWLEDGEMENT

Authors express their sincere thanks to Dr.hisao Kato and Mr.Kei-ichi
Enjyoji for the generous gifts of kininogens and the most helpful advices
and also to Dr.Masayasu Inoue and Dr.Nobukazu Watanabe of Kumamoto Univ.
for their kind help in measuring rat blood pressure.

REFFERENCES

1)K.Yamafuji, _Seikagaku_,58:629 (1986)
2)M.Watanabe,and K.Yamafuji, _Adv.Exp.Med.Biol._,198 PtA:19 (1986)
3)H.Okamoto,and L.M.Greenbaum, _Biochem.Biophys.Res.Commun._,112:702 (1983)
4)I.Hayashi, T.Ino, H.Kato, S. Iwanaga,T.Nakano,and S.Oh-ishi,
   Thromb.Res.,36:509 (1984)
5)A.J.Barrett, _Biochem.J._, 187:909 (1980)
6)A.Okamura, Y.Yasuhara,and T.Nakajima, _IYOUKIZAI Institute Report_,
   16:131 (1982)
7)S.F.Kato, A.Matsumoto, N. Kitamura,and S. Nakanishi, _J.Biol.Chem._,
   260:12054 (1985)
8)W.Sakamoto, A.Yokoyama, F.Sato, and S.Nagasawa, _Seikagaku_, 59:665 (1987)
9)T.Morita, h.Kato, S.Iwanaga, K.Takada, T.Kimura, and S. Sakakibara,
   J.Biochem.,82:1495 (1977)
10)H.Kato, N.Adachi, Y.Ohno, S.Iwanaga, K.Takada, and S.Sakakibara,
   J.Biochem.,88:183 (1980)

A NOVEL KININ, MET-ILE-SER-BRADYKININ(MET-T-KININ) IS RELEASED FROM T-

KININOGEN BY AN ACID PROTEINASE OF GRANULOMATOUS TISSUES IN RATS

Wataru Sakamoto, Fumihiko Satoh*, Shigeharu Nagasawa*,
Hiroshi Handa**, Shigenori Suzuki***, Soichiro Uehara****
and Akio Hirayama****

Department of Biochemistry, School of Dentistry, *Faculty
of Pharmaceutical Sciences, **the 2nd Department of Internal
Medicine and ***College of Medical Technology, School of
Medicine, Hokkaido University, and ****Tonan hospital
Sapporo, Japan

SUMMARY

Acid proteinase of granulomatous tissues in rats with carrageenin-
induced inflammation released two types of kinin from T-kininogen. The
kinin was identified as Ile-Ser-bradykinin(T-kinin) and a novel kinin,
Met-Ile-Ser-bradykinin(Met-T-kinin), from determination of its amino acid
composition and its immunoreactivity toward anti-bradykinin antiserum. The
release of T-kinin and Met-T-kinin from T-kininogen were found to occur by
consecutive cleavage by cathepsin D and 72 kDa protease.

INTRODUCTION

Previously, we reported that the release of T-kinin from T-kininogen
occurred by consecutive cleavage by cathepsin E-like proteinase and 72 kDa
proteinase in rat spleen(1). However, it has not yet been clarified whether
T-kinin could be released from T-kininogen by granulomatous tissue in rats
with carrageenin-induced inflammation, although T-kininogen and free T-
kinin have been reported to increase in the plasma and pouch fluid of rats
with carrageenin-induced inflammation(2, 3). In this paper, we report the
mechanism of T-kinin and a novel kinin, Met-T-kinin from T-kininogen by
granulomatous tissues in rats.

MATERIALS AND METHODS

Assay procedures – Cathepsin D and acid proteinase activities were
measured with hemoglobin(bovine, Sigma Chemical Co., U.S.A.) as substrate
by the method of Yamamoto et al.(4). Namely, the reaction mixture contained
2.0 ml 0.2 M sodium acetate buffer(pH 4.0), 1.0 ml 0.125 % hemoglobin, and
100 µl of enzyme solution. The liberated peptides were measured by absorbance
at 280 nm, and one unit(U) was defined as an increase of 1.0 in the absorbance per h. Protein was determined by the method of Lowry et al.(5).
Kinin-releasing activity was measured as described previously(1). The amount
of kinin liberated was determined by a bioassay and enzyme immunoassay. T-

kininogen(specific activity : 9.2 μg bradykinin equivalent/mg protein) was
prepared from rat plasma, as described previously(6).

<u>Amino acid analysis</u> - Samples to be analysed for amino acid composition
were hydrolysed with 6 N HCl at 110°C for 24 h in evacuated and sealed tubes.
The hydrolysates were evaporated and analysed in a Hitachi-835 amino acid
analyzer.

<u>Animals and carrageenin-induced inflammation</u> - Male Wistar rats,ap-
proximately 200 g body weight, were first injected with 8 ml of air(subcutaneously, dorsum), and then 1 day later with 4 ml of 2 %(w/v) carrageenin
(seakem No.402, Iwai Kagaku Yakuhin, Co., Ltd., Japan) solution in 0.9 %
NaCl. The rats were killed 3, 5, 10, 15 or 20 days after injection of
carrageenin.

<u>Measurement of T-kininogen levels in plasma and pouch fluid</u> - T-
kininogen levels in plasma and pouch fluid were determined by a single
radial immunodiffusion using purified T-kininogen as a standard, by the
method reported previously(1).

<u>Isolation of cathepsin D and 72 kDa protease from granulomatous
tissues in rats</u> - Cathepsin D and 72 kDa protease were isolated from granulomatous tissues, which were collected on day 5 - 20 after carrageenin injection into rats(2), by chromatography on DEAE-Sephadex A-50, Sephadex G-
100 and Pepstatin-Sepharose 4B, according to the method of Yamamoto et al.
(4) and our previous report(1).

<u>Isolation of kinin and kinin-containing peptides from T-kininogen
by acid proteinase and cathepsin D</u> - Purified T-kininogen was digested with
acid proteinase or cathepsin D in 0.2 M glycine-HCl buffer(pH 3.6) containing
2 mM EDTA. The reaction was terminated by acidifying the mixture to pH 2.5
with 1 N HCl. The liberated kinin and kinin-containing peptide were extracted
with n-butanol and subjected into reverse-phase HPLC(ODS-120T, Toyo Soda,
Japan).

RESULTS

<u>Changes over time in T-kininogen and granuloma after carrageenin injection
in rats</u>

As shown in Fig. 1, T-kininogen levels in plasma and pouch fluid were
maximum on day 5 after carrageenin injection, whereas granuloma was on day
10. Namely, the increase of T-kininogen was not in parallel with the marker
of the inflammatory conditions, the wet weight of granuloma.

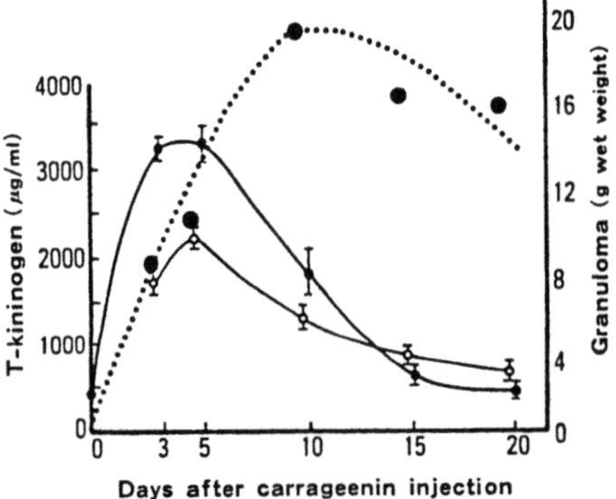

Fig. 1. Changes over time in
T-kininogen in plasma and pouch
fluid, and granuloma after
carrageenin injection in rats.
●-●, T-kininogen in plasma;
o-o, T-kininogen in pouch fluid;
●··●, wet weight of granuloma
(pouch fluid plus pouch wall).

Identification of T-kinin and a novel kinin, Met-T-kinin released from T-kininogen by acid proteinase in rat granuolatous tissues

As shown in Fig. 2, the acid proteinase in rat granulomatous tissues released two types of kinin(K-1 and K-2) from T-kininogen. The retention time(21.76 min) of K-1 was identified with that of synthetic T-kinin(Peptide Institute, Inc., Osaka, Japan), but the retention time(33.70 min) of K-2 differed from those of Met-Lys-bradykinin, Lys-bradykinin and bradykinin. The novel kinin, K-2 was identified as Met-Ile-Ser-bradykinin from determination of its amino acid composition and its immunoreactivity toward anti-bradykinin antiserum, as described previously(7).

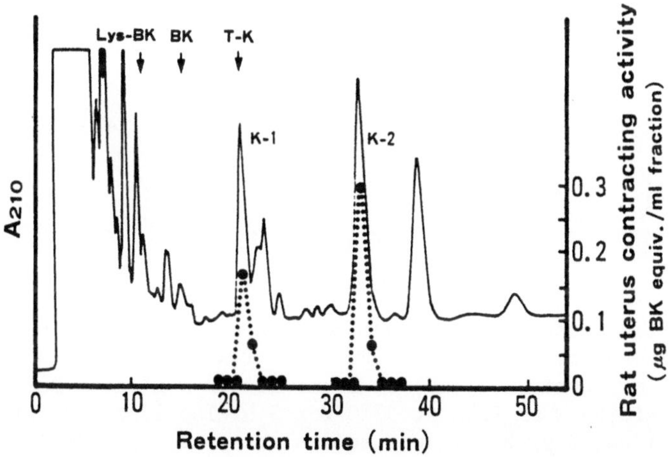

Fig. 2. Reverse-phase HPLC of kinin released from T-kininogen by acid proteinase and of synthetic kinins. Purified T-kininogen(2 mg) was digested with acid proteinase(0.4 U) at 37°C for 60 min in 12.0 ml of 0.2 M glycine-HCl buffer(pH 3.6) containing 2 mM EDTA. The released kinin(0.7 μg bradykinin equivalent) was injected into the reverse-phase column. The column was eluted isocratically with 20 % acetonitrile in 0.05 % trifluoroacetic acid at a flow rate of 1.0 ml/min. The arrows show the elution position of synthetic kinins. ●··●, rat uterus contracting activity.

Identification of kinin-containing peptides released from T-kininogen by cathepsin D

As shown in Fig. 3, cathepsin D released kinin-containing peptides from T-kininogen. Namely, two types of kinin-containing peptide(T-I and T-II) were eluted at 40 to 42 % of acetonitrile(retention time of 61.33 min and 62.45 min, respectively) on the reverse-phase HPLC. As shown in Table 1, T-I and T-II fractions had no biological activity on rat uterus contracting activity and the immunoassay using rabbit anti-bradykinin antiserum. However, T-I showed virtually equal rat uterus contracting activity and immunoreactivity to T-kinin and bradykinin by 72 kDa protease. The amino acid composition of T-I had one additional Leu residue in comparison with that of T-kinin(Table 2). From these results the amino acid sequence of T-I was identified as T-kinin-Leu. On the other hand, the retention time of T-II was identified with that of synthetic Met-T-kinin-Leu(Peptide Institute, Inc., Osaka, Japan). Therefore, T-II is assumed to be Met-T-kinin-Leu.

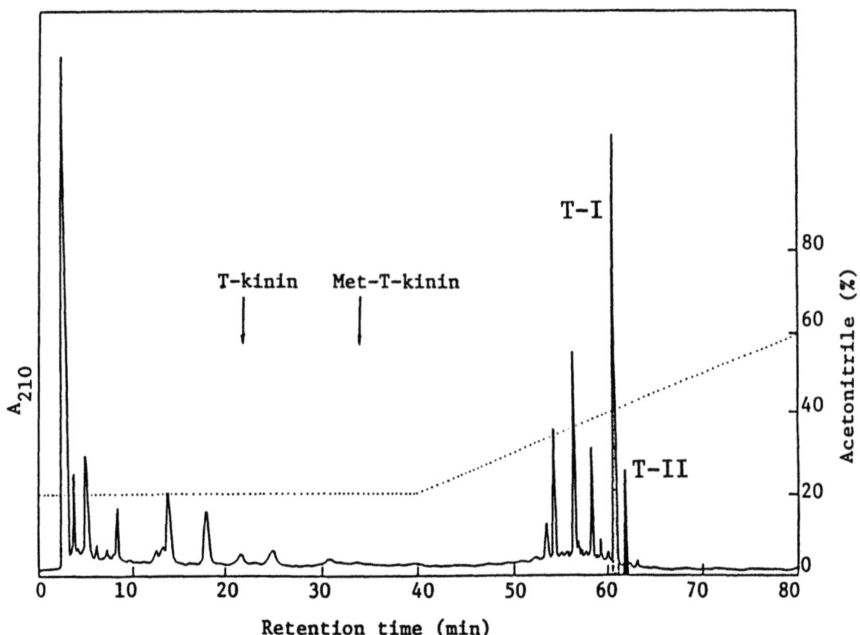

Fig. 3. Reverse-phase HPLC of kinin-containing peptides released from T-kininogen by cathepsin D. Purified T-kininogen(20 mg) was digested with cathepsin D(25 mU) in 18 ml of 0.2 M glycine-HCl buffer(pH 3.6) containing 2 mM EDTA at 37°C for 3 h. The liberated kinin-containing peptides(60 µg bradykinin equivalent) was injected into the reverse-phase column. The column was eluted with 20 % acetonitrile in 0.05 % trifluoroacetic acid for the first 40 min and then with a linear gradient from 20 to 60 % acetonitrile, at a flow rate of 1.0 ml/min. The arrows show the elution position of synthetic kinins. ...., acetonitrile.

Table 1. Kinin-release from kinin-containing peptides(T-I and T-II) by 72 kDa protease

	Rat uterus contracting activity (ng bradykinin equiv.)	Immunoreactivity to anti-bradykinin antiserum (ng bradykinin equiv.)
T-I		
Non-treatment	N.D.	N.D.
72 kDa protease	149	145
T-II		
Non-treatment	N.D.	N.D.
72 kDa protease	50	77

50 µl aliquots of T-I and T-II fractions were treated by 72 kDa protease (20 mU) in 450 µl of 0.2 M glycine-HCl buffer(pH 3.6) containing 2 mM EDTA for 60 min at 37°C. N.D., not detectable.

Table 2. Amino acid composition of kinin-containing peptide (T-I) released from T-kininogen by cathepsin D

| Amino acid | T-kinin-containing peptide (T-I) | | | T-kinin |
	nmol	mol/mol of Ile	Residue/molecule	Residue/molecule
Ser	7.7	2.0	2	2
Pro	10.5	2.7	3	3
Gly	5.8	1.5	1	1
Ile	3.9	1.0	1	1
Phe	7.2	1.8	2	2
Arg	7.1	1.8	2	2
Leu	4.5	1.2	1	—

Purified kinin-containing peptide(T-I)(5.8 µg bradykinin equivalent) was hydrolyzed with 6 N HCl at 110°C for 24 h in evacuated and sealed tube. The hydrolyzate was evaporated and analyzed in a Hitachi-835 amino acid analyzer.

DISCUSSION

Recently, we and other investigators have observed an increase in T-kininogen in plasma of rats following experimentally induced inflammation by Freund's adjuvant and carrageenin(1 - 3). On the other hand, T-kininogen appears to play a physiological role as an acute phase protein, cysteine proteinase inhibitor, and chemical mediator of inflammation(8 - 10). In this report, T-kininogen appears to be used a kinin precursor in granulomatous tissues with carrageenin-induced inflammation. Namely, it has been shown that T-kinin and the novel kinin, Met-T-kinin can be generated from T-kininogen by acid proteinase of the granulomatous tissues. In addition, the release of T-kinin and Met-T-kinin from T-kininogen were found to occur by consecutive cleavage by cathepsin D and 72 kDa protease, as described previously(1). Recently, Nakanishi et al.(11) have reported that T-kininogen harbors an Ile-Ser-bradykinin sequence preceded by the dipeptide Met-Met, from the results of nucleotide sequencing of rat T-prekininogen I mRNA. Therefore, cathepsin D of granulomatous tissues appears to cleave both Met-Met and Met-Ile bonds at the amino terminal position of Ile-Ser-bradykinin, and Leu-Val at the carboxy terminal.

ACKNOWLEDGEMENTS

This research was supported in part by grants from the Ministry of Education, Science and Culture of Japan and the Kanae Igaku Foundation.

REFERENCES

1. W.Sakamoto, K.Yoshikawa, A.Yokoyama, and M.Kohri, T-kinin is released from T-kininogen by consecutive cleavage by cathepsin E-like proteinase and 72 kDa proteinase, Biochim.Biophys.Acta, 884 : 607(1986).
2. W.Sakamoto, K.Yoshikawa, H.Handa, S.Uehara, and A.Hirayama, T-kininogen in rats with carrageenin-induced inflammation, Biochem.Pharmacol., 35 : 4283(1986).

3. A.Barlas, K.Sugio, and L.M.Greenbaum, Release of T-kinin and bradykinin in carrageenin induced inflammation in the rat, FEBS Lett., 190 : 268 (1985).

4. K.Yamamoto, N.Katsuda, and K.Kato, Cathepsin D of rat spleen - affinity purification and properties of two types of cathepsin D, Eur.J.Biochem., 92 : 499(1978).

5. D.H.Lowry, N.J.Rosebrough, A.L.Farr, and R.Randall, Protein measurement with folin phenol reagent, J.Biol.Chem., 193 : 265(1951).

6. W.Sakamoto, K.Yoshikawa, S.Uehara, O.Nishikaze, and H.Handa, Purification and characterization of rat low molecular weight kininogen, J.Biochem., 96 : 81(1984).

7. W.Sakamoto, F.Satoh, K.Gotoh, and S.Uehara, Ile-Ser-bradykinin(T-kinin) and Met-Ile-Ser-bradykinin(Met-T-kinin) are released from T-kininogen by acid proteinase of granulomatous tissues in rats, FEBS Lett., 219 : 437(1987).

8. A.Barlas, H.Okamoto, and L.M.Greenbaum, T-kininogen - the major plasma kininogen in rat adjuvant arthritis, Biochem.Biophys.Res.Commun., 129 : 280(1985).

9. T.Cole, A.S.Inglis, C.M.Roxburgh, G.J.Howlett, and G.Schreiber, Major acute x1-protein of rat is homologous to bovine kininogen and contains the sequence for bradykinin, FEBS LETT., 182 : 57(1985).

10. T.Sueyoshi, K.Enjyoji, T.Shimada, H.Kato, S.Iwanaga, Y.Bando, E.Kominami, and N.Katunuma, A new function of kininogens as thiol-proteinase inhibitors : inhibition of papain and cathepsin B, H and L by bovine, rat and human plasma kininogens, FEBS Lett., 182 : 193(1985).

11. S.Furuto-Kato, A.Matsumoto, N.Kitamura, and S.Nakanishi, Primary structures of the mRNA encoding the rat precursors for bradykinin and T-kinin, J.Biol.Chem., 260 : 12054(1985).

T-KININ IN HUMAN OVARIAN CARCINOMA ASCITES

G. Wunderer and I. Walter

1. Frauenklinik der Universität
Maistr. 11
D - 8000 München 2
(Director: Prof. Dr. G. Kindermann)

INTRODUCTION

Ascites is a frequent side-effect of malignant diseases in gynecological patients suffering from e.g. metastatic ovarian or breast carcinomas. The pathophysiology of ascites generation is not understood in detail.
In general, ascites results from the imbalance of abundant plasma exudation via peritoneum and of reduced resorption due to occluded lymph vessels. The tremendous plasma exudation into the peritoneal cavity seems to be the result of both necrosis of capillary vessels and of increased permeability. The latter effect is shown to be quantitatively more important [1]. In any case, it is more relevant because of its implications in therapeutic treatment. We therefore analysed a series of ascites samples for permeability factors.
The aim of our studies was to expand and to gain further evidence supporting the hypothesis of Greenbaum's leukokinin/ogen system in malignant ascites [2].

MATERIALS AND METHODS

Ascites

Ascitic fluid was obtained at laparotomy or by trans-peritoneal puncture from patients with metastatic ovarian or breast carcinomas, or other diseases (Table). An inhibitor cocktail containing aprotinin, benzamidine, EDTA, polybrene [3] and in addition pepstatin (100 nM final concentration) was added to the sample immediately to avoid further degradation. After centrifugation at 3000 rpm for 10 min at 4° C the supernatant was aliquoted, frozen in liquid nitrogen and stored at -22° C.

Abbreviation: PF = permeability factor

<u>Permeability testing</u>

Permeability tests were performed as published previously [4].
Bradykinin was used as reference substance and compared to synthetic T-kinin as shown in Fig.1.

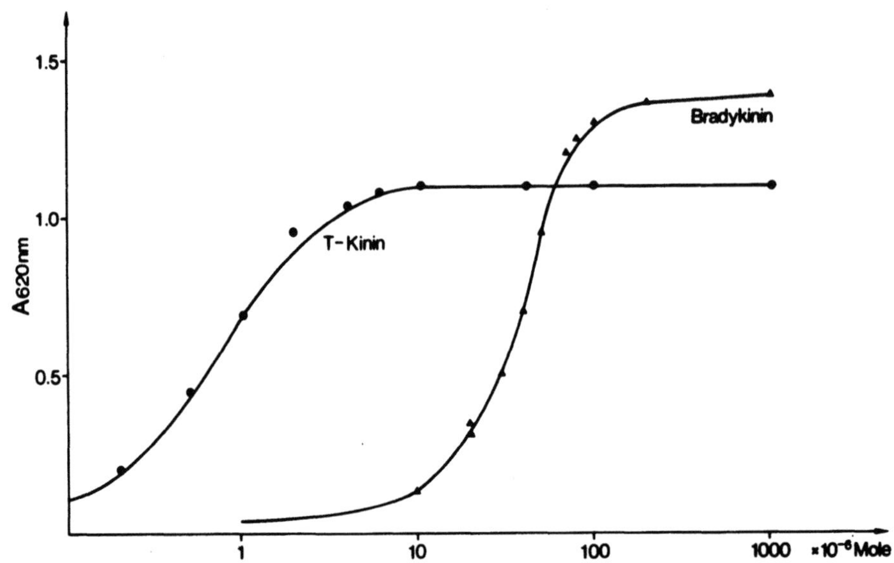

Fig. 1   Permeability increasing activity of T-kinin and of
          bradykinin. Samples of kinins were injected intra-
          cutaneously into the BS rat skin. Evans blue was
          injected i.v.. After 30 min. the rats were
          sacrificed and the blue areas were cut out. The blue
          dye was extracted with formamide and its absorption
          measured at 620 nm. The absorption (A 620 nm) is
          correlated to increasing amounts of kinins applied.

<u>Isolation Procedure</u>

Pretreated ascites (200 ml) was applied to an Ultrogel AcA 44 column (6x120 cm) in 25 mM Na_2HPO_4/25 mM NaCl buffer,pH 7.4, at 4°C, at a flow rate of 80 ml/h.
Two main fractions with permeability increasing activity were eluted (Fig. 2A). The first fraction eluted at a molecular mass of about 60 kDa. This material was allowed to stand 4 hours at room temperature. Thereafter, an aliquot was rechromatographed on another Ultrogel AcA 44 column (2.5x100cm) in 50 mM ammonium acetate buffer, pH 7.4, at 4°C, at a flow rate of 15 ml/h (Fig. 2B). Fractions were assayed for permeability factors.

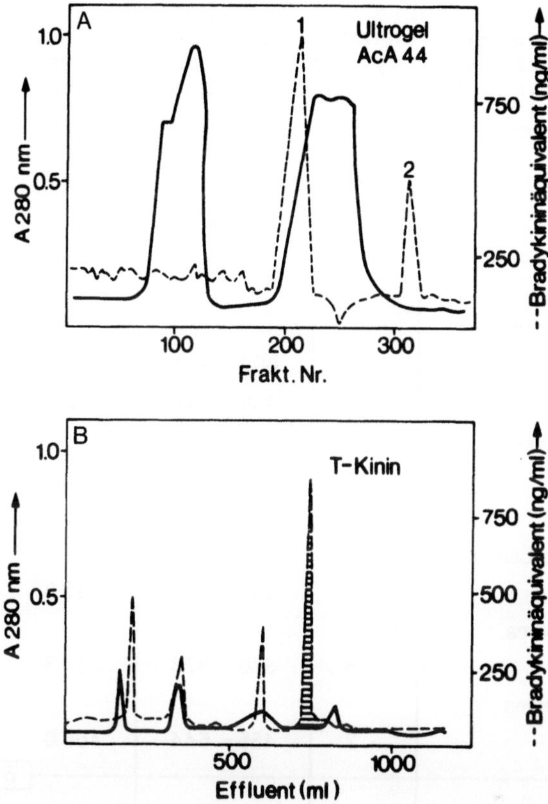

Fig. 2   Isolation of T-kinin by gel permeation chromatography

2A   Chromatography of pretreated ascites on Ultrogel
AcA 44 column (6x120cm), in 25 mM Na_2HPO_4/25 mM
NaCl buffer, pH 7.4, 4°C at a flow rate of 80 ml/h.
Fraction 1 corresponds to a molecular mass of
60 kDa, fraction 2 corresponds to about 1 kDa.

2B   Rechromatography of fraction 1 shown in Fig. 2A;
after 4 hours incubation at room temperature.
Column material:Ultrogel AcA 44; dimensions:
2.5x100 cm; solvent: 50 mM ammonium acetate pH 7.4;
flow rate: 15 ml/h; absorbance at 280 nm (full line);
PF (broken line).

Table 1   Permeability increasing activity of various
           fluids.
           Samples obtained from patients with malignant
           diseases contain significantly higher amounts of
           permeability factors than samples obtained from
           patients with non-malignant diseases.

Diagnosis	Number	Perm. factor Bradykinin – equivalent (ng/ml)		
		Range	Mean	
Ovarian Carcinoma				
– Ascites	161	602 –1241	873.6	
– Pleura	10	450 – 540	472.9	
Mamma Carcinoma				
– Ascites	49	480 – 950	600.6	
– Pleura	54	450 – 810	378.0	
Fallopian Tube Carcinoma				Malignant
– Ascites	3	506 – 605	530.8	MW = 700
Clitoris Carcinoma				SD = 210
– Ascites	3	360 – 373	334.3	n = 294
Cervix Carcinoma				
– Ascites	2	455 – 544	466.6	
			$p < 0.001$	
Livercirrhosis				
– Ascites	9	45 – 65	46.2	
Peritoneal Fluid	2	82 – 100	92.4	
Ovarian Cyst Fluid	7	68 – 135	94.5	Non-Malignant
Follicular Fluid	5	71 – 95	84.0	MW = 75.6
Hydrosalpinx	1		75.6	SD = 28.3
Fetal Ascites	1		138.0	n = 26
Liver Cyst (fetal)	1		134.0	

Permeability factors

Ascites samples obtained from patients with various diseases were tested for permeability factors by means of the rat skin test [4]. The results are depicted on the Table.
Permeability factors determined show significant differences between ascites corresponding to malignant diseases as compared to non-malignant diseases. Ascites, obtained from patients with ovarian carcinoma or metastatic breast carcinoma is very rich in PF.
Pleura exudate of both carcinomas is found to have minor amounts of PF. However, ascites from patients with liver cirrhose is inactive. In fact this ascites proved to be poor in protein and showed low inflammation factors, thus being considered as transudate. Setting an arbitrary limit of PF= 250 ng/ml bradykinin equivalents, it is evident that in the case of all ascites samples corresponding to malignant diseases the PF value lies above this limit, whereas samples corresponding to non-malignant diseases or other transudates are below this limit. This difference is significant on the $p < 0.001$ level. Consequently, the PF value permits distinguishing between these two forms of ascites.
Yet, this rule should be regarded critically, since the test used cannot distinguish between different PF's but only measure the overall effect, so it was inevitable to differentiate this permeability increasing activity. Based on previous reports by Greenbaum [2], we decided to characterize the major permeability factors involved in ovarian carcinoma ascites.

Isolation of T-kinin

When ascites was pretreated with inhibitors for proteinases and for carboxypeptidases the degradation of PF was found to be slower. We therefore choose pretreated ascites of patients with ovarian carcinoma for the isolation procedure. Ascites was separated by gel permeation chromatography on Ultrogel AcA 44 (Fig. 2A) and the effluent was tested for presence of PF by means of the rat skin test. The 60 kDa fraction was selected for further processing, since it contained the major part of the activity. To our surprise, however, we found that rechromatography of a 60 kDa aliquot which was allowed to stand 4 hours at room temperature, on a second Ultrogel column resulted in a shift of most of the PF activity towards an effluent corresponding to a considerably smaller molecular size (Fig. 2B). We observed this fact repeatedly in different ovarian carcinoma ascites samples. Analysis of the smallest PF showed that it was a pure peptide with the T-kinin sequence, Ile-Ser-bradykinin [4,5].
100 ml ascites obtained from a patient with papillary cystadenocarcinoma of the ovary, rendered 450 mmol (0.5 mg) T-kinin. This is an extremely high amount of PF, as compared to that of kininogen in plasma. HPLC analysis of the smaller fraction of the first Ultrogel chromatography (Fig. 2A) showed also high amounts of T-kinin , yet no bradykinin. T-kinin/ogen has been found in rats but not in human or bovine material, when analysed on the mRNAs level [6].

Thus, it was surprising to find T-kinin in ascites from
patients with ovarian carcinoma. As a consequence of this
finding the site and mechanism of release of T-kinin has to
be looked for. Our primary assumption was that T-kinin
derives from a third type of human kininogen, unknown till
now, in analogy to the T-kininogen systems in the rat [6].
However this hypothesis could not be substantiated until now,
so we should take another mode of generation into account.
T-kinin may be considered as a worthful candidate as marker
for malignant disease, since this substance has not been
found in a healthy person till now.

ACKNOWLEDGEMENT

The support by the Sonderforschungsbereich 207 of the
Deutsche Forschungsgemeinschaft is gratefully acknowledged.

REFERENCES

1.   K.   Hirabayashi, J. Graham, <u>Am. J. Obstet. Gynecol.</u>
          106 492-497 (1970).

2.   L.M. Greenbaum, "Handbook of Experimental Pharmacology"
          Vol. 25, Supplement, Erdös E.G. ed., Springer Verlag
          Berlin, pp. 91-102 (1979).

3.   W.   Müller-Esterl, M. Vohle-Timmermann, B. Boos,
          B. Dittmann, <u>Biochim. Biophys. Acta</u>
          706 145-152 (1982).

4.   G.   Wunderer, I. Walter, E. Müller, A. Henschen,
          <u>Biol. Chem. Hoppe-Seyler</u> 367 1231-1234 (1986).

5.   H.   Okamoto, L.M. Greenbaum, <u>Biochem. Biophys. Res. Commun.</u>
          112 701-708 (1983).

6.   R.   Kageyama, N. Kitamura, H. Ohkubo, S. Nakanishi,
          <u>J. Biol. Chem.</u> 260 12060-12064 (1985).

PLASMA KININ LEVELS IN EXPERIMENTAL HYPERTENSION IN RATS

Motoya Nakagawa and Alberto Nasjletti

Department of Pharmacology, University of Tennessee
Memphis, Tennessee and Department of Pharmacology
New York Medical College, Valhalla, New York

INTRODUCTION

The status of circulating kinin levels in relation to the development
of hypertension has not been clarified. In patients with essential
hypertension, the concentration of kinins in the peripheral venous plasma
was shown not to deviate from the values in normotensive subjects (1),
but the concentration of kinins in the renal venous blood was reported to
increase (2). In animals with experimental hypertension, the level of
kinins in arterial plasma was shown to fall in dogs with acute
renovascular hypertension (3), but the level of kinins in arterial blood
was reported to increase in rats with one clip-one kidney hypertension
(4). The aforementioned observations on the plasma concentration of
kinins (1,3) probably do not reflect the circulating level of kinins,
since the measures to prevent ex vivo kinin generation during blood
sampling were limited.

Reports that the plasma concentration of high molecular weight
kininogen is depressed in patients with malignant hypertension (5), and
that the concentration of arterial blood kinins is increased in rats with
severe one kidney-one clip hypertension (4), raise the possibility that
the vascular injury accompanying severe hypertension creates conditions
that are conducive to augmentation of blood kinin generation and levels
(6). If so, severe hypertension, regardless of the etiology, may be
expected to increase circulating kinins. Therefore, this study was
designed to compare the concentration of kinins in the arterial plasma of
normotensive rats and of rats with severe hypertension caused by chronic
angiotensin infusion or by treatment with desoxycorticosterone (DOC) and
increased dietary sodium.

METHODS

Studies were conducted on male Sprague-Dawley rats (Harlan
Industries, Indianapolis, IN). The animals were housed in group cages,
were fed ad libitum a standard chow (Ralston Purina, St. Louis, MO), and
had the systolic blood pressure determined at 4-7 day intervals by tail
sphygmography after warming in a chamber at $37^{\circ}C$ for 10 min.

<u>Angiotensin-Induced Hypertension</u>. An Alzet osmotic minipump (Model 2002, Alza Corporation, Palo Alto, CA) filled with isoleucine[5]-angiotensin II or I (Sigma Chemical Co., St. Louis, MO), or with vehicle only (0.01 N acetic acid), was placed through a 1-cm midline incision in the abdominal cavity of rats anesthetized with ether. The calculated infusion rate of angiotensin II and I was 125 ng/min and 150 ng/min, respectively. Animals in all groups had free access to tap water to drink throughout the study. The concentration of kinins in the arterial plasma was determined on the 12th day after the onset of angiotensin or vehicle infusion.

<u>DOCA-Salt Hypertension</u>. In all rats, the left kidney was removed via a left flank incision under ether anesthesia. One day after uninephrectomy, the animals were randomly divided into three groups. Throughout the study, rats in group 1 drank deionized water, rats in group 2 drank 1% NaCl (saline), and rats in group 3 drank 1% NaCl and received weekly subcutaneous injections of DOC (Percorten Pivalate, CIBA, Summit, NJ; 25 mg/kg body weight, sc). The concentration of kinins in the arterial plasma was determined on the 5th week after the onset of treatment.

<u>Assay of Kinins.</u> Rats were anesthetized with ether, the abdomen opened with a midline incision, and blood (4.0 ml) for assay of plasma kinins was rapidly drawn from the abdominal aorta into a chilled plastic syringe containing a mixture (0.4 ml) of kallikrein and kininase inhibitors (aprotinin 4,000 KIU, soy bean trypsin inhibitor 320 μg, 1,10-phenanthroline 4 mg, disodium ethylenediaminetetraacetate 8 mg, and hexadimethrine 1.6 mg). After centrifugation (2,000 rpm, 15 min, 4°C), the concentration of kinins in the plasma was measured by radioimmunoassay as described by Shimamoto et al. (7), after sample purification by the method of Ando and Shimamoto (8). The bradykinin antibody was a gift from Dr. Kazuaki Shimamoto, Sapporo Medical College, Sapporo, Japan, and ^{125}I-Tyr^8-bradykinin was obtained from New England Nuclear, Boston, MA. The recovery of unlabeled bradykinin added to blood at the time of sampling was 82.9±5.0%. The recovery of ^{125}I-Tyr^8-bradykinin added to each plasma sample before purification was 66.0±1.4%; the individual recovery values served to correct the estimates of the plasma kinin concentration for losses incurred during purification. The concentration of kinins in plasma is expressed as picograms per milliliter.

<u>Statistical Analysis</u>. Results are expressed as mean ± standard error of the mean. Comparisons among groups were made by student's t-test. The null hypothesis was rejected when the p value was less than 0.05.

RESULTS

Relative to values in vehicle infused rats, systolic blood pressure was increased by about 45 mmHg and 48 mmHg in rats infused with angiotensin II (125 ng/min) and angiotensin I (150 ng/min), respectively (Table 1). The concentration of kinins in the arterial plasma of rats with angiotensin II-induced hypertension did not differ from that in vehicle-infused controls (Table 1). In contrast, the concentration of kinins in the arterial plasma of rats with angiotensin I-induced hypertension was 87% higher than that in rats infused with vehicle only (Table 1).
DOC-treated rats (25 mg/kg per week) drinking 1% NaCl for 5 weeks had a higher systolic blood pressure than rats drinking either water or 1% NaCl without DOC treatment (Table 1). The concentration of kinins in the

arterial plasma of rats with DOC-salt hypertension was 50% lower than the
arterial plasma kinin concentration in water drinking rats (Table 1).
Rats drinking 1% NaCl without DOC treatment also had a lower arterial
plasma kinin concentration than normotensive control rats drinking water
(Table 1). But the arterial plasma kinin concentration of rats with
DOC-salt hypertension did not differ from that in normotensive rats
drinking 1% NaCl (Table 1).

Table 1. Systolic blood pressure and arterial plasma kinin concentration
in normotensive control rats and in rats with angiotensin II-induced
hypertension, angiotensin I-induced hypertension, and DOC-salt
hypertension.

Treatment Group	Blood Pressure (mmHg)	Kinin (pg/ml)
Vehicle (N=6)	123 ± 2	10.1 ± 1.0
Angiotensin II (N=6)	$168\pm12^{*}$	10.6 ± 2.8
Vehicle (N=5)	118 ± 5	12.0 ± 2.2
Angiotensin I (N=6)	$167\pm8^{*}$	$22.5\pm2.2^{*}$
Water Drinking (N=8)	138 ± 3	$14.0+1.4$
1% NaCl Drinking (N=10)	141 ± 3	$8.1\pm1.3^{*}$
DOC-1% NaCl Drinking (N=9)	$210\pm4^{*}$	$7.0\pm1.3^{*}$

Values are means $\pm$ S.E.; asterisks indicate $P<0.05$ relative to control.
See text for additional details.

DISCUSSION

Reports that the plasma concentration of high molecular weight
kininogen is depressed in patients with malignant hypertension (5), and
that the concentration of arterial blood kinins is increased in renal
hypertensive rats (4), raised the possibility that the vascular injury
accompanying severe hypertension creates conditions that are conducive to
augmentation of blood kinin generation and levels. Our study does not
support such a view, as the arterial plasma concentration of kinins,
irrespective of the level of blood pressure, was unchanged in rats with
angiotensin II-induced hypertension, increased in rats with angiotensin
I-induced hypertension, and diminished in rats with DOC-salt
hypertension. Accordingly, it would appear that the mechanisms
underlying the abnormal arterial plasma kinin levels observed in rats
with angiotensin I-induced hypertension and DOC-salt hypertension are
triggered by factors related to the specific etiology of the hypertension
rather than by the hypertension itself. In support of this view we found
that the concentration of arterial plasma kinins was decreased in
normotensive rats drinking 1% NaCl, suggesting that the lowering of
arterial plasma kinin levels in DOC-salt hypertensive rats is related to
the increased dietary sodium rather than to the excess of
mineralocorticoids or hypertension.

Recently, we reported that even during infusion of exogenous
bradykinin, to greatly diminish the relative contribution to circulating
kinin levels of endogenously produced kinin, DOC-salt hypertensive rats
and saline-drinking normotensive rats continued exhibiting diminished
arterial plasma kinin levels relative to the levels in water drinking

controls (9). We also reported that following treatment with captopril, to inhibit kinin degradation by kininase II (converting enzyme), the arterial plasma kinin level in DOC-salt hypertensive rats and in saline-drinking normotensive rats did not differ significantly from the values in water drinking normotensive controls (9). Collectively, these observations are compatible with the notion that the reduction of arterial plasma kinins in DOC-salt hypertensive rats and in saline-drinking rats may be due to augmentation of kinin degradation.

Bradykinin and related peptides are degraded by several peptidases including a peptidyldipeptidase, kininase II or converting enzyme, which also converts angiotensin I to angiotensin II (10). A competitive interaction between angiotensin I and kinins at the level of their metabolism by the peptidyldipeptidase is suggested by reports that angiotensin I and bradykinin can inhibit each other hydrolysis by the enzyme (11,12). But a role for angiotensin I in inhibiting the degradation of kinins in a physiological setting is open to questions because the preferred substrate for the peptidyldipeptidase is bradykinin rather than angiotensin I (13). Nonetheless, one still must consider the possibility that the diminution of angiotensin I levels accompanying increases in dietary sodium and DOC treatment creates a setting that favors the metabolism of plasma kinins by kininase II, thus reducing arterial plasma kinin levels. Conversely, in rats with angiotensin I-induced hypertension the increase in circulating angiotensin I levels may bring about inhibition of kinin degradation by kininase II, leading to augmentation of arterial plasma kinin levels.

In summary, this study demonstrates that the arterial plasma concentration of kinins is unaffected in rats with angiotensin II-induced hypertension, increased in rats with angiotensin I-induced hypertension, and diminished in rats with DOC-salt hypertension. We suggest that the abnormalities in arterial plasma kinin levels which are associated with angiotensin I-induced hypertension and DOC-salt hypertension are triggered by factors related, directly or indirectly, to the specific etiology of the hypertension rather than by the hypertension itself.

ACKNOWLEDGEMENT

This work was supported by USPHS Grant HL-18579.

REFERENCES

1. J.H. Mersey, G.H. Williams, R. Emanuel, R.G. Dluhy, P.Y. Wong, and T.J. Moore. Plasma bradykinin levels and urinary kallikrein excretion in normal renin essential hypertension. <u>J. Clin. Endocrinol. Metab</u>., 48:642 (1979).
2. L. Hulthen. Kinins in blood and urine with special reference to intrarenal kinin formation in normal and hypertensive individuals. <u>Acta. Endocr. Scand</u>., 94 (Suppl. 235):1 (1980).
3. J.J. Moore, J.A. Gagnon, P.S. Verma, G.E. Sander, and D.E. Butkus. Plasma kinin levels in acute renovascular hypertension in dogs. <u>Renal Physiol</u>., 7:102 (1984).
4. M.C.O. Salgado, S.F. Rabito, and O.A. Carretero. Blood kinin in one-kidney, one-clip hypertensive rats. <u>Hypertension</u>, 8 (Suppl. I): I-110 (1986).
5. A.B. Ribeiro, S.R. Schwarzwalder, M.A.S. Saragoca, F.A. Almeida, A. Voos, R.C.R. Stella, and O.L. Ramos. Malignant hypertension: A syndrome accompanied by plasmatic diminution of low and high molecular weight kininogens. <u>Hypertension</u>, 5 (Suppl. V):V-158 (1983).

6. R. Colman, and P.Y. Wong. Participation of Hageman factor dependent pathways in human disease states. Thromb. Haemost., 38:751 (1977).

7. K. Shimamoto, T. Ando, T. Nakao, S. Tanaka, M. Sakuma, and M. Myahara. A sensitive radioimmunoassay method for urinary kinins in man. J. Lab. Clin. Med., 91:721 (1978).

8. T. Ando and K. Shimamoto. A sensitive radioimmunoassay of blood and plasma kinin and its clinical applications. Sapporo Med. J., 82:453 (1983).

9. M. Nakagawa and A. Nasjletti. Plasma kinin levels in desoxycorticosterone (DOC)-salt hypertensive rats. Fed. Proc., 46:670 (1987).

10. E.G. Erdos and R.A. Skidgel. The unusual substrate specificity and the distribution of human angiotensin I converting enzyme. Hypertension, 8 (Suppl. I):I-34 (1986).

11. R. Igic, E.G. Erdos, H.S.J. Sorrels, and T. Nakajima. Angiotensin I converting enzyme of the lung. Circ. Res., 31 (Suppl. II):II-51 (1972).

12. A. Fitz, S. Wyatt, D. Boaz, and B. Fox. Peptide inhibitors of converting enzyme. Life Sci., 21:1179 (1977).

13. F.E. Dorer, J.R. Kahn, K.E. Lents, M. Levine, and L.T. Skeggs. Hydrolysis of bradykinin by angiotensin-converting enzyme. Circ. Res., 34:824 (1974).

ROLE OF RENAL KALLIKREIN IN THE REGULATION OF BLOOD PRESSURE IN THE RAT

REMNANT KIDNEY MODEL OF CHRONIC RENAL FAILURE

Masayuki Kanazawa, Keishi Abe*, Minoru Yasujima,
Kazunori Yoshida, Masahiro Kohzuki, Masaya Tanno, Yutaka Kasai,
Ken Omata, Makito Sato, Kazuhisa Takeuchi, Masao Hiwatari and
Kaoru Yoshinaga

The Second Department of Internal Medicine, and *Dept of
Clinical Biology and Hormonal Regulation, Tohoku University
School of Medicine, Sendai, Japan

ABSTRACT

We studied urinary excretion of active and inactive kallikrein every
day for 3 weeks in spontaneously hypertensive rats (SHR) and Wistar-Kyoto
rats (WKY) subjected to 5/6 nephrectomy (5/6), 1/2-nephrectomy (1/2) or
sham-operation (Sham). We determined urinary active and inactive
kallikrein by measuring kallikrein activity using a kininogenase assay
before and after treatment with trypsin (200 µg/ml). In the SHR group,
blood pressure was significantly elevated in 5/6-animals as compared with
1/2 or sham, whereas in the WKY group blood pressure was not changed after
either operation. Urinary active and total kallikrein excretion were
decreased in 5/6-SHR to 34 % and 59 %, respectively, as compared with
values of sham-SHR, and in 1/2-SHR to 70 % and 70 %, respectively.
Similarly, they were also decreased in 5/6-WKY to 36 % and 55 %,
respectively, as compared with values of sham-WKY. In 1/2-WKY urinary
active kallikrein excretion was decreased to 88 % as compared with the
value of sham-WKY, but urinary total kallikrein excretion was not
different from that of sham-WKY. Thus, the suppressed renal kallikrein
activity due to reduced renal mass was not associated with any significant
change in blood pressure in WKY, although it induced an elevation of blood
pressure in SHR. These results indicate that the decreased production of
renal active kallikrein may not play a significant role in the regulation
of blood pressure in the rat remnant kidney model of chronic renal
failure. In addition, it is suggested that the elevation of blood pressure
in this model of SHR may be due to other factors than renal kallikrein.

INTRODUCTION

The kidney is considered to be one of the most important organs in
the regulation of blood pressure and the impaired renal function may be
associated with an elevation of blood pressure.

Renal kallikrein is a serine protease which releases kinins, potent
vasodilator peptides, from substrates called kininogens and is a component
of the vasoactive peptide system called the kallikrein-kinin system. It is
also well known that renal kallikrein-kinin system exerts important
physiologic functions, including the regulation of blood pressure and

modulation of salt and water transport in the kidney (Levinsky.1979,
Carretero.1980).

Urinary kallikrein excretion is often decreased in patients and
animals with primary, or secondary hypertension without mineralocorticoid-
excess (Margolius et al.1974, Carretero et al.1978, Keiser et al.1976).
Furthermore, Mitas et al.(1978) reported that urinary kallikrein excretion
was markedly decreased in patients with renal parenchymal disease and
hypertension, and the severity of hypertension inversely correlated with
kallikrein excretion, suggesting that the reduced production of renal
kallikrein may be a factor in the pathogenesis of hypertension associated
with chronic renal failure. On the contrary, it was also reported that
urinary excretion of kallikrein is normal in experimental chronic
glomerulonephritis in rats (Godon et al.1974) and is normal or increased
in patients with chronic renal failure (Cannella et al.1973).

Although it has not yet been proved that the altered excretion of
kallikrein is one of the factors in the pathogenesis of hypertension,
there may be a possibility that renal kallikrein plays an important role
in the regulation of blood pressure in chronic renal failure. To
investigate this possibility, we studied urinary excretion of active and
total kallikrein in the rat remnant kidney model of chronic renal failure.

MATERIALS AND METHODS

Male spontaneously hypertensive rats (SHR) and Wistar-Kyoto rats
(WKY) were subjected to 5/6 nephrectomy (5/6)(SHR n=12, WKY n=12) by
infarction of 2/3 of the right kidney at 7 weeks of age and removal of the
left kidney at 8 weeks, or to 1/2 nephrectomy (1/2)(SHR n=8, WKY n=6) by
removal of the left kidney at 8 weeks or to sham operation (Sham)(SHR n=8,
WKY n=7) at 8 weeks as a control study. Animals were housed in individual
metabolic cages in a humidity- and temperature-controlled room and fed a
regular diet (Oriental CMF, 0.24 % of sodium, 0.69 % of potassium) and
were given ad libitum access to tap water. Studies were performed after a
7-day period of acclimatization to the housing, feeding and drinking
conditions and were continued for up to 3 weeks.

Daily systolic blood pressure was recorded in conscious rats by an
indirect tail-cuff method (Pfeffer et al.1971), and also daily urine
volume and urinary kallikrein excretion were determined.

At the end of the study rats were killed by rapid decapitation and
trunk blood was collected for determination of serum creatinine (Scr) and
blood urea nitrogen (BUN), and creatinine clearance (Ccr) was calculated.

The active kallikrein in urine samples was measured by its
kininogenase activity (kinin releasing capability) using the mothod of Abe
et al.(1979). Briefly, duplicate aliquots of 20 µl of urine samples were
incubated with 4 µg of purified bovine serum low molecular weight
kininogen as substrate (generously supplied by Dr H. Kato, Fukuoka, Japan)
in the presence of 1-10 phenanthroline (3 mmol/l), disodium ethylene
diaminetetraacetic acid (EDTA, 30 mmol/l) to inhibit kininases and
neomycin (0.1 %) as an antibacterial agent. The incubation volume was
adjusted to 400 µl with 0.1 mol/l phosphate buffer, pH 8.5. The samples
were incubated at 37 °C for 20 min and the reaction was stopped by heating
in a boiling water bath for 5 min. The samples were then diluted with 1 ml
of ice cold 0.1 mol/1 Tris-HCl buffer, pH 7.4, and the generated kinins
were radio-immunologically measured by a modification of the method of
Carretero et al.(1976). Rabbit antibradykinin serum was generously
supplied by Dr O.A. Carretero (Detroit, USA). Kallikrein activity is
expressed as the amount of kinin/ml urine as generated by the incubation
of urine samples with bovine serum low molecular weight kininogen for 20
min. Total kallikrein was determined by measuring the kininogenase
activity in urine samples after inactive kallikrein had been activated
with trypsin. To activate the inactive kallikrein, duplicate 10 µl

aliquots of urine samples were incubated with 2 µg trypsin for 30 min at 37 °C. The reaction was stopped by adding 100 µg soybean trypsin inhibitor (SBTI). The incubation volume was adjusted to 400 µl with 0.1 mol/l phosphate buffer, pH 8.5, and the mixture was incubated for more than 2h at room temperature. Kininogenase activity was then measured as described above. To determine the optimal amount of trypsin needed to activate urinary inactive kallikrein in the preliminary experiments, the pooled rat urine (10 µl) from 10 normal rats was incubated with trypsin at doses of 0.1, 0.5, 2, 5 and 10 µg for 30 min at 37 °C. The reaction was stopped by adding 100 µg SBTI. The maximum activation of urinary inactive kallikrein by trypsin was observed at a concentration of 0.2 µg/ml, and the dose of SBTI used completely inhibited the kininogenase activity of trypsin. Furthermore, we confirmed that the doses of trypsin and SBTI used in the present experiment did not affect the radio-immunoassay of kinins.

Scr and BUN were measured with an autoanalyzer.

Values are given as means ± standard error of the mean. Significance was assessed using analysis of variance and Student's t-test, and statistical significance was defined as $P < 0.05$.

RESULTS

Systolic Blood Pressure

Systolic blood pressure was significantly elevated in 5/6-SHR as compared with 1/2- or sham-SHR whereas in WKY systolic blood pressure was not changed in the three models throughout the 3 week experimental period. Four weeks after surgery average values of systolic blood pressure were 236 ± 9.3 mmHg in 5/6-SHR, 219 ± 11.4 mmHg (n.s.) in 1/2-SHR, 201 ± 1.0 mmHg (P<0.01) in sham-SHR and 134 ± 2.2 mmHg in 5/6-WKY, 138 ± 3.7 mmHg (n.s.) in 1/2-WKY, 132 ± 2.6 mmHg (n.s.) in sham-WKY.

Renal Function

Four weeks after surgery significantly higher concentration of Scr and BUN were found in 5/6-SHR than those of 1/2- or sham-SHR and similarly in 5/6-WKY than those of 1/2- or sham-WKY. Average Scr and BUN concentrations were 0.74 ± 0.05 mg/dl and 57.4 ± 10.4 mg/dl in 5/6-SHR, 0.32 ± 0.02 mg/dl (P<0.001) and 16.3 ± 0.8 mg/dl (P<0.01) in 1/2-SHR, 0.24 ± 0.04 mg/dl (P<0.001) and 12.2 ± 0.9 mg/dl (P<0.01) in sham-SHR, 0.71 ± 0.12 mg/dl and 45.8 ± 8.0 mg/dl in 5/6-WKY, 0.27 ± 0.03 mg/dl (P<0.05) and 8.3 ± 1.7 mg/dl (P<0.01) in 1/2-WKY, 0.17 ± 0.03 mg/dl (P<0.01) and 7.3 ± 0.03 mg/dl (P<0.01) in sham-WKY, respectively. Average values of Ccr were 0.71 ± 0.05 ml/min in 5/6-SHR, 1.79 ± 0.12 ml/min (P<0.001) in 1/2-SHR, 2.65 ± 0.26 ml/min (P<0.001) in sham-SHR, 0.89 ± 0.13 ml/min in 5/6-WKY, 1.99 ± 0.14 ml/min (P<0.001) in 1/2-WKY, 3.3 ± 0.52 ml/min (P<0.01) in sham-WKY. Markedly impaired renal function was found in 5/6-rats as compared with 1/2- or sham-rats both in SHR and WKY.

Urinary Excretion of Active and Total Kallikrein

Four weeks after surgery urinary excretion of active and total kallikrein were decreased in 5/6-SHR to 34 % and 59 %, respectively, and in 1/2-SHR to 70 % and 70 %, respectively, as compared with values of sham-SHR. Similarly, they were decreased in 5/6-WKY to 35 % and 55 %, respectively, as compared with values of sham-WKY. In 1/2-WKY urinary active kallikrein excretion was decreased to 88 % as compared with values of sham-WKY, but urinary total kallikrein excretion was not different from that of sham-WKY. Lower value of the ratio of active to total kallikrein were found in 5/6-SHR and WKY than those of sham-SHR and WKY. Average values of urinary active and total kallikrein excretion were 5.7 ± 0.9 µg/day and 15.1 ± 1.7 µg/day in 5/6-SHR, 11.7 ± 2.2 µg/day (p<0.05) and 18.1 ± 2.5 µg/day (n.s.) in 1/2-SHR, 16.7 ± 2.9 µg/day (P<0.05) and 25.7 ± 3.1 µg/day (P<0.05) in sham-SHR, respectively, and 3.6 ± 1.1 µg/day and

10.1 ± 1.6 µg/day in 5/6-WKY, 9.0 ± 3.2 µg/day (n.s.) and 20.7 ± 5.3 µg/day (n.s.) in 1/2-WKY, 10.2 ± 2.4 µg/day (P<0.05) and 18.3 ± 3.4 µg/day (P<0.05) in sham-WKY, respectively.

DISCUSSION

In the present study, lower values of urinary excretion of active and total kallikrein, and the ratio of active to total kallikrein were found in 5/6-SHR and WKY than those of sham-SHR and WKY. It may be postulated that the presence of protein in the urine has something to do with the lower value of urinary kallikrein in this model, since a large amount of protein is excreted into the urine in these animals. However, we could exclude this possibility by showing no influence of protein on the kininogenase assay in our method in preliminary experiments.

The decrease in urinary excretion of active kallikrein agrees with the finding of Croxatto et al.(1970), who reported that urinary kallikrein activity was decreased in uninephrectomized rats with a figure-of-8-ligature in the remnant kidney and in uninephrectomized rats as compared with the value of normal rats. Accordingly, it is suggested that in 5/6-SHR and WKY the renal ability to activate kallikrein may be attenuated due to reduced renal mass, and that in those rats the ability to produce kinins may be impaired, although the precise mechanisms remain to be determined.

Blood pressure was significantly elevated in 5/6-SHR but not in 5/6-WKY in the present study. However, Croxatto et al.(1970) reported that in uninephrectomized Wistar rats with a figure-of-8-ligature in the remnant kidney developed high levels of arterial blood pressure. Therefore, an inverse relationship between increase in blood pressure and urinary kallikrein was observed. At the moment, we have no explanation for this discrepancy in blood pressure between the present results and data reported previously.

Does this diminished activity of kallikrein contribute to the pathogenesis of hypertension in the rat remnant kidney model of chronic renal failure ? In the present study, the equally suppressed renal kallikrein activity due to reduced renal mass was not associated with any significant changes in blood pressure in WKY although it induced an elevation of blood pressure in SHR. These results indicate that the decreased production of renal active kallikrein may not play a significant role in the regulation of blood pressure in the rat remnant kidney model of chronic renal failure.

In conclusion, it is suggested that in the rat remnant kidney model of chronic renal failure the renal ability to produce kallikrein may be impaired and also the ability to activate kallikrein may be attenuated due to reduced renal mass. Furthermore, it is suggested that the decreased activity of urinary kallikrein may not be involved in the pathogenesis of hypertension in this model of rat and that the elevation of blood pressure in this model of SHR may be due to other factors than renal kallikrein although the exact mechanism of the impaired production and activation of renal kallikrein remains to be determined.

ACKNOWLEDGEMENTS

This study was supported by a Grant-in-Aid for Cardiovascular Disease (60-C-3) from the Ministry of Health and Welfare and for Scientific Research (61132005 and 62570376) from the Ministry of Education, Science and Culture, Japan, and by the Miyagi Prefectural Kidney Association. We wish to acknowledge the excellent technical assistance of Miss Keiko Shiraishi, Miss Michiko Okamoto, Miss Naeko Nakagawa, and the secretarial assistance of Miss Junko Okazaki.

REFERENCES

Abe, K., Kato, H., Sakurai, Y., Ito, T., Saito, K., Haruyama, T. , Otsuka, Y., and Yoshinaga, K.,1979, Estimation of urinary kininogenase activity using bovine serum low molecular weight kininogen, In Kinin II edited by Fujii, S., Moriya, H., Suzuki, T., New York: Plenum Publishing Corporation, pp 105-114.

Cannella, G., Baggio, B., Antonello, A., Favaro, S., Todesco, S., Borsatti, A., and Campanacci, L.,1973, L'escrezione urinaria di callicreina nella glomerulonefrite, Boll. Soc. Ital. Biol. Sper., 49:580-585.

Carretero, O.A., Oza, N.B., Piwonska, A., Ocholik, T., Scicli, A.G.,1976, Measurement of urinary kallikrein activity by kinin radioimmunoassay, Biochem Pharmacol, 25:2265-2270.

Carretero, O.A., Amin, V.M., Ocholik, T., Scicli, A.G., and Koch, J.,1978, Urinary kallikrein in rats bred for their susceptibility and resistance to the hypertensive effect of salt: a new radioimmunoassay for its direct determination, Circ. Res., 42:727-731.

Croxatto, H.R., San Martin, M.,1970, Kallikrein-like activity in the urine of renal hypertensive rats, Experientia, 26:1216-1217.

Godon, J.P., and Damas, J.,1974, The kallikrein-kinin system in normal and glomerulonephritic rats, Arch Int Physiol Biochem, 82: 273-277.

Keiser, H.R., Geller, R.G., Margolius, H.S., and Pisano, J.J.,1976, Urinary kallikrein in hypertensive animalmodels, Federation Proc., 35: 199-202.

Levinsky, N.G.,1979, The renal kallikrein-kinin system, Circ res, 44:441-451.

Margolius, H.S., Horwitz, D., Pisano, J.J., and Keiser, H.R.,1974b, Urinary kallikrein excretion in hypertensive man. Relationship to sodium intake and sodium-retaining steroids, Circ. Res., 35: 820-825.

Mitas, J.A., Levy, S.B., Holle, R., Frigon, R.P., and Stone, R.A.,1978, Urinary kallikrein activity in the hypertension of renal parenchymal disease, New England Journal of Medicine, 299:162-165.

Pfeffer, J.M., Pfeffer, M.A., and Frohlich, E.D.,1971, Validity of an indirect tail-cuff method for determining systolic arterial pressure in unanesthetized normotensive and spontaneously hypertensive rats, J Lab Clin MED, 78:957-962.

THE RENAL KALLIKREIN-KININ SYSTEM IN RENOPARENCHYMAL HYPERTENSION

Toshiaki Ando, Kazuaki Shimamoto, Nobuyuki Ura, Toyoharu
Yokoyama, Shuzaburo Fukuyama, Yasukazu Yamaguchi, Hidehisa
Nakagawa, Yoshihiro Mori, Hitoko Ogata, and Osamu Iimura

The Second Department of Internal Medicine, Sapporo Medical
College, S1 W16, Chuoku, Sapporo 060, Japan

SUMMARY

In order to investigate the pathophysiological role of renal kallikrein
(KK)-kinin system in renoparenchymal hypertension(RHT), urinary excretion of
KK was measured in 15 patients with RHT and compared with that in 16 normotensive subjects(NT). The urinary kininase excretion was also determined in
some subjects. KK quantity and activity was measured by direct radioimmunoassay and kininogenase assay, respectively. Kininase activity was determined
as a bradykinin-degradating activity. The urinary excretion of KK quantity
and activity as well as the fractional excretion of KK were significantly
lower in RHT than in NT. Significantly positive correlations were observed
between urinary excretion of KK quantity or KK activity and creatinine
clearance. The fractional excretion of kininase was significantly higher in
RHT than in NT while no significant difference was found in the urinary
kininase excretion between these groups. These results suggest that renal
KK-kinin system is suppressed not only in the whole kidney but in each
nephrone which is still functioning, and the suppression of this system may
contribute to the pathophysiology of RHT

INTRODUCTION

It is well known that the incidence of hypertension increases in
relation to the reduction of renal function in renoparenchymal diseases. The
pathogenesis of hypertension in renoparenchymal diseases has been
investigated in various fields, and it has been suggested that renin-
angiotensin system, extracellular fluid volume and vasodepressor systems,
such as kallikrein-kinin system or prostanglandins, may contribute to the
development of hypertension in this disease.

In this study, in order to investigate the pathophysiological role of
the renal kallikrein-kinin system, urinary excretion of kallikrein and
kininase were determined and contrasted to those in normotensive subjects.

SUBJECTS AND METHODS

Sixteen normotensive subjects (7 males and 9 females, aged 44.3+3.4
years, mean+SE) and 15 patients with renoparenchymal hypertension (7 with

chronic glomerulonephritis and 8 with diabetic nephropathy, 7 males and
8 females, aged 51.2+3.6 years) were employed in this study. All subjects
were hospitalized and received an unrestricted diet. A 24-hour collection of
urine was collected for three days in order to measure the urinary
kallikrein, kininase, creatinine and sodium. Urinary kallikrein was measured
by direct radioimmunoassay(Shimamoto et al., 1980) as an enzyme quantity,
and with kininogenase assay(Kondo et al., 1984) as an enzymatic activity.
Kininase was determined as a bradykinin-degradating activity(Ura et al.,
1985). A statistical analysis was performed by Student's t-test for unpaired
data, and correlation coefficients were obtained by linear regression
analysis. All values were expressed as the mean+SE.

RESULTS

    The comparisons of creatinine clearance, urinary sodium excretion and
urinary kallikrein excretion between normotensive subjects and patients with
renoparenchymal hypertension are shown in Fig.1. The creatinine clearance

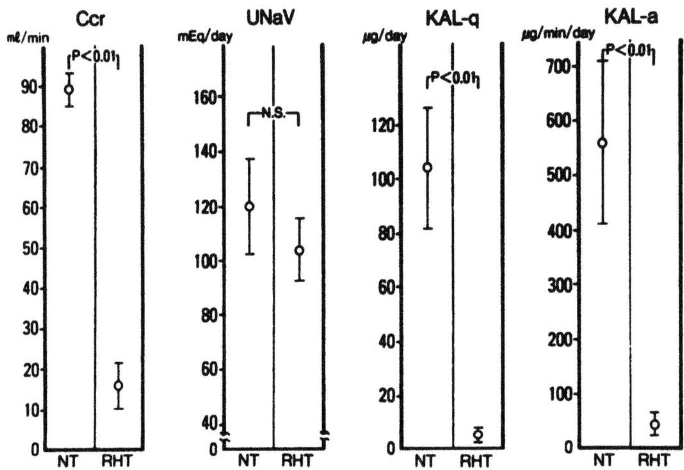

Fig.1. The comparison of creatinine clearance(Ccr), urinary Na
       excretion(UNaV), and urinary kallikrein excretion
       between normotensives(NT) and renoparenchymal hyperten-
       sives(RHT). KAL-q:kallikrein quantity, KAL-a:kallikrein
       activity.

(Ccr) in patients with renoparenchymal hypertension(16.1+5.7 ml/min) was
significantly lower than that in normotensive subjects(89.3+3.9 ml/min,
p<0.01). Urinary sodium excretion(UNaV) in patients with renoparenchymal
hypertension and that in normotensive subjects were 104.4+11.8 mEq/day and
119.9+17.5 mEq/day, respectively. There was no significant difference
between these two groups. The urinary excretion of KK quantity and activity
in normotensive subjects were 104.1+22.3 ug/day and 561.0+149.1 ug/min/day,
respectively. Patients with renoparenchymal hypertension showed a markedly
reduced urinary excretion of both KK quantity(6.3+2.7 ug/day) and
activity(44.6+20.2 ug/min/day) as compared to normotensive subjects. The
urinary KK excretion was significant and positively correlated with Ccr or
with urinary sodium excretion; Correlation coefficients were r=0.611 in KK
quantity vs Ccr, r=0.634 in KK activity vs Ccr(Fig.2), r=0.470 in KK
quantity vs UNaV, and r=0.593 in KK activity vs UNaV(Fig.3). All values were
statistically significant(p<0.01).

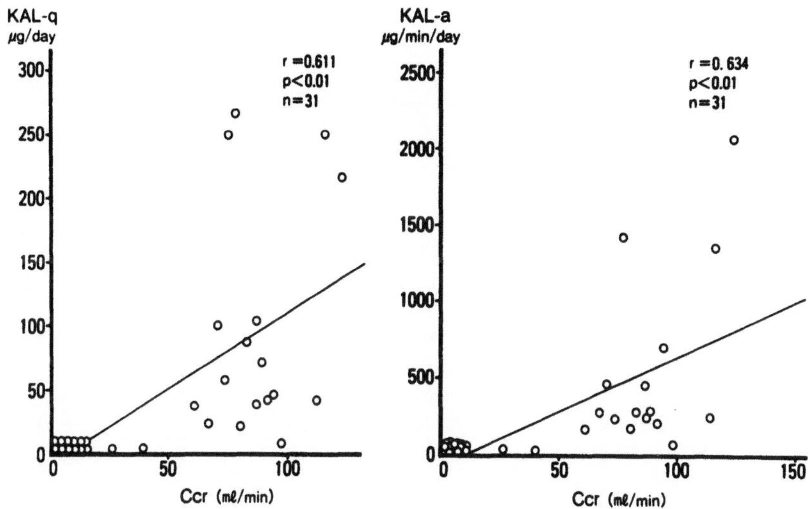

Fig.2. The correlation between creatinine clearance(Ccr) and urinary kallikrein excretion. Abbreviations are shown in Fig.1.

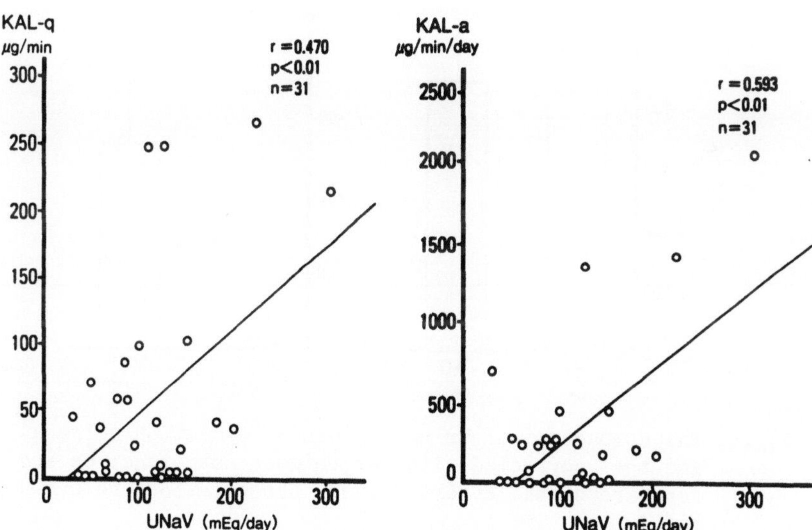

Fig.3. The correlation between urinary Na excretion(UNaV) and urinary excretion of kallikrein. Abbreviations are shown in Fig.1.

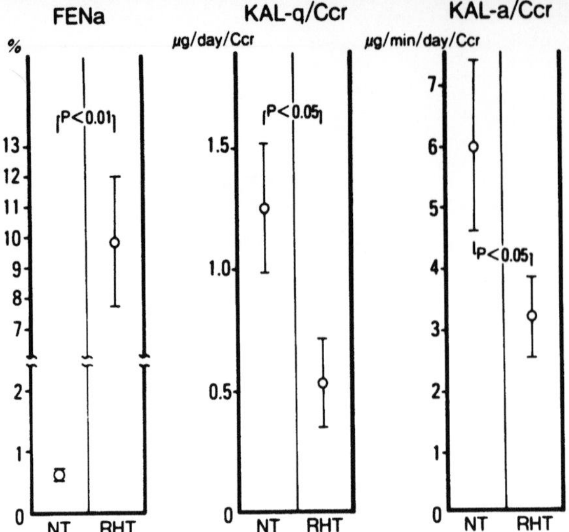

Fig.4. The comparison of fractional excretion of Na and urinary kallikrein excretion corrected with Ccr between NT and RHT. Abbreviations are shown in Fig.1.

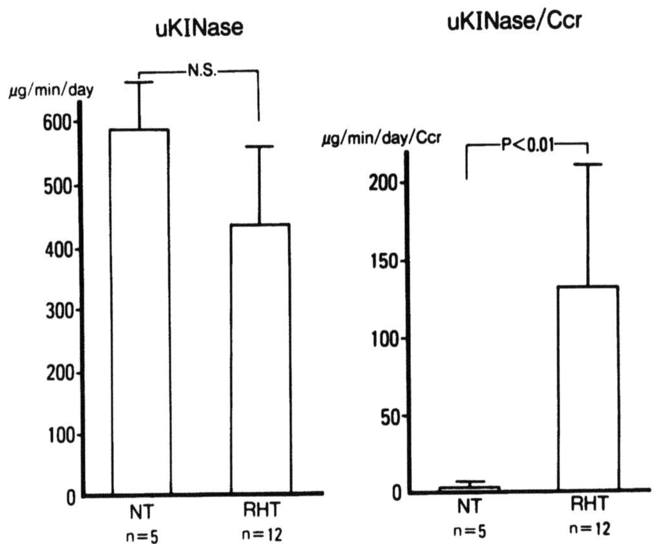

Fig.5. The comparison of urinary kininase excretion(uKINase) and that corrected with Ccr between normotensives and renoparenchymal hypertensives. Abbreviation are shown in Fig.1.

The values of urinary excretion of kallikrein quantity and activity corrected with Ccr were significantly lower in patients with renoparenchymal hypertension than in normotensive subjects, while the fractional excretion of sodium(FENa) in the patients was significantly higher than that in normotensive subjects(Fig.4).

Urinary kininase excretions were 598+167 ug/min/day in normotensive
subjects and 435+126 ug/min/day in the patients, respectively. A significant difference was not observed between them. However, the values of
urinary kininase excretion corrected with Ccr was significantly higher in
the patients than in normotensive subjects(Fig.5).

DISCUSSION

It has been reported that, in essential hypertension, the renal
kallikrein-kinin system was suppressed and suspected to be involved in the
development of high blood pressure(Margolius et al. 1971; Seino et al. 1975;
Shimamoto et al. 1981 & 1983). In this study, a clear suppresion of renal
kallikrein-kinin system was also observed in renoparenchymal hypertension.

Urinary kallikrein excretion was evaluated as the quantity and activity
by radioimmunoassay and kininogenase assay, respectively, and were
significantly decreased in patients with renoparenchymal hypertension. Since
urinary kallikrein excretion was significantly correlated with Ccr, the
decreased kallikrein excretion seemed to reflect the decreased renal
function. However, even when the urinary kallikrein excretion was corrected
with Ccr, this value was still lower in patients with renoparenchymal
hypertension than that in normotensive subjects. These findings were
compatible with that reported by Mitas et al.(1979), and may indicate that
the decrease of kallikrein excretion was due to not only a decrease of
functioning nephrones but also a lowering of the kallikrein excretion from
each of the functioning nephrones that remained. On the other hand, a marked
augmentation of FENa was observed in patients with renoparenchymal hypertension. This augmentation might be caused by pressure natriuresis mechanism,
to which kallikrein-kinin system in the kidney might not contribute since
the value of kallikrein excretion per functioning nephrone was clearly
decreased.

Kininase is another important factor in the kallikrein-kinin system.
The urinary kininase excretion in patients with renoparenchymal hypertension
was not significantly different from those in normotensive subjects.
However, the corrected value with Ccr was significantly higher in the
patient group. This increased kininase excretion from functioning nephrone
may indicate an increased degradation of kinin in each functioning nephrone
level.

Thus, in addition to the decrease of kallikrein excretion, an increase
of urinary kininase excretion was revealed in the patients with
renoparenchymal hypertension. This increase of kininase excretion may
contribute to the further suppression in the total activity of the renal
kallikrein-kinin system in this disease.

REFERENCES

Kondo,M., Shimamoto,K., Ura,N., Nishimiya,T., Mita,T., Nakagawa,M.,
     Maeda,T., Yamaguchi,Y., and Iimura,O. 1984, A simple and sensitive
     method for determination of human urinary kallikrein activity
     (kininogenase activity), using human low molecular weight kininogen.
     Endocrinol.Japon. 31:635
Margolius,H.S., Geller,R., Pisano,J.J., and Sjoerdsma,A. 1971, Altered
     urinary kallikrein excretion in human hypertension. Lancet,ii:1063
Mitas,J.A., Levy,S.B., Holle,R., Frigon,R.P., and Stone,R.A., 1978, Urinary
     kallikrein activity in the hypertension of renal parenchymal disease.
     N.Engl.J.Med. 299:162.
Seino,M., Abe,K., Otsuka,Y., Saito,T., Irokawa,N., Yasujima,M., Chiba,S.,
     and Yoshinaga,K. 1975, Urinary kallikrein excretion and sodium
     metabolism in hypertensive patients. Tohoku J.Exp.Med., 116:359

Shimamoto,K., Chao,J., and Margolius,H.S., 1980, The radioimmunoassay of
    human urinary kallikrein and comparisons with kallikrein activity
    measurements. J.Clin.Endocrinol.Metab., 51:840
Shimamoto,K., Ura,N., Tanaka,S., Ogasawara,A., Nakao,T., Nakahashi,Y.,
    Chao,J., Margolius,H.S., and Iimura,O., 1981, Excretion of human
    urinary kallikrein quantity measured by a direct radioimmunoassay of
    human urinary kallikrein in patients with essential hypertension and
    secondary hypertensive diseases. Jpn.Circ.J., 45:1092
Shimamoto,K., Nakao,T., Ura,N., Tanaka,S., Ando,T., Nishimiya,T., Mita,T.,
    Kondo,M., Nakagawa,M., and Iimura,O., 1983, The role of the renal
    kallikrein-kinin system in sodium metabolism in normal and low renin
    essential hypertension. Jpn.Circ.J., 47:1210
Ura,N., Shimamoto,K., Tanaka,S., Nishimiya,T., Mita,T., Nakagawa,M.,
    Maeda,T., Yamaguchi,Y., and Iimura,O., 1985, Urinary excretions of
    kininase I and kininase II activities in essential hypertension -
    A sensitive and simple method for its kinin-destroying capacity.
    J.Clin.Hypertens. 1:15

EFFECT OF ORAL POTASSIUM ON URINARY KALLIKREIN EXCRETION IN ESSENTIAL
HYPERTENSION

Eiki Murakami, Kunio Hiwada, Tatsuo Kokubu and Yoichi Imamura[*]

The 2nd Department of Internal Medicine, Ehime University
School of Medicine, Onsen-gun, Ehime 791-02, Japan
* The Department of Medicine, Matsuyama Red Cross Hospital
Matsuyama City, Ehime 791, Japan

INTRODUCTION

Renal kallikrein-kinin system is considered to play an important role
in the homeostasis of sodium and water balance in the kidney. Urinary
kallikrein originates from the kidney and the activity of kallikrein in
urine has been used as a marker of the activity of this system in the
kidney. Although many hormonal factors including aldosterone and antidiuretic hormone are known to stimulate the excretion of urinary kallikrein, the standard method to stimulate the release of kallikrein into the
urine is not available.

In this paper, we demonstrated that urinary potassium excretion was
more closely correlated with urinary kallikrein excretion than aldosterone
excretion both in dynamic and static sodium states in the body. We also
presented a useful releasing test for urinary kallikrein by oral supplement of potassium.

SUBJECTS AND METHODS

Subjects

The subjects were normotensive controls and essential hypertensive
patients aged 30 to 59 years. The essential hypertensive patients were
subgrouped as stage I and stage II by WHO stage classification. All
subjects were admitted to our hospital for examination. Informed consent
was obtained from each subject. All hypertensive patients were untreated
or withdrawn antihypertensive drugs for a minimum of 1 week before the
study.

Methods

Hypertonic saline infusion. The detailed test procedure was described
previously[1]. In summary, hypertonic saline (1.3 %, 525 ml) containing
120 mEq of sodium was administered to the subjects by 1 h-drip infusion.
Urine samples for measurements of kallikrein activity and potassium concentration and blood samples for plasma aldosterone concentration were
obtained before and after the saline infusion. The correlations between
urinary kallikrein and urinary sodium, potassium, volume or plasma aldosterone were compared.

<u>Oral sodium load</u>. The correlation of the change of urinary kallikrein with the changes of urinary electrolytes and aldosterone was examined in 3 different states of sodium intake. At the first period of 7 days, the subjects were plased on a mild salt restriction (Na: 120 mEq /day). Then, a low salt diet (Na: 30 mEq/day) was given for 5 days. After the low salt diet period, supplement of 290 mEq of sodium a day was given with a high salt diet and sodium tablets. On the last day of each period, the 24 h-urine sample for measurements of kallikrein activity, sodium, potassium and aldosterone concentrations was collected.

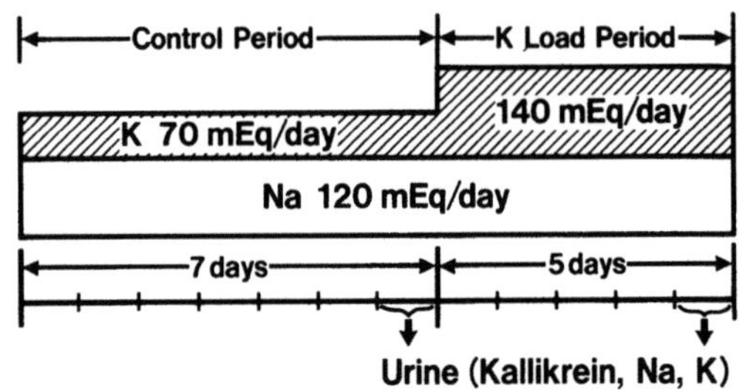

Fig. 1. The method of the releasing test for urinary kallikrein

<u>The releasing test for urinary kallikrein</u>. This study was performed in 7 normotensive control subjects (45 $\pm$ 4 years old), 10 stage I essential hypertensive patients (45 $\pm$ 3 years old) and 11 stage II essential hypertensive patients (47 $\pm$ 2 years old). Figure 1 shows the method of this study. After 7 days of control period when subjects took 120 mEq of sodium and 70 mEq of potassium a day, a supplement of another 70 mEq of potassium by taking potassium containing tablets (Slow K ®, Ciba-Geigy) was added to the control diet for next 5 days. The 24 h-urine sample for measurements of kallikrein, sodium and potassium was collected on the last day of the control and potassium load periods. Blood pressure in the supine position was measured on the final 2 days in each period.

<u>Analytical methods</u>. Sodium and potassium concentrations in the urine were measured by flame photometry. Urinary kallikrein activity was measured by colorimetric assay using prolyl-phenylalanyl-arginine-α -naphthylester as substrate, and kallikrein activity was expressed in terms of naphthol units (NU) by the method of Hitomi et al[2]. It was demonstrated that the esterase activity determined by this method correlated highly (r = 0.9) with both kininogenase activity and kallikrein concentration by direct radioimmunoassay in human urine in our laboratory. Linear regression analysis by the least-square method was used to evaluate correlations. The results were expressed as means $\pm$ S.E.M.. The significance of differences between mean values were evaluated by paired Student's t-test. Results with p<0.05 were cosidered statistically significant.

RESULTS

Correlation with urinary kallikrein

As shown in Table 1, the activity of urinary kallikrein was always
significantly correlated with urinary potassium both in acute sodium
load and oral sodium load. Aldosterone was significantly ($p < 0.05$) correlated with urinary kallikrein only in the static sodium state. The
excreted amount of urinary sodium and urinary volume did not correlate
with urinary kallikrein in the present study.

Table 1. Correlation with Urinary Kallikrein

	Urinary K	Plasma Aldosterone	Urinary Na	Urine Volume
Dynamic Na Load (Na Infusion) Before (n=48)	r = 0.60 (p 0.001)	r = 0.58 (p 0.001)	r = −0.39 (p 0.005)	r = −0.09 (NS)
After (n=48)	r = 0.63 (p 0.001)	r = 0.20 (NS)	r = 0.00 (NS)	r = 0.22 (NS)
	Urinary K	Urinary Aldosterone	Urinary Na	Urine Volume
Static Na Load (Oral Na Intake) (n=20)	r = 0.67 (p 0.001)	r = 0.37 (p 0.05)	r = 0.23 (NS)	r = 0.12 (NS)

r = correlation constant, n = number of dots evaluated,
NS = not significant

Effect of oral potassium load on urinary kallikrein excretion

As shown in Fig. 2, excreted amounts of urinary sodium and potassium
were similar in the 3 groups of subjects both in control and potassium
load periods. Basal level of urinary kallikrein was the highest in normotensive subjects, followed by stage II essential hypertensive patients.
The stage II patients showed the lowest value of basal urinary kallikrein.
In normotensives and stage I hypertensive patients, urinary kallikrein was
significantly ($p < 0.05$) increased accompanied with the increase in urinary
potassium excretion after oral potassium load. However, the stage II
hypertensive patients did not show any increase in urinary kallikrein
excretion by potassium load. Systolic and diastolic blood pressure in the
supine position did not significantly change in the 3 groups of subjects.

DISCUSSION

Aldosterone is considered to be the most important factor for
regulating urinary kallikrein excretion[3]. However, our result showed that
urinary kallikrein excretion more closely correlated with urinary potassium
excretion than with plasma aldosterone concentration and urinary aldosterone excretion. Zinner et al[4] first demonstrated the high correlation
between urinary kallikrein and urinary potassium. The site of urinary
kallikrein synthesis in the kidney is located at the distal and cortical
connective tubles[5] where potassium is excreted. The mechanism of stimulated excretion of renal kallikrein by potassium is not known. It is uncertain that potassium directly acts on the synthesis of kallikrein. In

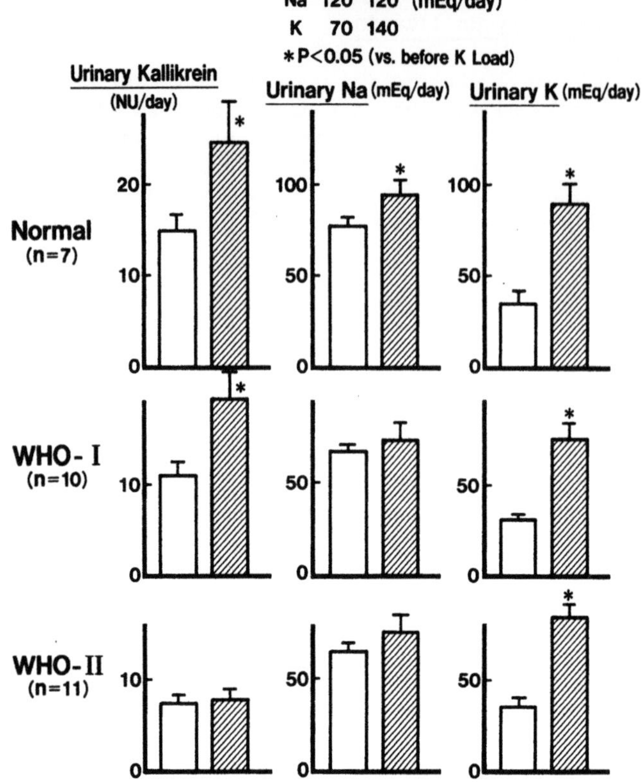

Fig. 2. Excretions of urinary kallikrein, sodium and potassium before and after oral potassium load. Values are means ± S.E.M.. n = number of subjects

all subjects in this study, supplementary potassium intake of daily 70 mEq to the control diet (120 mEq of sodium and 70 mEq of potassium) for 5 days was well tolerated without any side effects. Oral potassium load is seemed to be a convenient and useful method to see the reserved capacity of renal kallikrein synthesis.

The renal kallikrein-kinin system has been proposed to control the volume homeostasis by means of regulation of renal circulation and excretion of salt and water. Our previous study[1] indicated that WHO stage II essential hypertensive patients had exaggerated natriuretic and diuretic responses following a hypertonic saline infusion. The development of essential hypertension seems to induce a functional state that resembles expansion of extracellular fluid volume. Our present results suggest that the decreased functional role of renal kallikrein-kinin system may contribute to sodium and water retension in stage II essential hypertensive patients.

Zinner et al[4] observed that the children of hypertensive families excreted less kallikrein than the chidren of normotensive families and proposed the significance of the decreased function of renal kallikrein -kinin system in the pathogenesis of essential hypertension. Iimura et al[6]

reported that urinary kallikrein excretion was suppressed in essential
hypertension, especially in low renin groups of hypertension. They
considered that the suppression of renal kallikrein synthesis might
contribute to the etiological factor for low renin essential hypertension.
Renal damages caused by long duration of essential hypertension may
reduce kallikrein synthesis. We cannot assess from the present study
whether the decreased function of renal kallikrein-kinin system causes
blood pressure elevation in stage II essential hypertensive patients or
the long duration of blood pressure elevation produces the renal dysfunction with the reduced activity of renal kallikrein-kinin system in
advanced stage of essential hypertensive patients.

SUMMARY

Urinary kallikrein and potassium were excreted in parallel in not
only static but also dynamic sodium states. Oral potassium load stimulated
the release of urinary kallikrein in normotensive subjects and WHO stage
I essential hypertensive patients. Stage II essential hypertensive patients had the lowest value of basal level of urinary kallikrein and
showed no increase in urinary kallikrein by oral potassium load. These
results suggest that the functional activity of renal kallikrein-kinin
system decreases with the development of essential hypertension.

REFERENCES

1. T. Kokubu, K. Hiwada, T. Kobayashi et al, An exaggerated natriuretic
    response to hypertonic saline infusion in the stage II (WHO stage
    classification) essential hypertensive patients, Clin. Exp.
    Hypertens. A6:731 (1984).
2. Y. Hitomi, M. Ninobe and S. Fujii, A sensitive colorimetric assay for
    human urinary kallikrein, Clin. Chim. Acta 100:275 (1980).
3. M. Marin-Grez, Multihormonal regulation of renal kallikrein: The
    involvement of the renin-angiotensin-aldosterone system, the
    corticotropin-glucocorticoid system, antidiuretic hormone, cate-
    cholamines and prostaglandins, Biochem. Pharmacol. 31:3941 (1982).
4. S. H. Zinner, H. S. Margolius, B. Rosner et al., Familial aggregation
    of urinary kallikrein concentration in childhood: Relation to blood
    pressure, race and urinary electrolytes, Am. J. Epidemiol. 104:124
    (1976).
5. K. Omata, O. A. Carretero, A. G. Scicli et al, Localization of active
    and inactive kallikrein (kininogenase activity) in the micro-
    dissected rabbit nephron, Kidney Int. 22:602 (1982).
6. O. Iimura, K. Shimamoto, N. Ura et al, Study on the renal kallikrein
    -kinin system in normal and low renin subgroups of essential hyper-
    tension, J. Hypertens. 2(Suppl. 3):299 (1984).

THE EFFECTS OF AGING ON URINARY KALLIKREINS AND OTHER VASOACTIVE
SUBSTANCES IN ESSENTIAL HYPERTENSION

S. Fang, K. Abe*, K. Omata, M. Yasujima and K. Yoshinaga

The Second Department of Internal Medicine , *Department of
Clinical Biology and Hormonal Regulation , Tohoku University
School of Medicine 1-1,Seiryochyo, Sendai, Miyagi 980, Japan

INTRODUCTION

Previously we investigated the effects of aging on vasoactive substances
and other hormones which regulated the blood pressure in normal subjects.
The following is the result of that study. Although the level of renin
and aldosterone were decreased with aging, renin productivity was not
affected by aging. In addition, the synthesis of renal kallikrein and
renal prostaglandin decreased with aging in contrast to the increased
synthesis of renal thromboxane A_2 with aging.[1] It is uncertain of the
effects of aging on these substances in patients with essential
hypertension in comparison to normal subjects. In the present study, we
investigated the effects of aging on vasoactive substances and other
hormones related to regulating blood pressure in patients with essential
hypertension in comparison to normal subjects from young to elderly.

SUBJECTS AND METHODS

Studies were done in 90 patients with essential hypertension (47 men and
43 women), ranging in age from 20 to 93 yr. They were 4 patients in
stage I, 73 patients in stage II, and 13 patients in stage III of W.H.O
classification, and divided into 4 age-groups. All patients were
ambulatory and did not receive any medication at least for one week prior
to the study and allowed to take their regular diets. Blood pressure
was measured by the sphygmomanometer and blood sampling were performed in
fasting subjects kept in recumbent position of 2 hours in the morning. The
plasma samples were rapidly stored at -20°C in the freezer until the
measurment of plasma renin activity and plasma aldosterone concentration
and other laboratory examination. 24 hour urine was collected in the
refrigerator for consecutive three daysat 4°C. After measuring urine
volume, creatinine and electrolytes, urine samples were stored at -20°C in
the freezer until the measurement of urinary active kallikrein, total
kallikrein, prostaglandin E_2 and thromboxane B_2. Serum Na,K,Cl and
creatinine, and urinary Na,K,Cl and creatinine were measured by an
autoanalyzer (ASTRA-8,Beckman).
Plasma renin activity (PRA) was determined by means of radioimmunoassay
of angiotensin I (Abe et al.,1975)[2].
Plasma aldosterone concentration (PAC) was measured with a commercial
radioimmunoassay kit (Cer Ire Sorin).

Urinary active kallikrein excretion ($U_{A-K}V$) was measured as the kininogenase activity by the radioimmunoassay of generated kinin (Abe et al.,1978)[3]. Urine (20µl) was incubated with bovine low molecular weight kininogen (equal to 4000ng of generated kinin; supplied by Dr.Kato, Protein Research Institute, Osaka). After the incubation, the kinin generated during the incubation was determined by the method of Carretero et al.,(1976). In our method, the extraction procedure was not necessary, because low molecular weight kininogen had no cross reaction to our antiserum.

Urinary total kallikrein ($U_{T-K}V$) and inactive kallikrein ($U_{I-K}V$) were determined as following. Urine (10µl) was incubated with 10µg of trypsin at 37°C for 30 min, and also inactivated by 500µg of soy bean trypsin inhibiter (SBTI). After trypsin activation, $U_{T-K}V$ was determined by its kininogenase activity as same as $U_{A-K}V$. $U_{I-K}V$ was determined by the differance between $U_{T-K}V$ and $U_{A-K}V$.

Urinary prostaglandin E_2 excretion ($U_{PGE}V$) was measured as follows.

Urin (1ml) was acidified to pH 3.0-3.5 with 1N-hydrochrolic acid and extracted with 8 ml of ethylacetate. The dried organic extract was then chromatographed on a silicic acid column for prostaglandin (PG)E which was eluted by a mixture of benzene and ethylacetate according to Jaffe's method. The PGE fraction was dried and measured radioimmunologically using anti-PGE_2 antiserum (Pasteur Institute)[4].

Urinary thromboxane B_2 (TXB_2) was measured by radioimmunoassay[5]. 3 ml of urine was acidified to pH 2.4 with 1N-hydrochrolic acid and extracted with 4 volumes of chloroform. After evaporation of the organic phase, the dry residue was dissolved in 1ml of benzen / ethylacetate, 60:40 and applied onto a silicic acid column. TXB_2 was eluted with 4 ml of bezene / ethylacetate / methanol, 60:40:20.[2] After extraction, the samples were measured radioimmunologically by chacol method using anti-TXB_2 antiserum (perchased from Pasteur Institute).

RESULTS

The parameters of the subjects are shown in the Table. Urinary creatinine excretion ($U_{Cr}V$) was decreased with aging. Urinary sodium ($U_{Na}V$) and potassium (U_KV) excretion were decreased significantly in the age-group of 80 yr and above (p < 0.05) compared with age-group ranging in age from 40 to 59 yr. The level of serum creatinine was not different among each groups and was within normal limit. The level of blood urea nitrogen (BUN) tended to increase with aging within normal limit. Systolic and diastolic blood pressure in the age-group of 80 yr and above were significantly higher than that in the age-group of 40 to 59 yr. Creatinine clearance of 24 hour (Ccr24hrs) in the age-group of 80 yr and above was significantly lower than the age-group of 40 to 59 yr(p < 0.05).

Table 1. Comparison of parameters between different age-groups.

AGE(years)	20 − 39	40 − 59	60 − 79	80 −
Number	14	45	23	8
UcrV(g/day)	1.43 ± 0.15	1.08 ± 0.05	0.94 ± 0.05*	0.62 ± 0.11*
UNaV(mEq/day)	194.7 ± 16.4	231.7 ± 13.3	241.7 ± 26.3	152.6 ± 37.7*
UKV(mEq/day)	32.3 ± 4.5	39.4 ± 1.8	41.0 ± 3.7	26.8 ± 3.6*
SerumCr(mg/dℓ)	0.95 ± 0.05	0.94 ± 0.03	0.90 ± 0.04	0.91 ± 0.05
BUN(mg/dℓ)	12.6 ± 1.2*	15.5 ± 0.6	17.2 ± 0.9	19.0 ± 1.2*
SystBP(mmHg)	153.6 ± 7.3	144.9 ± 3.5	166.8 ± 3.5	173.8 ± 13.7*
DiastBP(mmHg)	93.3 ± 4.2	86.5 ± 2.1	92.6 ± 1.4	101.0 ± 6.9*
Ccr24hrs(ℓ/day)	128.2 ± 11.6	117.8 ± 4.9	111.7 ± 6.8	65.1 ± 3.7*

*p < 0.05

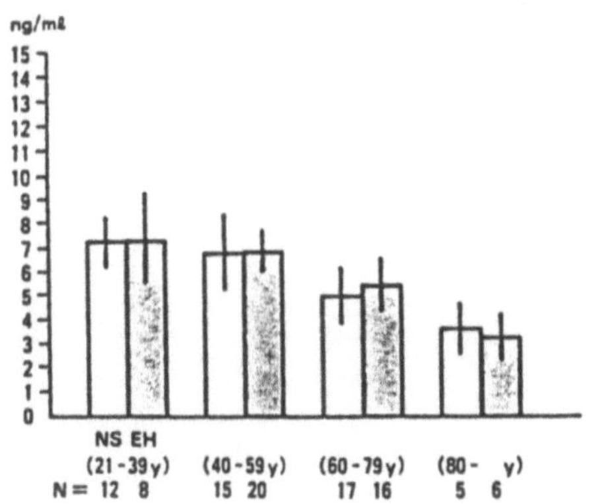

Fig. 1. Plasma renin activity in normal subject(NS) and essential hypertension(EH).

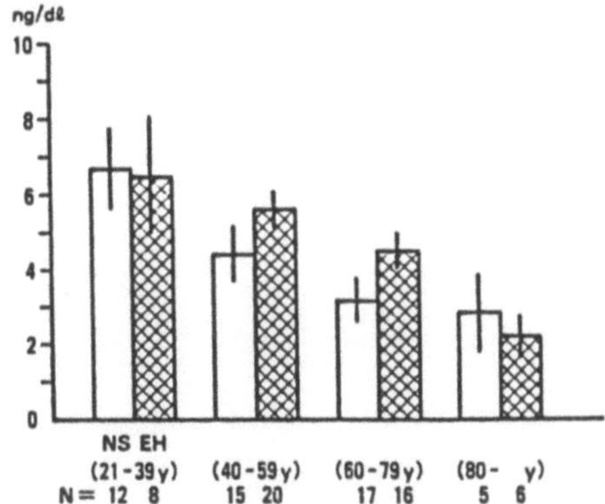

Fig. 2. Plasma aldosterone concentration in normal subject(NS) and essential hypertension(EH).

*open column;NS(normal subject), filled or hatched column;EH(essential hypertension)

Figure 1 to 6 show the results of humoral factors. PRA and PAC were investigated in the subjects whose urinary sodium excretion were above 150 mEq/day. PRA decreased with aging both in normal subjects and in the patients with essential hypertension. There was a significant reduction in PRA in the age-group of 80 yr and above compared with age-groups of 21 to 39yr and 40 to 59 yr, both in essential hypertension and in normal subjects.(Fig,1) The level of plasma aldosterone concentration (PAC) was also decreased with aging both in normal subjects and in essential hypertension,and there was no significant differance between them. (Fig,2)

Urinary excretion of total kallikrein ($U_{T-K}V$) decreased with aging in both groups and was also significantly lower in essential hypertension at the age-groups of 20 to 39 yr and 40 to 59 yr than those in age-matched normal subjects.(p<0.01, Fig,3) On the other hand, although the urinary excretion of active kallikrein ($U_{A-K}V$) was lower in the age-groups of 60 yr and above than younger groups in normal subjects, there was no significant age-related change in essential hypertension. Furthermore,in age-groups of 20 to 39 yr and 40 to 59 yr, urinary excretions of active kallikrein were significantly lower in essential hypertension than in age-matched normal subjects.(Fig,4) In addition, there were significant

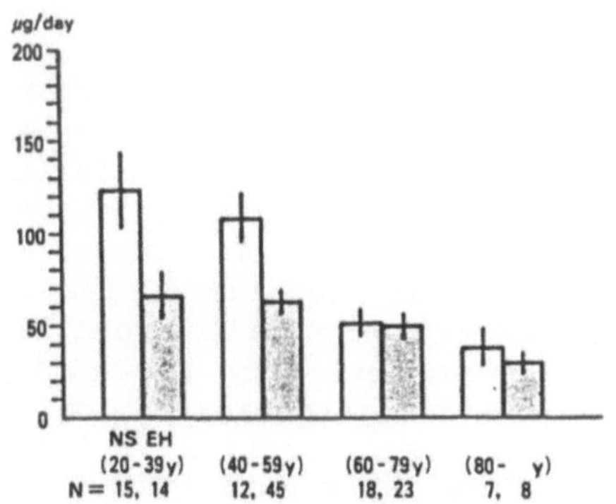

Fig. 3. Urinary excretion of total kallikrein in normal subject(NS) and essential hypertension(EH).

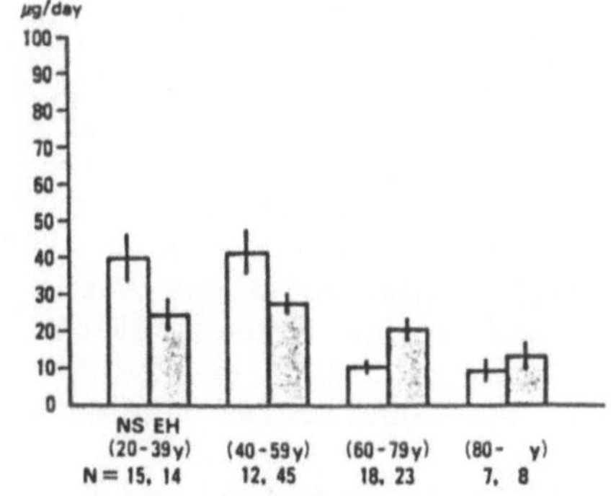

Fig. 4. Urinary excretion of active kallikrein in normal subject(NS) and essential hypertension(EH).

* open column;NS(normal subjects), filled column;EH(essential hypertension)

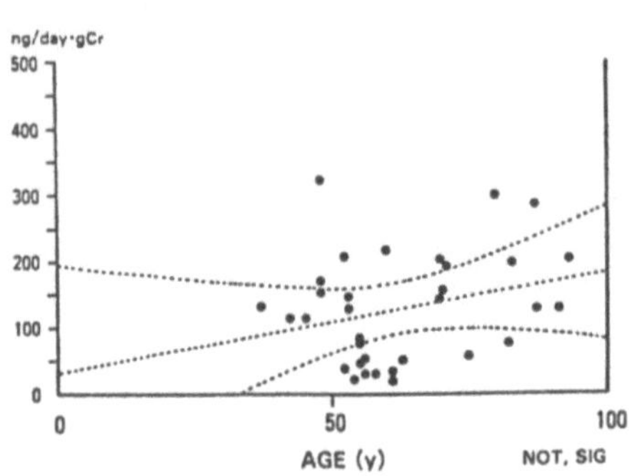
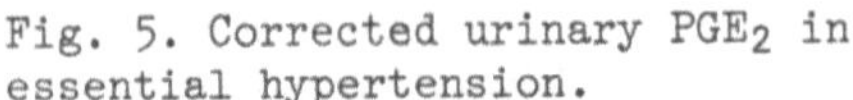

Fig. 5. Corrected urinary PGE₂ in essential hypertension.

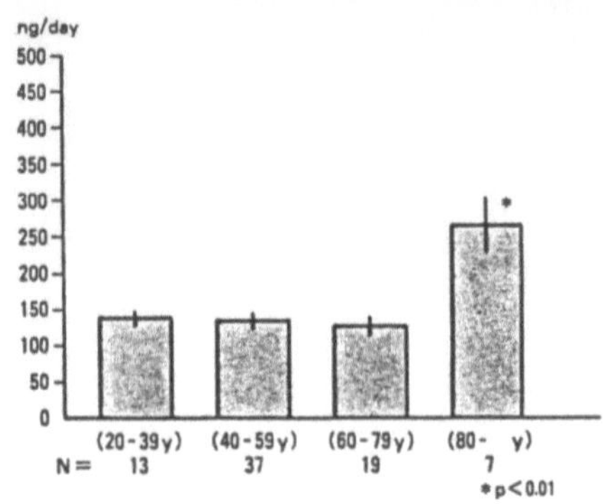

Fig. 6. Corrected urinary thromboxane B₂ in essential hypertension.

negative correlations with age in $U_{T-K}V$ and $U_{I-K}V$ (r=-0.23: p<0.05 , r=-0.24: p<0.05 respectively), and there was no age-related change of active kallikrein ratio which is the ratio of $U_{A-K}V$ to $U_{T-K}V$ in essential hypertension.

Since urinary PGE₂ is not a reliable indicater of renal PGE₂ synthesis in male subjects, we measured urinary PGE₂ only in female subjects (33 female patients, ranging in age from 37 to 93 yr) in the present study. As shown in Fig.5, there was no significant age-related changes in urinary excretion of PGE₂ in female patients with essential hypertension.

Since there is no sex differance in urinary excretion of thromboxane B₂ (TXB₂)corrected for urinary creatinine, we investigated 76 patients (39 men and 37 women, ranging in age from 20 to 93 yr) with essential hypertension. There was a significant positive correlation between age and urinary TXB₂ excretion (r=0.318; p<0.01),which was significantly higher in the group of 80 yr and above in patients with essential hypertension, that is almost consistent with our previous findings in normal subjects(data were not shown).

DISCUSSION

In the present study, we clearly demonstrated that plasma renin activity and plasma aldosterone concentration decreased with aging in patients with essential hypertension as well as in normal subjects. Since creatinine clearance decreased more markedly with aging than urinary sodium excretion, fractional sodium excretion increased with aging in consequence, and age related reduction of renin-angiotensin system may, at least in part, due to the increase of fractional sodium excretion[1]. In addition, as it is suggested that kallikrein is one of the factors stimulating renin secretion[6]-[7], age related reduction of R-A-A system may be influenced by the decrease of urinary kallikrein excretion in the elderly . Consequently the effect of aging on renin-angiotensin system were found in the patients with essential hypertension as same as in normal subjects. Since there is no age-related increase of plasma norepinephrine concentration in the elder patients with essential hypertension(Y.Miura et al., 1979), there might not exist the possibility that the function of the sympathetic β-receptors deteriorate in the elderly. It is interesting to note that urinary excretion of total kallikrein ($U_{T-K}V$)was already decreased from younger patients with essential hypertension. In addition, it is shown that the difference of $U_{T-K}V$ in subjects with essential hypertension and in normal subjects became small with aging. Urinary excretion of active kallikrein ($U_{A-K}V$) was not affected by aging and the difference of $U_{A-K}V$ in essential hypertension and in normal subjects also became small. However there was no age-related change in active kallikrein ratio in essential hypertension. It is known that aldosterone[8] and prostaglandin[9]-[10] are the factors to stimulate renal kallikrein synthesis. However, in this study, there was no difference in plasma aldosterone profiles between essential hypertension and normal subjects, plasma aldosterone might not contribute directly to this decrease of urinary kallikrein excretion in younger patients with essential hypertension. On the other hand, the decrease of urinary PGE_2 excretion might contribute to the decrease of urinary kallikrein excretion in young subjects with essential hypertension.

Renal PGE_2 excretion was not affected by aging and already decreased in younger patients with essential hypertension. This findings may suggest that aging process already advances in young patients with essential hypertension.

Renal TXB_2, which is the metabolites of renal TXA_2, increased with aging in essential hypertension as same as in normal subjects. Since it is suggested that renal TXA_2 plays an important role in developing the renal disease with increasing renal vascular resistance[11], it is conjectured that the level of urinary TXB_2 excretion in essential hypertension may be higher than that in normal subjects; however, further investigations may be required.

In conclusion, age-related changes in renal kallikrein, PGE_2 and TXB_2 synthesis might be involved in the pathogenesis of essential hypertension.

Acknowledgments

This work was supported by a Grant(No,62870011) from the Ministry of Education, Science and Culture and a Grant-in-Aid for Cardiovascular Disease from the Ministry of Health and Welfare(62-C-6) of Japan. The author is also indebted to Dr,M.Hayashi and staffs in Hiraka General Hospital for their assistance.

REFERENCES

1. K.ABE, M.YSUJIMA, K.OMATA, and K.TSUNODA , The Effect of Aging on Vasoactive Substances, Res.Rep.Takeda Med.Res,Found.,13,32-36(1986)
2. K.ABE, Y.OTSUKA, T.SAITO, C.SIANG, H.AOYAGI, N.IROKAWA, M.SEINO, S.MIYAZAKI, Y.MIURA, I.ONO, MINAI , Measurement of plasma renin activity by angiotensin-I radioimmunoassay. A modification of Haber's method. , Jpn.Circ.J 36. 741 (1972)
3. K.ABE, H.KATO, Y.SAKURAI, T.ITO, K.SAITO, T.HARUYAMA, Y.OTSUKA and K.YOSHINAGA , Estimation of urinary kininogenase activity using bovine serum low molrcular weight kininogen. In Kinins II , Biochemistry, Pathophysiology and Clinical Aspects, Edited by S.Fujii, H.Moriya, T.Suzuki, New York, Plenum Publishing Corporation,   105-114 (1979)
4. M.YASUJIMA, K.ABE, M.TANNO, K.YUTAKA, K.SATO, J.TAJIMA, K.KUDO, K.TSUNODA and K.YOSHINAGA , Renal Prostaglandin E in the Hypotensive Mechanism of MK-421 in conscious Rats. , Journal of Hypertension 2, 623-629, 1984
5. S.CHIBA, K.ABE, K.KUDO, K.OMATA, M.YASUJIMA, M.SATO and K.YOSHINAGA , Sex and age-related differences in the urinary excretion of TXB_2 in normal human subjects: A possible pathophysiological role of TXA_2 in the aged kidney. , Prostaglandins Leucotriens and Medicine 16,347 (1982)
6. Beierwaltes,W.H.et al. , Stimulation of renin by kallikrein and kinin isolated glomeruli., Physiologist 25(40):318,(1982)

7. Yun,J.et al., Role of prostaglandins in the control of renin secretion in the dog , <u>Circ.Res</u>.40:459,(1977)

8   Malgolius,H.S., Horowitz,D., Geller,R.G., Alexander,R.W., Gill,J.R., Pisano,J.J.,and Keiser,H.R., Urinary kallikrein excretion in normal man: relationship to sodium intake and sodium retaining steroids. , <u>Circ.Res</u>.,35,812(1974)

9. Mills,I.H., Kallikrein kininogen and kinins in control of blood pressure , <u>Nephron</u> 23:61(1979)

10. Nasjletti,A.et al. , Relationships between the kallikrein-kinin and prostaglandin system , <u>Life Sci</u>.25:99(1979)

11 K.KUDO, K.ABE, M.SEINO, M.YASUJIMA, M.SATO, K.OMATA, M.TANNO, M.KOTSUKI, K.YOSHINAGA and S.CHIBA , The urinary excretion of TXB_2 in normal human subjects: Sex and age differences. , <u>Japanese Journal of Medicine</u>. 75:626-632 (1986)

RENAL KININASES IN PRIMARY ALDOSTERONISM

Nobuyuki Ura, Kazuaki Shimamoto, Hitoko Ogata, Toru Sakakibara,
Toshiaki Ando, Shuzaburo Fukuyama, Motoya Nakagawa,
Shigeyuki Saito, Shigemichi Tanaka and Osamu Iimura

The Second Department of Internal Medicine, Sapporo Medical
College, S-1 W-16, Sapporo, Japan

SUMMARY

In order to further clarify the role of renal kallikrein-kinin (K-K)
system in primary aldosteronism (PA), daily urinary excretions of renal K-K
system components including kallikrein (KAL), kinin (KIN), total kininase
(K-ase), K-ase I, K-ase II and neutral endopeptidase (NEP) were measured in
PA and normotensives (NT). In this study, a new method for the simultaneous
determination of human urinary K-ase I, II and NEP was established and employed. The daily excretions of KAL was significantly higher in PA than
that in NT, while no difference was found in KIN between PA and NT. On the
other hand, total K-ase in PA (897 ± 258 µg/min/day) was significantly higher
than that in NT (209 ± 6). NEP was also significantly higher in PA (262 ± 22
µg/min/day) than that in NT (127 ± 6), whereas there were no differences in
K-ase I and K-ase II between PA and NT. The relative contributions of K-ase
I, II and NEP to total K-ase in NT were 14, 27 and 59 %, while those in PA
were 12, 17 and 36 %, respectively. As a result, these three K-ase contributed only 64 % to the total K-ase in PA. These findings suggested that 1)
NEP may play a major role in the catabolism of renal KIN in human, 2) NEP is
accerelated in PA, 3) unknown K-ase, different from K-ase I, II or NEP, may
exist in PA, and 4) accerelated renal K-ase activity may play some role on
the disorder of renal water-sodium metabolism and high blood pressure in PA.

INTRODUCTION

Recently, several reports have shown that the urinary kallikrein excretion does not necessarily reflect the true intrarenal kinins (1,2), known
as biological active substances of the renal kallikrein-kinin system.
Kinins are rapidly metabolized by enzymes collectively called kininases (3)
and renal tissue and urine both contain such kininases (3-6). Thus, the
intrarenal concentration of kinins may depend on both the production and
destruction of this peptide. Therefore, it is very important to determine
renal kallikrein, kinins and kininases, simultaneously for evaluation of the
renal kallikrein-kinin system. NEP (enkephalinase A), which cleaves to
kinins (7), is present in human (8,9) and porcine (7) kidneys and rat urine
(10), together with kininase I and II.
In this study, we established a method of simultaneous determination
for human urinary kininase I, kininase II and NEP, and estimated urinary

kininase I, II and NEP in patients with primary aldosteronism and normotensives, in addition to the measurements of urinary kallikrein and kinins,
to further elucidate the role of the renal kallikrein-kinin system in the
pathophysiology of primary aldosteronism.

MATERIALS AND METHODS

Subjects consist of twenty-one normotensives (NT) and eight patients
with primary aldosteronism (PA). All subjects were hospitalized and placed
on a regular diet containing 120 mEq/day of sodium and 75 mEq/day of
potassium without any medication for at least two weeks prior to examination. Twenty-four hour urine samples were collected daily for 3 days to
measure the renal kallikrein-kinin system components. Urine samples were
divided equally into two parts. Half the volume was put in a bottle with
400 μg of pepstatin dissolved in 10 ml of hydrochrolic acid for the measurement of urinary kinins, and the other half was put into a bottle without any
reagents for measurement of other components. In all subjects, renal function was within the normal range, as shown by the creatinine clearance of
more than 70 ml/min.

The urinary kallikrein (11) and kinins (12,13) were measured by direct
radioimmunoassay as reported by us. The details of the measurement of
urinary total kininase, kininase I, kininase II and NEP activities are shown
in Figure 1. Human urinary kininase was determined by measuring the hydrolysis of synthetic bradykinin and intact bradykinin was measured by kinins'
radioimmunoassay (12,13). The urine was desalted on a Sephadex G-25 fine
column. Thirty μl of a desalted urine sample and 50 μl of 0.1 M tris buffer

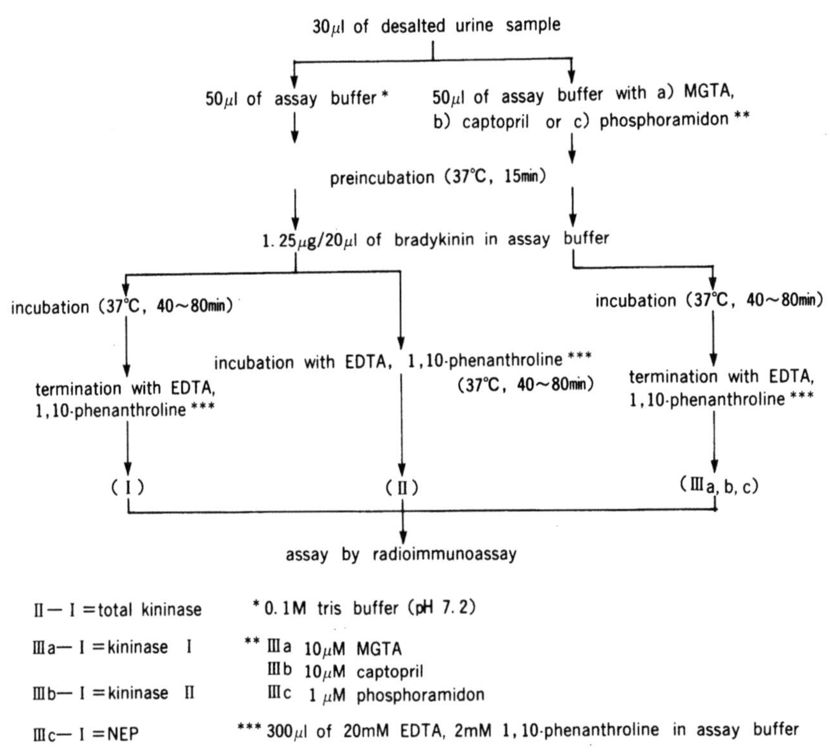

Fig. 1. Assay procedure for human urinary kininase I, kininase II and NEP
determination.

(pH 7.2) were mixed in a polypropylene tube, and preincubated at 37°C
for 15 min. Prewarmed 12.5 µg of synthetic bradykinin in 20 µl of assay
buffer was added to each tube to initiate the reaction. The mixture was
incubated for 40 to 80 min at 37°C. The reaction was terminated by the
addition of 300 µl of assay buffer containig 20 mM EDTA and 2 mM 1,10-
phenanthroline. Total kininase was calculated as the difference in kinin
concentration between the kininase inhibited and uninhibited sample.
Kininase I, II or NEP activity was determined by using their specific inhibitors; 2-mercaptomethyl-3-guanidinoethylthiopropanoic acid, captopril or
phosphoramidon.

All values were expressed as the mean+SEM. Statistical analysis was
performed with a student's t-test.

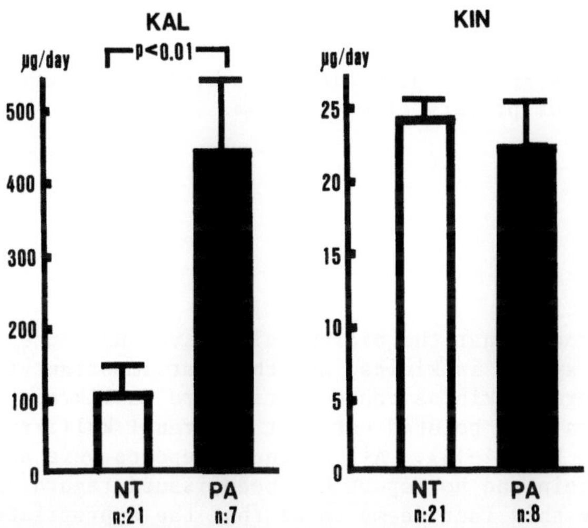

Fig. 2.   Urinary excretions of kallikrein and kinin in normotensives or
primary aldosteronism.

RESULTS

The daily excretions of kallikrein and kinin in NT or PA are shown in
Figure 2. Kallikrein was significantly higher in PA (445.3±93.5 µg/day)
than that in NT (127.6±17.7 µg/day), while there was no difference in kinins
between PA (22.6±2.6 µg/day) and NT (24.5±1.0 µg/day). Total kininase was
obviously higher in PA (836.9±198.9 µg/min/day) than that in NT (265.8±35.9
µg/min/day). In NT, urinary kininase I, kininase II and NEP were 36.1±4.4,
72.4±12.5 and 155.1±17.6 µg/min/day, and in PA, they were 101.9±28.6, 133.7±
27.6 and 261.7±21.6 µg/min/day, respectively (Fig. 3). Thus in PA, NEP was
significantly higher than that in NT, while no difference was observed in
kininase I or II between NT and PA. The relative contributions of kininase
I, II and NEP to total kininase are shown in Figure 4. In NT, kininase I,
II and NEP contributed 14±2m, 27±2 and 59±2% to total kininase, whereas they
contributed 12±2, 17±4 and 36±7% to total kininase in PA. As a result,
these three kininases contributed only 64% of the total kininase and not
100% in PA, while they contributed almost 100% in NT.

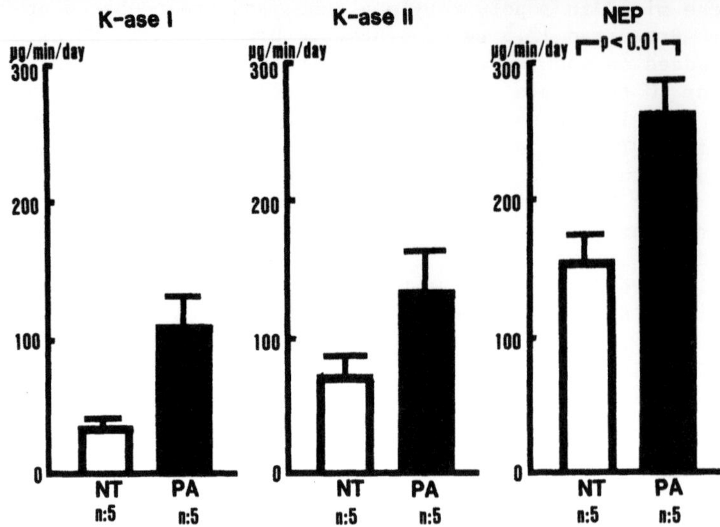

Fig. 3. Urinary excretions of kininase I, kininase II and NEP in normotensives or primary aldosteronism.

DISCUSSION

It is well known that the biological active substance in the
kallikrein-kinin system is kinins, and the most important factors that determine the intrarenal kinins concentration are kallikrein and kininases.
Some investigators have pointed out that the renal kallikrein-kinin system
is accelerated in PA (14-16). All of these reports were acomplished by
measuring kallikrein and no report has been issued regarding kininases. One
of the causes for this fact seems to be that the appropriate method for the
determination of urinary kininases has not been made available. Previously,
we reported a method to measure human urinary kininase I and kininase II
activities with bradykinin as a substrate (17); however, the technique employed has some limitations. First, kininase I activity was calculated by
subtracting the value of kininase II from that of the total kininase.
Second, phosphate buffer was employed as an incubation buffer, which may
act to suppress urinary NEP activity. Human (8,9) and animal (7,10) kidneys
are rich in NEP.

In this study, a very sensitive and specific assay system for human
urinary kininase I, II and NEP activities was established by using their
specific inhibitors. Unexpectedly, NEP contributed 59 % to total kininase
activity indicating that NEP is a major kininase also in normotensives, the
same as in the rat. Moreover another kininase, other than kininase I, II or
NEP may not exist in normotensives.

In primary aldosteronism, urinary kinins excretion remained within the
normal range in spite of accelerated urinary kallikrein excretion. Accelerated urinary NEP may be one of the causes for the discrepancy between urinary kallikrein and kinins excretions. Therefore, the renal kallikrein-
kinin system may not correlate with the acceleration of kallikrein excretion in PA (14-16). Moreover, almost one-third of kininase activity may be
due to an unknown kininase different from kininase I, kininase II or NEP.
Although accelerated plasma aldosterone or stimulated renal kallikrein may
be concerned with the mechanism of the acceleration of NEP or unknown
kininase, it is still remains unknown.

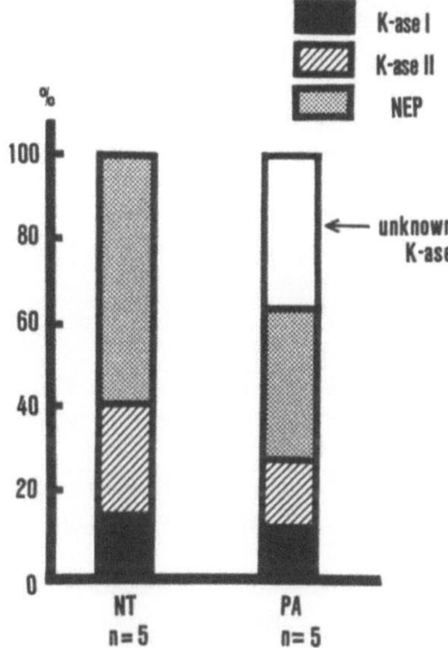

Fig. 4. Summation of relative contributions of kininase I, kininase II and NEP to total kininase in normotensives and primary aldosteronism.

From these results, it was suggested that accelerated renal kininase activity may play some role in the disorder of renal water-sodium metabolism and high blood pressure in primary aldosteronism.

ACKNOWLEDGEMENTS

The authors wish to thank Miss M. Mori, Miss R. Chiba and Miss M. Toyooka for their technical assistance.

REFERENCES

1. J. H. Vinci, R. H. Zusman, J. L. Izzo, R. E. Bowden, D. Horwitz, J. J. Pisano and H. R. Keiser, Human urinary and plasma kinins: relationship to sodium-retaining steroid and plasma renin activity, Circ. Res., 44:228-238 (1979).
2. A. G. Scicli, S. Rabito and O. A. Carretero, Blood and urinary kinins in human subjects during normal and low sodium intake, Proc. Int. Conf. Kinins. Adv. Exp. Med. Biol., 156A:877-882 (1982).
3. E. G. Erdos, Kinins, in bradykinin, kallidin and kallikrein, in: "Handbook of experimental pharmacology," E. G. Erdos, ed., Springer-Verlag, Heiderberg (1978).
4. T. Kokubu, I. Kato, K. Nishimura, K. Hiwada and E. Ueda, Angiotensin I-converting enzyme in human urine, Clin. Chim. Acta, 89:375-379 (1978).
5. R. A. Skidgel, R. M. Davis and E. G. Erdos, Purification of a human urinary kininase: a carboxypeptidase distinct from carboxypeptidase A, B or N, Anal. Biochem., 140:520-531 (1984).
6. E. Werle and E. G. Erdos, Über rine neue blutdrucksenkende, darm und uteruserregende Substanz in menschlichen, Urin. Arch. Exp. Pathol. Pharmakol., 223:234-243 (1954).

7. R. A. Mumford, P. A. Pierzchala, A. W. Strauss and M. Zimmerman, Purification of a membran-bound metalloendopeptidase from porcine kidney that degrades peptide hormones, Biochemistry, 78:6623-6627 (1981).

8. J. T. Gafford, R. A. Skidgel, E. G. Erdos and L. B. Hersh, Human kidney "enkephalinase", a neutral metalloendopeptidase that cleaves active peptides, Biochemistry, 22:3265-3271 (1983).

9. R. A. Skidgel, W. W. Schulz, L. T. Tam and E. G. Erdos, Human renal angiotensin I converting enzyme and its "helper enzyme", Kidney Int., (suppl 20) 31:S45-S48 (1987).

10. N. Ura, O. A. Carretero and E. G. Erdos, Role of renal endopeptidase 24.11 in kinin metabolism, Kidney Int., 32:507-513 (1987).

11. K. Shimamoto, J. Chao and H. S. Margolius, The radioimmunoassay of human urinary kallikrein and comparison with kallikrein activity measurements, J. Clin. Endocrinol. Metab., 51:840-848 (1980).

12. K. Shimamoto, T. Ando, T. Nakao, M. Sakuma and M. Miyahara, A sensitive radioimmunoassay method for urinary kinins in man, J. Lab. Clin. Med., 91:721-728 (1978).

13. K. Shimamoto, T. Ando, S. Tanaka, Y. Nakahashi, T. Nishitani, S. Hosoda, H. Ishida and O. Iimura, An improved method for the determination of human blood kinin levels by sensitive kinin radioimmunoassay, Endocrinol. Jpn., 29:487-494 (1982).

14. H. S. Margolius, R. Horwitz, J. J. Pisano and H. R. Keiser, Urinary kallikrein excretion in hypertensive man: relationship to sodium intake and sodium retaining steroid. Circ. Res., 35:820-825 (1974).

15. B. D. Holland, J. M. Chud and H. Braunstein, Urinary kallikrein excretion in essential and mineralocorticiod hypertension, J. Clin. Invest., 65:347-356 (1980).

16. K. Shimamoto, N. Ura, S. Tanaka, A. Ogasawara, T. Nakao, Y. Nakahashi, J. Chao, H. S. Margolius and O. Iimura, Excretion of human urinary kallikrein quantity measured by a direct radioimmunoassay of human urinary kallikrein in patients with essential hypertension and secondary hypertensive diseases, Jpn. Circ., 45:1092-1097 (1981).

17. N. Ura, K. Shimamoto, S. Tanaka, T. Nishimiya, T. Mita, M. Nakagawa, T. Maeda, Y. Yamaguchi and O. Iimura, Urinary excretions of kininase I and kininase II activities in essential hypertension: a sensitive and simple method for its kinin-destroying capacity, J. Clin. Hypertens., 1:15-22 (1985).

PURIFICATION AND IMMUNOLOGICAL PROPERTIES OF HUMAN URINARY KALLIKREIN AND
PROKALLIKREIN

Akiko Irie, Saori Takahashi, Yoshiaki Katayama,
Yukio Shibata*, and Yoshihiro Miyake

National Cardiovascular Center, Fujishiro-dai, Suita, Osaka
565, Japan. *Aichi Medical University, Nagakute, Aichi
480-11, Japan

SUMMARY

Human urinary prokallikrein and kallikrein have been purified from
the same source of urine simultaneously. The anti-kallikrein and anti-
prokallikrein antibodies were raised in rabbits using the purified
preparations. With respect to solid phase enzyme immunoassay (EIA),
immunoaffinity column chromatography, and single radial immunodiffusion,
reactivity of each antibody with kallikrein was distinctly different from
that with prokallikrein. Kallikrein could be determined by anti-
kallikrein antibody-immobilized EIA below 20 ng per ml, whereas
prokallikrein was undetectable. Prokallikrein became detectable at higher
concentrations, although it was less reactive than kallikrein. The
anti-prokallikrein antibody-immobilized EIA detected both kallikrein and
prokallikrein with the same sensitivity. However, the binding capacity
for kallikrein was about one-third less than that for prokallikrein. The
results show that kallikrein in human urine may be determined directly
and selectively. Similar difference in reactivity was observed with
immunoaffinity column chromatography and single radial immunodiffusion.
The presence of 3-4 antigenic sites per molecule was indicated by
quantitative precipitin reaction, and it is suggested from analysis of
amino acid sequence of kallikrein by the method of Hopp and Woods[1] that
four hydrophilic regions exist in kallikrein molecule.

Introduction

Tissue-type kallikrein in human urine is generally measured on the
basis of its hydrolytic activity toward ester bonds with kininogens or
synthetic substrates. The low specificity of the methods used, however,
prevents the accurate estimation of kallikrein. Moreover, the methods
cannot measure prokallikrein directly. Radioimmunoassay (RIA) and enzyme
immunoassay (EIA) procedures have thus designed as specific and sensitive
methods[2-4]. However, the results as to the reactivities of prokallikrein
in the immunoassays were contradictory. Therefore, it is necessary to
analyze the reaction using the purified prokallikrein. The reaction of
the anti-prokallikrein antibody with prokallikrein and kallikrein is also
important to solve the problem. As both human urinary kallikrein and
prokallikrein have been purified[5-10], it is now possible to study the
problems in detail.

In the present study, we have purified kallikrein and prokallikrein from the same source of human urine simultaneously and investigated the immunochemical properties using rabbit antibodies to solve the conflicting results regarding RIA and EIA of human urinary prokallikrein and kallikrein.

MATERIALS AND METHODS

Materials

Beta-galactosidase from E. coli was purchased from Boehringer Mannheim Co., TPCK-trypsin, soybean tryspin inhibitor and pepsin from Cooper Biochemical, and CNBr-activated Sepharose 4B from Pharmacia Fine Chemicals. Human urinary prokallikrein and kallikrein were purified by the procedure of Irie et al[10]. A typical preparation is shown in Table I. Rabbit anti-human urinary prokallikrein and kallikrein antisera were prepared by the procedure described previously[4]. Immunoglobulin in the antisera was purified by the method of Fudenberg[11] or with protein A Sepharose according Pharmacia's instruction. Immobilization of immunoglobulin to CNBr-activated Sepharose 4B was also performed according to Pharmacia's instruction.

Assays

Kallikrein activity was measured using Pro-Phe-Arg-MCA as a substrate. Single radial immunodiffusion was performed on a 1% agar gel plate containing 10 mM Tris-HCl, pH 7.5, 0.15 M NaCl, 0.02% NaN_3, 0.5%

Table I. Purification of Human Urinary (A) Prokallikrein and (B) Kallikrein

Step	Total Protein (mg)	Specific Activity (nmol/mg/min)	Purification (fold)	Yield (%)
(A) Prokallikrein				
1. Concentrated urine	1,520	22.3	1	100
2. DEAE-Sepharose	92.4	271	12.2	73.9
3. Aprotinin-Sepharose	79.8	256	11.5	60.3
4. IgG-Sepharose	1.25	10,600	475	39.1
(B) Kallikrein				
1. Concentrated urine	1,520	14.9	1	100
2. DEAE-Sepharose	96.7	131	8.79	56.0
3. Aprotinin-Sepharose	0.98	12,300	826	53.2

Prokallikrein and kallikrein were separated briefly by DEAE-Sepharose column chromatograly. Accordingly, purification was performed separately from Step 3. The activity of prokallikrein was measured after tryptic digestion .

sodium cholate and 5% antiserum by the method of Mancini et al.[12] The
reaction was carried out for 48 h at room temperature. Enzyme immunoassay
was performed by the procedure described previously[4]. Briefly, immunoglobulin fraction, $F(ab')_2$, was isolated from antiserum and then reduced,
β-galactosidase was labelled to the reduced immunoglobulin fraction,
$F(ab')$. $F(ab')_2$-coated polystyrene beads were prepared by immersing the
beads (6.5 mm) in 10 mM sodium carbonate buffer, pH 8.5, containing
$F(ab')_2$ overnight. With EIA, prokallikrein or kallikrein was reacted with
a $F(ab')_2$-coated bead for 4 h at 37°C with stirring and then overnight at
4°C. The bead was then reacted with β-galactosidase-labelled $F(ab')$ for 6
h at 25°C. Finally, β-galactosidase reaction was carried out at 37°C for
10 min. For immunoaffinity column chromatography, a solution containing
both purified prokallikrein and kallikrein was reacted with the antibody-
immobilized Sepharose in 10 mM phosphate buffer, pH 7.2, containing 0.15
M NaCl at 4°C overnight. The mixture was allowed to settle in a column.
The column was then washed with the same buffer containing 0.5% polyethylene glycol #6000. Next, the column was equilibrated with 0.1 M
acetate buffer, pH 5.8, containing 1 M NaCl and 0.5% polyethylene glycol
#6000, and then pH-gradient column chromatography was performed. Quanti-
tative precipitin reaction was performed by the procedure descirbed
previously[13]. Hydrophilic values of kallikrein molecule were estimated by
the method of Hopp and Woods[1] using amino acid sequence of human urinary
kallikrein (S. Takahashi et al., this proceedings).

RESULTS AND DISCUSSION

EIA of Prokallikrein and Kallikrein

With anti-kallikrein antibody-immobilized EIA (HUK-EIA), the dose
responce curve for kallikrein increased with increasing the concentration
of kallikrein, whereas that for prokallikrein was increased slightly and
almost undetectable below 20 ng per ml (Fig. 1A). At higher concentrations, the curve for kallikrein tended to reach the maximum between 50
and 100 ng per ml, and that for prokallikrein increased gradually up to
2,000 ng per ml, thus hard to observe the maximum. On the other hand,
with anti-prokallikrein antibody-immobilized EIA (HUPK-EIA), both curves
were close each other below 20 ng per ml (Fig. 1B). However, the slop of
the curve for kallikrein became less than that for prokallikrein with
increasing the concentration further. In the case of HUPK-EIA, the dose
responce curves for prokallikrein and kallikrein both almost reached the
maximum at around 50 ng per ml, and the fluorescence intensity with
kallikrein at saturation level was about one-third less than that with
prokallikrein. The results in Fig. 1 indicate that kallikrein in human
urine may be determined directly and selectively, and the conflicting
results that have been reported for determination of prokallikrein in
urine by RIA and EIA using the immobilized anti-kallikrein antibody may
be explained by the difference in reactivity of the anti-kallikrein
antibody for prokallikrein and kallikrein as shown in Fig. 1.

Immunoaffinity Column Chromatography and Single Radial Immunodiffusion

The elution profile of prokallikrein and kallikrein by pH-gradient
immunoaffinity column chromatography also differed. With anti-kallikrein
antibody-immobilized Sepharose column, prokallikrein was eluted as a
broad band with decreasing pH, whereas kallikrein was hardly eluted until
pH had decreased to 2.7. On the other hand, kallikrein was eluted as a
sharp band from anti-prokallikrein antibody-immobilized column when the
pH had decreased slightly from 5.8, and, in this case, prokallikrein was
eluted as a very broad band. With single radial immunodiffusion also,
kallikrein formed precipitin rings on the gel containing the anti-

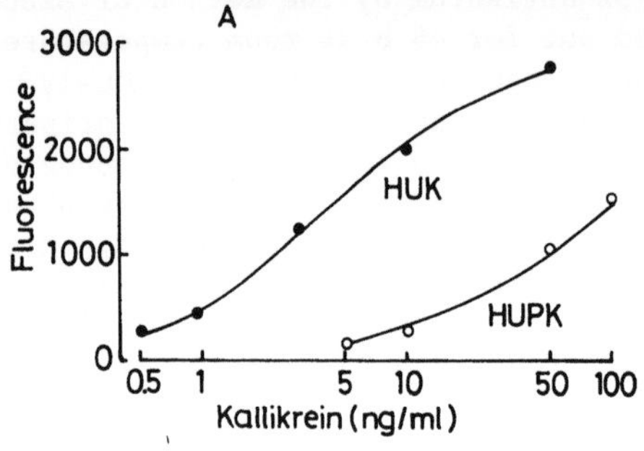

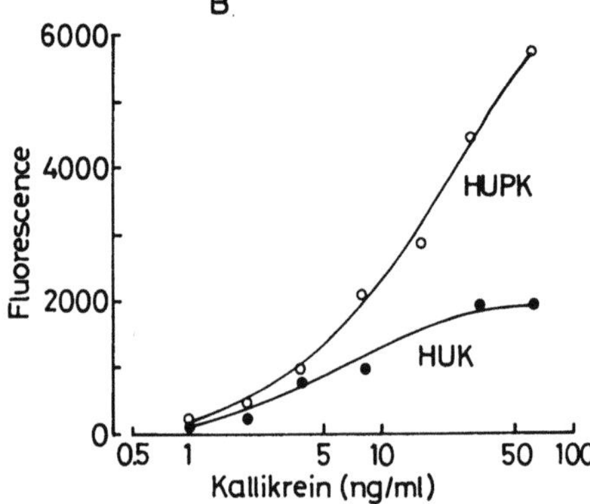

Fig. 1. Dose response curves for kallikrein (–●–) and prokallikrein (–○–)
on (A) HUK-EIA and (B) HUPK-EIA. The ordinate represents
fluorescence intensity with an arbitrary scale. HUK, human
urinary Kallikrein; HUPK, Human urinary prokallikrein.

kallikrein antiserum, and the density and diameter of the ring were
proportional to the amount of added kallikrein (20-200 ng), while prokallikrein did not produce any ring. In contrast, prokallikrein formed
precipitin rings on the gel containing the anti-prokallikrein antiserum
of which density and diameter were also dependent upon the concentration
of prokallikrein used (21-205 ng). The precipitin ring of kallikrein on
the gel containing anti-prokallikrein antiserum was small and faint in
the same concentration range. These results show that reactivities of
prokallikrein and kallikrein toward each antibody differ distinctly, as
was observed with EIA.

Quantitative Precipitin Reactions of Prokallikrein and Kallikrein

The results of quantitative precipitin reactions of prokallikrein and
kallikrein are shown in Fig. 2. Each curve was then analyzed in the zone
of antibody excess. As shown in the insets, plots of r/(A) against r
showed a straight line, where r and (A) represent the number of molecules of antibody bound per mol of antigen and the concentration of
uncombined antibody, respectively, and the apparent association constant
(K) of antigen and antibody and the number of antigenic site per molecule (n) were obtained from the slope of the line and the intercept on
abscissa. The results were shown in the insets of Fig. 2. No distinct

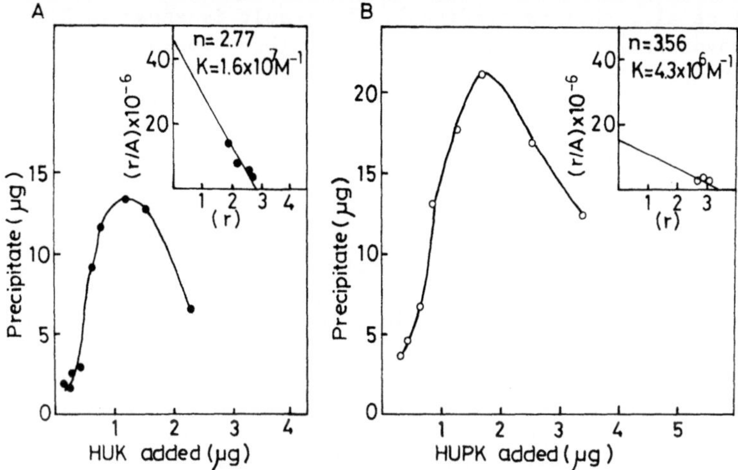

Fig. 2. Quantitative precipitin curves of the reactions of (A) HUK with anti-HUK IgG and (B) HUPK with anti-HUPK IgG. The inset, plots of r/(A) against r.

difference were noted between prokallikrein and kallikrein, although there are some difference in the values between the two.

Hydrophilic Regions of Kallikrein Molecule

In connection with the number of antigenic site of prokallikrein and kallikrein, hydrophilic regions of kallikrein molecule were analyzed by the method of Hopp and Woods[1]. Amino acid sequence of human urinary kallikrein that we have recently determined was used for the anaysis (S.

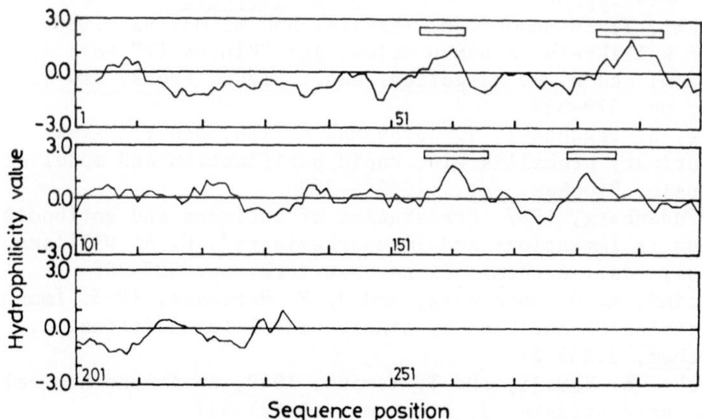

Fig. 3. Hydrophilic values of human urinary kallikrein by the procedure of Hopp and Woods[1]. Open boxes represent hydrophilic regions of kallikrein molecule.

Takahashi et al., this proceedings). The result is shown in Fig. 3. Four distinct hydrophilic regions were observed (Open boxes). As human urinary and porcine pancreatic kallikreins showed about 70% sequence homology, we constructed a model structure of human urinary kallikrein using computer graphics based on three dimensional structure of porcine pancreatic kallikrein[14]. In the model, it was shown that all of the four hydrophilic regions were oriented at the surface of the molecule.

REFERENCES

1. T. P. Hopp, and K. R. Woods, 1981, Prediction of protein antigenic determinants for amino acid sequences, Proc. Natl. Acad. Sci. USA, 78:3824-3828
2. M. R. Silver, O. ole-MoiYoi, K. F. Austen, and J. Spragg, 1980, Active site radioimmunoassay for human urokallikrein and demonstration by radioimmunoassay of a latent form of the enzyme, J. Immunol., 124:1551-1555
3. N. B. Oza, W. Lieberthal, D. B. Bernard, and N. G. Levinsky, 1981, Antibody that recognizes total human urinary kallikrein: Radio-immunological determination of inactive kallikrein, J. Immunol., 126:2361-2364
4. A. Irie, Y. Katayama, K. Ito, S. Takahashi, and Y. Miyake, 1985, Determination of human urinary kallikrein by an enzyme immunoassay method, Jap. J. Clin. Chem., 14:27-33
5. R. Geiger, K. Mann, and T. Bettels, 1977, Isolation of human urinary kallikrein by affinity chromatography. Determination of human urinary kallikrein, I, J. Clin. Chem. Clin. Biochem., 15:479-483
6. O. ole-MoiYoi, J. Spragg, and K. F. Austen, 1979, Structural studies of human urinary kallikrein (urokallikrein), Proc. Natl. Acad. Sci. USA, 76:3121-3125
7. A. Irie, H. Kushiro, J. Kodama, M. Ohta, and Y. Miyake, 1982, Isolation and properties of human urinary kallikrein and urokinase, in: "Recent Progress on Kinins," H. Fritz, G. Dietze, F. Fiedler, and G. L. Harberland, eds., Birkhauser, Basel Boston Stuttgart, pp. 131-136
8. Y. Takada, R. A. Skidgel, and E. G. Erdös, 1985, Purification of human urinary prokallikrein. Identification of the site of activation by the metalloproteinase thermolysin, Biochem. J., 232:851-858
9. K. Kizuki, Y. Shimamoto, M. Ikekita, and H. Moriya, 1986, An inactive form of kallikrein in human urine, in: "Kinins IV" Part A, L. M. Greenbaum, and H. S. Margolius, eds., Plenum Press, New York and London, pp. 329-337
10. A. Irie, S. Takahashi, Y. Katayama, K. Ito, and Y. Miyake, 1986, Human urinary prokallikrein: Rapid purification and model activation by trypsin, Biochem. Int., 13:375-382
11. H. H. Fudenberg, 1967, Preparation of antigens and antibodies, in: "Methods in Immunology and Immunochemistry", C. A. Williams, and M. W. Chase, eds., Academic Press, New York, pp. 307-385
12. G. Mancini, A. O. Carbonara, and J. F. Heremans, 1965, Immunochemical quantitation of antigens by single radial immunodiffusion, Immunochem, 2:235-254
13. Y. Miyake, K. Yamaji, and T. Yamano, 1969, An immunochemical study of D-amino acid oxidase, J. Biochem., 65:531-537
14. W. Bode, Z. Chen, K. Bartels, C. Kutzbach, G. Schmidt-Kastner, and H. Bartunik, 1983, Refined 2 Å X-ray crystal structure of porcine pancreatic kallikrein A, a specific trypsin-like serine proteinase. Crystallization, structure determination, crystallographic refinement, structure and its comparison with bovine trypsin, J. Mol. Biol., 164:237-282

CHARACTERIZATION OF N-LINKED OLIGOSACCHARIDES OF HUMAN

URINARY KALLIKREIN MOLECULES

Masahiko Ikekita, Kazumasa Aoki, Masafumi Kamada,
Kazuyuki Kizuki and Hiroshi Moriya

Department of Biochemistry, Science University of
Tokyo, Shinjuku-ku, Tokyo 162, Japan

SUMMARY

The micro-heterogeneity due to varied N-linked oligosaccharides
of both active- and pro-types of human urinary kallikrein (HUK) in
normal subjects and some patients were investigated by the methods
of serial lectin affinity chromatography and crossed affino-
immunoelectrophoresis. In the case of both types of normal HUK, the
species carring tri- and/or tetra-antennary oligosaccharide(s), core-
fucosylated bi-antennary oligosaccharide(s), and bi-antennary
oligosaccharides containing outer galactose residues and an N-
acetylglucosamine residue linked β1,4 to a β-linked mannose residue
(bisecting N-acetylglucosamine residue) amounted to approximately
36, 33 and 17% of the total of each type of HUK, respectively. On
the other hand, in some diseases, i.e. essential hypertension, Bartter's
syndrome and acute pancreatitis, alterations of the chromatographic
and electrophoretic patters were observed and are assumed to correspond
to glycosylation changes in each HUK molecule.

INTRODUCTION

In the case of Bartter´s syndrome, the HUK showed the same
immunoreactivities as normal HUK against anti-normal HUK antibody,
but the electrophoretic mobility of the HUK was slower than that of
normal HUK(1). These preliminary results suggest that in Bartter's
syndrome, the transformational change(s) were induced mainly in the
carbohydrate moieties of the HUK molecule.

It has recently been reported that changed patterns of micro-
heterogeneity and/or structures of oligosaccharides of glycoproteins
such as α-fetoprotein(2), γ-glutamyltranspeptidase(3), chorionic
gonadotropin(4) and thyroglobulin(5) were induced by malignant
transformation. HUK is also expected to be one of the useful markers
for the diagnosis of renal disease and there has been considerable
interest in the study of the carbohydrate structures and/or the micro-
heterogeneity of HUK from patients.

This paper deals with the pattern of micro-heterogeneity and
the carbohydrate structures of both active- and pro-types of HUKs
derived from normal subjects and some patients as elucidated by serial
lectin affinity chromatography and crossed affino-immunoelectrophoresis.

The results obtained from normal subjects and some patients are compared and discussed.

MATERIALS AND METHODS

Materials

Concanavalin A (Con A) and wheat germ agglutinin (WGA) were purified from jack bean meal and wheat germ, respectively and coupled to carboxyl-Sepharose 4B(6). Erythroagglutinating phytohemagglutinin (E-PHA)-, leukoagglutinating phytohemagglutinin (L-PHA)- and lentil lectin-agarose were purchased from E.Y Laboratories, San Mateo, USA. α-Methyl-D-glucose (α-MeGlc) was from Nakarai Chemicals, Kyoto, Japan. Trypsin (type III-S) and soybean trypsin inhibitor (type I-S, SBTI) were from Sigma Chemical, St. Louis, USA. Prolyl-Phenylalanyl-arginine -4-methylcoumaryl-7-amide (H-Pro-Phe-Arg-MCA) was from the Protein Research Foundation, Osaka, Japan. Anti-HUK antibody was prepared as described previously(1). Seakem Agarose (ME) was from Marine Colloids, Rockland, USA. Other chemicals were of guaranteed reagent grade.

Methods

Kallikrein Assay ----Amidolytic activity of HUK toward H-Pro-Phe-Arg-MCA was determined by a slight modification of the method of Iwanaga et al(7). The amount of active HUK was determined as differential activity in the absence and presence of anti-HUK antibody. After activation with trypsin(8), differential activity in the absence and presence of the antibody was measured as total (active plus pro) HUK activity, and the pro-HUK activity was defined as differential activity between total and active HUK(6).

Preparation of HUKs ---- Individual samples of normal (HUK-Na, -Nb, -Nc and -Nd) and patients HUKs were partially purified from fresh urine (each 5-7 l) of normal subjects (Na, Nb, Nc and Nd, respectively) and patients by the following steps, i,e, DEAE-Sephadex A-50 adsorption and elution (batch method) after dialysis against tap water and ammonium sulfate precipitation (80% saturation precipitate). The precipitate was dissolved in deionized water and dialyzed against TBS (0.01M Tris, 0.15M NaCl, 1mM CaCl$_2$, 1mM MgCl2, 0.02%(W/V) NaN3, pH 8.0) for 24 h at 4°C.

Sugar analysis of kallikreins, lectin affinity chromatography and crossed affino-immunoelectrophoresis were done according to our previously described methods with minor modification(6,9). Other methods with kallikrein were carried out as previously reported (1,10).

RESULTS AND DISCUSSION

Active HUK purified from urine of healthy males is a glycoprotein with a carbohydrate content of 23.5%(W/W), and as the main amino sugar is N-acetylglucosamine, the oligosaccharides bound to the HUK molecule might be mainly Asn-linked type(s)(6). Furthermore, preliminary observations obtained from analysis of the sugar moieties of active-type HUK showed that the charge heterogeneity of HUK may arise from micro-heterogeneity in the sugar moiety of this enzyme. In order to obtain a better understanding of the nature of heterogeneity in both active- and pro-types of HUK, we have developed procedures of serial lectin affinity chromatography and lectin affino- immuno-electrophoresis for the detection and fractionation of molecular variants depending on the differences in the affinities of Asn-linked oligosaccharides for lectins. Lectins have been widely used for the study of the structures and functions of glycoproteins. Previous studies from a number of laboratories have established that Asn-linked oligosaccharides can be effectively fractionated on columns of immobilized lectins(11,12).

Analysis of the Pattern of Heterogeneity of Normal HUK by Using Immobilized Lectins

In this study, we showed that the majority of the Asn-linked oligosaccharides of both active- and pro-types of HUK can be fractionated by serial chromatography on Con A-, E-PHA-, lentil lectin- and WGA-agarose columns, according to the method of Cummings and Kornfeld(11). This method of fractionation is simple, rapid and sensitive, and allows for quantitative estimates of the component Asn-linked oligosaccharide(s) of active- and pro-types of HUK. For example, in the case of active HUK in normal subjects, the species containing tri- and/or tetra-antennary oligosaccharide(s) account for approximately 36%, the species containing core-fucosylated bi-antennary oligosaccharide(s) account for 33%, and the species containing bi-antennary oligosaccharides with outer galactose residues and an N-acetylglucosamine residue linked β1,4 to a β-linked mannose residue (bisecting N-acetylglucosamine residue) account for 17% of the total active type HUK. The profiles of micro-heterogeneity found by serial lectin affinity chromatography of the pro-type HUK in normal subjects were similar to those of the active-type HUK. These data are summarized in Fig. 1 and Table I.

Analysis of the Pattern of Heterogeneity of Normal HUK by Crossed Affino-immunoelectrophoresis

Normal HUKs (HUK-Na, -Nb, -Nc, and -Nd) were also analyzed by crossed affino-immunoelectrophoresis with Con A. The electrophoregrams

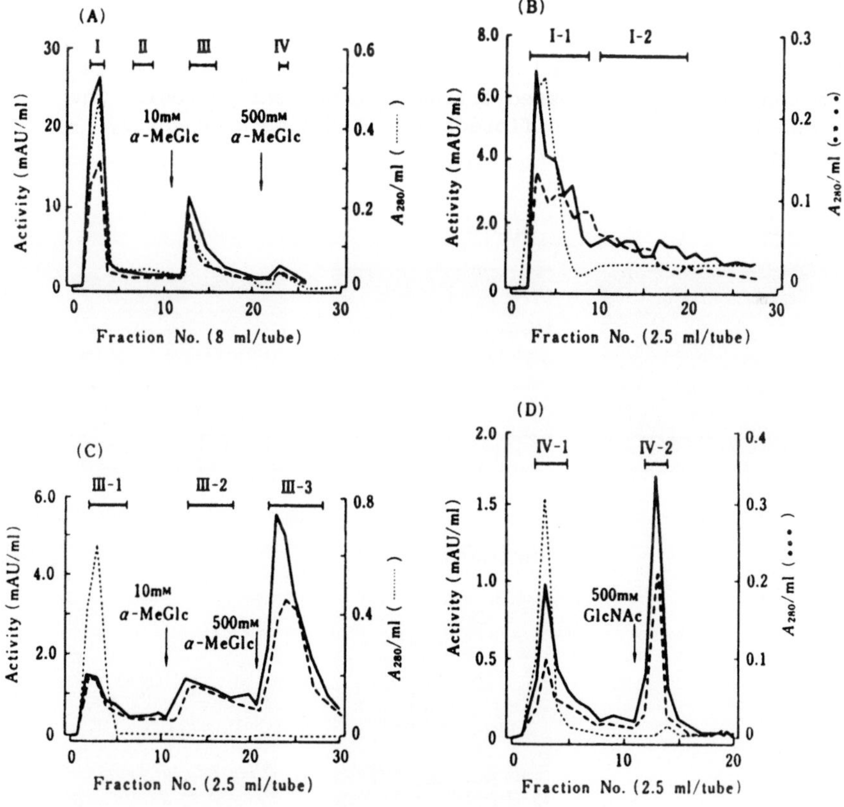

Fig. 1. Lectin-Agarose Affinity Chromatography of HUK from One Normal Individual(HUK-Na). Partial purified HUK-Na was applied to Con A-Sepharose(A), E-PHA-agarose (B), lentil lectin-agarose(C) and WGA-Sepharose(D) columns as described in Materials and Methods and Results. Activity: - - -, active HUK; ——, pro HUK.

Table 1. Patterns of Micro-heterogeneity of Active- and Pro-Types of Normal
HUKs Determined by Serial Lectin Affinity Chromatography.

Fraction	Proportion (%) Active (Pro)	Characteristics of oligosaccharides bound to HUKs
I-1	36 (36)	Tri- or tetra-antennary
I-2	17 (17)	Bi-antennary with bisecting GlcNAc
II	9 (8)	
III-1	6 (6)	Bi-antennary without fucose
III-2	9 (10)	Bi-antennary with fucose
III-3	24 (23)	
IV-1	3 (4)	High-mannose type
IV-2	3 (3)	Hybrid type

are shown in Fig. 2. The conventional crossed immunoelectrophoresis
of normal HUK (HUK-Na) with a second-dimensional gel impregnated with
monospecific anti-HUK antibody gave a single precipitation peak (Fig.
2, control HUK-Na). Including free Con A in the first-dimensional
gel leads to the appearance of two main peaks (peaks A and B) which
reflect different degrees of interaction and/or different numbers
of binding sites between the Con A and HUK molecules (containing
active and pro HUKs) (Fig. 2, Na-Nd). It was found that peak A
included nonreactive HUK, and that peak B corresponded to weakly and
strongly reactive HUKs (data not shown). In individual normal HUKs,
fractions A and B accounted for 36%-52% and 48%-57% of the tatal HUK,
respectively. In the case of HUK-Nc, a small nonmigrating fraction
(peak C) was observed (Fig. 2).

The analysis of affinity for Con A was carried out by two methods,
i.e. the enzymochemical method of affinity chromatography and the
immunochemical method of crossed affino-immunoelectrophoresis. The
results obtained by the two different analytical methods mostly
coincided well with each other.

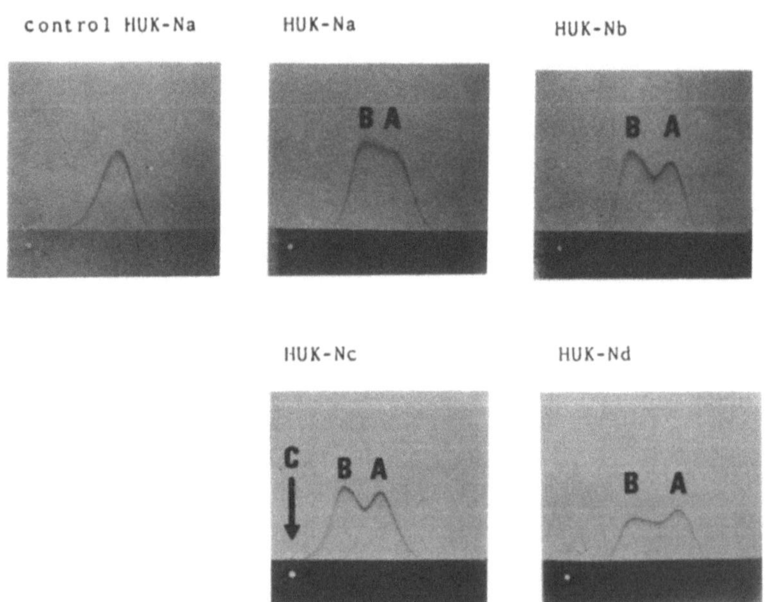

Fig. 2. Crossed Affino-immunoelectrophoresis of HUKs from Normal Individuals.
Experimental details are given in the text.[6] Control HUK-Na was subjected to electrophoresis without free Con A in the first-dimensional
gel and other procedures were similar to those applied to the test
samples.

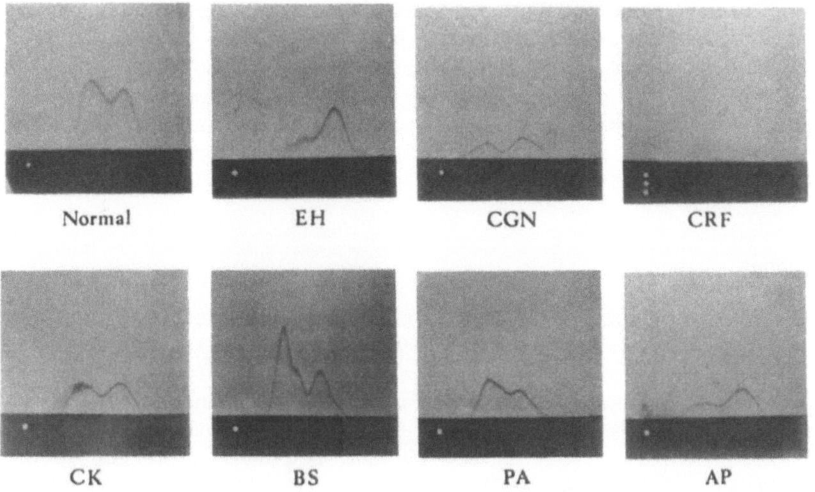

Fig. 3. Crossed affino-immunoelectrophoresis of HUKs excreted from a normal
subject and some patients. In analysis of CRF-HUK, three times volume
of sample solution was applied. AP; acute pancreatitis, EH; essential
hypertension, CGN; chronic glomerulonephritis, CRF; chronic renal
failure, NS; nephrotic syndrome, CK; polycystic kidney, BS; Bartter's
syndrome, PA; primary aldosteronism.

Analysis of Sugar Moieties of Patients Individual HUKs

The investigations of characteristics of HUK in diseased states
are necessary to elucidate the relationships between HUK and diseases.
The results obtained from two analytical methods coincided with each
other, i.e. in EH, CRF and AP, the radio of Con A unbound or nonreactive HUK was increased in each analytical method (Fig. 3). The
carbohydrate structures of Con A unbound glycoprotein is thought to
possess bi-antennary complex type sugar chains with bisecting N-
acetylglucosamine and/or tri- or more branched complex type sugar
chains(13). So that it was suggested that the ratio of such sugar
chains was increased in EH-, CRF- and AP-HUK.

In the analysis of EH-HUK by E-PHA-agarose column, altered
chromatographic patterns found in half of the four EH patients
suggested alterations of the sugar moieties. These two patients had
relatively lower blood pressures (case 1, 166/90mmHg; case 2, 146/86mmHg
than the other EH patients.

In the cases of BS and PA, the proportion of Con A weakly bound
HUK, which is thought to possess the bi-antennary complex type sugar
chain without bisecting N-acetylglucosamine(13), was increased (Fig.
3). These facts suggested the possibility that excess aldosterone
might influence the processing of sugar moieties of kallikrein, as
for sample, it might decrease the activity of N-acetylglucosamine
transferase III which transfers bisecting N-acetylglucosamine residue.

Some investigators have attempted to apply the alterations of
heterogeneity of glycoproteins to clinical diagnosis(2). Namely, it
might be useful for differential diagnosis to investigate the difference
in crossed affino-immunoelectrophoretic pattern of α-fetoprotein from
patients with hepatoma and yolk sac tumor(2). As concerns HUK,
detailed investigations of the alterations might lead to a new method
for differential diagnosis or early detection in some extent.

However, it is impossible to draw any such conclusion from our
present results because our obseration has been based on a small
number of patients.

In this paper, we succeeded in fractionating both active- and
pro-types of HUK molecules. Because of their simplicity, serial

lectin agarose chromatography and crossed affino-immunoelectrophoresis
are expected to provide a powerful general approach for detection
of subtle changes of oligosaccharides of both active and pro HUKs
that might occur in various disorders. Studies of carbohydrate micro-
heterogeneity in HUKs from various patients with various renal disorders
is in progress. This work could help to solve the problem of the
physiological and/or pathological significance of the tissue kallikreins.

<u>References</u>

1. M. Ikekita, K. Kizuki and H. Moriya, Immunological Relationships
   of the Glandular Kallikrein, <u>Chem. Pharm. Bull.</u>, 31, 2466(1983).
2. J. Breborowicz and A. Mackiewicz, Application of Lectin Affinity
   Electrophoresis for Studies of Microheterogeneity of Human
   Alphafefetoprotein "<u>Lectins-Biology, Biochemistry, Clinical
   Biochemistry</u>," Vol. 1, ed. by T.C. Bog-Hansen, Walter de Gruyter,
   Berlin, 1981, pp.303-314.
3. K. Yamashita, A. Hitoi, N. Taniguchi, N. Yokosawa, Y. Tsukada
   and A. Kobata, Comparative Study of the Sugar Chains of -
   Glutamyltranspeptidases Purified from Rat Liver and Rat AH-
   66 Hapatoma Cells, <u>Cancer Res.</u>, 43, 5059 (1983).
4. T. Mizuochi, R. Nishimura, C. Derappe, T. Taniguchi, T. Hamamoto,
   M. Mochizuki and A. Kobata, Structures of the Asparagine-linked
   Sugar Chains of Human Chorionic Gonadortopin Produced in
   Choriocarcinoma, <u>J. Biol. Chem.</u>, 258, 14126 (1983).
5. K. Yamamoto, T. Tsuji, O. Tarutani and T. Osawa, Structural Changes
   of carbohydrate Chains of Human Thyroglobulin Accompanying
   Malignant Transormations of Thyroid Glands, <u>Eur. J. Biochem.</u>,
   143, 133 (1984).
6. M. Ikekita, T. Masunaga, K. Kizuki and H. Moriya, Human Urinary
   Kallikrein.II. Analysis of Asparagine-Linked Oligosaccharides
   by Using Lectins, <u>Chem. Pharm. Bull.</u>, 35, 2071 (1987).
7. S. Iwanaga, T. Morita, H. Kato, T. Harada, N, Adachi, T. Sugo,
   I. Maruyama, K. Takada, T. Kimura and S. Sakakibara, Fluorogenic
   Peptide Substrates for Proteases in Blood Coagulation, Kallikrein-
   Kinin and Fibrinolysis System, "<u>Advances in Experimental Medicine
   and Biology; NININS-II</u>", Vol. 120A, ed. by S. Fujii, H. Moriya
   and T. Suzuki, Plenum Press, New York, 1979, pp. 147-163.
8. K. Kizuki, M. Ikekita, Y. Shimamoto and H. Moriya, Porcine
   Pancreatic Prokallikrein. I. Its Partial Purification and
   Effects of Various Proteases on its Activation, <u>Chem. Pharm.
   Bull.</u>, 31, 1052(1983).
9. T. Masunaga, K. Yamanoue, K. Aoki, M. Kamada, M. Ikekita, K.
   Kizuki, H. Moriya, K. Kimura, T. Ikari and Y. Atomi, Observation
   of the Varied Micro-Heterogeneous Forms of Human Urinary
   Kallikrein Individually Excreted in Some Diseases, <u>Jap. J.
   Clin. Chem.</u>, 16, 8 (1987).
10. M. Ikekita, H. Moriya, S. Ozawa and K. Kizuki, Studies on
    Heterogeneous Components of Hog Pancreatic Kallikrein.
    "Possible Role of the Neuraminic Acid Residues", <u>Chem. Pharm.
    Bull.</u>, 29, 545(1981).
11. R. D. Cummings and S. Kornfeld, Fractionation of Asparagine-linked
    Oligosaccharides by Serial Lectin-Agarose Affinity Chromatography
    <u>J. Biol. Chem.</u>, 257, 11235 (1982).
12. E. P. Cowan, R.D. Cummings, B.D. Schwartz and S.E. Cullen, Analysis
    of Murine Ia Antigen Glycosylation by Lectin Affinity
    Chromatography, J. Biol. Chem., 257, 11241 (1982).
13. K. Kornfeld, M.L. Reitman and R. Kornfeld, The Carbohydrate-
    binding Specificity of Pea and Lentil Lectins. <u>J. Biol. Chem.</u>,
    256, 6633 (1981).

RAT SUBMANDIBULAR GLAND KALLIKREINS A AND B: ISOLATION, PURIFICATION AND
PROPERTIES

Audrey H.I. Salgado*, Glênio R.T. Siqueira**, Luis Juliano***
and Amintas F.S. Figueiredo*

*Departamento de Bioquímica e Imunologia do ICB da UFMG, Caixa
Postal 2486, 31270 Belo Horizonte, MG, Brazil. ** Departamento
de Fisiolgoia e Biofísica do ICB da UFMG, Belo Horizonte, MG
Brazil. ***Departamento de Biofísica, Escola Paulista de
Medicina, São Paulo, SP, Brazil

INTRODUCTION

Kallikreins (EC.3.4.21.8) are a group of serine proteinases with
specific and limited proteolytic activity. They release vasoactive peptides,
kinins, from the substrates, kininogens, present in plasma, lymph and
interstitial fluid in mammals (Schachter, 1980). There are two kinds of
kallikreins - glandular kallikreins, derived from glandular sources - and
plasma kallikreins - present in plasma or serum (Webster, 1970). Three
types of kininogens have already been described: high - molecular - mass
kininogen, low-molecular - mass kininogen and T-kininogen (Müller - Esterl
et al, 1986). The last one seems to be present only in the rat (Barlas et
al, 1985) Glandular kallikreins are found in salivary glands, pancreas,
small and large intestine, kidney, urine and plasma or serum (Geiger and
Fritz, 1981).

The submandibular gand is one of the richest source of kallikrein in
the organs of the rat (Orstavik, 1972).

An interesting biological property of rat glandular kallikrein is the
contraction of the isolated rat uterus that it causes, without the addition
of kininogen, observed for the first time by Beraldo et al (1966) and whose
mechanism remains uncertain. Pure rat submandibular gland kallikrein is
needed for further characterization of the enzyme and for studies in order
to explain the mechanism of the kallikrein - induced rat uterus contraction.

In the present wook we describe a purification procedure which
permited us to completely purify two forms of rat submandibular gland
kallikreins and a comparison of some of their properties.

MATERIALS AND METHODS

Kinin-releasing activity. Substrate preparation. Rat substrate was
prepared by a modification of the method of Henriques and Allan (1972).
For this purpose, rat plasma was heated at 61°C/1 h and centrifuged at
805 g/1 h. The supernatant was made 1 mM in Na$_2$EDTA and precipitated with
ammonium sulfate at 50% saturation. The mixture was centrifuged at 7500 g/
1 h and the precipitate was dialyzed and freeze dried. A 20 mg/ml in
200 mM Tris-HCl pH 8.2, 1 mM in NaCl was used in the assay of kinin-

release. The incubation mixture containing 300 ul of substrate plus 20 ul
of an appropriate kallikrein solution was incubated 1 min at 37°C and the
reaction was stopped by the addition of 10 ul of Trasylol (Bayer). The kinin
released was determined through biological assay using isolated rat uterus
according to Geiger and Fritz (1981). Bradykinin (Departamento de Biofísica,
Escola Paulista de Medicina, São Paulo, SP, Brazil at a 100 ug/ml solution
in saline was used as standard.

Amidasic activity with Acetyl-Phe-Arg-p-nitroanilide (APApNA, Juliano
and Juliano, 1985, Departamento de Biofísica, Escola Paulista de Medicina,
São Paulo,SP, Brazil). The amidasic activity with APApNA as substrate was
performed according to Erlanger et al (1961) and Mares-Guia (1968). The
incubation mixture contained 1 mM APApNA and 50 ul of an appropriate
kallikrein solution. After 30 min at 37°C the reaction was stopped by the
addition of 50 ul of 60% (v/v) acetic acid solution. The absorbance of the
reaction was read at 405 nm.

Protein determination. Protein was determined by the method of Lowry
et al (1951).

SDS/Polyacrylamide gel electrophoresis (SDS/PAGE). SDS/PAGE was
performed in 10% acrylamide (Bio-Rad) gels containing 0.1% SDS(Sigma)
according to the method of Laemmli(1970).

Isoelectric focusing. Isoelectric points were determined by
electrofocusing kallikreins at 200 V for 18 h at room temperature, in 5%
acrylamide gels containing 5% ampholine (LKB), pH 3.0 - 6.0, according to
Figueiredo et al (1983).

Analytical gel filtration. The apparent molecular weight of
kallikreins were determined by gel filtration on a calibrated column of
Sephadex G-100 (Pharmacia).

Purification of kallikrein. All the steps of this purification were
carried out at 4°C. Kallikrein was purified from rat submandibular gland
of female Wistar rats (180 - 200 g). The glands were minced and homogeneized
in a Tri-R-Stirr homogeneizer model 563 C in 10 mM sodium phosphate pH 7.0
containing 0.1 % Triton-X. The misture was centrifuged at 2000 g/90 min.
The supernatant, was fractionated with ammonium sulfate at 30 - 80%
saturation. The mixture was centrifuged at 5000 g/1 h and the precipitate
was disolved and dialyzed in 10 mM sodium phosphate pH 6.0, 100 mM in
NaCl. The kallikrein solution was applied to a column (2.4 x 20 cm) of DEAE-
-Cellulose DE-52 (Whatman) washed and eluted according to Nustad and Pierce
(1974). The kallikrein pool was applied to a column (2.1 x 6.0 cm) of
aprotinin-Sepharose (Sigma) which was washed and eluted according to Geiger
and Fritz (1981). The kallikrein pool was applied twice to the same column
of Sephadex G-100. The kallirein pool from the second gel filtration
chromatography was stored frozen.

RESULTS

Purification of kallikrein. Results of purification of kallikrein are
summarized in Table I.
By the six-step procedure, a 760 - fold purification was attained with
a yield of 14%. Figure 1 shows the gel filtration chromatography which
separated 2 kallikrein components (RSGK-A and RSGK-B).
The second gel filtration of RSGK-A and RSGK-B on Sephadex G-100
column are shown in Figures 2 and 3 respectively.

Table I. Purification of Rat Submandibular Gland Kallikreins(RSGK-A, RSGK-B)

purification steps	total protein (mg)	specific activity [ug of bradykinin equivalents(mg of protein)$^{-1}$.min^{-1}]a	total activity [ug of bradykinin equiv. min^{-1}]	x-fold purification	yield %
(1) Crude extract	840	23.6	19824	1	100
(2) Ammonium sulfate fractionation (30-80% saturation)	168.2	82.7	13908	3.5	70
(3) DEAE-Cellulose	24.8	351.7	8723	15	44
(4) Aprotinin-Sepharose	1.72	2,935.4	5049	124	25
(5) Sephadex G-100					
RSGK-A	0.52	3,196.8	1662	135	8
RSGK-B	0.26	7,684.6	1998	325	10
(6) Twice Sephadex G-100					
RSGK-A	0.15	10,589.8	1536	448	8
RSGK-B	0.10	17,846.1	1285	756	6

a-treated rat plasma

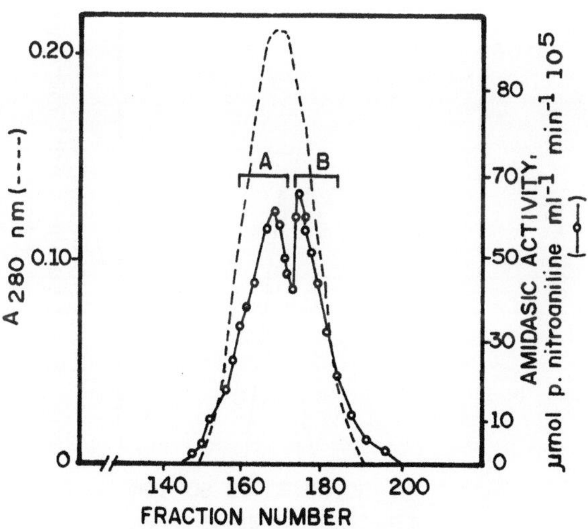

Figure 1. Gel filtration over Sephadex G-100: 1.72 mg of protein applied to a 1.2 x 114 cm column, equilibrated with 25 mM sodium phosphate, pH 7.0, 500 mM in NaCl. Elution took place with the same buffer; fraction volume 1.8 ml; activity was determined with APApNA/as in Material and Methods.

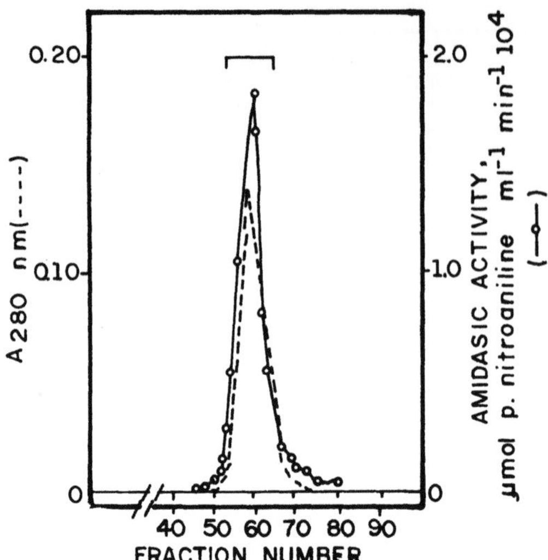

Figure 2. Gel filtration over Sephadex G–100: 0.52 mg in protein of RSGK–A applied to a 1.2 x 114 cm column, equilibrated with 25 mM sodium phosphate pH 7.0, 500 mM in NaCl. Elution took place with the same buffer; fraction volume 1.8 ml; activity was determined with APApNA as in Material and Methods.

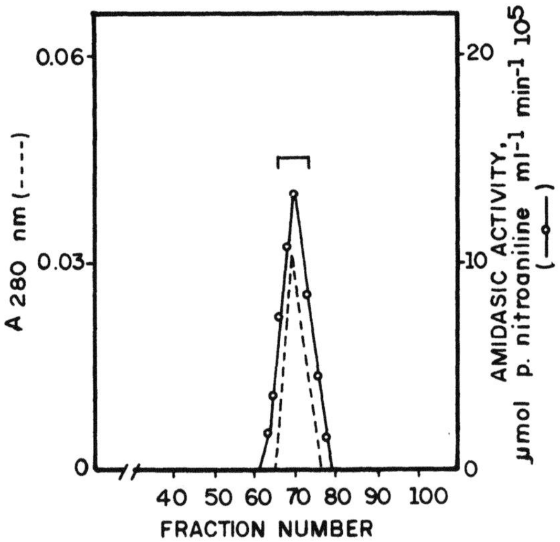

Figure 3. Gel filtration over Sephadex G–100: 0.26 mg in protein of RSGK–B applied to a 1.2 x 114 cm column, equilibrated with 25 mM sodium phosphate pH 7.0, 500 mM in NaCl. Elution took place with the same buffer; fraction volume 1.8 ml; activity was determined with APApNA as in Material and Methods.

<u>Molecular properties</u> - Table II shows the physicochemical properties of rat submandibular gland kallikreins.

Table II. Physicochemical Properties of Rat Submandibular Gland
Kallikreins (RSGK-A, RSGK-B)

| Kallikrein | Apparent Molecular Weight | | pI |
	Filtration	SDS/PAGE	
RSGK-A	33884	31623	4.02
RSGK-B	21380	19840	4.13

DISCUSSION

The six-step procedure used in this work allowed us to completely purify rat submandibular gland kallikrein. Two kallikrein components RSGK-A and RSGK-B homogenous on SDS/PAGE and on isoelectric focusing were obtained. Tunes et al (1984) also isolated and purified two components (α and β) from rat urinary kallikrein.

The specific kinin-releasing activities determined for RSGK-A and RSGK-B using rat substrate, are the highest already reported for glandular kallikreins. An interesting result was found when the specific kinin--releasing activities of RSGK-A and RSGK-B were compared with their apparent molecular weights.

Thus, RSGK-A which has the highest apparent molecular weight, shows the smallest specific kinin-releasing activity. On the other hand, RSGK-B which has the smallest apparent molecular weight shows the highest specific releasing activity. Completely different results were obtained in this laboratory with human urinary kallikreins which showed a direct correlation between specific kinin-releasing activity and apparent molecular weight.

The pI values determined for RSGK-A and RSGK-B agree with those found by Brandtzaeg et al (1976) for rat submandibular gland kallikrein.

The results described here emphasize the important point that futher chemical, physicochemical and biological studies with these kallikreins are necessary for better assess about differences and similarities on their properties.

ACKNOWLEDGEMENTS

This work was supported by grants from CPq/UFMG No 230072, 062635/85; CNPq Proc. 408243/85-BF, FINEP /Bioquímica-552 and PADCT/FINEP-558.

REFERENCES

Barlas, A., Okamoto, K., and Greenbaum, L.M., 1985, T-Kininogen. The major plasma kininogen in rat adjuvant arthritis, <u>Biochem. Biophys. Res. Commun.</u>, 129: 280.

Beraldo, W.T., Araujo, R.L., and Mares-Guia, M., 1966, Oxytocic esterase in rat urine. Am. J. Physiol., 211: 975.

Brandtzaeg, P., Gautvik, K.M., Nustad, K., and Pierce, J.V., 1976, Rat submandibular gland kallikrein: Purification and cellular localization. Br. J. Pharmac., 56: 155.

Erlanger, B.F., Kokowsky, N. and Cohen, W., 1961, The preparation and properties of two new chromogenic substrates of trypsin, Arch. Biochem. Biophys., 95: 271.

Figueiredo, A., Takii, Y., Tsuji, H., Kato, K., and Inagami, T., 1983, Rat Kidney renin and cathepsin D: purification and comparison of properties, Biochemistry, 22: 5476.

Geiger, R., and Fritz, H., 1981, Human urinary kallikrein, in: Methods in Enzymol., Academic Press, Inc. New York, 80: 466.

Henriques, O.B. and Allan, L., 1972, Glass activated kallikrein from human plasma, Biochem. Pharmacol., 21: 3163.

Juliano, M.A. and Juliano, L., 1985, Synthesis and kinetic parameters of hydrolysis by trypsin of some acyl-arginyl-p-nitroanilides and peptides containing arginyl-p-nitroanilides, Brazilian J. Med. Biol. Res., 18: 435.

Laemmli, U.K., 1970, Cleavage of structural proteins during the assembly of the head of bateriophage T4, Nature, 227: 680.

Lowry, O.H., Rosebrough, N.J., Farr, A.L., and Randall, R.J., 1951, Protein measurement with the Folin phenol reagent, J. Biol. Chem., 193: 265.

Mares-Guia, M., 1968, Hydrophobic interactions in the trypsin active center. The sensitivity of the hydrophobic binding site to side chain modifications in competitive inhibitors of the amidinium type, Arch. Biochem. Biophys., 127: 317.

Müller-Esterl, W., Iwanaga, S., and Nakanishi, 1986, Kininogens revisited, Trends Biochem. Sci., 11: 336.

Nustad, K. and Pierce, J.V., 1974, Purification of rat urinary kallikreins and their specific antibody, Biochemistry, 13: 2312.

Orstavik, T.B., 1978, The distribution and secretion of kallikrein in some organs of the rat, Acta Physiol. Scand., 104: 431.

Schachter, M., 1980, Kallikreins (kininogenases) – A group of serine proteases with bioregulatory actions, Pharmacol. Rev.., 31:1.

Tunes, H., Silva, and Mares-Guia, M., 1983, Alpha-and Beta-rat urinary kallikreins: chemical and physicochemical properties, Brazilian J. Med. Biol. Res., 16: 193.

Webster, M.E., 1970, Recommendations for nomenclature and units, in: Handbook of Experimental Pharmacology, Ed. Erdös, E., Springer-Verlag, New York, Vol. 25: 659.

HUMAN SALIVARY KALLIKREIN AND SUBMAXILLARY GLANDS KALLIKREINS

Yoshifumi Matsuda,* Yukio Fujimoto,** Yasuhiro Watanabe,**
Tadashi Obara*** and Sumiyuki Akihama*

*Department of Biochemistry, Meiji College of Pharmacy
Tokyo 154, **Department of Clinical Biochemistry, Hokkaido
Institute of Pharmaceutical Sciences, Otaru 047-02 and
***Central Research Laboratories, Yamanouchi Pharmaceutical
Co. Ltd, Tokyo 174, Japan

INTRODUCTION

Glandular kallikreins (EC 3.4.21.35) are known to be members of a
closely related subfamily of serine proteases, which cleave the substrate
kininogen, and release the vasoactive peptides of kinins. On the other
hand, certain kallikreins seemed process biologically active peptides and
some protein precursors. Mason et al.[1] have reported that the kallikrein
gene family of male mouse submaxillary glands comprises highly homologous
genes that encode specific proteases involved in the processing of
biologically active peptides.

Recently, Nakanishi's group has reported that the amino acid
sequence of human pancreatic kallikrein was deducible from the cloned
cDNA sequence, and that it was identical with human urinary kallikrein.[2]
Furthermore, they have shown, by means of blot-hybridization technique
that human pancreatic kallikrein mRNA is expressed not only in the kidney
but also in the sublingual glands.

Human salivary kallikrein is apparently secreted from the salivary
glands, i.e., glandula submaxillaris, sublingualis and parotis. We are
very interested in human salivary glands kallikrein and its related
enzymes, if any, and its secreted form in the saliva. In the present
study, we first purified human salivary kallikrein and then compared the
determined sequence with those of other kallikreins. Then, we performed
the partial purification of the kallikrein obtained from submaxillary
glands, and examined some properties of the submaxillary glands kallikrein, of the kallikrein-like esteropeptidase, and of the purified human
salivary kallikrein.

MATERIALS AND METHODS

<u>Materials</u>. Human saliva was collected from healthy adults of both sexes.
Human submaxillary tissues with no pathological changes observed at
autopsy were kindly provided, after chemical and histological examinations, by the Department of Pathology, Sapporo Medical College.

Enzyme assays. Esterolytic activity was determined by both colorimetry and spectrophotometry.[3] Amidolytic activity was assayed according to a modification of the method of Amundsen et al.[4] The assaying of kallikrein activity on the basis of vasodilation was performed as described previously.[3]

Electrophoresis. Polyacrylamide gel electrophoresis was performed in the presence of SDS according to the method of Laemmli.[5] Isoelectric focusing was performed using Ampholine system with a carrier ampholyte of pH 3.5 to 5.0.

Amino acid analyses and amino acid sequence determination. The amino acid composition was determined by the conventional method, using Hitachi amino acid analyzer, model 835. The amino-terminal amino acid sequence was determined with a gas phase protein sequencer (model 470A; Applied Biosystem Inc., U.S.A.) and a high performance liquid chromatograph (model 8100; Spectra Physics, U.S.A.).

RESULTS

Purification of kallikrein from human saliva

We essentially followed the conventional purification procedures we adopted earlier,[6,7] except for a few modification as follows. Firstly, instead of acetone-precipitated powder used earlier, the freshly collected human saliva was utilized as the starting material. The collected and pooled saliva (14.1 l) was diluted with tap water until the conductivity of the solution was below 1 mS/cm and was adjusted to pH 7.5. Secondly, we omitted the hydroxyapatite chromatography step from the purification procedure to avoid the possible loss of the enzyme activity.

The specific activity of the purified kallikrein (HSK; activity, 31.5 µmoles/min/A_{280}) showed 2,400 times higher esterolysis of N-α-tosyl-L-arginine methyl ester (Tos-Arg-Me) than in the case of the mixed raw saliva. The protein recovery at the final stage was 0.03 % and the esterolytic activity 70 % over that the starting material, respectively. The vasodilator activity was 1,100 KU/mg protein. The absorbancy at

Human salivary kallikrein (this work)
```
    1        5          10         15          20
    I V G G W E X E Q X S Q P W Q A A L Y X F X ...
```

Human urinary kallikrein (Lottspeich et al.[8])
```
    1        5          10         15          20
    I V G G W E X E Q X S Q P W Q A A L Y (H) F X ...
```

Human pancreatic kallikrein (Fukushima et al.[2])
```
    1        5          10         15          20
    I V G G W E C E Q H S Q P W Q A A L Y H F S ...
```

Rat submaxillary (PS) kallikrein (Ashley and MacDonald[9])
```
    1        5          10         15          20
    V V G G Y N C E M N S Q P W Q V A V Y Y F G ...
```

Fig. 1. Comparison of the amino acid sequence of mammalian kallikreins. The partial amino-terminal amino acid sequence of human kallikreins of saliva and urine origin are aligned with the reported sequence of human pancreatic kallikrein and rat submaxillary glands kallikrein deducing from the cloned cDNA sequences.

280 nm of 1 mg/ml of the final preparation in a 1 cm width cubette was 1.33±0.03 (n=5). HSK was revealed to comprise a single polypeptide chain with a molecular weight of 33,000 daltons on SDS-polyacrylamide gel electrophoresis, although it was determined to be 28,000 daltons on Sephadex G-75 gel filtration. Most of its chemical and biological properties coincided well with those reported previously,[6,7] except some differences noted in pI value (4.20±0.05: n=3, instead of 4.0) and in the optimal pH range (9.5-9.8 instead of 8.0). The amino-terminal sequence of 21 residues of HSK is presented in Fig. 1 in comparison with those of other kallikreins.

Partial purification of human submaxillary glands kallikreins

Step 1. Human submaxillary glands (169 g) were minced, frozen over-night and then thawed. Distilled water was added to the minced tissues (2 ml per 1 g original wet weight), followed by vigorous shaking and then standing overnight at 4°C. Suspension of the tissues was then homogenized in cold saline with a porcelain motor, and centrifuged at 7,000 x g for 30 min. The supernatant was dialyzed overnight against distilled water. After removal by centrifugation of the precipitates formed during the dialysis, the supernatant was used for further purification. The total protein and activity was 19,460 A_{280} and 786 EU, respectively. One EU is defined as the hydrolysis of one μmol of Tos-Arg-Me per min.

Step 2. The dialyzed tissue-extract was diluted with water as described for the saliva. DEAE-cellulose (50 g) was added to the diluted solution and then the slurry was introduced into a column after 2 hrs adsorption. The column was washed with 0.05 M Tris-HCl buffer, pH 7.5 (buffer A), and then eluted with buffer A containing 1 M NaCl. The eluted fractions which showed Tos-Arg-Me esterolytic activity were pooled and then dialyzed against buffer A overnight. The solution was applied to a DEAE-cellulose column (1.5 x 70 cm) which had been equilibrated with the same buffer. After the column had been washed, a NaCl linear gradient from 0 to 0.5 M, in buffer A (500 ml in total) was applied. By this exchange chromatography, two peaks showing esterolytic activity were found in the fractions corresponded to the NaCl concentrations around 0.15 M and 0.25 M. They were pooled separately and tentatively called the former as Pool B and the latter as Pool A, respectively. In this study, Pool A was used further purification of kallikrein. It was dialyzed against buffer A containing 0.05 M NaCl. Recoveries of the protein and the activity were 350 A_{280} and 130 EU, respectively.

Step 3. The dialyzed solution above was concentrated and loaded on a Sephadex G-100 column (2.0 x 60 cm) and then eluted with buffer A. This procedure yielded two peaks showing esterolytic activity (Fig. 2). The material corresponding to the first one was arbitrarily called kallikrein-like esteropeptidase (KLEP) and that of second peak was designated as human submaxillary glands (HSG)-kallikrein, respectively, and they were collected separately. The protein recovery of HSG-kallikrein was 10.1 A_{280} with 9.8 EU of the activity. On the other hand, total absorbancy at 280 nm of the KLEP preparation was 30.7 with the activity of 20.4 EU.

Step 4. The pooled fractions of KLEP and HSG-kallikrein were sepa-rately applied to a QAE-Sephadex A-50 column (1.5 x 70 cm) which had been equilibrated with buffer A containing 0.05 M NaCl. The active fractions showing an esterolysis were pooled and then dialyzed against buffer A overnight. Recovery of HSG-kallikrein was 0.77 A_{280} with 3.6 EU and of KLEP was 5.0 A_{280} with 6.1 EU, respectively. KLEP was further applied to the Sephadex G-150 column (2.0 x 60 cm) before its use in the following experiment. The resultant activity was 3.39 EU/A_{280}.

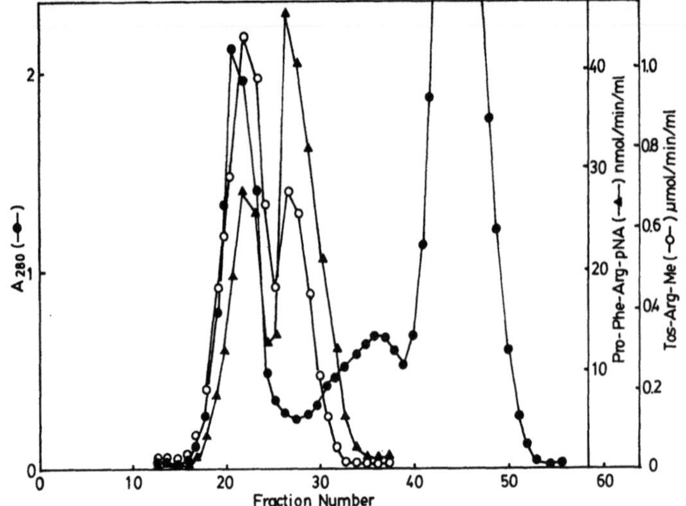

Fig. 2.   Sephadex G-100 gel filtration of the protein obtained on ion exchange chromatography. The volume of each fraction was 3.5 ml.

Partially purified HSG-kallikrein and KLEP

The molecular weights of HSG-kalkrein and KLEP were estimated to be about 30,000 daltons and 54,000 daltons, respectively, on Sephadex G-100 gel filtration. However, SDS-polyacrylamide gel electrophoresis revealed the presence of some minor bands in addition to the main broad band for each enzyme. This indicated that a few more purification steps were necessary to achieve complete purification of HSG-kallikrein and KLEP. Both enzyme exhibited the pH optimum of around 10.

Some properties of the purified HSK, and of the partially purified HSG-kallikrein and KLEP

Substrate specificity and kinetics. The relative rates of esterolysis and amidolysis by the purified HSK, and of the partially purified HSG-kallikrein and KLEP are shown in Table 1. As can be seen, a substrate Ac-Phe-Arg-Me was hydrolyzed most rapidly by these enzymes. The kinetics parameters of HSK were determined from Lineweaver-Burk plots at various pHs. For Bz-Arg-Et, the activity was determined by spectrophotometry, measuring the increase in absorbance at 254 nm and 25°C. The K_m (mM) and V_{max} (μmol/min/A$_{280}$) were estimated to be 0.31 and 11.5, 0.31 and 17.7, and 0.32 and 14.3, at pHs 8.0, 9.0 and 10.4, respectively. On the other hand, the K_m (μM) and V_{max} (μmol/min/A$_{280}$) values of HSK toward S2266 (Val-Leu-Arg-pNA) were found to be 50 and 2.4, 51 and 3.9, 50 and 5.6, and 52 and 4.6, at pHs 8.0, 9.0, 10.0 and 11.0, respectivery.

Effect of protease inhibitors. The effects of several protease inhibitors of plasma, plant and microbial origin, and of some chemical inhibitors were examined. Mixtures of the designated inhibitors and enzymes were incubated at 30°C for 30 min at pH 8.0, and then the remaining activity was determined by the amidolytic assay with the S2266 as a substrate. No inhibition was observed of all three enzymes when following inhibitors were used in the range of 1-100 µg: trypsin inhibitors of soybean (SBTI), lima bean (LBTI) and ovomucoid (OTI), anti-thrombin III (dissolved in heparin), hirudin (the peptidic protease inhibitor obtained from the salivary glands of Hirudo medicinalis) and bovine macroglobulin. PCMB and EDTA, in the range of 10^{-7}-10^{-4} M, failed likewise to inhibit

Table 1. Substrate specificities of the purified HSK, and the partially purified HSG-kallikrein and KLEP

Substrate	HSK	HSG-kallikrein	KLEP
Tos-Arg-Me[a]	31.5	4.78	3.39
Bz-Arg-Me	21.8	6.69	3.38
Ac-Phe-Arg-Me	379.0	7.17	8.81
Tos-Lys-Me	18.0	3.25	2.44
Ac-Lys-Me	4.30	3.15	2.34
Ac-Gly-Lys-Me	27.0	3.49	2.47
ε-Cbz-Lys-Me	0.63	-[c]	-[c]
α-Z-Lys-Me	8.37	3.49	2.27
ε-Z-Lys-Me	0.76	3.11	2.03
Lys-Me	-[c]	3.11	2.20
Bz-Cit-Me	12.6	2.49	1.63
Ac-(Ala)$_3$-Me	1.40	-[c]	-[c]
Ac-Phe-Me	3.57	-[c]	-[c]
Val-Leu-Arg-pNA[b]	2.42	0.398	0.168
Val-Leu-Lys-pNA	1.02	0.059	0.055
Pro-Phe-Arg-pNA	0.33	0.372	0.017
Bz-Pro-Phe-Arg-pNA	0.077	-[c]	-[c]
Tos-Gly-Pro-Phe-Arg-pNA	0.199	0.070	0.001
Z-Gly-Pro-Arg-pNA	0.123	0.034	0.002
Tos-Gly-Pro-Phe-Lys-pNA	0.110	-[c]	-[c]
Z-Phe-Val-Arg-pNA	0.082	0.013	0.006
Cbz-Arg-pNA	0.022	0.020	0.004

[a] Esterolytic activity was determined by the colorimetric method with chromotropic acid, at pH 8.0 and 30°C. The substrate concentration was 20 mM in each case.

[b] Amidolytic activity was assayed with a substrate concentration of 1 mM each at pH 8.0 and 30°C. Both activity (a and b) is expressed in terms of μmol/min/A$_{280}$.

[c] (-) indicates that activity was not measured.

the enzyme activity. Neither were microbial inhibitors such as pepstatin, chymostatin and antipain effective. Human α_1-antitrypsin had inhibitory effect slightly. However, aprotinin caused considerable inhibition. The IC$_{50}$ value of aprotinin for HSK was estimated to be 6 KIU/ml.

DISCUSSION

Recently, Fukushima et al.[2] have reported on the amino acid sequence of the human pancreatic kallikrein deduced from the cloned cDNA sequence, and have pointed out that the pancreatic preprokallikrein consists of 262 amino acid residues with a calculated molecular weight of 28,889 daltons, containing the corresponding signal sequence and profragment of 24 amino acids. The 31 residues of the pancreatic kallikrein have been reported to be exactly corresponding with the amino-terminal sequence of the human urinary kallikrein.[8] Fujimoto et al.[6] previously estimated the molecular weight of HSK to be 28,000 daltons and 23,500 daltons on gel filtrations and on ultracentrifugation, respectively. In the present study, we determined the amino acid composition of the currently purified HSK. Inconsistently with our previous data,[6] the result corresponded well with that obtained by way of deducing from the cloned nucleotide sequence of human pancreatic kallikrein[2] (data not shown). The molecular weight of HSK obtained by SDS-polyacrylamide gel electrophoresis in the present study suggests that the human salivary kallikrein is the glycosylated form of the glandular kallikrein gene product. The analysis of the 21 amino-terminal sequence of HSK was consistent with reported by Fukushima et al.[2,8] and that of the amino-terminal sequence of human urinary kallikrein (Fig. 1). It has been reported earlier that the source of the urinary kallikrein is the kidney[10] and that mRNA is expressed in the renal tissue.[2] However, the current results suggest strongly that the urinary kallikrein is composed not only of kidney kallikrein but also of the kallikrein derived from salivary glands and/or the pancreas excreted from kidney, without fundamental structural metabolical modification, although it still remains to be seen, how many of the kallikreins are from salivary glands and how many of pancreatic and/or renal origin.

The kallikreins of mouse and rat were reported to be encoded by a large gene family.[11] Although the number of the gene seemed to be less in the human DNA than that of the murine DNA, it has been suggested that human kallikrein is also encoded by a multigene family.[2] Up to now, there has been no report on the purification of kallikrein and its related enzymes obtained from human salivary glands. As reported in this paper, we identified at least the two distinct molecules having kallikrein-related enzyme activity. And further, in addition to the enzymes, we found the third enzyme (Pool B in Step 2), which should be clarified in the near future. Although it is not yet certain, whether these three activities are mutually related at the gene basis, it is of great interest to identify the amino acid sequence of these enzymes when it comes to determining the mechanism of the gene expression in the different tissues and/or organs of the multi-kallikrein gene family of the human salivary glands.

ACKNOWLEDGEMENTS

We are grateful to Dr. Kokichi Kikuchi, Professor and Chairman of the Department of Pathology, Sapporo Medical College, for his kind supply of materials. We wish to thank Professor Dr. Shin-ichi Ishii, Hokkaido University, for his help in the amino acid analyses. We also thank Professor Dr. Hiroshi Moriya, Science University of Tokyo, for his encouragement.

REFERENCES

1. A. J. Mason, B. A. Evans, D. R. Cox, J. Shine and R. I. Richards, Structure of mouse kallikrein gene family suggests a role in specific processing of biologically active peptides, Nature, 303: 300-307 (1983).

2. D. Fukushima, N. Kitamura and S. Nakanishi, Nucleotide sequence of cloned cDNA for human pancreatic kallikrein, Biochemistry, 24: 8037-8047 (1985).

3. Y. Matsuda, S. Akihama and Y. Fujimoto, Rat submaxillary gland kallikrein: Purification and some properties, Jpn. J. Clin. Chem., 15: 131-139 (1986).

4. E. Amundsen, J. Putter, P. Friberger, M. Knos, M. Larsbranten and G. Claseson, Methods for the determination of glandular kallikrein by means of colorimetric tripeptide substrate, in: "Adv. Exp. Med. Biol.", vol. 120A, S. Fujii, H. Moriya and T. Suzuki eds., Plenum Press, New York, pp. 83-95 (1979).

5. U. K. Laemmli, Cleavage of structural protein during the assembly of the head of bacteriophage T, Nature, 227: 680-685 (1970).

6. Y. Fujimoto, H. Moriya and C. Moriwaki, Studies on human salivary kallikrein I. Isolation of human salivary kallikrein, J. Biochem., 74: 239-246 (1973).

7.   Y. Fujimoto, C. Moriwaki and H. Moriya, Studies on human salivary kallikrein II. Properties of purified salivary kallikrein, J. Biochem., 74: 246-252 (1973).

8.   F. Lottspeich, R. Geiger, A. Henschen and C. Kutzbach, N-terminal amino acid sequence of human urinary kallikrein, Z. Physiol. Chem., 360: 1947-1950 (1979).

9.   P. L. Ashley and R.J. MacDonald, Kallikrein-related mRNAs of the rat submaxillary gland: Nucleotide sequence of four distinct types including tonin, Biochemistry, 24: 4512-4520 (1985).

10. M. Schachter, Kallikrein (Kininogenases)-A group of serine proteases with bioregulatory actions, Pharmacol. Rev., 31: 1-17 (1980).

11. G. H. Swift, J. -C. Dagorn, P. L. Ashley, S. W. Cumings and R. J. MacDonald, Rat pancreatic kallikrein mRNA: Nucleotide sequence and amino acid sequence of the encoded preproenzyme, Proc. Natl. Acad. Sci., 79: 7263-7267 (1982).

CHARACTERIZATION OF HUMAN PANCREATIC KALLIKREIN

H. Terashima[a], Y. ATomi[a], N. Ohnishi[a], A. Kuroda[a], Y. Morioka[a],
M. Ikekita[b], K. Aoki[b], M. Kamada[b], K. Kizuki[b] and H. Moriya[b]

1st Department of Surgery, Faculty of Medicine, University of
Tokyo, Bunkyo-ku, Tokyo, Japan (a) Department of Biochemistry
Science University of Tokyo, Shinjuku-ku, Tokyo, Japan (b)

SUMMARY

Human pancreatic kallikrein (H.Panc.K.) was purified from human pancreas by ion exchange chromatography on DEAE-cellulose, affinity chromatographies on p-aminobenzamidine Sepharose 6B and aprotinin aminocellulofine, followed by gel filtration on Sephacryl S-200. The final preparation had a specific activity of 9.2 AU/A_{280} (AU; amidase unit for H-Pro-Phe-Arg-MCA) and its N-terminal sequence coincided with the reported sequence for H.Panc. K.. In HPLC (gel filtration), one symmetrical peak corresponding to a molecular weight of 48,000 was obtained. In SDS-PAGE without 2-mercaptoethanol (2-ME), one band corresponding to a molecular weight of 52,000 was obtained, but with 2-ME, 2 bands, 52,000 and 30,000, were obtained. Km value for MCA was 4.9 x 10^{-2} mM. Proteinase inhibitor specificities of H.Panc.K. were the same as those of human urinary kallikrein (HUK) and hog pancreatic kallikrein (hog Panc.K.), while anti-HUK antibody inhibited the activities of H.Panc.K. and HUK, but not that of hog Panc.K.. From the analysis of affinity for concanavalin A (Con A) and erythroagglutinating phytohemagglutinin (E-PHA), the carbohydrate parts of H.Panc.K. are relatively rich in biantennary complex type sugar chains with bisecting GlcNAc compared with those of human salivary kallikrein (H.Saliv.K.) and HUK.

INTRODUCTION

Glandular kallikreins (EC 3.4.21.35) are serine proteinases secreted from various organs, such as salivary glands, pancreas, kidney etc. They are glycoproteins and their enzymic functions in vivo are limited to hydrolysis of kininogen to kinin. To date, many studies have been done on H.Panc.K.[1,2] and other glandular kallikreins[3]. The identity of the protein parts of HUK and H.Panc.K. was indicated by the coincidence between partially elucidated amino acid sequence of HUK and overall amino acid sequence of H.Panc.K. from cloned cDNA sequence analysis[4]. The discrimination regarding the origin of glandular kallikrein is assumed to be derived from the difference in carbohydrate moieties. As for HUK, its carbohydrate structure was partially clarified[5], but that of H.Panc.K. has not yet been reported. In this paper we report the purification procedures of kallikrein from human pancreas and add some data to previously reported properties of this enzyme.

MATERIALS AND METHODS

Chemicals

The followings were obtained commercially; H-Pro-Phe-Arg-4-methyl-coumaryl-7-amide (MCA) and antipain (Peptide Research Foundation, Osaka, Japan), soy bean trypsin inhibitor (SBTI), lima bean trypsin inhibitor (LBTI) and p-aminobenzamidine (p-AB, Sigma Chemical Co., St. Louis, USA), aprotinin (Bayer Co., Leverkusen, Germany), DEAE-cellulose (Brown Co., Berlin, USA), p-AB Sepharose 6B and Sephacryl S-200 (Pharmacia Fine Chemicals Co., Uppsala, Sweden), E-PHA agarose (E-Y Laboratories Co., San Mateo, USA). Aprotinin aminocellulofine was kindly provided by Seikagaku Kogyo Co., Tokyo, Japan. HUK and hog Panc.K. were purified according to the method of Ikekita et al[5]. H.Saliv.K. was partially purified from 200 ml of one normal human saliva with aprotinin aminocellulofine. Anti-HUK antibody and Con A Sepharose 4B was prepared in the laboratory of Science University of Tokyo[5,6]. Other chemicals were of analytical reagent grade.

Starting Materials

For the purpose of systemic lymph nodes dissection in surgery for gastric cancer, the tails of the pancreas are sometimes resected. The resected pancreases are usually cancer-free and discarded. We obtained 100g of these organs, and stored them until use at -20°C.

Activity and Inhibition Measurement

The amidolytic activity of kallikrein toward MCA was determined by the method of Iwanaga et al[7]. Inhibition measurement was performed as follows; Mixture of 20 µl of enzyme solution (approximately 0.2 AU/A_{280}), 20 µl of inhibitor solution and 10 µl of 1M Tris-HCl pH 8.0 was incubated at 30°C for 30 min with the same mixture not containing inhibitor solution but 0.05 M Tris-HCl buffer as substitute. Enzyme-linked immunosorbent assay (ELISA) using anti-HUK antibody was carried out as descrived by Suzuki et al[8].

Other Methods

Polyacrylamide gel electrophoresis with sodium dodecyl sulfate (SDS-PAGE) was carried out with Pharmacia's automatical equipment for electrophoresis, "Phast System". Molecular weight was determined by SDS-PAGE and HPLC (gel filtration, one column of Shodex WS-803 and two columns of Shodex WS-802.5 (Showa Denko Co., Tokyo, Japan) were directly connected.)

N-terminal sequence was analyzed with the protein-peptide sequencer, model 477A/120A, Applied Biosystems, Co., Tokyo, Japan.

Carbohydrate structures of H.Panc.K., H.Saliv.K. and HUK were analyzed by lectin affinity chromatographies on Con A Sepharose 4B and E-PHA agarose acorrording to the method of Cumming and Kornfeld[9].

Purification Procedures

The pancreas (100g) was thawed and homogenized with Polytron homogenizer in 400ml of 0.05M phosphate buffer pH 7.2, then stirred at 4°C for 4 hours. After centrifugation (7000 x g, 30min), precipitate was stirred in 400ml of the same buffer and centrifuged once more in the same manner. To each supernatant solution, ammonium sulfate was added and fraction of 40%-75% sat. was dissolved in distilled water (164ml and 52ml each), then dialyzed against distilled water. Each dialysate was mixed and DEAE-cellulose (15g, dry weight) was added to the mixture. Then it was stirred at 4°C for 4 hours, and packed in a column (3.4 x 50cm). Elution was done with 40 m mho/cm ammonium acetate pH 6.0. Active fractions were collected and dialyzed against 0.05M Tris-HCl pH 8.0 containing 1 mM $CaCl_2$ at 4°C for 2 hours. Then, the dialysate was applied to p-AB Sepharose 6B column (2.1 x 17cm) equilibrated with the same buffer, and eluted with 0.1M CH_3COONa pH4.0 containing 0.5M NaCl. The eluate was neutralized immediately. After dialysis against 0.05M Tris-HCl pH 8.0, the enzyme was applied to aprotinin aminocellulofine column (1.5 x 10cm) equilibrated with 0.05M Tris-HCl pH 8.0 containing 0.1M NaCl. The column was washed with the same buffer, followed by washing with 0.05M Tris-HCl pH 8.0 containing 0.2M NaCl. Kallikrein was eluted with 0.1M CH_3COONa pH4.0 containing 0.5M NaCl, then the eluate was neutralized immediately. Active fractions were collected and dialyzed against distilled water. The sample was applied to Sephacryl S-200 column (1.4 x 115cm) equilibrated with 0.1M Tris-HCl pH 8.0 containing 0.15M NaCl at a flow rate 6 ml/h. Fractions with high specific activity were collected and pooled as a final preparation.

RESULTS

Purification of Kallikrein

Aprotinin aminocellulofine chromatogram showed 2 peaks of activity. (Fig. 1) Both of them were not inhibited by SBTI. ELISA using anti-HUK antibody reacted only to the enzyme in the second peak. The purification is summarized in Table 1. The final preparation was homogeneous on SDS-PAGE without 2ME (Fig. 2) and HPLC (gel filtration).

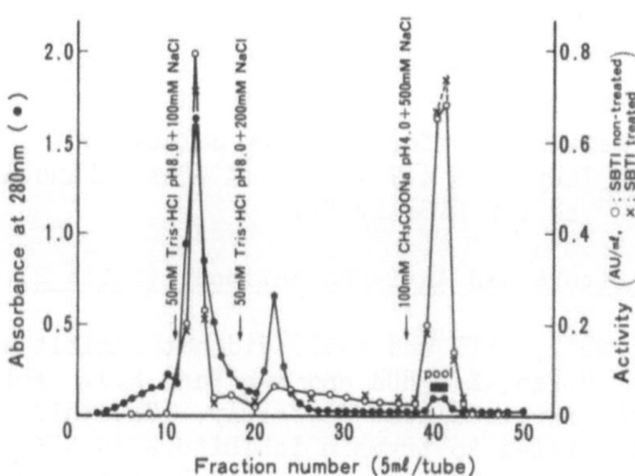

Fig. 1.
Aprotinin aminocellofine column was equilibrated with 0.05M Tris-HCl pH 8.0 containing 0.1M NaCl.
Eluants are shown by arrows. Fraction No.13 and 41 were assayed with ELISA using anti-HUK antibody. Only in the second peak existed the enzyme which was immunologically related with HUK.

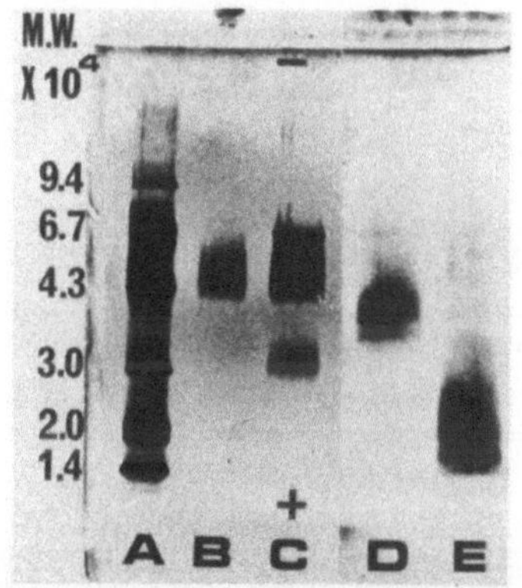

Fig. 2. SDS-PAGE
A: molecular mass standards
B: H.Panc.K. without 2-ME
C: H.Panc.K. with 2-ME
D: HUK
E: hog Panc.K.

Table 1. Purification of Human Pancreatic Kallikrein

	total A_{280}	total activity*	specific activity**	yield	purification factor
phosphate buffer extract	69,200	38.4	5.5×10^{-4}		1
ammonium sulfate precipitate	24,800	33.0	1.3×10^{-3}	0.86	2.4
DEAE-cellulose (batch method)	1,150	34.2	3.0×10^{-2}	0.89	55
p-AB Sepharose 6B	400	16.9	4.2×10^{-2}	0.44	76
aprotinin aminocellulofine	0.87	6.0	6.9	0.16	12500
Sephacryl S-200	0.051	0.47	9.2	0.012	16700

* AU (amidase unit; μM/min for MCA) with SBTI treated   ** AU/A_{280}

Molecular Weight

The molecular weight of H.Panc.K. was estimated to be 48,000 by HPLC
(gel filtratin), and 52,000 by SDS-PAGE without 2-ME, while, another protein
band corresponding to 30,000 emerged in SDS-PAGE with 2-ME. In various concentrations of 2-ME (from 5% to 20%), the results were identical and the
original band (52,000) did not move nor disappear. Purified HUK and hog
Panc.K. were also submitted to SDS-PAGE and compared with H.Panc.K.. The
migration distances were significantly different among them (Fig. 2).

Enzymic Properties

The Km values of three human kallikreins for MCA were calculated
through Lineweaver-Burk's diagram. They were 4.9×10^{-2} mM for H.Panc.K.,
1.8×10^{-2} mM for HUK and 1.7×10^{-2} mM for H.Saliv.K..

Effects of Various Proteinase Inhibitors and Anti-HUK Antibody (Table 2)

Trypsin inhibitors (antipain, SBTI, LBTI and p-AB) did not inhibit any
of these three types of kallikrein (H.Panc.K., HUK and hog Panc.K.). While,
aprotinin inhibited all types of kallikrein almost perfectly. So, this
purified enzyme has the same specificities to trypsin inhibitors as HUK and
hog Panc.K.. Anti-HUK antibody inhibited the activites of H.Panc.K. and
HUK, but not that of hog Panc.K.. This means that H.Panc.K. has a immunological relationshop with HUK, but not with hog Panc.K..

N-terminal Sequence

N-terminal sequence was determined as H-Ile-Val-Gly-Gly-Trp-Glu-(?)-Glu
-Gln-His-Ser-Gln-Pro-. Moreover, H-Gln-Ala- was detected in a small amount.

Table 2. Inhibition Assay (residual activity(%))

	antipain		SBTI		LBTI		aprotinin		p-AB		anti-HUK Ab
	1μM	10μM	1μM	10μM	1μM	10μM	10U	100U	1μM	10μM	
H.Panc.K.	102	100	112	112	108	106	88	7	93	104	14
HUK	93	114	104	130	110	81	90	6	75	97	14
hog Panc.K.	115	104	118	131	102	126	75	4	102	121	81

<u>Carbohydrate Analysis</u>

In Con A affinity chromatography analysis, almost all activities of
H.Panc.K. (over 90%) were detected in unbound fractions. The behavior of
H.Saliv.K. was similar to that of H.Panc.K.. By contrast, the increased
ratio of weakly bound HUK was observed. Further analysis of affinity for
E-PHA revealed that greater parts of H.Panc.K. were detected in the retarded
fractions compared with H.Saliv.K.. The results are summarized in Fig.3.
and Table 3.

DISCUSSION

In a preliminary experiment, we found that a large amount of amidase
activity of pancreas extract, not inhibited by SBTI, had been lost spontaneously, although stored at 4°C. Since glandular kallikreins were known
to be stable at this temperature, we guessed that large parts of this activity were attributed to some other enzyme. To date, mesotrypsin has been
reported as such an enzyme[10]. We tried to separate kallikrein from mesotrypsin using immobilized p-AB. However, the ion exchange effect rather
than affinity effect did not allow the separation. It was achieved by
aprotinin aminocellulofine (Fig. 1). In this chromatogram, the existence of
an enzyme distinct from both trypsin and kallikrein was suggested.

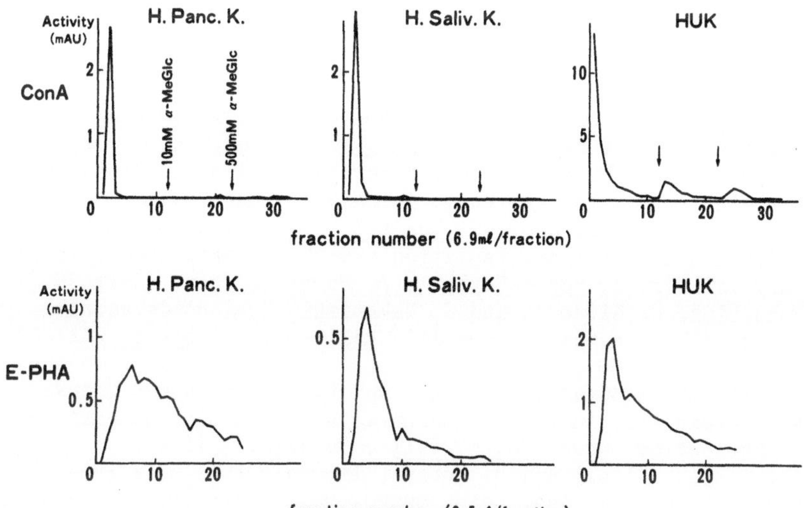

Fig. 3. Con A Sepharose 4B columns were equilibrated with TBS(0.01M
Tris, 0.15M NaCl, 1mM $CaCl_2$, 1mM $MgCl_2$, 0.02%(w/v) NaN_3, pH 8.0).
Eluants are shown by arrows. Three groups (unbound, weakly bound,
strongly bound, 11fractions /group, 6.9ml/fraction) were collected
each. The flow rate was 10ml/h. E-PHA agarose columns were equilibrated with PBS(0.14M NaCl, 2.7mM KCl, 1.5mM KH_2PO_4, 8.1mM Na_2HPO_4,
0.02%(w/v) NaN_3, pH 7.4). Kallikreins were eluted with PBS (25
fractions, 2.5ml/fraction). The flow rate was 12ml/h.

Table 3. Fractination of Three Human Kallikreins by Con A (n=2)

	unbound	weakly bound	strongly bound
H.Panc.K.	94(%)/ 97(%)	3.5(%)/ 1(%)	2.5(%)/ 2(%)
H.Saliv.K.	92 / 85	3 / 4	5 / 11
HUK	74 / 74	17 / 22	9 / 4

In SDS-PAGE with 2ME, the molecular weight of newly emerged protein band was as about half as that of the original one. Even in stronger conditions (up to 20% of 2ME), there appeared no other protein band and the original band did not move nor disappear. The possible explanation for this is that the final preparation was a mixture of single chain molecules and double chain molecules (connected with S-S bond(s)). This was supported by N-terminal sequence analysis. We suppose that the original H.Panc.K. molecule was single chain, but in some molecules purification procedures themselves brought a nick at nearly a half length of the chain.

Asn-linked oligosaccharides of glycoproteins can be analyzed by lectin affinity chromatographies. This approach is based on the fact that each lectin has its own specific affinity for some oligosaccharides. Lectin affinity analysis of this study revealed that the carbohydrate parts of H. Panc.K. are relatively rich in biantennary complex type sugar chains with bisecting GlcNAc and those of H.Saliv.K. are rich in tri- or more branched sugar chains, on the other hand, those of HUK are relatively rich in biantennary complex type sugar chains with or without fucose compared with other two kallikreins. These findings explain the different behaviors in SDS-PAGE between H.Panc.K. and HUK. And they support the hypothesis that the origin of HUK is different from those of H.Panc.K. and H.Saliv.K.. Furthermore, they will be of help to know the origins of glandular kallikreins in serum or other body fluids, and to clarify the physiological and pathophysiological roles of glandular kallikreins.

REFERENCES

1. H. Moriya, J. V. Pierce and M. E. Webster, Purification and some properties of three kallikreins, Ann. N. Y. Acad. Sci., 104;172 (1963).
2. M. Amouric and C. Figarella, Characterization and purification of a kallikrein from human pancreatic juice and immunological comparison with other kallikreins, Hoppe-Seyler's Z. Physiol. Chem., 360;157 (1979).
3. W. Hofmann and R. Geiger, Isolation and characterization of human salivary kallikrein, Hoppe-Seyler's Z. Physiol. Chem., 364;425 (1983).
4. D. Fukushima, N. Kitamura and S. Nakanishi, Nucleotide sequence of cloned cDNA for human pancreatic kallikrein, Biochem., 24;8037 (1985).
5. M. Ikekita, T. Masunaga, K. Kizuki and H. Moriya, Human urinary kallikrein. II. Analysis of asparagin-linked oligosaccharides by using lectins, Chem. Pharm. Bull., 35(5);2071 (1987).
6. M. Ikekita, K. Kizuki and H. Moriya, Immunological relationships of the glandular kallikreins, Chem. pharm. Bull., 31(7);2466 (1983).
7. S. Iwanaga, T. Morita, H. Kato, T. Harada, N. Adachi, T. Sugo, I. Maruyama, K. Takada, T. Kimura and S. Sakakibara, Fluorogenic peptide substrates for proteases in blood coagulation, kallikrein-kinin and fibrinolysis systems, in: "Advances in Experimental Medicine and Biology, Kinin II," vol.120A, S. Fujii, H. Moriya and T. Suzuki, ed., Plenum Press, N. Y. (1979).
8. S. Suzuki, M. Ikekita, K. Kizuki and H. Moriya, Abstract of papers, Proceeding of the 26th annual meeting of Jap. Society of Clin. Chem. vol. 26;86 (1986).
9. R. D. Cummings and S. Kornfeld, Fractination of asparagin-linked oligosaccharides by serial lectin-agarose affinity chromatography, J. Biol. Chem., 257;11235 (1982).
10. H. Rinderchnecht, I. G. Rennen, S. B. Abramson and C. Carmark, Mesotrypsin: A new inhibitor-resistant protease from a zymogen in human pancreatic tissue and fluid, Gastroenterology, 86;681 (1984).

IMMUNOCYTOCHEMICAL IDENTIFICATION OF GLANDULAR KALLIKREIN IN THE RAT

ANTERIOR PITUITARY

Carlos P. Vío(1), Ricardo H. Silva(2) and C. Andrew Powers(3)

(1) Departamento de Fisiología, Pontificia Universidad
Católica de Chile, (2) Institutos de Fisiología y Medicina
Interna, Universidad Austral de Chile, (3) Department of
Pharmacology, New York Medical College, Valhalla, NY, USA

INTRODUCTION

Glandular kallikrein (EC 3.4.21.35) is a trypsin-like serine protease
characterized by an ability to generate kinins from kininogens (inactive
plasma glycoproteins) with a high degree of specificity. Although classical-
ly postulated to play a role in local blood flow regulation via the
generation of kinins (potent vasodilatory peptides), this enzyme has increas-
ingly been proposed to possess a multiplicity of functions (for review see
1,2). In particular, glandular kallikrein has recently been recognized to
cleave precursor molecules other than kininogen in vitro (3,4,5). Further,
the glandular kallikrein gene is the prototypical member of a large gene
family coding for a number of highly homologous trypsin-like serine
proteases (6,7). Certain other products of this gene family have been
linked to growth factor processing-suggesting that the glandular kallikrein
gene family may play a role in processing of diverse biologically active
peptides (8).

Recently, a kininogenase indistinguishable from glandular kallikrein
has been detected in the anterior and neurointermediate lobes of the rat
pituitary (9,17). Glandular kallikrein in the anterior pituitary is ten
to twenty times higher in females than in males (10,11,13,17) owing to
powerful hormonal induction by ovarian estrogens (13,16,17). This estrogen
induction is mediated by increased gene expression since glandular
kallikrein mRNA levels are also estrogen dependent (17,18,9). Additionally,
glandular kallikrein enzyme and mRNA levels are modulated by inhibitory
dopaminergic mechanisms (16,29). This dual estrogen and dopaminergic
regulation of anterior pituitary glandular kallikrein parallels the
regulation of PRL (for review see 20,21) suggesting a possible functional
association. Indeed, glandular kallikrein levels are markedly elevated
in pituitary tumors induced in F344 rats by estrogen implants (22). Such
tumors are well known to arise from lactotroph proliferation suggesting
that rat anterior pituitary glandular kallikrein derives from lactotrophs.

The purpose of the present study was to establish the presence
cellular of glandular kallikrein in the anterior pituitary using immunocytochemistry.

MATERIALS AND METHODS

Female Sprague-Dawley rats weighing 200 to 250g were treated with 10 ug estradiol benzoate every 48 h for 10 days as previously described (13) to induce anterior pituitary glandular kallikrein. Rats were then anesthetized with sodium pentobarbital (50 mg/kg). Pituitaries were fixed with either one of the following methods: transcardial perfusion with saline followed by perfusion with Bouin's fluid and then dissection, or rats were decapitated, the pituitaries removed, bisected, and immersed in Bouin's fluid. In both cases, the dissected pituitaries remained immersed in Bouin's fluid for 24 to 48 h and gave equivalent immunostaining for glandular kallikrein.

Pituitaries were embedded in paraffin (Paraplast-Plus; Brunswick Labs, St. Louis, MO). For Paraplast-Plus embedding, tissues were dehydrated in a graded series of ethanol solutions followed by n-butanol and then Paraplast-Plus; sections 5 to 7 u thick (semi-thick sections) were then cut and mounted on glass slides.

Immunostaining

The immunostaining procedure employed was the unlabeled antibody method of Sternberger (23) as previously modified to describe the cellular localization of glandular kallikrein in the rat nephron (24,25,26). All antisera and peroxidase-antiperoxidase (PAP) complexes were diluted in 0.05 M Tris-phosphate (pH 7.8) containing 0.7% lambda carrageenan, and 0.5% Triton X-100 (27). The antiserum dilutions used for glandular kallikrein were: 1:3,000 to 1:10,000. Immunostaining was accomplished by incubating the tissues mounted on glass slides for 18 to 72 h in glass staining jars containing the primary antiserum at 22°C, followed by a 30 min incubation with rabbit antiserum against sheep IgG (1:500). Slides were then incubated with second antibody (goat antiserum against rabbit IgG; 1:150) for 30 min, followed by PAP complex (1:150) for 30 min, and then incubated with a solution containing 0.2% 3,3 diaminobenzidine tetrachloride and 0.01% H2O2 in 0.05 M Tris-phosphate (pH 7.8) for 15 min. Between incubations slides were washed with buffer. After staining, slides were dehydrated, cleared with xylene and coverslipped.

The antisera employed were obtained from the following sources: sheep antiserum against rat urine glandular kallikrein (Dr. J.J. Pisano, National Heart Lung and Blood Institute, NIH, Bethesda, MD, USA), and the following supplies were obtained commercially: rabbit antiserum against sheep IgG, (Cappel Laboratories, Westchester, PA, USA): goat antiserum against rabbit IgG, normal rabbit serum, normal goat serum, PAP complex of rabbit origin (Sternberger-Meyer, Jarrestville, MD, USA).

Replacement of the primary antiserum by antiserum preabsorbed with purified rat urinary kallikrein or the use of preimmune serum served as controls.

RESULTS

Glandular kallikrein was readily detected by the immunostaining procedure of semi-thick (7 u) paraffin sections in cells of the anterior pituitary (Fig. 1). The immunoreactive kallikrein was not distributed over the entire cytoplasm but, mostly concentrated in the perinuclear area (Fig. 1, inset). Antiserum preabsorbed with purified glandular kallikrein produced no detectable staining of the sections (Fig. 2), no staining was observed either when the primary antiserum was replaced by nonimmune serum.

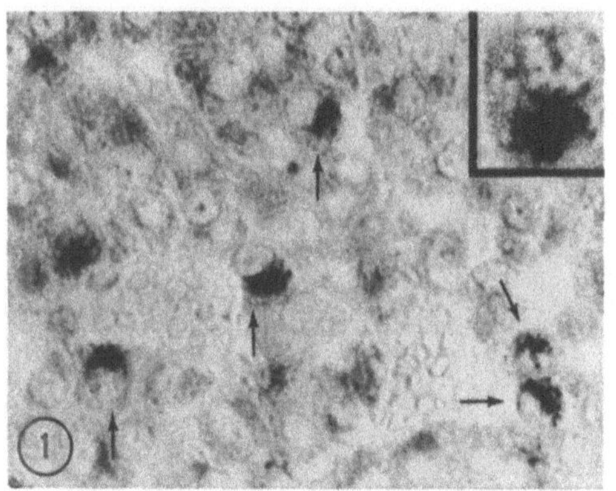
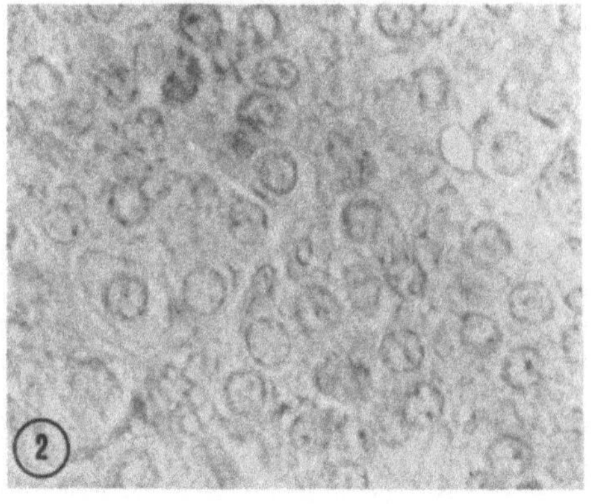

Figure 1. Paraplast section (8 u) of anterior pituitary immunostained for glandular kallikrein. Some of the several kallikrein containing cells are pointed by arrows. Kallikrein immunoreaction is concentrated in the perinuclear area (X 400). Inset: shows at higher manification the concentration of kallikrein in the perinuclear area (X 1200).

Figure 2. Paraplast section (8 u) of anterior pituitary immunostained with antiserum against glandular kallikrein preabsorbed with purified kallikrein (X 400).

DISCUSSION

It has been known for over 50 years that highly specific kininogenases (kallikreins) are abundant in a variety of exocrine glands and their excretions (e.i. pancreas and pancreatic juice, submandibular gland and saliva, kidney and urine) (1,2). These enzymes have been widely designed as "glandular kallikreins" ever since it was recognized that kallikrein from different glands were enzymatically and immunologically indistinguish-able, whereas plasma kallikrein is a distinct entity. Glandular kallikreins have been identified in a number of nonexocrine tissues (i.e. vascular tissue, spleen, brain) (31,32,33). However, only recently have glandular kallikreins or similar enzymes been reported in endocrine glands, first by immunocytochemistry in the B-cells of human pancreatic islets (34), and later by enzymatic assays in the rat thyroid gland (35), and rat and pig pituitary (10,11,36,37). Most recently, glandular kallikrein has been reported in the pineal gland using radioimmunoassay and cDNA probes for its mRNA (18). The existence of glandular kallikrein in pancreatic islet tissue has been questioned due to the failure of different groups to detect glandular kallikrein in such tissue using immunocytochemistry (38, 39). However, the existence of glandular kallikrein in the rat pituitary is now firmly established by virtue of multiple reports from independent laboratories confirming enzymatic activity, immunologic activity, and mRNA coding for glandular kallikrein in the anterior and neurointermediate lobes of the rat pituitary (9,19).

The cell of origin of glandular kallikrein in the neurointermediate lobe of the rat pituitary was determined in previous studies by dis-section of the lobe into its components - the pars intermedia and pars nervosa. Glandular kallikrein activity was almost exclusively localized to the pars intermedia while the pars nervosa contained little or no activity (9,14,15). The pars intermedia is essentially a pure population of melanotrophs (producing alfa-MSH and B-endorphin) with negligible connective, vascular, or other tissue elements (37,38), thus, the distribution of glandular kallikrein in the neurointermediate lobe seems to be localized within melanotrophs. This finding was corroborated by the inhibitory dopaminergic regulation of glandular kallikrein activity and mRNA levels in the neurointermediate lobe (12,15,19), such inhibitory regulation is a characteristic feature of pituitary melanotrophs.

Determination of the cell origin of glandular kallikrein in the rat anterior pituitary is more problematic. The lobe contains at least 5 distinct hormone-producing cell types interspersed throughout the tissue. However, the estrogen induction of glandular kallikrein in the anterior pituitary (10,13,17,18), its inhibitory dopaminergic regulation (16,19), and its high levels in estrogen-induced lactotroph tumors (22) argued for a localization in lactotrophs. Ongoing studies using two color double immunoperoxidase staining of consecutive thin sections with alternating series of antisera against kallikrein and pituitary hormones, and ultra-structural immnocytochemistry will give further information on the cellular localization and subcellular distribution of kallikrein in the rat anterior pituitary.

It should be noted that glandular kallikrein in the anterior or neurointermediate lobes of the pituitary appears indistinguishable from glandular kallikrein in the kidney or urine on the basis of their kininogenase activity, synthetic substrate specificity, inhibitor sensitivity, pH optima, immunoprecipitation curves and radioimmunoassay curves (9,13,14,17,22). Moreover, nucleotide sequencing and restriction endonuclease analysis of glandular kallikrein cDNA cloned from anterior or neurointermediate lobe mRNA has established that the true glandular kallikrein gene is expressed in these sites (19), rather than distinct but closely related gene products which may exhibit similar enzymatic and immunological activity. Thus, glandular kallikrein has now been associated with two different cell types producing peptides other than kinins. Identification in such sites lends support to the often stated hypothesis that glandular kallikrein may function in the processing of peptides other than kinins (1,6,8,39). Nonetheless, much more work is needed to elucidate the functional role of glandular kallikrein in the rat pituitary. In any event, the vascular anatomy of the pituitary makes it virtually impossible for glandular kallikrein to exercise its classical-ly postulated function - the regulation of local blood flow and vascular permeability via kinins (40). The anterior pituitary receives the venous drainage of the hypothalamus which feeds into a network of fenestrated sinusoids devoid of smooth muscle (41,42), such a low pressure, low resistance circuit is all suited for flow or permeability regulation by vasoactive agents. Further, the pars intermedia is essentially avascular (40).

Clearly, novel functions for glandular kallikrein are likely in the rat pituitary.

ACKNOWLEDGEMENTS

This work was supported by Grants from the American Cancer Society BC597, DIUC 202/86, DIUACH S 85-38, NIH DK 32782 and a Sinsheimer Scholar Award to Dr Powers. The authors wish to acknoledge to Mrs Eliana Lira and Silvia Troncoso for the technical assistance.

REFERENCES

1. M. Schachter, Kallikreins (kininogensas) - a group of enzymes with bio regulatory actions. Pharmacol Rev 31:1 (1980).
2. P. J. Fuller, J. W. Funder, The Cellular physiology of glandular kallikrein. Kidney Int 29:953 (1986).

3. O. Ole-MoiYoi, G. S. Pinkus, D. C. Seldin, J. Spragg, K. F. Austen, Sequencial cleavage of proinsulin by human pancreatic kallikrein and a human pancreatic kininase. Proc Nat Acad Sci USA 76:3612 (1979)
4. E. S. Prado, L. Prado de Carvalho, M. S. Araujo-Viel, N. Ling, J. Rossier A met-enkephalin-containing peptide, BAM 22P, as a novel substrate for glandular kallikreins. Biochem Biophys Res Commun 112:366 (1983)
5. M. G. Currie, D. M. Geller, J. Chao, H. S. Margolious, P. Needleman, Kallikrein activation of a high molecular weight atrial peptide. Biochem Biophys Res Commun 120:461 (1984)
6. A. J. Mason, B. A. Evans, D. R. Cox, J. Shine, R. I. Richards, Structure of the mouse kallikrein gene family suggests a role in specific processing of biologically active peptides. Nature 303:300 (1984)
7. P. L. Ashley, R. J. MacDonald, Kallikrein-related mRNAs of the rat submaxillary gland: nucleotide sequences of four distinct types including tonin. Biochemistry 24:4512 (1985)
8. M. A. Bothwell, W. H. Wilson, E. M. Shooter, The relationship between glandular kallikrein and the growth factor processing proteases of the mouse submaxillary gland. J Biol Chem 254:7287 (1979)
9. C. A. Powers, A. Nasjletti, A kininogenase resembling glandular kallikrein in the pars intermedia of the rat pituitary. Endocrinology 112:1194 (1983)
10. C. A. Powers, A. Nasjletti, A major sex differences in kallikrein -like activity in the rat anterior pituitary. Endocrinology 114:1841 (1984)
11. C. A. Powers, P. G. Baer, A. Nasjletti, Reduced glandular kallikrein-like activity in the anterior pituitary of the New Zealand genetically hypertensive rat. Biochem Biophys Res Commun 119:689 (1984)
12. C. A. Powers, Dopamine receptor blockade increases glandular kallikrein-like activity in the neurointermediate lobe of the rat pituitary. Biochem Biophys Res Commun 127:668 (1985)
13. C. A. Powers, Anterior pituitary glandular kallikrein: trypsin activation and estrogen regulation. Mol Cell Endocrinol 46:163 (1986)
14. C. A. Powers, Trypsin activation, partial characterization, and distribution of kallikrein-like and thrombin-like proteases in the neurointermediate lobe of the rat pituitary. J Neurochem 47:145 (1986)
15. C. A. Powers, Dopaminergic regulation of glandular kallikrein in the intermediate lobe of the rat pituitary. Neuroendocrinology 43:368 (1986)
16. C. A. Powers, M. A. Hatala, Dopaminergic regulation of the estrogen-induced glandular kallikrein in the rat anterior pituitary. Neuroendocrinology 44:462 (1986)
17. J. Chao, L. Chao, C. C. Swain, J. Tsai, H. S. Margolius, Tissue kallikrein in rat brain an pituitary: regional distribution and estrogen induction in the anterior pituitary. Endocrinology 120:475 (1987)
18. J. A. Clements, P. J. Fuller, M. McNally, I. Nikolaidis, J. W. Funder, Estrogen regulation of kallikrein gene expression in the rat anterior pituitary. Endocrinology 119:268 (1987)
19. D. B. Pritchett, J. L. Roberts, Dopamine regulates expression of the glandular-type kallikrein gene at the transcriptional level in the pituitary. Proc Nat Acad Sci USA, in press (1987)
20. P. S. Dannies, Control of prolactin production by estrogen. In: Litwack G (ed) Biochemical Actions of Hormones, Vol XII. Academic Press, New York, pp 289 (1985)
21. J. Tuomisto, P. Mannisto, Neurotransmitter regulation of anterior pituitary hormones. Pharmac Rev 37:249 (1985)
22. C. A. Powers, Elevated glandular kallikrein in estrogen-induced pituitary tumors. Endocrinology 120:429 (1987)

23. L. A. Sternberger, Immunocytochemistry, 2nd ed, J. Wiley & Sons, New York, (1979)

24. C. D. Figueroa, I. Caorsi, J. Subiabre, C. P. Vío, Immunoreactive kallikrein localization in the rat kidney: An immuno-electron microscopic study. J. Histochem Cytochem 32:117 (1984)

25. C. P. Vío, C. D. Figueroa, Subcellular localization of renal kallikrein by ultrastructural immunocychemistry. Kidney Int 28:36 (1985)

26. C. P. Vío, C. D. Figueroa, Evidence for a stimulatory effect of high potassium diet on renal kallikrein. Kidney Int 31:1327 (1987)

27. W. Sofroniew, U. Schrell, Long-term storage and regular repeated use of diluted antisera in glass staining jars for increased sensitivity, reproducibility, and convenience of single-and two-color light microscopic immunocytochemistry. J. Histoch Cytochem 30:504 (1982)

28. H. Nolly, A. G. Scicli, G. Scicli, O. A. Carretero, Characterization of a kininogenase from rat vascular tissue resembling tissue kallikrein. Cir Res 56:816 (1985)

29. J. Chao, C. Woodly, L. Chao, H. S. Margolius, Identification of tissue kallikrein in brain and in the cell-free translation product encoded by brain mRNA. J Biol Chem 258:1517 (1985)

30. J. Chao, L. Chao, H. S. Margolius, Isolation of tissue kallikrein in rat spleen by monoclonal antibody affinity chromatography. Biochem Biophys Acta 801:244 (1984)

31. O. Ole-MoiYoi, G. S. Pinkus, J. Spragg, K. F. Austen, Identification of human glandular kallikrein in the beta cell of the pancreas. New Eng J Med 300:1289 (1979)

32. K. Uchida, H. Kushiro, J. Kodama, Y. Hitomi, M. Niinobe, S. Fujii, Rat thyroid kallikrein: its purification and properties. Agents Actions Suppl 9:167 (1982)

33. E. Polivka, M. Maier, B. R. Binder, Purification and characterization of a kallikrein-like kininogenase from pig pituitary glands. Agents Actions Suppl 9:153 (1982)

34. C. A. Powers, A. Nasjletti, A novel kinin-generating protease (kininogenase) in the porcine anterior pituitary. J Biol Chem 257:5594 (1982)

35. T. B. Ortstavik, P. Brandtzaeg, K. Nustad, J. V. Pierce, Immunocytochemical localization of kallikrein in human pancreas and salivary glands. J Histochem Cytochem 28:557 (1981)

36. P. Lechene de la Porte, M. Amouric, C. Figarella, Immunolocalization of kallikrein in porcine pancreas at the ultrastructural level. Hoppe Seyler's Z Physiol Chem 362:439 (1981)

37. A. Howe, D. S. Maxwell, Electron microscopy of the pars intermedia of the pituitary gland in the rat. Gen Comp Endocrinol 11:169 (1968)

38. F. J. Tilders, P. G. Smelik, Effects of hypothalamic lesions and drugs interfering with dopaminergic transmission on pituitary MSH content of rats. Neuroendocrinology 25:275 (1978)

39. K. D. Bhoola, R. May Yi, J. Morley, M. Schachter, Release of kinin by an enzyme in the accessory sex glands of the guinea-pig. J Physiol (Lond) 163:269 (1962)

40. S. M. Hilton, The physiological role of glandular kallikreins. In: Erdos EG (ed) Handbook of Experimental Pharmacology. Springer, Berlin, vol 25:389 (1970)

41. J. D. Green, The compartive anatomy of the hypophysis with special reference to its blood supply and innervation. Amer J Anat 88:225 (1951)

42. J. F. Reinhart, M. G. Farquhar, The fine vascular organization of the anterior pituitary gland. An electron microscopic study with histochemical correlations. Anat Rec 121:207 (1955)

LOCALIZATION OF KALLIKREIN IN HUMAN MALE GENITAL ORGAN

Yoshiaki Kumamoto, Seiichi Saito, Naoki Ito, Kazuaki
Shimamoto and Osamu Iimura

Department of Urology and The Second Department of
Internal Medicine, Sapporo Medical College, S-1,W-16
Chuo-ku, Sapporo 060, Japan

SUMMARY

Male genital organs (testis, epididymis, seminal vesicle and vas
deferens) were stained by the peroxidase-antiperoxidase (PAP) method to
clarify the localization of kallikrein. Sertoli cells of the testis,
epithelial cells of the epididymis, and adenocytes of the prostate gland
were specifically stained showing that endogenous kallikrein was localized
in these cells.

INTRODUCTION

It is known that the spermatogenesis in the testis is controlled by
hormones such as luteinizing hormone (LH),follicle-stimulating hormone
(FSH),and testosterone(1),however,its mechanism has not been elucidated
completely. The concern of the other substances besides hormones with the
spermatogenesis is considerable. Recently,it has been reported that
kallikrein accelerates the spermatogenesis,the metabolism of sperm and
the sperm motility(2). The correlation between male genital organs and
kallikrein has been noted,while the secretory site and action mechanism
of kallikrein remain to be obscure.
We clarified the localization of kallikrein in male genital organs
by using the enzyme antibody method and examined the secretory site of
kallikrein.

MATERIALS AND METHODS

Materials were testis,epididymis,vas deferens,prostate,seminal vesicle,and kidney that were obtained at various urological operations.
Tissue pieces of them were fixed for 48 hours in the formalin fixative (4% formalin in 0.05 M phosphate buffer,pH7.2). After fixation,PAP
method were performed as described previously(3).
The localization of kallikrein was indicated by the production of
the water-insoluble reddish brown color. It was produced by oxidation
reaction catalyzed by peroxidase that was bound to the antigen site.

RESULTS

In order to confirm the specificity of the antibody,renal tissue
where the presence of kallikrein had already been reported was stained.
As shown in Fig.1, lumen surface of the distal uriniferous tubule
having many nuclei was stained,which was similar to previous reports.
From this results,the specificity of the antibody was confirmed.
Fig.2 shows stained tissue pieces of the testis. Only Sertoli cells
were stained. The germinal cells and Leydig cells were not stained.
This observation showed that kallikrein was localized in Sertoli cell in
the testis.

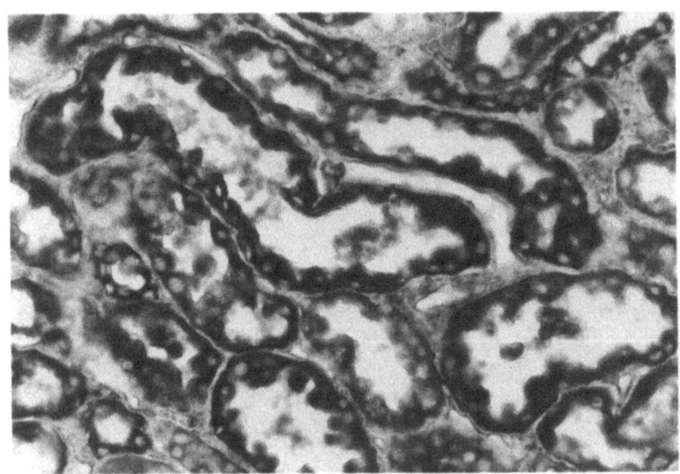

Fig.1 Kidney (x280): Positive staining is demonstrated
in the distal tubules specifically.

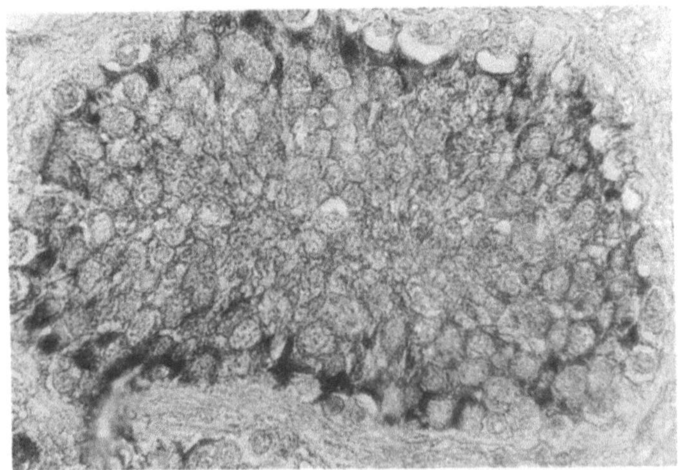

Fig.2 Testis (x448): Sertoli cells in seminiferous
tubules are stained specifically,but germinal
cells,Leydig cells and others are not stained.

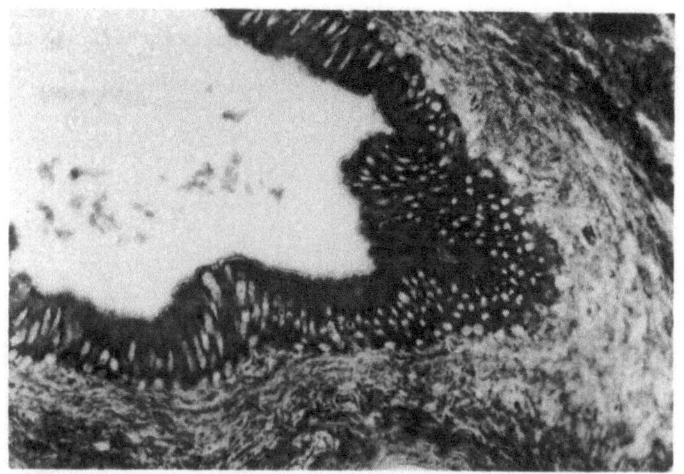

Fig.3 Epididymis (x112): Epithelial cells,especially
     in the portions of body to tail, are stained
     specifically.

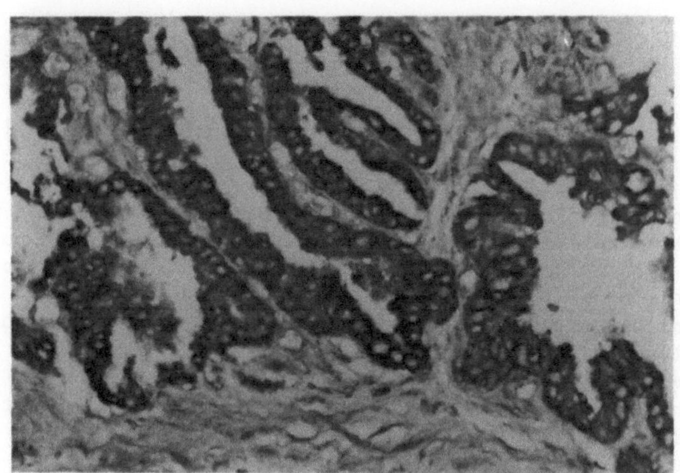

Fig.4 Prostate (x280): Adenocytes of the prostate,
     especially cytoplasma, are stained specifically.

Fig.3 and Fig.4 show stained tissue pieces of the epididymis and of the prostate gland,respectively. Epithelial cells in the epididymis and adenocytes of the prostate were specifically stained,which showed the localization of kallikrein in these cells.

But kallikrein was not found in the seminal vesicle and vas deferens (data not shown).

The summary of above observations was shown in Fig.5: kallikrein was localized in Sertoli cells of the testis,epithelial cells of the epididymis,and adenocytes of the prostate gland.

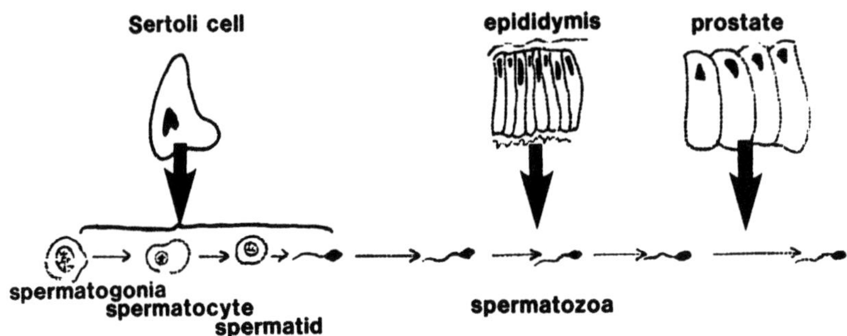

Fig.5 Secretory portions of kallikrein in human male genitalia.

DISCUSSION

Examining the localization of kallikrein in renal tissues using the first antibody which was obtained by immunizing rabbits with human urine kallikrein proved the specificity of the antibody(4). Using the stop-flow method,Scicli et al.(5) estimated that kallikrein was secreted from the distal uriniferous tubule. Using the fluorescent antibody technique, Orstavik et al.(6) showed that kallikrein was localized in the lumen surface of the distal uriniferous tubule. Simson(7) demonstrated the same result using the PAP method. With using our antibody,the same region was specifically stained.

We studied the localization of kallikrein in male genital organs by PAP method using the antibody refered to above. Sertoli cells of the testis,epithelial cells of the epididymis,and adenocytes of the prostate gland were specifically stained,showing the localization of kallikrein in these regions.

As to the study of the reproducing function,Fink et al.(8) reported the presence of kallikrein in the human semen. They pointed out that since a great amount of kallikrein was contained in the first fraction of the fractional ejaculation,kallikrein was possibly secreted from the prostate gland or the epididymis. Our studies using the staining method also showed the possibility that it was secreted from the prostate gland

and the epididymis because these two organs were stained,and furthermore
the secretion from the testis was suggested.

Concerning the effects of the kallikrein-kinin system on male genital organs,since Stuttgen(9) reported the increase of the number of spermatozoa after administering kallikrein to patients with oligozoospermia, many researchers(10-12) reported the increased number of spermatozoa,the improvement of sperm motility,and the decrease of the ratio of abnormal spermatozoa after administering kallikrein to patients with sterility.

Our finding of the presence of kallikrein in Sertoli cells of the seminiferous tubule strongly suggested that direct concern of endogenous kallikrein with the process of spermatogenesis. In the epididymis,spermatozoa are matured,the cytoplasmic droplet is falls off,and components of the membrane are eliminated. Kallikrein was also considered to influence these process. The possibility exists that kallikrein is secreted from the epididymis and also is transited from the blood flow.

Since the mechanism of its secretion from the testis and epididymis has not been clarified,further studies are necessary.

In this report,we stated the presence of kallikrein in the testis, the epididymis,and the prostate gland. Kallikrein localized in these organs seems to play an important role in the reproducing function. Its mechanism should be studied further.

REFERENCES

1. Steinberger,E.: Hormonal control of mammalian spermatogenesis. _Physiol. Rev_. 51:1-22 (1971)
2. Schill,W.E.,Wallner,O.,Palm,S. and Fritz,H.: Kinin stimulation of spermatozoa motility and migration in cervical mucus. _In_: Human semen and fertility regulation in men. Edited by E.S.E.Hafez,pp442 (1976)
3. Saito,S.,Kumamoto,Y.,Shimamoto,K.,and Iimura,O.: Kallikrein in the male reproductive system. _Arch. Androl_. 19:133-147 (1988)
4. Shimamoto,K.,Mayfield,R.K.,Margolius,H.S.,Chao,J.,Stroud,W. and Kaplan, A.P.: Immunoreactive tissue kallikrein in human serum. _J.Lab.Clin.Med_. 103:731-738 (1984)
5. Scicli,A.G.,Carretero,O.A.,Hamptom,A.,Cortes,P. and Oza,N.B.: Site of kininogenases secretion in dog nephron. _Am.J.Physiol_. 230:533-536 (1976)
6. Orstavik,T.B.,Nustad,K.,Brandtzaeg,P. and Pierce,J.V.: Cellular origin of urinary kallikreins. _J.Histochem.Cytochem_. 24:1037-1039 (1976)
7. Simson,A.,Spicer,S.S.,Chao,J.,Grimm,L. and Margolius,H.S.: Kallikrein localization in rodent salivary glands and kidney with the immuno-peroxidase bridge technique. _J.Histochem_. 27:1567-1576 (1979)
8. Fink,E.,and Schill,W.B.: Tissue kallikrein in human seminal plasma. _Adv.Exp.Med.Biol_. 156:1175-1180 (1983)
9. Stuttgen,G.: Clinical substitution of the effects of kallikrein. Kininogenases-Kallikrein 1. Schattauer,Sttutgart. New York: 189-192 (1971)
10. Schill,W.B.: Improvement of sperm motility in patients with asthenozoospermia by kallikrein treatment. _Int.J.Fertil_. 20:61-63 (1975)
11. Schill.W.B.: Recent progress in pharmacological therapy of male subfertility-review. _Andrologia_ 11:77-107 (1979)
12. Schirren,C.: Clinical experiences with kallikrein on subfertile males. Kininogenases-Kallikrein 4. Schattauer,Sttutgart. New York: 247-250 (1978)

ISOLATION AND PARTIAL CHARACTERIZATION OF RABBIT URINARY KALLIKREIN

R.C.R. Stella, P.C. Duarte, M.S. Araujo-Viel, M.U. Sampaio
and C.A.M. Sampaio

Departamento de Bioquimica, Escola Paulista de Medicina
Caixa Postal 20372, 04034, S.Paulo, SP, Brazil

INTRODUCTION

Tissue kallikrein (E.C.3.4.21.35) usually splits mammalian high-
and low-molecular weight kininogens [1] releasing lysyl-bradykinin,
differently from plasma kallikrein (E. C. 3.4.21.34), that releases
bradykinin [2], mainly from high molecular weight kininogen [3]. However,
rat urinary kallikrein is known to release bradykinin, instead of
lysyl-bradykinin from homologous kininogen [4], which occurs as three
different molecular species, low- and high-molecular weight, and
T-kininogen [5,6].

Urinary kallikrein from other rodents, and close to rodent
mammalians, is not as well characterized as rat kallikrein, and concerning
kininogen, it has been reported that rabbit and human kininogen levels are
comparable, being the T-kininogen content much lower than in rat [5].

The recent report on kallikreins discrimination, based upon
hydrolysis of synthetic tetrapeptide substrates [7], shows that rat
urinary kallikein does not discriminate Ac-Phe-Arg-Arg-Val-NH2 from
Ac-Phe-Arg-Arg-Pro-NH2, as do horse and human urinary, and also porcine
pancreatic kallikrein.

This report describes the isolation of kallikrein from rabbit
urine, and some of its enzymatic properties.

MATERIALS AND METHODS

Tosyl-arginine methyl ester (TAME) was from Merck. The chromogenic
p-nitroanilide substrate H.D.Val-Leu-Arg-pNA (S-2266) was from Kabi, and
Ac-Phe-Arg-pNA (APANA) was a kind gift of Dr. Luis Juliano, Departamento
de Biofisica, Escola Paulista de Medicina, who also provided the
tetrapeptide substrates Ac-Phe-Arg-Arg-Val-NH2 and Ac-Phe-Arg-Arg-Pro-NH2.
DEAE-Sephacel was from Pharmacia, and Aprotinin-Sepharose was prepared by
Aprotinin (Bayer) coupling to CNBr-activated Sepharose 4B (Pharmacia) [8].

Bovine trypsin was from Sigma, and benzamidine was from Aldrich. HPLC
column was a Microbondapack C-18 from Waters [7].

Rabbit urine concentration and salt precipitation: 11.5 L rabbit
urine, were concentrated to 426 mL, in a Pellicon System (Millipore).
Solid NaCl was added under stirring to the concentrate, at room
temperature, up to 0.6 M final concentration, and following pH adjustment
to 5.6 with 1 M HCl, the mixture was left at 4°C for about 16 hours. The
precipitate material was separated by centrifugation at 5,000 x g, for 20
min, at 4°C and discarded. The supernatant, that bears a dark brown color,
was dyalyzed successively against distilled water and 0.01 M sodium
phosphate buffer, pH 7.0, containing 0.05 M NaCl, and final volume was
460 mL.

DEAE-Sephacel ion-exchange chromatography: entire volume of
dyalyzed material was chromatographed on DEAE-Sephacel column (4 x 32 cm)
equilibrated with 0.01 M sodium phosphate buffer, pH 7.0, containing 0.1 M
NaCl. Following extensive washing with equilibrium buffer (absorbance at
280 nm 0.1), elution was carried out with stepwise NaCl concentration,
0.15, 0.25 and 0.35 M, in the same buffer system, being 10.0 mL fractions
collected at 120 mL/hour, at room temperature. Protein and activity
elutions were followed by A 280 and TAME hydrolysis, respectively. The
three eluted peaks, with kinin-releasing activity, were pooled (112 mL),
and concentrated on cellulose nitrate filter (Sartorius, SM 13200 E), to a
final volume of 28 mL (peak C).

Aprotinin-Sepharose chromatography: Peak C (volume of 28 mL) was
chromatographed on Aprotinin-Sepharose, equilibrated with 0.01 M sodium
phosphate buffer, pH 7.0, containing 0.25 M NaCl. Resin was washed with
the same buffer until A 280 was 0.2, and bound material was eluted with 1
M benzamidine, in the same buffer, in 20 mL effluent, which was dyalyzed
against distilled water.

Protein determination, carried out following benzamidine dyalysis
removal, was performed according to a modified Lowry procedure [9].

Activity assay upon TAME was based on a described procedure [10].
Amidolytic activity was followed spectrophotometrically at 405 nm[11],
and peptide bond cleavage was followed by HPLC [7].

Enzyme inhibition was studied with benzamidin and Aprotinine upon
TAME hydrolysis.

Kinin bioassay was performed on isolated guinea pig ileum [12] by
incubation of 250 uL rabbit plasma (pre-heated for 30 min at 60 C) with
rabbit urinary enzyme in the tissue chamber, and elicited contractions
were compared to standard bradykinin, alternatively, rabbit heat-treated
plasma, containing 5 mM 1,10 phenantroline, was incubated with enzyme (40
mUTAME/mL plasma) and aliquots withdrawn at different time intervals were
assayed as before.

Molecular weight of rabbit urine enzyme was estimated by gradient
polyacrylamide-gel electrophoresis (10 - 20%), under the conditions
described by Laemmli [13], and staining was performed with either
Coomassie Blue or silver nitrate [14].

One unit (U) rabbit urinary kallikrein was defined as the amount
that hydrolysis 1 umol TAME/min/mg enzyme.

RESULTS

Rabbit urinary kallikrein was purified from concentrated urine into at least three esterase and kinin-yielding materials by DEAE-Sephacel chromatography, A, B and C. Only C was further characterized as rabbit urinary kallikrein, since A and B contained other proteolytic contaminants (as plasminogen activator) and most of the dark brown pigment. Table 1 shows the purification steps.

TABLE 1

PURIFICATION OF RABBIT URINARY KALLIKREIN

MATERIAL		VOLUME	TOTAL ACTIVITY (U)	TOTAL PROTEIN (mg)	SPECIFIC ACTIVITY (mU/mg)	PURIFICATION	YELD (%)
URINE concentrate		426	151	19500	8	(1)	(100)
NaCl fraction		460	110	7300	15	1.9	73
DEAE-Sephacel	A	122	31	670	50	5.8	20
	B	250	47	950	50	5.8	31
	C	112	12	700	17	2.1	8
Aprotinin-Sepharose	C	39	9	23	400	50.0	6

Rabbit urinary kallikrein, as seen by polyacrylamide gel electrophoresis (not shown) appears as a 30,000 molecular weight diffuse band (unreduced).

Both incubation procedures for kinin release produced 0.7 to 1 ug bradykinin equivalents/mL rabbit plasma (not shown).

The kinetic parameters of rabbit urinary kallirein hydrolysis of synthetic substrates are shown in Table 2.

TABLE 2

KINETIC CONSTANTS FOR HYDROLYSIS OF Ac-Phe-Arg-pNA AND

H.D.Val-Leu-Arg-pNA (S-2266) BY RaUK.

SUBSTRATE	Km (M)	kcat (sec-1)	kcat/Km (M-1 x sec-1)	RATE (ug eq.BK/ min.ug)
H.D.Val-Leu-Arg-pNA	29 x 10-6	0.28	932	-
Ac-Phe-Arg-pNA	11 x 10-5	0.08	727	-
Kinin releasing activity	-	-	-	0.09

Table 3 shows the relative activity of rabbit urinary kallikrein upon tetrapeptide substrates, Ac-Phe-Arg-Arg-Val-NH2 and Ac-Phe-Arg-Arg-Pro-NH2.

Benzamidine and Aprotinin inhibition of rabbit urinary kallikrein is seen in table 4.

TABLE 3

TETRAPEPTIDE HYDROLYSIS BY RABBIT URINARY KALLIKREIN

PEPTIDE	RATE OF HYDROLYSIS nmol/min/enzyme unit
P2 P1 P'1 P'2	
Ac-Phe-Arg-Arg-Val-NH2	46.6
Ac-Phe-Arg-Arg-Pro-NH2	0.62

TABLE 4

INHIBITION OF RABBIT URINARY KALLIKREIN BY

BENZAMIDINE AND APROTININ

INHIBITOR	Ki (mM)
Aprotinin	0.09
Benzamidine	0.45

Aprotinin inhibition (0.02 - 0,08 mM) with 16,8 ug enzyme, in 0.05 M tris-HCl, pH 8.0, 30°C.
Benzamidine inhibition (0.25 - 2.0 mM) was measured in 2.5 mM and 5.0 mM TAME, in a pH-stat, pH 8.0, 30°C.

DISCUSSION

Kinin maximally released by rabbit urinary kallikrein, approximately 1 ug bradykinin equivalents/ mL rabbit plasma, would correspond to 3 - 4 ug lysyl-bradykinin assayed upon isolated guinea pig ileum[15]. These data are in agreement with our results (unpublished), on the amount of kinin maximally released by trypsin from rabbit heat-treated plasma (aproximately 4 ug bradykinin/mg trypsin/mL plasma). However, such an amount of kinin corresponds to about half of the bradykinin content reported by Okamoto and Greenbaum, for acid diluted plasma[5].

The tetrapeptide discrimination system, used as substrate for rabbit urinary kallikrein, adds evidence to support its characterization as a tissue-type kallikrein, comparable to human and horse urinary, and also porcine pancreatic kallikrein, but differing from rat urinary kallikrein[7]. Rabbit urinary kallikrein hydrolysis rate of Ac-Phe-Arg-Arg-Val-NH2 is 75 times faster than that of Ac-Phe-Arg-Arg-Pro-NH2, while for rat urinary kallikrein the reported rate ratio is 1.5, approximately[7].

In vitro inhibition of rabbit urinary kallikrein, especially that of Aprotinin (Ki = 10-5 M, approximately) distinguishes this enzyme from other tissue kallikreins, that are much more efficiently inhibited, as horse (Ki = 0.41 x 10-9 M, Dr. E.S. Prado, personal communication), or human (Ki = 10-10 M, approximately)[16]. The importance of inhibition of tissue kallikreins remains to be seen, since it is not clear yet if there is any physiologically active inhibitor for these enzymes[17].

The reported data on rabbit urinary kallikrein, isolated by a relatively simple procedure, show that it shares functional similarities with other mammalian tissue kallikreins, but not with rat urinary kallikrein.

REFERENCES

1 - H. Kato, S. Nagasawa and S. Iwanaga, HMW and LMW kininogens, Methods Enzymol. , 80: 172 (1981).
2 - E.S. Prado, M.E. Webster and J.L. Prado, Kallidin (lysilbradykinin), the kinin formed, from horse plasma by horse urinary kallikrein, Biochem. Pharmacol., 20: 2009 (1971).
3 - M.L. Oliva, M.U. Sampaio and C.A.M. Sampaio, Properties of highly purified human plasma kallikrein, Agents Actions, 9: 52 (1982).
4 - H. Kato, K. Enjyoji, T. Miyata, I. Hayashi, S. Oh-ishi and S. Iwanaga, Demonstration of argynyl-bradykinin moiety in rat HMW kininogen:direct evidence for liberation of bradykinin by rat glandular kallikreins, Biochem. Biophys. Res. Comm., 127: 289 (1985).
5 - H. Okamoto and L.M. Greenbaum, Kininogen substrates for trypsin and cathepsin D in human, rabbit and rat plasmas, Life Sciences, 32: 2007 (1983).
6 - I. Hayashi, T. Ino, H. Kato, S. Iwanaga, T. Nakano and S. Oh-ishi, Demonstration of the third kininogen in high and low molecular weight kininogens-deficient brown norway katholiek rat, Thrombosis Res., 36: 509 (1984).
7 - E.S. Prado, M.S. Ara|jo-Viel, M.A. Juliano, R.C.R. Stella and C.A.M. Sampaio, Tetrapeptide substrates for discrimination among kallikreins and other trypsin-like serine proteinases, Biol. Chem. Hoppe-Seyler, 367: 199 (1986).
8 - P. Cuatrecasas, Protein purification by affinity chromatography, J. Biol. Chem., 245: 3059 (1970).
9 - M.A.K. Markwell, S.M. Hass, L.L. Bieber and N.E. Tolbert, A modification of the Lowry proceduce to simplify protein determination in membrane and lipoprotein samples, Anal. Biochem., 87: 206 (1978).
10- C.A.M. Sampaio and D. Grisolia, Human plasma kallikrein. Preliminary studies on hydrolysis of proteins and peptides, Agents Actions, 8: 125 (1978).
11- M. A. Juliano and L. Juliano, Synthesis and kinectic parameters of hydrolysis by trypsin of some acyl-arginyl-p-nitroanilide, Brazilian J. Med. Biol. Res. 18: 435 (1985).
12- C.A.M. Sampaio, S.T. Nunes, M.G.N. Mazzacoratti and J.L. Prado, Inactivation of kinins by chymotrypsin, Biochem. Pharmacol., 25: 2391 (1976).
13- U.K. Laemmli, Cleavage of structural proteins during the assembly of the head of bacteriophage T4, Nature, 227: 680 (1970).
14- J.H. Morrissey, Silver stain of protein polyacrilamide gels:a modified procedure with enhanced uniform sensitivy, Anal. Biochem., 117: 307 (1981).
15- M.R. Reis, L. Okino and M. Rocha e Silva, Comparative pharmacological actions of bradykinin and related kinins of larger molecular weights, Biochem. Pharmacol., 20: 2935 (1971).
16- R. Geiger, U. Stuckstedte and H. Fritz, Isolation and characterization of human urinary kallikrein, Biol. Chem. Hoppe-Seyler, 361: 1003 (1980).
17- H.S. Margolius, The kallikrein-kinin system and the kidney, Ann. Rev. Physiol., 46: 309 (1984).

TISSUE KALLIKREINS OF THE GUINEA-PIG

Gabriele Mayer, Kanti D. Bhoola[*], and Franz Fiedler

Department of Clinical Chemistry and Clinical Biochemistry, Surgical Clinic, University of Munich
Munich, FRG, and [*]Department of Pharmacology, University of Bristol, Bristol, UK

INTRODUCTION

Several years ago, we reported on the properties of
tissue kallikrein (EC 3.4.21.35) purified from submandibular
glands of the guinea-pig (1). This enzyme was found to be
similar to a kininogenase which had previously been isolated
from coagulating glands of this animal (2), but seemed to be
distinctly different. In the meantime, the existence of
numerous enzymes with tissue kallikrein-like sequences has
been demonstrated in rats and mice (3,4, and references cited
therein). As many as 8 to more than 17 genes (or pseudogenes)
encoding such sequences were found in the rat (5,6) and 25 to
30 in the mouse (7). These spectacular findings suggested a
role for tissue kallikrein-like enzymes in the specific processing of biologically active peptides (7).

This exciting possibility would require the occurrence
of a multigene tissue kallikrein family in all mammals. In
submandibular glands of rats and mice, several members of the
tissue kallikrein family are expressed, and a number of peaks
with arginine esterase or amidase activities can be separated
by chromatography on DEAE ion exchangers (8,9). At the outset
of a study aimed at the comparative investigation of tissue
kallikrein-like enzymes from various organs of the guinea-
pig, attention was therefore directed to the possible occurrence of multiple enzymes with arginine esterase activity.
DEAE-Sephadex chromatography of tissue extracts was used as
the first step of the purification procedure. All column
eluates in this and subsequent purification steps were
assayed with the sensitive tissue kallikrein substrate Ac-
Phe-ArgOEt (10).

MATERIALS AND METHODS

Submandibular glands, the coagulating gland/prostate
complex, or pancreata of male guinea-pigs (all tissues stored

frozen before use) were homogenized with 5 parts of water. After centrifugation, 1/20 volume of 1 M Tris/HCl pH 7.5 was added, and the extracts were applied to pre-equilibrated columns of DEAE-Sephadex A-50. All procedures were performed at 0-6°C.

Esterase activity of the extracts and column eluates was assayed with Ac-Phe-ArgOEt (Bachem AG, Bubendorf, Switzerland) as substrate (10). Soybean trypsin inhibitor (final concentration, 3 mg/ml) was added when the samples contained trypsin. Kininogenase activity was determined with bovine LMW kininogen as substrate, the released kallidin being identified by HPLC (11).

RESULTS

Tissue Kallikrein from Guinea-Pig Submandibular Glands

All arginine esterase activity from extracts of guinea-pig submandibular glands was eluted from a column of DEAE-Sephadex by a sodium chloride gradient in a single, though rather broad peak with severe tailing (Fig. 1A). The breakthrough and the washings with 3 M sodium chloride contained at most 0.01% and 0.02% of the total esterase activity. This result is quite different from that obtained with rat submandibular glands (8) where under similar conditions there appeared several well-resolved esterase peaks with comparable activities. Rechromatography of the whole peak of guinea-pig submandibular esterase under the same conditions gave a much sharper single peak of esterase activity in the same position (Fig. 1B). Evidently, extracts of submandibular glands contain material which perturbs chromatography.

In the course of further purification (starting with larger amounts of tissue) that comprised gel filtration and chromatography on hydroxyapatite (1), all fractions collected from the various columns were also meticulously assayed with Ac-Phe-ArgOEt. No evidence for esterase activity existed outside the single main peak of each of the columns. The arginine esterase activity did not increase on purification or on treating homogenates with trypsin. So it seems most unlikely that another similar enzyme might have existed in the precursor form and thus escaped detection. The specific activity of the final peak recovered from hydroxyapatite was essentially constant accross the peak, a fact also indicating uniformity of the enzyme preparation. Submandibular glands of male guinea-pigs, in contrast to those of rats and mice, appear to contain only a single arginine esterase. Its tissue kallikrein nature demonstrated previously (1) was confirmed by the release of kallidin from pure bovine LMW kininogen.

Tissue Kallikrein from Guinea-Pig Coagulating Gland/Prostate Complex

Chromatography of extracts of the guinea-pig coagulating gland/prostate complex under the same conditions also revealed only a single peak of arginine esterase activity, in a similar position and of comparable width as the peak of submandibular kallikrein on rechromatography (Fig. 1C). The esterase content of the complex, 3600 U/g frozen tissue, is

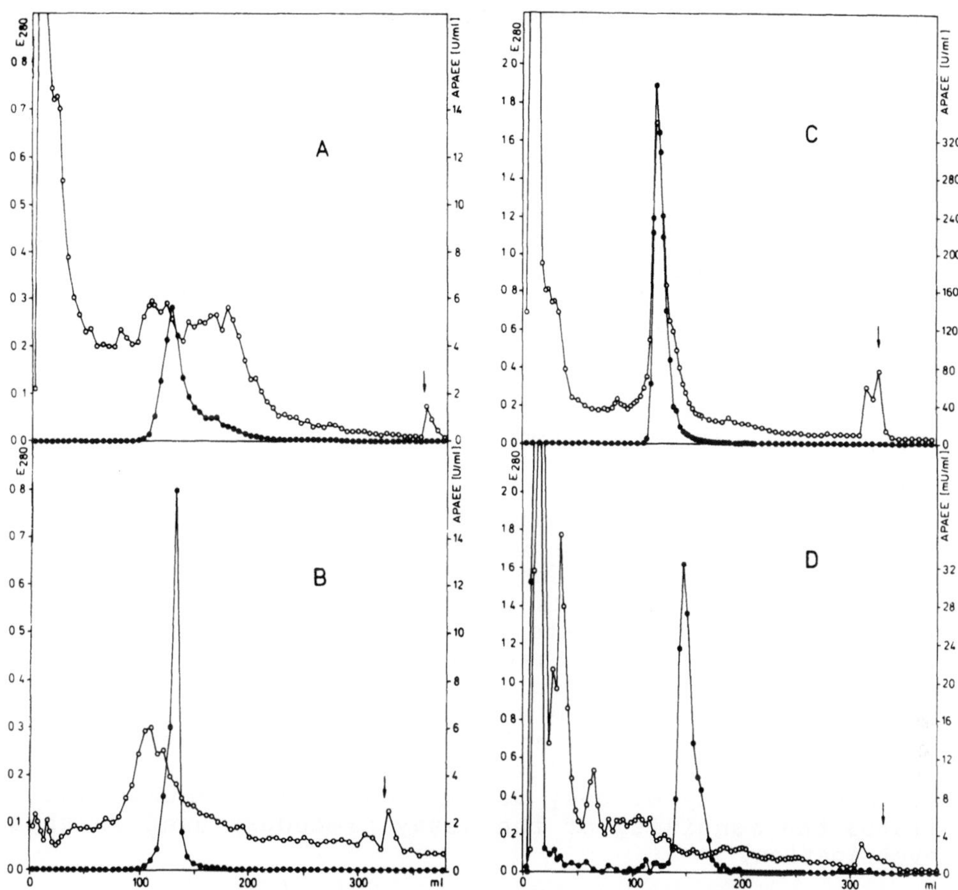

Fig. 1   Chromatography of extracts of tissues from male
          guinea-pigs on a column of DEAE-Sephadex A-50
          (0.7 x 22 cm). (A), 1g submandibular glands;
          (B), rechromatography of the fractions from 88
          to 302 ml; (C), 1g coagulating gland/prostate
          complex; (D), 1.6 g pancreas.
          Linear gradient from 0 to 0.6 M NaCl in 50 mM
          Tris/HCl, pH 7.5. At the arrow, washing with 3
          M NaCl in the same buffer was begun. o, E_{280nm};
          ●, activity determined with Ac-Phe-ArgOEt as
          substrate.

much higher than that of submandibular glands (210 U/g), and
was also not increased on trypsin treatment. Further purification by the steps outlined above also revealed only a
single type of enzyme activity, with a specific activity
(with Ac-Phe-ArgOEt) similar to that of the submandibular
enzyme. This arginine esterase from the coagulating
gland/prostate complex of the guinea-pig has also the properties of a tissue kallikrein as evident from the release of
kallidin from bovine LMW kininogen. However, it distinctly
differs from guinea-pig submandibular kallikrein by a much
slower rate of kallidin liberation. These observations confirm the previous reports of kallidin release from a dog
plasma pseudoglobulin fraction by the coagulating gland enzyme (12) and its relatively low kininogenase activity (2).

Extracts of guinea-pig pancreas contain an arginine esterase which is not inhibited by soybean trypsin inhibitor, as would be expected for a tissue kallikrein. Only homogenates prepared in the presence of this inhibitor do not show this activity, but it appears in the course of the assay. This phenomenon is in contrast to observations on pancreatic prokallikrein of the rat which is difficult to activate (13), but reminescent of the easy activation of porcine pancreatic prokallikrein (14). The remarkably low level of this activity, 0.4 Ac-Phe-ArgOEt units/g frozen pancreas, does not further increase on prolonged incubation, not even when massive activation of endogenous trypsinogen occurs after standing for 24 h at room temperature. On DEAE-Sephadex chromatography of a freshly prepared extract of guinea-pig pancreas (Fig. 1D), considerable arginine esterase activity is found in the first, not retained fractions and most probably represents the developing activity of cationic trypsin. The position of the main esterase peak eluted from the column with the sodium chloride gradient corresponds to that of the other tissue kallikreins, and its size is similar to the amount of esterases in the homogenate not inhibited by soybean trypsin inhibitor. The main peak therefore most probably represents pancreatic kallikrein, even though final proof is still pending. The other peaks are very minor, and at least one of them could be due to beginning activation of anionic trypsinogen. The ease with which the main peak, with a total esterase activity of only 0.6 U, could be detected demonstrates the sensivity of the assay procedure used in this investigation.

DISCUSSION

Our preliminary results on the properties of submandibular and of coagulating gland/prostate kallikreins of the guinea-pig demonstrate their similarities, but also their distinct differences. A recent report on the amino acid sequence of guinea-pig prostate kallikrein (15) allows comparison with the sequence of the 31 N-terminal amino acids of submandibular kallikrein determined previously (1). Only three of these amino acids are found to differ. It is suggested that enzymes with the amino acid sequence of submandibular kallikrein be referred to as guinea-pig tissue kallikrein I and the coagulating gland kallikrein/prostate enzyme as tissue kallikrein II, in analogy to the nomenclature for trypsins. The arginine esterase with the chromatographic properties of a tissue kallikrein detected in low amounts in guinea-pig pancreas might well have the same protein part as the submandibular enzyme, as shown previously for the porcine tissue kallikreins (16), and thus be of type I.

Of especial interest appears the finding that in spite of all efforts only a single arginine esterase could be detected in each, guinea-pig submandibular glands and the coagulating gland/prostate complex. This is of course no rigid proof that the guinea-pig owns not more than two different enzymes of the tissue kallikrein family, but is nevertheless in striking contrast to the numerous similar activities found to occur in submandibular glands of rats and mice. The present results conform to the reports of only 2-3 tissue kallikrein genes in the hamster (17) and a much lower number of such genes in man than in the rat (18), probably only two or three (19). The numerous tissue kallikrein-like enzymes of the rat and mouse appear to represent peculiarities of these closely related species even among the rodents, and so the importance of their surmised physiological roles as specific releasers of a multitude of effectors is doubtful. It would be interesting to determine the number of genes of the tissue kallikrein family in guinea-pigs as well as in other species.

Both tissue kallikreins of the guinea-pig release kallidin from kininogen, as is characteristic for such enzymes. Only rat tissue kallikreins have hitherto been found to liberate bradykinin (20), a property of a number of other proteinases. The tissue kallikrein/kinin system of the guinea pig thus resembles much more that of human and other species than that of the rat. The smaller number of tissue kallikrein-like enzymes occurring in the guinea-pig provide specificity to the determination of tissue kallikrein activities in tissues and body fluids. The specific release of kallidin could be used as a valuable marker for assessing the importance of the tissue kallikrein/kinin system in health and disease. Consequently, the guinea-pig would appear to be more suitable an animal model for studying the physiological and clinical relevance of tissue kallikreins and kinins.

REFERENCES

1. F. Fiedler, M. J. C. Lemon, C. Hirschauer, G. Leysath, F. Lottspeich, A. Henschen, W. Gau, and K. D. Bhoola, Purification and properties of guinea-pig submandibular-gland kallikrein, Biochem. J. 209:125 (1983).
2. C. Moriwaki, N. Watanuki, Y. Fujimoto, and H. Moriya, Further purification and properties of kininogenase from the guinea pig's coagulating gland, Chem. Pharm. Bull. 22:628 (1974).
3. P. L. Ashley and R. J. MacDonald, Kallikrein-related mRNAs of the rat submaxillary gland: nucleotide sequences of four distinct types including tonin, Biochemistry 24:4512 (1985).
4. B. H. van Leeuwen, B. A. Evans, G. W. Tregear, and R. I. Richards, Mouse glandular kallikrein genes. Identification, structure, and expression of the renal kallikrein gene, J. Biol. Chem. 261:5529 (1986).
5. P. L. Ashley and R. J. MacDonald, Tissue-specific expression of kallikrein-related genes in the rat, Biochemistry 24:4520 (1985).
6. W. L. Gerald, J. Chao, and L. Chao, Immunological identification of rat tissue kallikrein cDNA and characterization of the kallikrein gene family, Biochim. Biophys. Acta 866:1 (1986).
7. A. J. Mason, B. A. Evans, D. R. Cox, J. Shine, and R. I. Richards, Structure of mouse kallikrein gene family suggests a role in specific processing of biologically active peptides, Nature 303:300 (1983).
8. P. Brandtzaeg, K. M. Gautvik, K. Nustad, and J. V. Pierce, Rat submandibular kallikreins: purification and

cellular localization, <u>Br. J. Pharmac.</u> 56:155 (1976).

9. W. H. Wilson and E. M. Shooter, Structural modification of the NH_2 terminus of nerve growth factor: purification and characterization of ß-nerve growth factor endopeptidase, <u>J. Biol. Chem.</u> 254:6002 (1979).

10. F. Fiedler, R. Geiger, C. Hirschauer, and G. Leysath, Peptide esters and nitroanilides as substrates for the assay of human urinary kallikrein, <u>Hoppe-Seyler's Z. Physiol. Chem.</u> 359:1667 (1978).

11. F. Fiedler, H. Hinz., and F. Lottspeich, Individual reaction steps in the release of kallidin from kininogen by tissue kallikrein, <u>Adv. Exp. Med. Biol.</u> 198 A:283 (1986).

12. K. Kizuki, C. Moriwaki, and H. Moriya, Kinin-converting activity in the dog pseudoglobulin fraction from heated plasma and kinin liberation from dog kininogen by guinea-pig coagulating gland kallikrein (CGK), <u>Chem. Pharm. Bull.</u> 28:42 (1980).

13. K. M. Yusoff, D. Proud, R. Matsas, and G. S. Bailey, The existence of a trypsin inhibitor-prekallikrein complex in rat pancreatic homogenates, <u>Biochem. Intern.</u> 2:211 (1981).

14. F. Fiedler, C. Hirschauer, and E. Werle, Anreicherung von Präkallikrein B aus Schweinepankreas und Eigenschaften verschiedener Formen des Pankreaskallikreins, <u>Hoppe-Seyler's Z. Physiol. Chem.</u> 351:225 (1970).

15. J. C. Dunbar and R. A. Bradshaw, Amino acid sequence of guinea pig prostate kallikrein, <u>Biochemistry</u> 26:3471 (1987).

16. F. Fiedler, E. Fink, H. Tschesche, and H. Fritz, Porcine glandular kallikreins, <u>Methods Enzymol.</u> 80:493 (1981).

17. P. N. Howles, D. P. Dickinson, L. L. DiCaprio, M. Woodworth-Gutai, and K. W. Gross, Use of a cDNA recombinant for the γ-subunit of mouse nerve growth factor to localize members of this multigene family near the TAM-1 locus on chromosome 7, <u>Nucleic Acids Res.</u> 12:2791 (1984).

18. D. Fukushima, N. Kitamura, and S. Nakanishi, Nucleotide sequence of cloned cDNA for human pancreatic kallikrein, <u>Biochemistry</u> 24:8037 (1985).

19. A. R. Baker and J. Shine, Human kidney kallikrein: cDNA cloning and sequence analysis, <u>DNA</u> 4:445 (1985).

20. H. Kato, K. Enjyoji, T. Miyata, I. Hayashi, S. Oh-Ishi, and S. Iwanaga, Demonstration of arginyl-bradykinin moiety in rat HMW kininogen: direct evidence for liberation of bradykinin by rat glandular kallikreins, <u>Biochem. Biophys. Res. Commun.</u> 127:289 (1985).

PRESENCE OF IMMUNOREACTIVE TISSUE KALLIKREIN IN HUMAN POLYMORPHONUCLEAR

(PMN) LEUCOCYTES

C.D. Figueroa, A.G. MacIver[*], P. Dieppe[†], J.C. Mackenzie[**]
and K.D. Bhoola

Departments of Pharmacology, Pathology[*], Rheumatology[†] and
Nephrology[**], Medical School, University of Bristol
Bristol BS8 1TD, England

SUMMARY

The presence of tissue kallikrein in polymorphonuclear (PMN)
leucocytes from normal human blood and from patients with rheumatoid
arthritis and pyelonephritis was investigated. Immunoreactive tissue
kallikrein was specifically detected in neutrophil leucocytes. PMN
leucocytes displayed a granular staining. In the synovial membrane and
kidney, the cells were aggregated into pockets as part of an inflammatory
infiltrate. The presence of immunoreactive tissue kallikrein in human
PMN leucocytes may provide a new insight into the importance of this
enzyme in inflammation.

INTRODUCTION

Two distinct families of kininogenases have so far been found in
preparations of human PMN leucocytes isolated from blood [1-4]. One
group are leukokinin-forming enzymes with similar properties to cathepsins,
that act on leukokininogen to produce leukokinins, bioactive peptides of
21-25 amino acids [1]. The second group are neutral proteases that can
liberate methionyl-lysyl-bradykinin or bradykinin from plasma kininogen
[2-4]. The availability of specific antibodies to human tissue kallikrein
led us to investigate, whether in addition to the known kininogenases,
tissue kallikrein is also present in PMN leucocytes in human blood and in
two different pathological processes, namely rheumatoid arthritis and
pyelonephritis.

MATERIALS AND METHODS

Human blood from normal donors was used to prepare cellular pellets
and smears. Synovial samples and synovial fluid were obtained from
patients with rheumatoid arthritis (American Rheumatism Association
critera). Tissue samples were also obtained from kidneys affected by
acute pyelonephritis.

Pellet preparation

Synovial fluid was centrifuged in a refrigerated microcentrifuge

(Burkard, Koolspin, England) at 15,000 r.p.m. for 5 min. The resultant
pellet was fixed with 4% formal-saline and left in the tube with fixative
overnight. Normal human blood, collected in the presence of sodium
citrate was centrifuged and the buffy coat was fixed overnight. Pellets
and kidney samples were embedded in paraffin wax.

Smears

Air dried smears prepared from normal human blood were fixed for
5 min with a mixture of picric acid - 2% paraformaldehyde-0.1% glutaralde-
hyde [5] for 5 min at room temperature and processed for immunocytochemistry.

Immunocytochemistry

Antibodies to human urinary and salivary kallikrein were produced
in rabbits in our laboratory; their specificity had been previously
established [6]. Serial sections from paraffin wax embedded samples were
immunostained according to the peroxidase-anti-peroxidase method [7].
Prior to incubation with antibodies, the sections were treated with
methanol and hydrogen peroxide to block endogenous pseudoperoxidase
activity [8]. Controls included preabsorption of the primary antiserum
with purified human urinary kallikrein (40 µg/ml) and omission of the
primary antiserum to confirm the absence of any residual pseudoperoxidase
activity after the treatment with methanol and hydrogen peroxide. After
staining the sections were counterstained with Giemsa or haematoxylin and
eosin.

RESULTS

PMN from normal human blood

PMN leucocytes showed an intense staining for human tissue kallikrein
in contrast to other blood cells, such as monocytes, lymphocytes and
erythrocytes that were unstained (Fig. 1). The counterstaining of immunostained pellets and smears with Giemsa or haematoxylin and eosin showed
that neutrophil leucocytes contained demonstrable tissue kallikrein whereas
eosinophil leucocytes did not (Fig. 1). However, this technique does not
resolve the question whether tissue kallikrein is present in basophil
leucocytes. PMN leucocytes consistently displayed a granular pattern of
cytoplasmic immunoreactivity, especially in blood smears (Fig. 1).

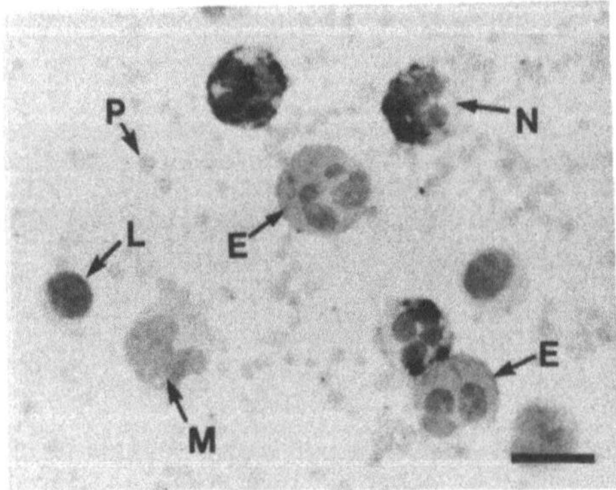

Fig.1. Blood smear.
Neutrophils (N) show
immunoreactive tissue
kallikrein. M, monocyte;
L, lymphocyte; E, eosinophil;
P, platelets. Bar = 7 µm.

<u>PMN leucocytes in rheumatoid arthritis</u>

Immunoreactive PMN leucocytes were numerous in the pellets from
synovial fluid (Fig. 2a), but they were scarce in the inflammatory
infiltrate of synovial membranes (Fig. 2b). At both sites, PMN leucocytes
were the only cell type that contained immunoreactive tissue kallikrein.

<u>PMN leucocytes in pyelonephritic kidneys</u>

Numerous PMN leucocytes containing immunoreactive tissue kallikrein
could be seen in the glomerular capillaries and in other renal blood
vessels. They were also found in the lumen of some renal tubules and in
the interstitium as part of the inflammatory reaction (Fig. 2c).

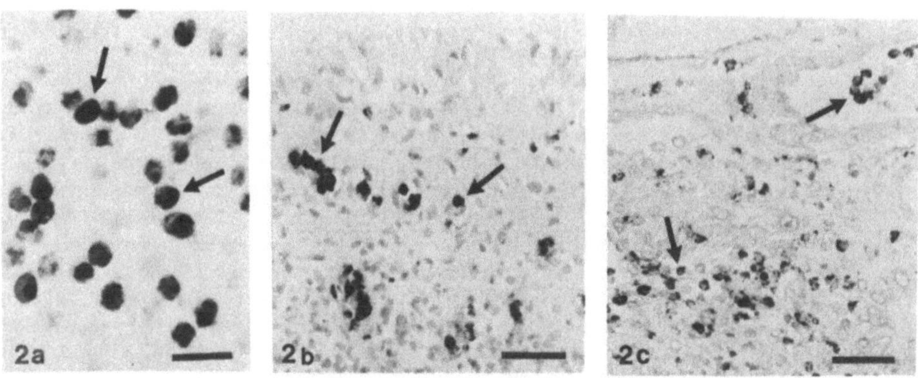

Fig. 2.
Immunoreactive tissue kallikrein in PMN leucocytes can be seen
(arrowed) in a pellet from synovial fluid (a), Bar = 12 μm;
and as part of the inflammatory infiltrate in synovial samples (b),
Bar = 28 μm; and pyelonephritis (c), Bar = 28 μm.

When the antisera to tissue kallikrein were absorbed with purified
human urinary kallikrein no immunostaining was observed in the PMN
leucocyte or any other cell type.

DISCUSSION

Immunoreactive tissue kallikrein is contained in human neutrophil
leucocytes and those involved in rheumatoid arthritis and pyelonephritis.
PMN leucocytes participate actively in inflammation, especially in the
early stages. Together with the accumulation of PMN leucocytes at the
site of inflammation, there is a characteristic increase in vascular
permeability [9]. Kinins produced by the action of plasma kallikrein on
kininogens are considered to act as mediators of the inflammatory response.
The presence of immunoreactive tissue kallikrein in PMN leucocytes suggests
an additional pathway for the generation of kinins during the inflammatory
response, especially if chemotactic factors draw PMN leucocytes to the
inflamed site. Immunoreactive PMN leucocytes are also present in synovial
fluid and in the inflammatory infiltrate of synovial membranes from
patients with rheumatoid arthritis. Furthermore, low molecular weight
kininogen has been identified in synovial fluid obtained from rheumatoid
patients by bioassay [10] and by immunocytochemistry [11]. Therefore,
tissue kallikrein from PMN leucocytes could be responsible, at least in
part, for the production of kinins in rheumatoid joints.

ACKNOWLEDGEMENTS

We wish to thank the Bristol Kidney Unit Research Fund and the Special Trustees of the United Bristol Hospital Fund (Bristol and Weston Health Authority) for financial support. We are grateful to Dr. Charles Hutton for performing some of the synovial biopsies.

REFERENCES

1. L.M. Greenbaum, Kininogenases of blood cells (Alternate kinin generating systems), in: "Bradykinin Kallidin and Kallikrein" E.G. Erdös, ed., Springer Verlag, Berlin (1979).

2. K.L. Melmon, M.J. Cline, Interaction of plasma kinins and granulocytes, Nature, 213:90 (1967).

3. H.Z. Movat, F.M. Habal, D.R. MacMorine, Neutral proteases of human PMN leukocytes with kininogenase activity, Int. Archs. Allergy Appl. Immunol., 50:257 (1976).

4. U. Lüpke, W. Rautenberg, H. Tschesche, Kininogenase from human polymorphonuclear leucocytes, Agents and Actions (Suppl.), 9:308 (1982).

5. C.D. Figueroa, J. Subiabre, I. Caorsi, C.P. Vio, Immunoreactive kallikrein localization in the rat kidney. An immunoelectron microscopic study, J. Histochem. Cytochem., 32:117 (1984).

6. A.F. Bagshaw, K.D. Bhoola, M.J.C. Lemon, J.T. Whicher, Development and characterization of a radioimmunoassay to measure human tissue kallikrein in biological fluids, J. Endocrinol., 101:173 (1984).

7. L.A. Sternberger, The unlabeled antibody peroxidase-antiperoxidase (PAP) method, in: "Immunocytochemistry" J. Wiley & Sons, New York (1979).

8. J.G. Streefkery, Inhibition of erythrocyte pseudoperoxidase activity by treatment with hydrogen peroxide following methanol. J. Histochem. Cytochem., 20:829 (1972).

9. G. Majno, G.E. Palade, Studies in inflammation.I. The effect of histamine and serotonin on vascular permeability. An electron microscopic study, J. Biophys. Biochem. Cytol., 11:571 (1961).

10. K. Sawai, S. Niwa, M. Katori, The significant reduction of high molecular weight-kininogen in synovial fluid of patients with active rheumatoid arthritis, in: "Kinins II Advances in Experimental Medicine and Biology", S. Fuji, H. Moriya, T. Suzuki, eds., Plenum Press, New York, 120B:195 (1979).

11. C.D. Figueroa, P. Dieppe, K.D. Bhoola, (unpublished).

ENZYME-LINKED IMMUNOSORBENT ASSAYS FOR HUMAN TISSUE KALLIKREIN AND

ANALYSIS OF IMMUNOREACTIVE KALLIKREIN IN THE PLASMA BY THEM

Kazuyuki Kizuki, Satoru Suzuki, Kazumasa Aoki, Masafumi
Kamada, Masahiko Ikekita, Toshimori Inaba and Hiroshi Moriya

Department of Biochemistry, Faculty of Pharmaceutical
Sciences, Science University of Tokyo, 12, Ichigaya-
Funakawara-machi, Shinjuku-ku, Tokyo 162, Japan

SUMMARY

In order to study immunoreactive tissue kallikrein (TK) in human
plasma, three kinds of enzyme-linked immunosorbent assay (ELISA) systems
for human urinary kallikrein (HUK) were developed. All three types of
TK in the plasma, i.e., active kallikrein, prokallikrein and kallikrein-
$\alpha_1$antitrypsin (α_1AT) complex, could be measured by the competitive ELISA
(C-ELISA). However, the sandwich ELISA (S-ELISA) showed more strict
specificity. Namely, both active and prokallikreins were able to be
measured by the S-ELISA, while kallikrein-α_1AT complex was hardly
measurable. Measurement of this kallikrein-α_1AT complex was made
possible by using horseradish peroxidase (HRP)-labeled anti-α_1AT IgG
instead of HRP-labeled anti-HUK Fab' as the second antibody (HS-ELISA).

Using these ELISAs we studied TK in plasma and the following
observations were made. 1) The greater part of TK in the plasma was
found in a form of a complex with α_1AT. 2) The amount of free type TK
was very small and the most part of this type TK in normal plasma was
prokallikrein.

INTRODUCTION

It has been reported that TKs are present in the plasma of many
mammals, although the organs that secrete TK into the blood vessels or the
significance of TK in the plasma etc. are not clear as yet. The concentration of TK in the plasma is very low, so that the development of very
sensitive methods that can specifically detect immunoreactive kallikrein
in the plasma, such as radioimmunoassay and ELISA, are essential to the
analysis of the physiological or pathological significance of TK in plasma.

However, at least three different types of TK could be detected in
human plasma, i.e., active kallikrein, prokallikrein and kallikrein
bound to protease inhibitor(s). Therefore, the analysis of TK in the
plasma in physiological or pathological states may not be simple.

In the present work, the authors developed three kinds of useful
ELISA systems for HUK to study TK in plasma.

Anti-HUK Rabbit IgG. The HUK preparation purified in our laboratory by DEAE-Sepharose CL-6B chromatography, affinity chromatography on an Aprotinin-immobilized Sepharose 4B column and gel filtration on a Sephacryl S-200 column, which showed a single band on SDS-polyacrylamide gel electrophoresis and had a specific activity of 11.8 AU/mg was used for the preparation of anti-HUK rabbit serum as an antigen. The anti-HUK IgG fraction was prepared from the heated (56°C, 30 min) serum by the usual ways, viz., ammonium sulfate fractionation and DEAE-cellolose chromatography.

HRP-labeled Anti-HUK Fab' and HRP-labeled HUK. Anti-HUK IgG was treated with pepsin and the anti-HUK F(ab')$_2$ was prepared. Then, it was treated with 2-mercaptoethylamine and anti-HUK Fab' was obtained. The anti-HUK Fab' (4 mg) was conjugated with 4 mg of HRP according to the method of Ishikawa et al.[1]

HRP-labeled HUK was prepared according to the method of Nakane et al.[2]

Other Chemicals. Horseradish peroxidase (Type VI) and human α_1AT were purchased from Sigma Chemicals Co. (St. Lois, MO., U.S.A.). Anti-human α_1AT goat IgG and HRP-labeled anti-human α_1AT IgG were obtained from Kent Laboratories Inc. (Redmond, WA., U.S.A.) and Cappel Laboratories Inc. (Malvern, PA., U.S.A.), respectively. H-Pro-Phe-Arg-MCA was from Peptide Institute Inc. (Osaka, Japan). The E.I.A. microtitration plate (Linbro®, 96 wells) from Flow Laboratories Inc. (Mclear, VA., U.S.A.) was also used.

Kallikrein Activity Assay. H-Pro-Phe-Arg-MCA hydrolyzing activity of kallikrein was measured according to the method of Kato et al.[3] with slight modifications. One amidase unit (AU) was defined as the amount of enzyme that can hydrolyze 1 μmol of substrate per min at 30°C, pH 8.0. The amount of prokallikrein was estimated after the treatment with trypsin.[4]

ELISAs (Fig. 1). a) C-ELISA; Step 1. One hundred μl of anti-HUK IgG solution diluted to 2.0 μg/ml with 0.05 M carbonate buffer, pH 9.6, was added to each well of a microtiter plate and stood overnight at 4°C. After removing the solutions, 100 μl of 0.01 M phosphate buffer, pH 7.4, containing 1% (w/v) bovine serum albumin (BSA) was added to the wells and further incubated for 30 min at room temperature. The wells were then washed 3 times with 0.01 M phosphate buffer, pH 7.4, containing 0.1% BSA, 0.05% (v/v) Tween 20 and 0.15 M NaCl (washing buffer). Step 2. Fifty μl of sample solution or standard HUK solutions were added to the wells and 50 μl of HRP-labeled HUK solution (1 mPU/ml, PU; Pyrogallol Unit) was further added to each well. After stirring, the plate stood for 16 hr. at 4°C or 5 hr. at room temperature. Then, the wells washed 4 times with the washing buffer mentioned above. Step 3. One hundred μl of the substrate solution (0.8 mg/ml o-phenylenediamine and 0.006% H$_2$O$_2$ in 0.1 M citrate-phosphate buffer, pH 5.0) were added to the wells and incubated at room temperature in the dark. After 20 min. the enzyme reaction was stopped with the addition of 50μl of 4N HCl.

The absorbance at 492 nm was automatically recorded by a spectrophotometer (Corona Electric Co., Model MP-22, Japan). The amount of TK in the sample solution was calculated from the standard surve obtained.

b) S-ELISA; Step 1. Identical with the case of the C-ELISA. Step 2. One hundred μl of the sample solution or standard HUK solutions were added to the wells of the microtiter plate and incubated for the same time as the C-ELISA. After washing the wells with the washing buffer (4 times), 100 μl of HRP-labeled anti-HUK Fab' solution (3 mPU/ml) was added to the wells. After 2 hr incubation at room temperature, the wells were washed well with the washing buffer (4 times). Step 3. Identical with the C-ELISA.

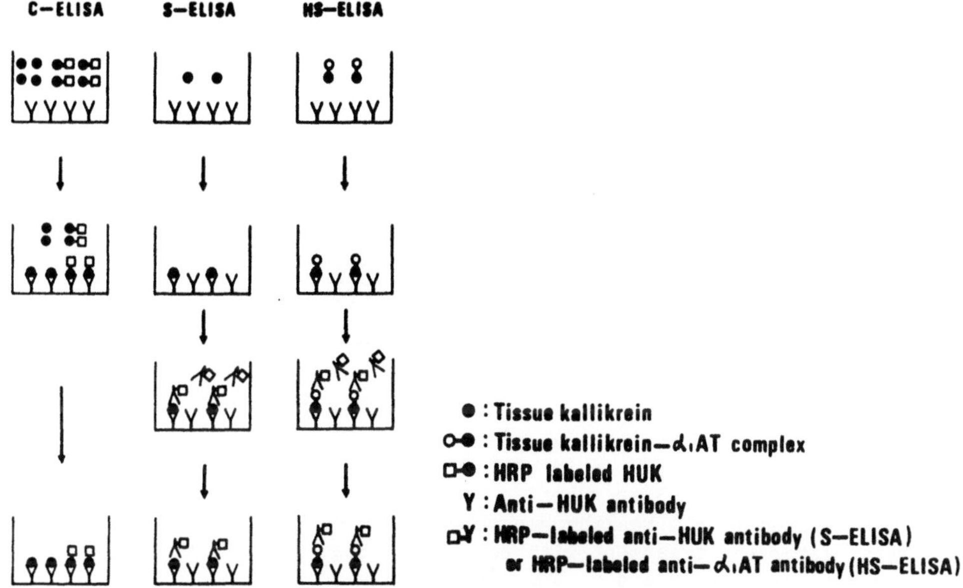

Fig. 1   Three ELISA Systems for Determination of TK

c) HS-ELISA; In step 2 in the S-ELISA, HRP-labeled anti-human α_1AT goat IgG was used instead of HRP-labeled anti-HUK Fab'.   Other procedures were identical with those of the S-ELISA.   Standard curves in the HS-ELISA were obtained by using HUK-α_1AT complex which had been prepared by the following ways.   Two hundred µl of HUK solution (0.1 mg/ml) was added to the same volume of α_1AT solution (10 mg/ml in 0.05 M of Tris-HCl buffer, pH 8.0) and incubated for 24 hr at 37°C.   After the confirmation that the H-Pro-Phe-Arg-MCA hydrolyzing activity of HUK was completely inhibited by α_1AT, this incubation mixture (50 µg HUK eq./ml) was used.   In this incubation mixture, an excess amount of free α_1AT remained.   However, this free α_1AT was completely removed by the washing procedure carried out in step 2.   Therefore, the second antibody (HRP-labeled anti-α_1AT IgG) reacted only with HUK-α_1AT complex on the solid phase.

In these ELISAs, dilutions of authentic HUK, HUK-α_1AT complex and sample solutions were carried out with 0.01 M phosphate buffer, pH 7.4, containing both 0.1% BSA and 0.15 M NaCl.

RESULTS AND DISCUSSIONS

Dose-Response Curves. Fig. 2 shows the typical standard curves obtained with authentic HUK in the C- and the S-ELISAs.   As shown in the figure, 0.3 - 100 ng/ml (0.015 - 5 ng/well) and 0.1 - 30 ng/ml (0.01 - 3 ng/well) of HUK solutions were able to be measured in the C- and the S-ELISA systems, respectively.

Specificity. The slopes of the dilution curves of human plasma, saliva, pancreatic juice, gastric juice and urine were well agreed with those of the standard curves of HUK prepared by using 1 - 100 ng/ml (C-ELISA) and 0.1 - 10 ng/ml (S-ELISA) of its solutions. Human albumin and plasma kallikrein, rat submandibular kallikrein and porcine pancreatic kallikrein did not react in both ELISAs.   Therefore, these two ELISAs seemed to be able to specifically detect human TK in the biological fluids.

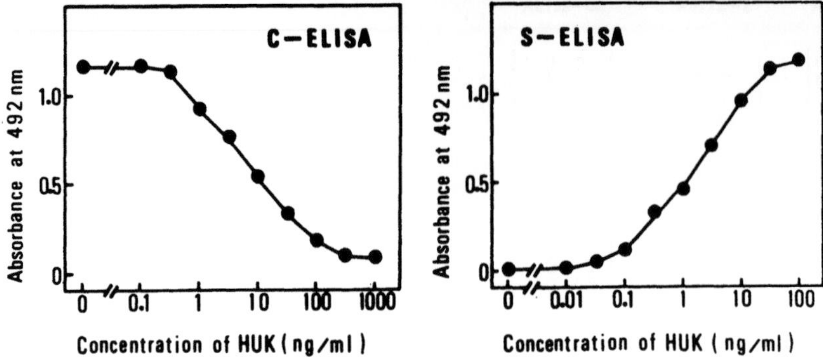

Fig. 2 Dose-Response Curves for HUK in C- and S-ELISAs

Prokallikrein. Next, we investigated whether prokallikrein is detectable by these ELISAs or not.   At first, prokallikrein contents in urines collected from 6 healthy men were determined by the H-Pro-Phe-Arg-MCA assay after the treatment with trypsin.   The prokallikrein contents in urines 1, 2, 3, 4, 5 and 6 shown in Fig. 3 were determined to be 76, 72, 61, 80, 70 and 78%, respectively.   Then, the amounts of kallikrein in these urines were separately determined by the S-ELISA (Fig. 3).   The abscissa in the figure is the incubation time with the first antibody. The open and the closed symbols are the urines before (nontreated) and after the treatment with trypsin, respectively.   As shown in the figure, before the 4 hr incubation periods, the amounts of kallikrein in the nontreated urines determined were slightly lower than those in the trypsin treated urines.   On the other hand, if the incubation times were prolonged to 8 and 16 hr, almost the same values were obtained. Therefore, we concluded that prokallikrein was also detectable by our S-ELISA in our experimental conditions.
The same observations were also obtained in the case of C-ELISA.

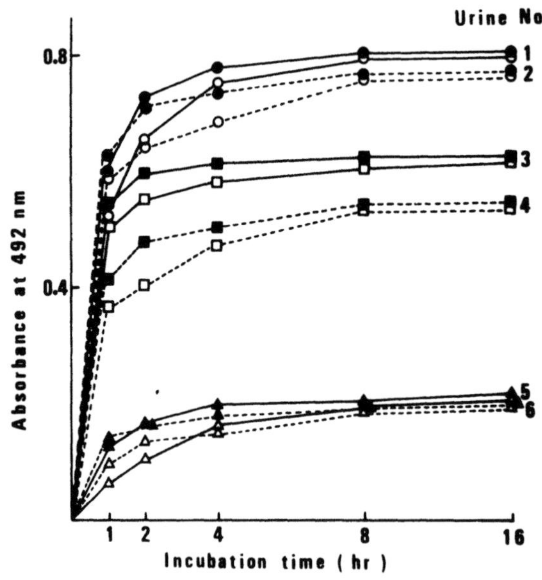

Fig. 3 Determination of Kallikrein in Urines before and
after the Treatment with Trypsin by the S-ELISA

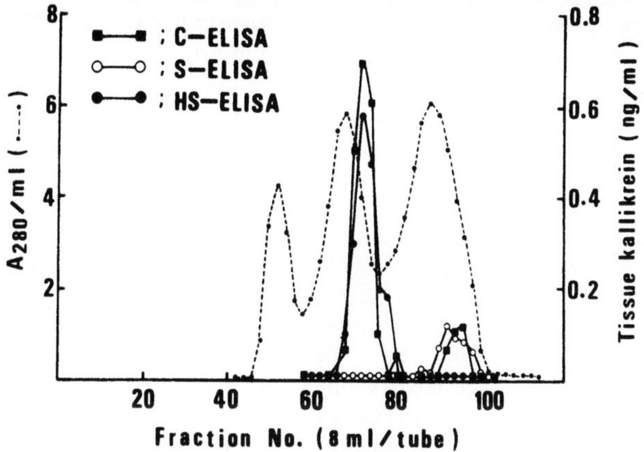

Fig. 4   Analysis of TK in Human Plasma after the Gel
Filtration on a Sephacryl S-200 Column

    <u>Quantitation and Analysis of TK in the Plasma</u>.   The contents of TK in
the plasma of healthy men determined by the C- and S-ELISAs were 1.39 ±
0.39 ng/ml (n=24) and 0.28 ± 0.14 ng/ml (n=24), respectively.   In order
to analyze this difference, the plasma (20 ml) was gel filtered on a column
of Sephacryl S-200 (4 X 130 cm) and the kallikreins in the fractions were
determined by the ELISAs; 10 times concentrated fractions by Minicon® B15
(Amicon Co., Danvers, MA., U.S.A.) were used for the ELISAs.   As shown in
Fig. 4, when the amounts of kallikrein were determined by the C-ELISA, two
peaks were observed, i.e., a large peak (M.W., 10 X 10^4) and a small one
(M.W., 4 X 10^4).   On the other hand, only one peak which eluted the same
position as the small peak observed in the C-ELISA was detected by the
S-ELISA.   The elution volume of the small peak was the same as that of
purified HUK.

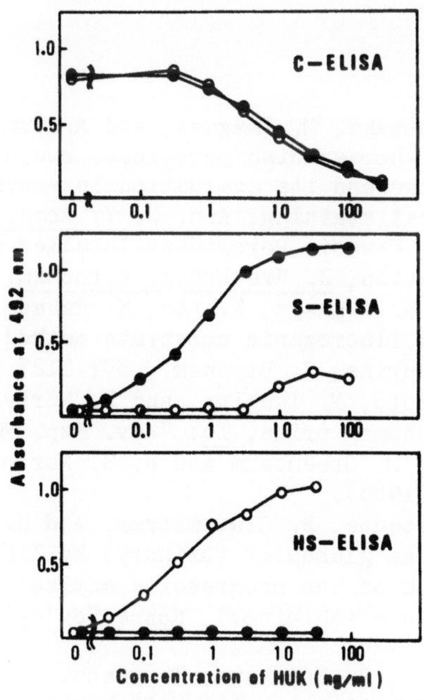

Fig. 5   Standard Curves obtained by the C-, S- and HS-ELISAs
for HUK (●—●) and HUK-α_1AT Complex (○—○)

Judging from these observations, the greater part of TK in the plasma
seemed to be present as a complex with some protease inhibitor(s) in the
plasma and the difference observed above between C- and S-ELISAs was
considered to indicate that our S-ELISA could not detect this complex type
kallikrein, probably due to some steric hindrance (second antibody hardly
reacted with the antigen-antibody complex on the solid phase). This
hypothesis was confirmed by the next observations. First, it had been
already reported that the main plasma protease inhibitor of TK is α_1AT,[5,6]
so we developed the HS-ELISA (see MATERIALS AND METHODS) and the amounts
of kallikrein in the fractions in Fig. 4 were determined by this method.
As shown in Fig. 4, only one peak corresponded to the large peak observed
in the C-ELISA was obtained by it. Second, as shown in Fig. 5, standard
curves for HUK and HUK-α_1AT complex obtained by the C-ELISA were nearly
identical. However, the reactivity of HUK-α_1AT complex was extremely
lower than that of HUK in the S-ELISA, and HUK-α_1AT complex was specifically measured by the HS-ELISA.

From these results, we concluded that the measured values by our
C-ELISA mainly represented the total amount of TK, while those by the
S- and HS-ELISAs reflected the amount of free type kallikrein (i.e.,
active and prokallikreins) and kallikrein-α_1AT complex in the plasma,
respectively.

Next, 50 ml of fresh human plasma was gel filtered on the same column
as Fig. 4 and the same gel filtrations were repeated 12 times (total plasma,
600 ml). The fractions corresponded to the small peak shown in Fig. 4 in
each gel filtration were pooled and the TK in this pooled fraction was
concentrated by an affinity column of anti-HUK IgG immobilized Sepharose 4B.
Then, the content of prokallikrein was determined by the H-Pro-Phe-Arg-MCA
assay. By this assay, content of prokallikrein in this pooled fraction
was determined to be 83%, while nearly equal values were obtained between
non-treated and trypsin treated samples by the S-ELISA. Therefore, the
most part of free type kallikrein in normal plasma was considered to be
prokallikrein.

REFERENCES

1. E. Ishikawa, S. Yoshitake, M. Imagawa, and A. Sumiyoshi, Preparation
   of monomeric Fab'-horseradish peroxidase conjugate using thiol
   groups in the hinge and its evaluation in enzyme immunoassay and
   immunohistochemical staining, Ann. N. Y. Acad. Sci., 420: 74 (1983).
2. P. K. Nakane, and A. Kawaoi, Peroxidase-labelled antibody. A new
   method of conjugation, J. Histochem. Cytochem., 22: 1084 (1974).
3. H. Kato, N. Adachi, S. Iwanaga, K. Abe, K. Takada, T. Kimura, and S.
   Sakakibara, A new fluorogenic substrate method for the estimation
   of kallikrein in urine, J. Biochem., 87: 1127 (1980).
4 K. Kizuki, Y. Shimamoto, M. Ikekita, and H. Moriya, An inactive form
   of kallikrein in human urine, in: "Adv. Exp. Med. Biol.; Kinins
   IV," Vol. 198, L. M. Greenbaum and H. S. Margolius, eds., Plenum
   Press, New York (1986).
5. R. Geiger, U. Stuckstedte, B. Clausmitzer, and H. Frits, Progressive
   inhibition of human glandular (urinary) kallikrein by human serum
   and identification of the progressive antikallikrein as α_1-anti-
   trypsin (α_1-protease inhibitor), Hoppe-Seyler's Z. Physiol. Chem.,
   362: 317 (1981).
6. K. Hirana, Y. Okumura, S. Hayakawa, T. Adachi, and M. Sugiura,
   Inhibition of human tissue kallikrein by α_1-protease inhibitor,
   Hoppe-Seyler's Z. Physiol Chem., 365: 27 (1984).

GLANDULAR KALLIKREIN-LIKE ENZYME IN ADRENAL GLANDS

G. Scicli**, H. Nolly*, O.A. Carretero, and A.G. Scicli

Hypertension Research Division, Henry Ford Hospital, Detroit
MI, USA, *Consejo Nacional De Investigaciones Cientificas y
Tecnicas (Conicet) and School of Medicine, University of Cuyo
Mendoza, Argentina

ABSTRACT

A kallikrein-like kininogenase was identified in the rat adrenal
gland. Most of the enzyme was present in an inactive form, since pre-
incubation with trypsin markedly increased kininogenase activity from
54.8 ± 11.8 to 230 ± 23.0 pg bradykinin/mg protein/min. Adrenal
kininogenase was inhibited 90% by phenyl methyl sulfonyl fluoride, 92% by
D-Phe-Phe-Arg-chloromethylketone, 91% by aprotinin, and only 15% by
soybean trypsin inhibitor. Pre-incubation with antibodies against rat
urinary kallikrein resulted in 85% inhibition. The apparent molecular
weight of adrenal kininogenase on gel filtration chromatography was 33 Kd.
The enzyme was strongly adsorbed to immobilized rat urinary kallikrein
antibodies and required drastic conditions for elution. In canine adrenal
glands, we found that there was no difference in the cortical and medullary
distribution of active and inactive SBTI resistant kininogenase activity.
We conclude that an enzyme which closely resembles glandular kallikrein is
present in adrenal glands.

INTRODUCTION

Glandular kallikrein belongs to a family of serine proteinases that
may be involved in bio-regulatory functions[1,2] either by generating kinins
or by processing peptide hormones[3,4]. Furthermore, kinins can stimulate the
release of catecholamines from adrenal medulla. The purpose of this study
was to determine whether a glandular kallikrein-like enzyme is present in
the adrenal gland. This study was performed using glands from rats. Canine
adrenal glands were used to determine whether kallikrein was present in the
cortex and/or medulla. We found that: 1) a glandular kallikrein-like
enzyme present in rat adrenals is predominantly in an inactive form

---

** To whom correspondence should be addressed.
Supported by NIH Grant HL28982

(trypsin-activatable kininogenase); and 2) the enzyme is present at similar concentrations in the cortical and medullary regions of canine adrenal glands.

MATERIALS AND METHODS

Reagents. The following materials were obtained from commercial sources: Molecular weight markers (Bio Rad), ultrogel AcA$_{54}$ (LKB); trypsin and soybean trypsin inhibitor [SBTI] (Worthington), aprotinin (Bayer); phenyl methyl sulfonyl fluoride [PMSF], (Sigma), and D-Phe-Phe-Arg-chloromethylketone (Calbiochem). All reagents used were analytical grade.

Preparation of Tissue Extracts. The adrenal glands were removed and cleaned from fifty male Wistar rats (250-300 g). After washing, the glands were frozen (-20°C) and thawed four times and then homogenized.

Whole adrenal glands or their cortical and medullary portions from mongrel dogs of either sex were homogenized in 0.1 M Tris-HCl, 0.25 M sucrose, 3 mg/ml Na$_2$ EDTA and 0.1% Triton X-100, pH 7.4.

Kininogenase Activity. Kinin-generating activity was determined by incubation of 200-400 μl of tissue extract or column eluate for 4 hours at 37°C with 200 μl of partially purified dog kininogen (2000 ng of kinin releasing capability). The kinins generated were measured by RIA[5].

Trypsin Activation. The adrenal homogenate was incubated with trypsin to determine the presence of inactive adrenal kininogenase. A fixed amount of tissue was pre-incubated for 30 minutes at 37°C with varying concentrations of trypsin ranging from 0.05 to 1.0 μg/mg wet tissue in 500 μl of 0.1 M Tris-HCl buffer, pH 8.5, to establish the best ratio on a weight basis between adrenal tissue and trypsin. The reaction was then stopped by adding 100 μl of SBTI (1 mg/ml). A ratio of trypsin to tissue equal to 0.2 μg/mg tissue was found to optimally activate SBTI-resistant kininogenase and was subsequently used.

The concentration of inactive adrenal kininogenase was calculated as the difference between kininogenase activity before and after trypsin treatment.

Inhibition Studies. Different aliquots of adrenal homogenates were pre-incubated (30 min. at 37°C) with the following inhibitors (final concentrations): SBTI (4 X 10^{-6} M); PMSF (2 X 10^{-3}M); aprotinin (1,000 KIU); D-Phe-Phe-Arg-Chloromethylketone (1 x 10^{-6}M). Inhibition of activity was accomplished with 10 μg of globulins purified from antiserum against rat urinary kallikrein using purified normal serum as control globulins. A similar protocol was performed with purified rat submandibular gland kallikrein (0.2 ng). After the pre-incubation period, the kininogenase activity was determined, always in the presence of excess SBTI.

Immunoreactive kallikrein was determined by RIA[6].

Gel Filtration on Ultrogel AcA$_{54}$. Supernatant of rat adrenal gland homogenate was applied to an Ultrogel AcA$_{54}$ column (100 x 1 cm) equilibrated with 0.1 M phosphate buffer, pH 7.4, and eluted using the same buffer. Fractions (3 ml) were collected and kininogenase activity was monitored in each sample. For molecular weight determination, the elution volume of the adrenal kininogenase was compared with that of the following molecular weight standards: Bovine albumin (MW. 67,000), ovalbumin (MW. 43,000), chymotrypsinogen (MW. 25,000), and myoglobin (MW. 17,000).

Rat submandibular kallikrein was purified using a modification of a previously described method[7], and released 1.2 μg of kinin per 1 μg protein per minute when incubated with semi-purified dog kininogen[7].

Protein was determined by the method of Bradford[8].

RESULTS

Active and inactive (trypsin activatable) SBTI-resistant kininogenase are present in the adrenal gland homogenates. Kallikrein antibodies inhibited 85% of the kininogenase activity (Table 1).

Table 1. Kininogenase Activity in Rat Adrenal Gland

	Kininogenase Activity (pg BK/mg/min)	% Inhibition by UKK Antibodies
Active:	55 ± 12 (n=9)	85 (n=5)
Trypsin-Activatable	230 ± 23 (n=12)	85 (n=5)

Kininogenase activity was measured using 200 μl of gland homogenate before and after activation with trypsin. Samples were pre-incubated for 30 minutes at 37°C with 10 μg of either globulins purified from normal rabbit serum or from glandular kallikrein antiserum. Incubations of submandibular gland kallikrein (0.2 ng) with kallikrein antibodies resulted in 90% inhibition of kininogenase activity.

Sensitivity of adrenal SBTI-resistant kininogenase and glandular kallikrein to various proteinase inhibitors is similar (Table 2).

Immunoreactive kallikrein was measured after gel filtration and was 30.7 ± 4.8 ng/mg protein (n=11). The apparent molecular weight of adrenal kininogenase on gel filtration was calculated as 33 Kd (Fig. 1). Adrenal kininogenase was strongly adsorbed to immobilized rat urinary kallikrein antibodies. The kininogenase bound to the immunoaffinity gel was not eluted by washing with buffer containing 1 M NaCl. The enzyme could be eluted by lowering the pH to 3.5 (Fig. 2). Figure 3 shows that similar concentrations of active and inactive (trypsin-activatable) forms of the enzyme were present in the medulla and cortex of canine adrenals.

DISCUSSION

This study demonstrates that an enzyme able to release kinins from kininogen is present in the adrenal gland. Several data indicate that this kininogenase resembles tissue kallikrein. Both the adrenal enzyme and glandular kallikrein are resistant to inhibition by SBTI, while kininogenases such as plasma kallikrein, trypsin and plasmin are inhibited by SBTI. Estimation of molecular weight by gel filtration indicated that both the adrenal SBTI-resistant kininogenase and rat glandular kallikrein have an apparent molecular weight of 33,000 daltons. The sensitivity to proteinase inhibitors of the adrenal kininogenase is similar to that of glandular kallikrein. Identification of the adrenal enzyme as glandular kallikrein is strengthened by the inhibition of the kininogenase activity by pre-incubation with antibodies against rat urinary kallikrein. Together, these data suggest that glandular kallikrein or an enzyme closely resembling glandular kallikrein is present in the adrenal gland. Most of the enzyme appears to be in an inactive form since incubation with trypsin resulted in a four-fold increase in the SBTI-resistant kininogenase of the adrenal homogenates. Both active and inactive SBTI-resistant kininogenase were also found in dog adrenals and preliminary data indicate that pig adrenals also contained the enzyme (unpublished data). In addition, the present data indicate that this glandular kallikrein-like enzyme is present in the adrenal medulla and also in the cortex.

The precise function of adrenal kallikrein is unknown at this time.

Table 2. Sensitivity to Serine Protease Inhibitors of Rat Adrenal Kininogense and Submandibular Gland Kallikrein

	Percent Inhibition	
Inhibitor	Rat Adrenal Kininogenase	Rat Submandibular Gland Kallikrein
Aprotinin		
100 KIU	79 ± 0.82	86 ± 1.15
1,000 KIU	91 ± 1.73	84 ± 1.10
Soybean trypsin inhibitor		
4×10^{-7} M	5 ± 1.20	0.6 ± 0.2
4×10^{-6} M	15 ± 1.22	3.0 ± 0.82
D-Phe-Phe-Arg-chloromethyl ketone		
1×10^{-6} M	92 ± 2.05	91 ± 1.23
Phenyl-methy-sulfonyl fluoride		
2×10^{-3} M	90 ± 0.41	91 ± 2.1

Kininogenase activity was measured in homogenates pre-incubated with the different proteinase inhibitors for 30 min. at 37°C. A similar protocol was performed with purified rat submandibular gland kallikrein (0.2 ng). The values represent the mean of three determinations.

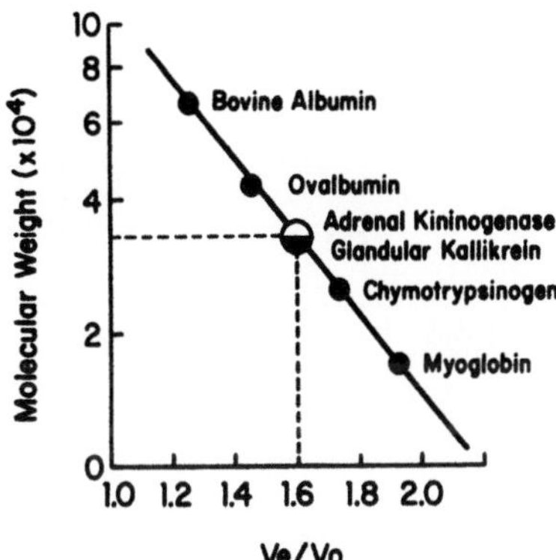

Fig. 1. *Molecular weight determination of the adrenal kininogenase on a calibrated column of ultrogel AcA$_{54}$. Standards were monitored by A280 and the adrenal enzyme was monitored by its SBTI-resistant kininogenase activity. Elution volume was taken as that of the maximum of each peak.*

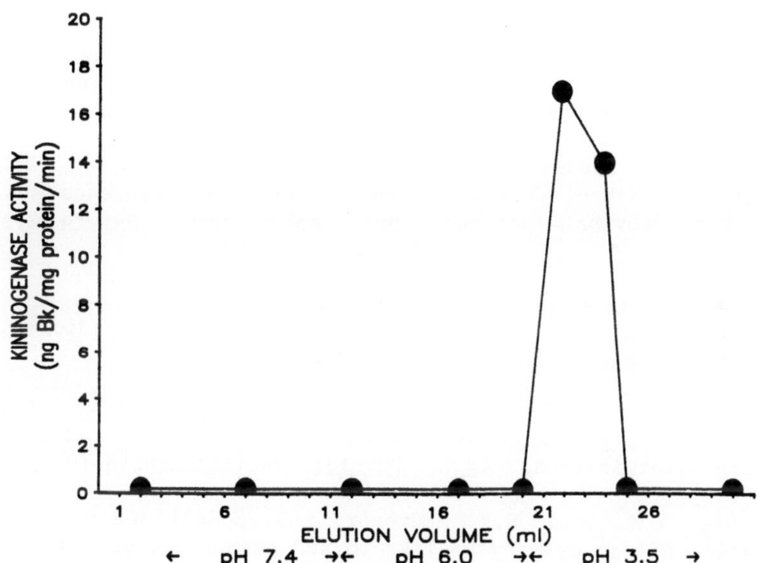

Fig. 2. *Immuno-affinity chromatography of adrenal homogenate on antikallikrein-CH-sepharose. The gel and the sample were equilibrated with 0.1 M sodium phosphate buffer pH 7.4, and mixed overnight at 4°C. After washing the gel with equilibrating buffer, weakly bound proteins were eluted with 0.1 M sodium phosphate, 1M sodium chloride, pH 6.0. The adrenal kininogenase was eluted with 0.1 M sodium acetate, 1 M NaCl, pH 3.5.*

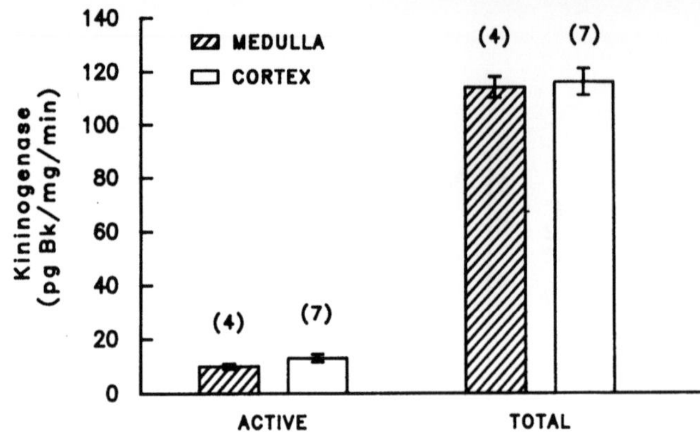

Fig. 3.   *Active   and   total   (after trypsin activation)   SBTI-resistant kininogenase   activity   in   homogenates   of   the   cortical   and medullary regions of canine adrenal glands.*

REFERENCES

1.   M. Schachter. Kallikreins (Kininogenase) - A group of serine proteases with bio-regulatory actions. Pharmacol. Rev. 31:1-17 (1980).

2.   O.A. Carretero and A.G. Scicli.   Possible role of kinins in circulatory homeostasis. Hypertension 3 (Suppl. I):I4-I12 (1981).

3.   L.E. Eiden, R.L. Eskay, J. Scott, H. Pollard and A.J. Hotchkiss. Primary cultures of bovine chromaffin cells synthesize and secrete vasoactive intestinal polypeptide (VIP). Life Sci. 33:687-693 (1983).

4.   M. Noda, Y. Furutani, H. Takahashi, M. Toyosato, T. Hirose, S. Inayama, S. Nakanishi and S. Numa. Cloning and sequence analysis of cDNA for bovine adrenal preproenkephalin. Nature 295:202-208 (1982).

5.   O.A. Carretero, N.B. Oza, A. Piwonska, T. Ocholik, and A.G. Scicli. Measurement of urinary kallikrein activity by kinin radioimmunoassay. Biochem. Pharmacol. 25:2265-2270 (1976).

6.   S.F. Rabito, A.G. Scicli, V. Kher and O.A. Carretero. Immunoreactive glandular kallikrein in rat plasma: A radioimmunoassay for its determination. Am. J. Physiol. 242(11):H602-H610 (1982).

7.   N.B. Oza, V.M. Amin, R.K. McGregor, A.G. Scicli and O.A. Carretero. Isolation of rat urinary kallikrein and properties of its antibodies. Biochem. Pharmacol. 25:1607-1612 (1976).

8.   M.M. Bradford. A rapid and sensitive method for the quantitation of microgram quantities of protein utilizing the principle of protein-dye binding. Anal. Biochem. 72:248-254 (1976).

FURTHER CHARACTERIZATION OF MONOCLONAL ANTIBODIES AGAINST RAT PLASMA

KALLIKREIN, RAT LOW MOLECULAR WEIGHT KININOGEN AND SYNTHETIC BRADYKININ

Gurrinder S. Bedi and Nathan Back

Department of Biochemical Pharmacology
State University of New York, Buffalo, NY 14260

INTRODUCTION

Complimentary biochemical and immunochemical techniques provide
very valuable information about the structure-function relationships of
biologically active molecules. Monoclonal antibodies offer advantages
over polyclonal antibodies with regard to fixed affinity, specificity
and unlimited availability. They thus very often make better reagents
for the development of immunoassays. Additionally monoclonal antibodies
are useful in rapid and specific immunoaffinity purification procedures.
This report summarizes further characterization of monoclonal antibodies produced by hybridoma cells against rat plasma kallikrein (1),
rat plasma low molecular weight kininogen (2) and synthetic bradykinin
(3).

MATERIALS AND METHODS

Rat plasma kininogen (4) and rat plasma kallikrein (5) were
purified as described earlier. Kallikrein from porcine pancreas, human
urine and human plasma were procured from Bayer AG (West Germany). Rat
urinary kallikrein was a gift from Dr. N. Oza (Boston, MA). Pristane
and polyethylene glycol was obtained from Aldrich Chemical Co.
(Milwaukee, WI). Thymidine, hypoxanthine, aminopurine, HEPES, Tris and
o-phenylenediamine were purchased from Sigma Chem. Co. (St. Louis, MO).
Peroxidase conjugated anti-mouse immunoglobulins were obtained from
Cappel Labs. (Cochranville, PA). Dulbecco's modified Eagle's medium,
horse serum and antibiotics were products of Gibco (Grand Island, NY).

Bradykinin (BK) was obtained from Vega Pharmaceuticals (Tucson,
AZ), lysyl-bradykinin (Kallidin) and methionyl-lysyl-bradykinin from
Sigma; [Tyr^1]-kallidin, from Beckman (Palo Alto, CA), des-Arg^1-
bradykinin, des-Arg^9-bradykinin and other bradykinin fragment
peptides from Serva Fine Biochemicals (Garden City Park, NY) respectively.
Bradykinin was coupled to carrier proteins ovalbumin and bovine serum
albumin (BSA) using 1-ethyl-3-(3-dimethylamine propyl) carbidiimide
by the procedure of Goodfriend et al (6). Bioassays for the
determination of kinin were performed on an isolated rat uterus
preparation perfused with modified de Jalon solution as described

previously (7). For the release of kinin from kininogen, samples were
incubated at 37 for 1 hr with 50 ug TPCK-treated trypsin in Tris-HCl
buffer, pH 7.8, in the presence of 0.02 M EDTA and 0.01 M o-phenanthroline to inhibit kininase activity. To prepare affinity adsorbants,
purified monoclonal antibodies were coupled covalently to cyanogen bromide-
activated Sepharose-4B according to the procedure of Cuatrecasas (8).

   <u>Preparation of Monoclonal Antibodies</u>. BALB/c mice (6-8 weeks of
age) were immunized by four subcutaneous injections of 100 ug of the
appropriate antigen emulsified with Freund's adjuvant, complete for the
first injection and incomplete for the subsequent weekly injections.
Three days prior to fusion donor animals received an intraperitoneal
injection of 50 ug of antigen in phosphate buffered saline. The spleen
of the immune mouse was removed aseptically and disaggregated by passing
it through a mesh screen into a Petri dish containing 10 ml Dulbecco's
Modified Eagle's Medium (DME). After centrifugation the cell pellet was
resuspended in 10 ml of cold 0.83% ammonium chloride and kept on ice for
5 min. Cells were pelleted, washed twice with DME and counted for
viability. Spleen cells ($1x10^8$) were fused with mouse P3x63-AG8.653
myeloma cells ($2x10^7$) in the presence of polyethylene glycol 4000 in
DME buffered with N-2-hydroxyethyl piperizine-N'-(2-ethane sulfonic
acid) (HDME) for 1.5 min at room temperature. Fused cells were washed
once gently with 10 ml HDME and resuspended in 25 ml DME and 10% fetal
calf serum. After 30 min, 25 ml of selective growth medium consisting
of 1000 x HAT (100 mM hypoxanthine, 0.4 mM aminopterin and 48 mM
thymidine) were added and cells distributed into two 24-well coaster
culture plates. Positive hybrids surviving HAT selective growth medium
were identified by enzyme-linked immunosorbent assay (ELISA) and subcloned
by limiting dilution in P-3 conditioned medium at a dilution of
<1 cell/well. Antibody-secreting hybrids were expanded and grown as
ascites tumor by injection of $5x10^6$ cells into the peritoneal cavity
of male Balb/c mice primed with 2,6,10,14-tetramethylpentadecane.
Mouse immunoglobulins (IG) were purified from ascites fluid on columns of
DEAE-Affigel Blue, packed and equilibrated with 0.02 M potassium
phosphate buffer, pH 7.2 and eluted with a linear NaCl gradient.

   <u>Enzyme-Linked Immunosorbent Assay (ELISA)</u>. Vinyl microtiter
plates (Costar) were coated with 10 ug/ml of appropriate antigen in 0.1
M sodium bicarbonate buffer, pH 9.6, at 37 for 1 h and then at 4
overnight. Non-specific binding to the microtiter plates was blocked
by soaking the wells in 1% bovine serum albumin in bicarbonate buffer.
After 5 washings with phosphate buffered saline (PBS), the plates were
incubated for 2 h at 37 with culture medium or ascites fluid diluted in
PBS. Unbound antibodies were removed and microtiter plates washed 5
times with wash buffer (0.02 M Tris-HCl, pH 8.0, containing 0.2%
Tween-20). The specifically-bound antibodies then were reacted for 1 h
with 100 ul of 1:3000 dilution of peroxidase-conjugated goat anti-mouse
immunoglobulin. Excess conjugate was removed and the plates washed 8
times with wash buffer prior to the addition of substrate (o-phenylene
diamine containing 0.03% H_2O_2 in 65 mM phosphate - 17 mM citrate
buffer, pH 4.5). The reaction was stopped by the addition of 50 ul of
4.0 M H_2SO_4 and read at 495 nm.

RESULTS AND DISCUSSION

   Independent fusions of spleen cells from mice immunized with
purified rat plasma kallikrein, kininogen and synthetic bradykinin (BK)
coupled to ovalbumin produced positive clones that secreted antigen
specific antibodies. The positive clones were subcloned and expanded

for use in the production of ascites tumor and the specificity of the
monoclonal antibodies (MAbs) established by ELISA using microtiter
plates coated with respective antigen. The isotype of the immunoglobulin fraction of each ascites fluid was characterized by double
immunodiffusion against class-specific antibodies. The antibody titers
of these antibodies at 50% ELISA values and the type characteristics
of these antibodies are shown in Table 1. None of the antibodies reacted
with microtiter plates coated with BSA. Higher anti-BK antibody titers
were noted when ELISA was performed on plates coated with BK-BSA conjugate. Apparently small peptides bind poorly to polysterene assay plates.

Table 1. Characteristics of monoclonal antibodies against rat plasma
kallikrein (KK), rat plasma kininogen (KNG) and synthetic bradykinin
(BK).

Monoclonal Antibody	Antibody Type		Titer[a]
	Heavy Chain	Light Chain	
KK-B3C9	IgG_1	k	5,000
KNG-C4G7	IgG_1	λ	80,000
KNG-D6H7	IgG_1	k	90,000
KNG-B5H10	IgG_1	k	150,000
KNG-B2E2	IgG_{2a}	k	150,000
KNG-B3F4	IgM	k	500
BK-B6C9	IgG_1	k	350 (20,000)[b]
BK-A3D9	IgG_1	k	7,000 (215,000)[b]
BK-D6A5	IgG_1	k	2,000 (90,000)[b]
BK-D2C7	IgG_1	k	8,000 (110,000)[b]

[a] Amount of dilution required to obtain half maximal ELISA value.

( )[b] Antibody titers on plates coated with bradykinin-BSA.

<u>Specificity of the Monoclonal Antibodies</u>. Increasing amounts of
MAbs were pre-incubated with purified rat plasma kallikrein and the
activity remaining in the supernatant measured on B_3-pro-phe-arg-pNA
substrate. About 75% of the enzyme activity could be immunoprecipitated
with 30 ug of IG from ascites fluid KK-B3C9, Fig. 1.

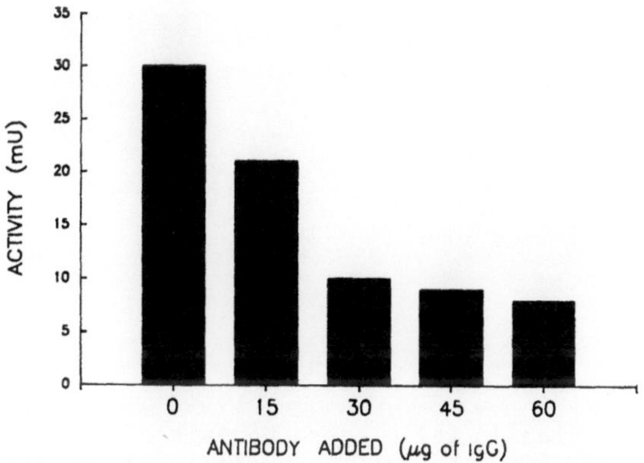

Fig. 1. Immunoprecipitation of rat plasma kallikrein with anti-rat
plasma kallikrein monoclonal antibodies.

The oxytocic response to BK was inhibited by pre-incubation
of bradykinin with MAbs BK-D6A5,BK-B6C9 and BK-A3D9. The uterine
contractile activity of the bradykinin-MAb complex was restored
by heating the complex in boiling water for 5 min, Fig. 2.

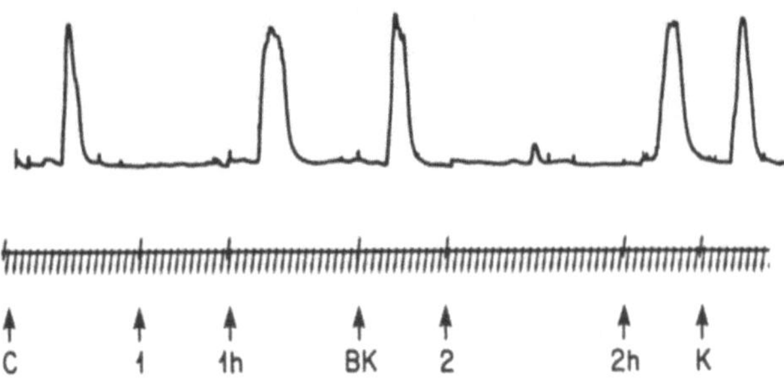

Fig. 2. Inhibition of bradykinin (BK) oxytocic response on isolated rat
uterus by anti-bradykinin MAbs BK-B6C9 (1), BK-A3D9(2). (C = untreated
BK control; 1 h, 2 h = heated BK antigen-antibody complex; K =
kallikrein antigen-antibody complex).

The antibody specificity of the MAbs to rat plasma kininogen was
confirmed by the immunoprecipitation of kininogen from a crude plasma
preparation by MAb coupled to Sepharose-4B. SDS-polyacrylamide gel
electrophoresis of the bound material, diluted later with 0.1 M
glycine-HCl buffer, pH 2.5, showed a single protein band with
electrophoretic mobility similar to that of purified kininogen, Fig. 3.

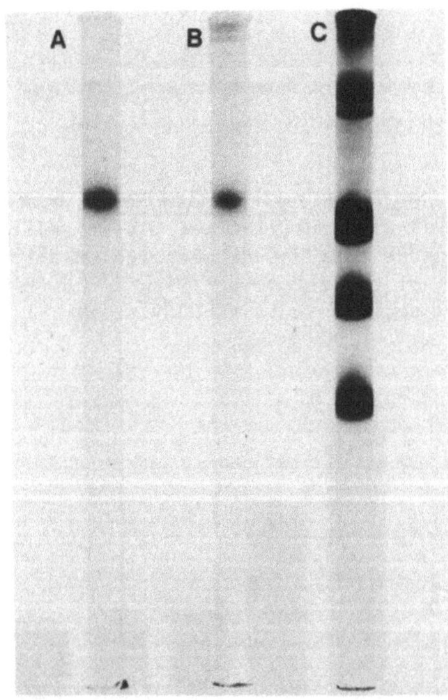

Fig. 3. SDS-polyacrylamide gel electrophoresis of rat plasma kininogen
purified by immunoaffinity chromatography (A), and by conventional
multistep purification procedure (B). Molecular weight markers shown in
(C) are: Transferrin (90,000), bovine serum albumin (68,000), ovalbumin
(45,000) and chymotrypsinogen A (25,000).

<u>Cross-Reactivity Studies</u>. The antigenic specificity of the MAbs
was evaluated further by ELISA. Anti-kallikrein MAbs KK-B3C9
cross-reacted strongly with human plasma kallikrein but not with human
or rat urinary kallikrein, rat salivary kallikrein or porcine
pancreatic kallikrein. Anti-kininogen MAbs also cross-reacted with
Murphy-Sturm lymphosarcoma tumor kininogen. All four anti-BK MAbs
cross-reacted with purified rat plasma kininogen as well as tryptic
digest of plasma kininogen, Fig. 4.

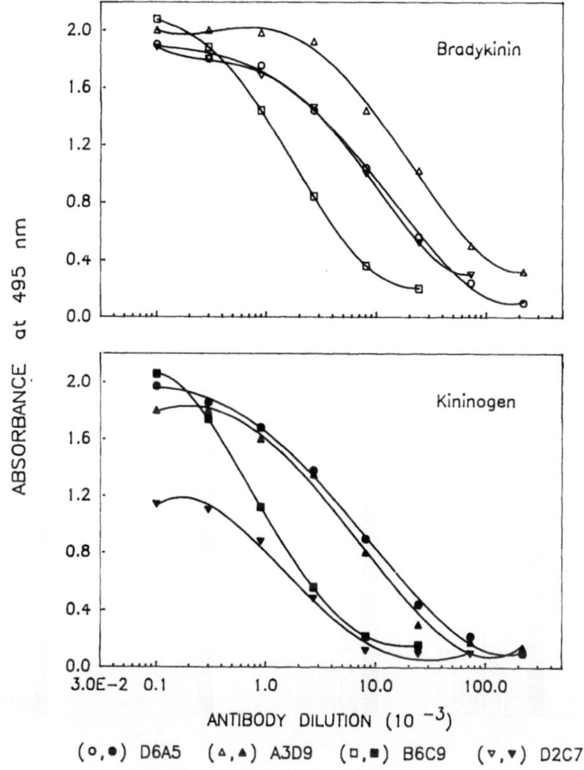

Fig. 4. Reactivity of bradykinin and rat plasma kininogen with
anti-bradykinin monoclonal antibodies.

However, none of the MAbs prepared against intact kininogen
cross-reacted with BK or BK-BSA conjugate. Though the kinin moiety in
intact kininogen molecule is exposed so as to be recognized by anti-BK
antibodies, it is not immuno-dominant.

The immunologic cross-reactivity of anti-BK MAbs with BK analogues
was evaluated by a competitive radio-immunoassay. Since all four MAbs
against BK bound 35-45% of the [Tyr[1]]-kallidin, the BK analogues and
fragments were tested for antibodies with [^{125}I-Tyr[1]]-kallidin. The
relative binding affinities were determined by comparing the
concentration of analogue with that of BK required to inhibit 50%
binding of the labeled antigen to MAbs. Except for binding to MAb
BK-B6C9, no significant difference was observed in the inhibition
profiles with BK, Lys-BK or Met-Lys-BK, Fig. 5. A five-fold higher
concentration of des-Arg[9]-BK was required for 50% inhibition of
binding of radioligand to MAbs BK-B6C9 and BK-D6A5 and a 20-25 fold
higher concentration for MAbs BK-A3D9 and BK-D2C7. Des-Arg[1]-BK showed
equivalent or better binding inhibition with MAbs BK-A3D9 and BK-D2C7. It
would appear that the arginine terminal at the NH$_2$-terminal of the

nonapeptide BK is critical for binding to all the MAbs whereas binding
to MAb BK-A3D9 and BK-D2C7 is not affected by removal of the
COOH-terminal arginine.

   <u>Applications: Enzyme-Linked Immunoassays</u>. A checkerboard
titration helped determine the optimal concentrations of MAbs and
microtiter plate antigen coating to develop a less tedious and cumbersome
enzyme-linked immunosorbent assay (ELISA). Standard curves for BK
obtained by ELISA as described under Methods showed the effective range
of BK determination to be 5-150 ng/sample. A linear standard curve was
obtained for the rat plasma kallikrein ELISA at concentrations between
0.1 and 10.0 ug/ml when the fraction of absorbance at 495 nm $A-N/A_O-N$
(A = absorbance, A_O = maximal absorbance with excess rat plasma
kallikrein and N = absorbance of blank) was plotted against the
concentration of rat plasma kallikrein in a logit-log mode, Fig. 6.

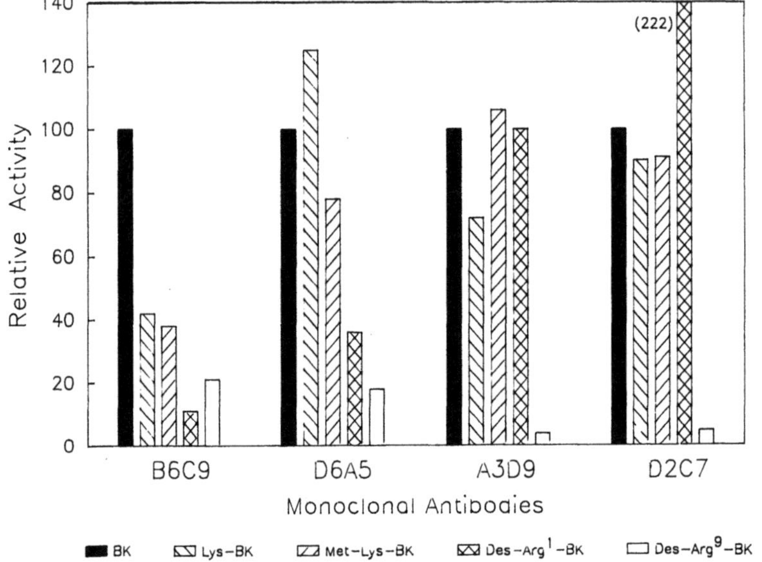

Fig. 5. Relative cross-reactivity of bradykinin, bradyklinin analogues
and fragments with anti-bradykinin monoclonal antibodies.

   The dose-response curves obtained with BK and kallikrein confirmed
the utilization of these MAbs in the development of enzyme-linked
immunoassays for components of the kallikrein-kininogen-kinin system.

   <u>Immuno-Affinity Purification</u>. An immunoadsorbent was prepared by
coupling the purified MAb KNG-B2E2 to cyanogen bromide activated
Sepharose-4B. Partially purified kininogen from citrated rat plasma
was mixed with immunoadsorbent in 0.1 M sodium phosphate buffer, pH 7.5.
Non-specifically bound proteins were washed extensively from the
adsorbent column with 0.5 M NaCl in 0.1 M phosphate buffer, pH 7.5, and
bound kininogen appearing as a single peak eluted by lowering the pH to
3.0 with glycine-HCl buffer. The eluted material was identified as
kininogen by bioassay technique on the isolated perfused rat uterus
preparation.

Our laboratory first reported in 1983 the successful production of
MAbs to rat plasma kallikrein (9) and then in 1984 to rat plasma
kininogen and synthetic bradykinin (10,11). Subsequent publications
described in more detail the production methodology and initial
characterization of these MAbs (1-3). Further characterization has been
provided in the present report. MAbs to human tissue kallikrein (12),
rat glandular kallikrein (13) and high molecular weight human plasma
kininogen (14) have been reported recently. Schmaier, et al (15) also
developed monoclonal antibodies to the heavy and light chains of high
molecular weight kininogen in normal human plasma. The recent increased
use of MAbs against components of the kallikrein-kininogen-kinin system
has been directed toward the development of immunoassays, component
purification and cellular localization as well as further characterization of individual components and their respective complexes (see
presentations of Veloso, et al; Oh-Ishi, et al; Chao, et al; Okubo,
et al; this volume).

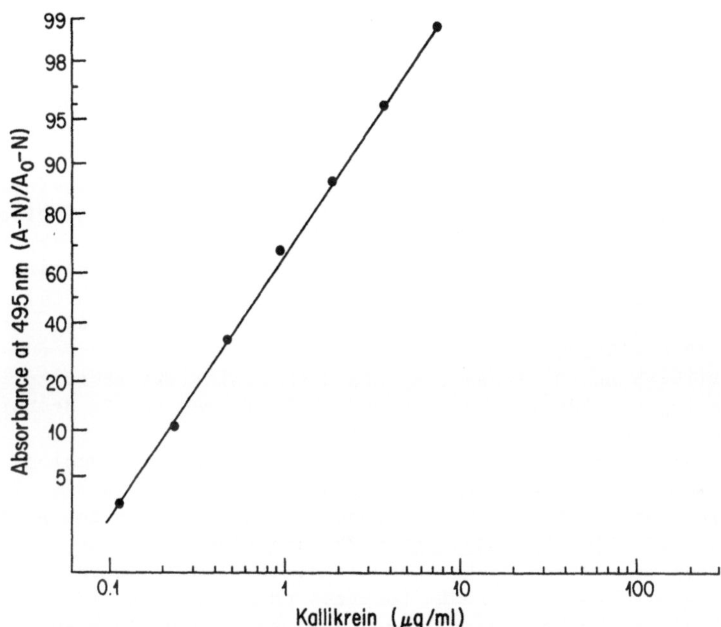

Fig. 6. Standard curve for the estimation of rat plasma kallikrein by
ELISA utilizing anti-kallikrein monoclonal antibodies.

SUMMARY

Monoclonal antibodies (MAbs) to rat plasma kallikrein, rat plasma
low molecular weight kininogen and synthetic bradykinin were
characterized further. The MAbs were obtained after the immunization of
BALB/c mice with the purified reagents and synthetic bradykinin coupled
to ovalbumin. The MAbs were very useful in characterizing components of
the kallikrein-kininogen-kinin system.

Plasma kallikrein MAbs bound specifically to both rat and human plasma kallikrein but did not interact immunologically with either rat or human glandular kallikrein. The MAbs immunoprecipitated about 75% of the kallikrein enzyme activity. Five stable hybridomas were obtained that produced MAbs against bradykinin. These MAbs cross-reacted with bradykinin, bradykinin analogues, purified rat plasma kininogen and tryptic digests of rat plasma kininogen. The MAbs also neutralized the smooth muscle contractile activity of bradykinin. The specificity of MAbs against rat plasma kininogens was confirmed by immuno-precipitation of ^{125}I-kininogen with MAbs followed by SDS-PAGE.

These MAbs were used successfully to develop immunoassays (ELISA) and immunoadsorbents to purify components of the kallikrein-kininogen-kinin system.

ACKNOWLEDGEMENT: Supported by the National Institutes of Health, National Cancer Institute Grant No. 5R01CA3827002.

REFERENCES

1. G.S. Bedi and Nathan Back: Monoclonal antibody to rat plasma kallikrein. _Hybridoma_ 3: 287-292 (1984).
2. G.S. Bedi and Nathan Back: Production and characterization of monoclonal antibodies to rat plasma kininogen. _Hybridoma_ 6: 521-526 (1987).
3. G.S. Bedi and Nathan Back: Monoclonal antibodies to bradykinin inhibit smooth muscle contractile action of bradykinin. _Biochem. Biophys. Acta_. 842: 90-99 (1985).
4. G.S. Bedi, J. Balwierczak and Nathan Back: Rodent kinin-forming enzyme system. I. Purification and characterization of plasma kininogen. _Biochem. Pharmacol_. 32: 2061-2069 (1983).
5. G.S.Bedi and Nathan Back: Purification and characterization of rat plasma kallikrein. _Preparative Biochem_. 14: 257-279 (1984).
6. T.L. Goodfriend, L. Levine and G.D. Fasman. _Science_ 144: 1344-1346 (1964).
7. H.J. Wilkens and R. Steger: Agents with kinin-like activity. _in_: Screening Methods in Pharmacology. R.A. Turner and P. Hebborn (eds.) Academic Press, NY p. 61-73 (1971).
8. P.O. Cuatrecasas and C.B. Enfinson _in_: Methods in Enzymology Vol. 22. W.D. Jakoby, ed. Academic Press, NY. pgs. 345-378 (1971).
9. G.S. Bedi and Nathan Back: A monoclonal antibody to rat plasma kallikrein. _The Pharmacologist_ 25: 405 (1983).
10. G.S. Bedi and Nathan Back: Monoclonal antibodies to rat plasma kininogen. Proc. Internat. Congress on Kinins. pg. 17 (1984).
11. G.S. Bedi and Nathan Back: Monoclonal antibodies to bradykinin. _Fed. Proc_. 43: 2143 (1984).
12. J. Chao, L. Chao, D.M. Tillman, Cheryl M. Woodley and Harry S. Margolius: Characterization of monoclonal and polyclonal antibodies to human tissue kallikrein. _Hypertension_ 7: 931-937 (1985).
13. R. T. Savoy-Moore, M. Khullar, K. Swartz, A.G. Scicli and O.A. Carretero: Characterization of monoclonal antibodies against rat glandular kallikrein. _J. Immunol. Methods_. 88: 45-51 (1986).
14. M. Berrettini, B. Lämmie, T. White, M.J. Heeb, H.P. Schwarz, B. Zuraw, J.Curd and J.H. Griffin: Detection of in vitro and in vivo cleavage of high molecular weight kininogen in human plasma by immunoblotting with monoclonal antibodies. _Blood_ 68: 455-462 (1986).
15. A.H. Schmaier, D. Schutsky, A. Farber, L.D. Silver, H.N. Bradford and R.W. Colman. Determination of the bifunctional properties of high molecular weight kininogen by studies with monoclonal antibodies directed to each of its chains. _J. Biol. Chem_. 262: 1405-1411 (1987).

AN ENZYME-LINKED IMMUNOSORBENT ASSAY (ELISA) FOR KININS IN TRYPTIC

DIGESTS

Kalyan Rao Anumula, Raymond P. Schulz and Nathan Back

Department of Biochemical Pharmacology
State University of New York, Buffalo, NY 14260

INTRODUCTION

Kinins are released from kininogens by proteolytic action of
kininogenases in tissues and biologic fluids (1,2). Released kinins
act on specific receptors (3) mediating potent pharmacologic responses
(4). The recent discovery that kininogens are cysteine proteinase
inhibitors has increased the need for a more specific and sensitive
quantitative method to estimate both kinins and kininogens (5,6).
Traditionally kinins are determined by bioassay utilizing an appropriate isolated smooth muscle preparation perfused in a tissue bath
(7). Other recently developed methods include radioimmunoassay (RIA)
(8) and separation of kinins by high-performance liquid chromatography
(HPLC) followed by RIA (9). This communication reports on a rapid and
specific enzyme-linked immunosorbent assay (ELISA) for kinins released
from rat and human plasma and purified kininogen subjected to a modified
tryptic digestion. In addition a simple solvent system for complete
separation of native kinins on an HPLC C-18 reversed phase column will
be described.

MATERIALS AND METHODS

Bradykinin (BK), Lys-BK, Met-Lys-BK, Ileu-Ser-BK, Tyr-BK,
[Tyr^5]-BK, [Tyr^8]-BK, and Des-Arg^9-BK were purchased either from
Chemical Dynamics or Sigma Co. Polystyrene ELISA plates were obtained
from Costar. Bovine serum albumin ((BSA) and γ-globulins (95% - 99%
pure) were Sigma products. TPCK-treated trypsin was provided by
Worthington Co. Citrated (0.38%) normal rat plasma either was
purchased from Pel-Freeze or collected from the abdominal aorta and
frozen. Mouse monoclonal antibodies to bradykinin and BSA-BK conjugates
were prepared in our laboratory as reported previously (10) and in
these Proceedings (11). Goat anti-mouse immunoglobulin horse radish
peroxidase conjugate was purchased from Zymed Laboratories. Kininogens
were purified from plasmas on a papain affinity column followed by
DEAE-Trisacryl column chromatography (12).

Release of Kinins by Trypsin Digestion. Samples of 50 µl plasma
were mixed with 50 µl 1.0 M NaCl and 0.9 ml of 0.5% HCl in 2-propanol,
boiled for 10 min and centrifuged for 2 min. The protein precipitates
were suspended in 0.25 ml of 0.05 M Na phosphate containing 0.15 M

NaCl, 5 mM EDTA and 2 mM 1,10 phenanthroline, pH 11 (final pH 8.0).
Trypsin (TPCK treated), 50 µl of 10 mg/ml in the above (pH 8.0) buffer,
was added, incubated at 37° for 1 h, and the trypsin inactivated by
boiling for 10 min. To make the samples compatible with the ELISA
incubation buffer, 50 µl of an inhibitor-protein mixture was added
consisting of 21 mM benzamidine-HCl, 14 mM EDTA, 1.4% Tween-20, 0.7%
BSA, 14 mM 1,10 phenanthroline, 7 mM NEM and 0.7% bovine Y-globulin,
pH 7.4. Digests were centrifuged at maximum speed for 5 min and the
kinins in the supernatant determined by ELISA. Kininogen preparations
were digested with trypsin as described above and after boiling for 10
min assayed without adding HCl/2-propanol.

ELISA of Kinins. ELISA manipulations were carried out
according to Monroe (13) and Ngo (14) with optimum concentrations
determined as suggested by Engvall (15). The kininase inhibitor 1,10
phenanthroline (2 mM) was included in all ELISA solutions.

HPLC of Kinins. Native and PITC kinins were separated on a C-18
reversed phase µ-Bondapak (Waters) 3.9 mm x 30 cm column and detected
at 214 and 254 nm respectively. The mobile phase for native kinins
consisted of A: 0.2% TFA in non-organic water and B: 0.15% TFA in
acetonitrile gradient starting at 17% to 35% at 40 min at a 2 ml/min
flow rate. The HPLC system consisted of a Waters M-45 pumps, Model 441
UV detector and a solvent mixer between the U6K injector and mixed
solvent outlet from the pumps. The gradient programs, data acquisition
and analyses were carried out with a Chromatochart-PC system from
Interactive Microwave on a Zenith-148 computer. HPLC reagents were
obtained from Pierce and solvents from either Fisher or J.T. Baker.

RESULTS

Kinin Determination in Tryptic Digests by ELISA. Properties of
the mouse monoclonal antibodies to BK prepared in our laboratory, D6A5,
D6C9 and A3D9 have been described (10,11). Incubation of various kinin
analogues with a mixture of monoclonal antibodies in the ELISA system
yielded similar curves with BK, Lys-BK, Met-Lys-BK, Ileu-Ser-BK and
Tyr-BK. Poor interaction was obtained with [Tyr^5]-BK,and [Tyr^8]-BK
(Fig. 1). Intact kinins in the range of 10-200 ng could be quantitated
by this ELISA procedure.

ELISA determination of total kinins generated from tryptic
digestion of rat and human plasmas showed that about 75% were released
within 30 min and no further increase after 2 h. Plasma kinin levels
determined as BK for normal rats, rats treated with turpentine and
normal human were 7.8 µg/ml, 80 µg/ml and 3.6 µg/ml respectively. In
the case of low molecular weight rat plasma kininogen (L-kininogen, MW
68,000), the kinin content as determined by ELISA was estimated at
18.5 µg/mg kininogen.

ELISA also was used to detect and quantitate kinins during the
course of purification of plasma kininogen from the papain affinity
(16) and DEAE-Trisacryl columns. A major protein peak showing kinin
immunologic activity in ELISA was L-kininogen as confirmed by SDS-PAGE
and papain inhibitory effect.

Resolution of Kinins by HPLC. Natural kinins were separated
completely on a µ-Bondapak C-18 reversed phase column within 20
minutes with the following retention times (in minutes): BK, 14.5;
Lys-BK, 12.9; Met-Lys-BK, 16.0; Ileu-Ser-BK, 17.4; [Tyr^5]-BK , 7.6;
[Tyr^8]-BK, 8.9 (Fig. 2). Synthetic Tyr-BK separated poorly from

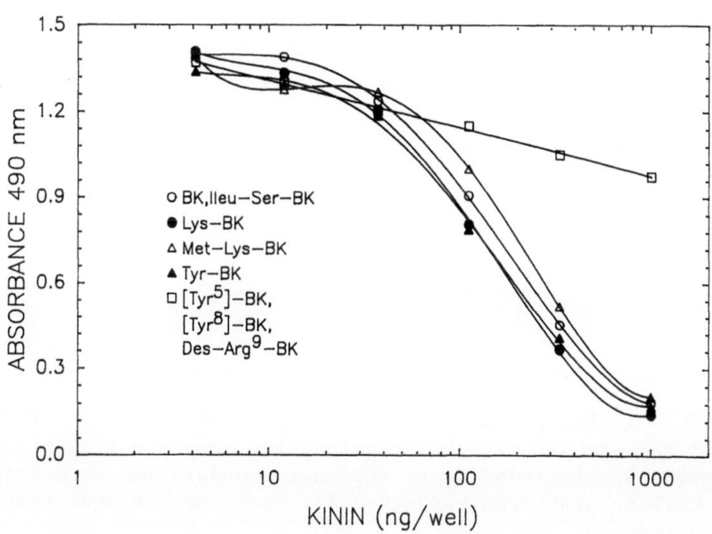

Fig. 1. Standard curves with synthetic bradykinin and bradykinin analogues in the ELISA using a mixture of monoclonal antibodies D6A5, B6C9, and A3D9.

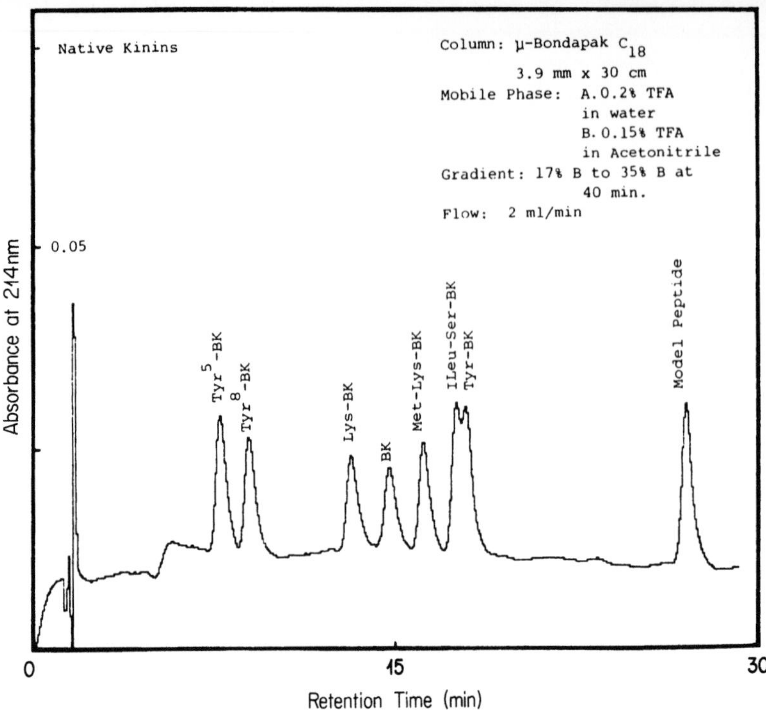

Fig. 2. Separation of standard mixture of native kinins by HPLC carried out on a μ-Bondapak C-18 reversed phase column. Kinins (1 μg each) were injected and absorbance recorded at 214 nm.

Ileu-Ser-BK. Trifluoroacetic acid concentrations of 0.15% or more in both water and acetonitrile was required for complete separation. A model peptide was included as an internal standard for both retention times as well as peak area reference for computer for peak identification and area determinations.

DISCUSSION

Determination of kinins is carrried out routinely by bioassay, an inconvenient and time-consuming method in which kinin-stimulated contractions of an isolated perfused smooth muscle (most often rat uterus) are measured. Radioimmunoassays and HPLC of kinins also have been reported (8,9). Homogenous enzyme immunoassay has been reported for the differential estimation of high and low molecular weight kininogens but this method was not suitable for the measurement of Ileu-Ser-BK in the rat (17). The published reports on an ELISA methods for kinins were limited only to standard curves (16).

The procedures developed for tryptic digestion of test samples and the subsequent ELISA of kinins presented in this report allow for the rapid estimation of kinins in biologic material as well as kininogen preparations. Treatment of plasma samples with 0.5% HCl in 2-propanol followed by boiling for 10 min was necessary for highly reproducible kinin estimates since plasma proteins were precipitated quantitatively under these conditions. Extraction of the plasma with hot HCL/2-propanol assured complete inactivation of proteinases as well as preliminary clarification of the sample for future derivatization of peptides and HPLC analysis.

Relatively high concentrations of trypsin (10 mg/ml plasma) were
necessary for complete release of kinins from rat plasma collected from
rats pre-treated 48 h before with turpentine, 0.5 ml/100 g body weight.
Such pretreatment in the rat elevated, by as much as 10-20 fold (17),
the levels of a third kininogen identical to a major acute phase plasma
protein and cysteine proteinase inhibitor (18). The release,
presumably from this third kininogen, of a vasoactive peptide with the
novel Ileu-Ser-amino terminus was reported first by Bedi, et al. (19)
and further determined as Ileu-Ser-BK (T-kinin) by Okamoto and
Greenbaum (20). Our kinin estimates from plasma of both normal and
turpentine-treated rats are in accord with the accepted kininogen/kinin
levels obtained under similar conditions (17,21-23). Use of hog
pancreatic kallikrein (200 μg/ml plasma) in place of trypsin yielded
kinin levels in normal plasma similar to those with trypsin; however,
plasma from turpentine-treated rats yielded only 14 μg kinin/ml plasma.
These results indicate that the hog pancreatic kallikrein was capable
of releasing only relatively small amounts (~10%) of the total
available Ileu-Ser-BK from the increased L-kininogen levels in the rat
"Turpentine" plasma. Previous studies in our laboratory showed that
rat plasma L-kininogen, purified by a single-step passage through an
anti-rat plasma L-kininogen monoclonal antibody immunoaffinity column
(24), was resistant to hog pancreatic kallikrein, human urinary
kallikrein as well as both rat and human plasma kallikrein (25). Thus
the ELISA system described could be used for differential estimation of
kininogens in plasma. From results with normal human and rat plasmas
it is demonstrated that high concentrations of trypsin during digestion
did not affect the released kinins.

ELISA conditions were optimized to give about 1.0 absorbance unit
in 30 min of color development in non-competing wells. The entire
ELISA procedure can be completed within 3-4 h. Proteinase inhibitors
and bovine γ-globulins were included in the ELISA buffers to prevent
the degradation of kinins during the 37° incubation and also prevent
color background. In some preparations of goat second antibody-enzyme
conjugates, addition of 0.01% goat γ-globulins to the incubation buffer
reduced the non-specific background color. Sensitivity of the assay
was in the 10-200 ng range, suitable for kinin measurement in normal
plasma tryptic digests. The kinin ELISA procedure is useful for
monitoring the immunologic kinin activity in fractions obtained during
either the purification of kininogens or the separation of kinins on
HPLC columns.

Methods for the HPLC resolution of kinin have employed complex
mixtures of solvents with limited success in complete separation
(26-28). In contrast the solvent systems developed in the current
study are simple utilizing only TFA as an additive. TFA concentrations
of 0.15% or more were critical for the complete separation of these
basic peptides, most probably due to effective ion pairing/ion exchange
with C-18 matrix at this concentration.

Detection of peptides at 214 nm was quite non-specific and also
subject to various interferences including solvent impurities
accumulating and eluting from the column with the gradient, and changes
in the refractive indices of the solvents in the flow cell. Specific
detection of kinins was improved when monitored at 254 nm following
PITC (12). This procedure was designed for the extraction of basic
peptides into upper aqueous-methanol phase. HPLC profiles of PITC
peptides obtained from plasma tryptic digests are complex and respective
kinin regions seriously overlapped. Retention times of such peptides
at best can be shortened by the use of small columns or cartridges.
Efforts continue to determine kinins directly in tryptic digests by

HPLC rather than identify and quantitate kinins in the eluted fractions
by ELISA or RIA.

   The procedures described for tryptic digestion, ELISA of kinins
and HPLC separation of kinins should prove useful in the continued
study of the kallikrein-kininogen-kinin system.

ACKNOWLEDGEMENTS

   We express our appreciation and gratitude to Dr. G.S. Bedi for the
preparation of the monoclonal antibodies used for the ELISA studies.
This study was supported by the National Institutes of Health, National
Cancer Institute, Grant No. 5RO1CA3827002.

REFERENCES

1. V. Eisen, New aspects of kinin formation, _Trends in Pharm._
    Sciences, 69: 190-191 (1985).
2. J.L. Prado, "Proteolytic enzymes as kininogenases". Handbook of
    Experimental Pharmacology, E.G. Erdos ed., Springer Verlag, New York
    pgs. 156-192 (1970).
3. D. Regoli and J. Barabe, Pharmacology of bradykinin and related
    kinins, _Pharmacological Rev._, 32: 1-36 (1980).
4. D.H. Miller and H.S. Margolius, Kallikreins and kinins. _in_
    Endocrinology. L.J. DeGroot and C.F. Cahill, Jr. Grune and Stratton,
    Orlando, FL. 2nd Edition, In Press. (1988).
5. A.J. Barrett, N.D. Rawlings,M.E. Davies, W. Machleidt, G. Salvesen
    and V. Turk,"Cysteine proteinase inhibitors of the cystatin
    superfamily" _in_: Proteinase Inhibitors", A.J. Barrett and G.
    Salvesen eds., Elsevier, Amsterdam. pgs. 515-569 (1986).
6. W. Müller-Esterl, S. Iwanaga and S. Nakanishi, Kininogens
    revisited, _Trends. Biochem. Sci._ 11: 336-339 (1986).
7. H.J. Wilkens and R. Steger, "Agents with kinin-like activity" _in_:
    Screening Methods in Pharmacology, Vol. 2, Academic Press, New York
    pgs. 61-73 (1971).
8. T.L. Goodfriend and C.E. Odya, "Bradykinin" _in_: Methods of
    Hormone Radioimmunoassay, B.M. Jaffe and H.R. Behrmann eds.,
    Academic Press, New York pgs. 909-923 (1979).
9. G. Fejes - To'th, A. Naray-Fejes and J.C. Fröhlich, Measurement
    of urinary kinins by HPLC-radioimmunoassay, _Clin. Chim. Acta_,
    140: 21-29 (1984).
10. G.S. Bedi and N. Back, Monoclonal antibodies to bradykinin inhibit
    smooth muscle contractile action of bradykinin, _Biochim. Biophys._
    Acta 842: 90-99 (1985).
11. G.S. Bedi and N. Back, Further characterization of monoclonal
    antibodies against rat plasma kallikrein, rat low molecular weight
    kininogen, and synthetic bradykinin. Kinins V, Adv. Exptl. Med. and
    Biol. (1988).
12. K.R. Anumula, R. Schulz and N. Back, Unpublished data.
13. D. Monroe, Enzyme immunoassay, _Anal. Chem._, 56: 920A-929A (1984).
14. T.T. Ngo, "Enzyme mediated immunoassay; an overview" _in_: Enzyme
    Mediated Immunoassay. T.T. Ngo and H.M. Lenhoff eds. Plenum Press, New
    York. pgs. 3-32 (1985).
15. E. Engvall, "Enzyme immunoassay ELISA and EMIT," _in_: Methods in
    Enzymology, H.V. Vunakis and J.J. Langone eds. Vol. 70A, Academic
    Press, New York, pgs. 419-439 (1980).

16. R. Geiger and W. Miska, Determination of bradykinin by enzyme
    immunoassay. Adv. Exp. Med. Biol., 198B: 531-536 (1986).
17. F. Esnard and F. Gauthier, Rat α-$_1$-cysteine proteinase inhibitor,
    J. Biol. Chem., 258: 12443-12447 (1983).
18. T. Cole, A.S. Inglis, C.M. Roxburgh, G.J. Howlett and G. Schreiber,
    Major acute phase -protein of the rat is homologous to bovine
    kininogen and contains the sequence for bradykinin: its synthesis is
    regulated at the mRNA level. FEBS Lett. 182: 57-61 (1985).
19. G.S. Bedi, J. Balwierczak and N. Back, A new vasopeptide formed
    by the action of a Murphy-Sturm lymphosarcoma acid protease on rat
    plasma kininogen. Biochem. Biophys. Res. Commun. 112: 621-628
    (1983).
20. H. Okamoto and L.M. Greenbaum, Isolation and structure of
    T-kinin. Biochem. Biophys. Res. Commun. 112: 701-708 (1983).
21. Y. Uchida, M. Majima and M. Katori, A method of determination of
    human plasma HMW and LMW kininogen levels by bradykinin enzyme
    immunoassay, Pharm. Res. Commun. 18: 831-846 (1986).
22. H. Okamoto and L.M. Greenbaum, Kininogen substrates for trypsin and
    cathepsin D in human, rabbit and rat plasma, Life Sci., 32: 2007-2013
    (1983).
23. A.D. Gounaris, M.A. Brown and A.J. Barrett, Human plasma α-cysteine
    proteinase inhibitor, Biochem. J. 221: 445-452 (1984).
24. G.S. Bedi and N. Back, Production and characterization of
    monoclonal antibodies to rat plasma kininogen. Hybridoma. 6:
    521-526 (1986).
25. G.S. Bedi and N. Back, Single-step purification of "kallikrein-
    resistant" kininogen from rat plasma using monoclonal antibody
    immunoaffinity chromatography. Prep. Biochem. 15: 159-169 (1985).
26. T.K. Narayanan and L.M. Greenbaum, Determination and quantitation
    of fluorescamine-labeled bradykinin, its analogues and metabolites
    using HPCL, J. Chrom. 306, 109-116 (1984).
27. I. Hayashi, H. Kuto, S. Iwanaga and S. Oh-ishi, Rat plasma high
    molecular weight kininogen, J. Biol. Chem. 260, 6115-6123 (1985).
28. T. Mindroiu, G. Scicli, F. Perini, O.A. Carretero and A. G. Scicli,
    Identification of a new kinin in human urine, J. Biol. Chem.
    261, 7407-7411 (1986).

16. K. Geiger and K. Miosga, Determination of bradykinin by enzyme
    immunoassay. Adv. Exp. Med. Biol., 120?, 21-29 (19??).

17. R. Zaneld and P. Geuskiel, Rat brain protease protiease inhibitor,
    J. Biol. Chem., 256: 1043-1047 (1981).

18. T. Cole, A.S. Inglis, C.M. Roxburgh, C.I. Howlett and G. Schreiber,
    Major acute phase α-protein of the rat is homologous to bovine
    Kininogen and contains the sequence of bradykinin. Its synthesis is
    regulated at the mRNA level. FEBS Lett., [illegible].

19. [illegible]

HYDROLYSIS OF SYNTHETIC PEPTIDES AND NATURAL SUBSTRATES BY PLASMA

KALLIKREIN AND ITS LIGHT CHAIN

Guacyara Motta, Misako U. Sampaio and Claudio A.M. Sampaio

Departamento de Bioquimica, Escola Paulista de Medicina
Caixa Postal 20372
CEP 04034 S. Paulo, SP, Brasil

INTRODUCTION

Human plasma kallikrein (E.C. 3.4.21.34) is synthetized as a single-chain precursor with 619 amino-acid residues; following activation, it is split between residues 371 and 372 (Arg-Ile) [1] . A heavy chain and a light chain are formed during the activation process. Heavy chain is responsible for the interaction of kallikrein with high-molecular weigth kininogen, and light chain contains the enzyme active site; light chain can be found as two variants, molecular weight 36,000 or 33,000 [2].

Two forms of active plasma kallikrein were described recently: α-kallikrein, formed during the activation of prokallikrein, contains intact heavy and light chains; and β-kallikrein, that shows an extra cleavage in the heavy chain, thus forming two chains of approximately 30,000 and 20,000 each, kept linked by disulfide bridges [3,4].

Plasma kallikrein shows esterolytic activity towards arginine derivatives, but also cleaves amide bonds in peptide derivatives of p-nitroaniline. The study of the specificity of plasma kallikrein on tetrapeptides has shown that the enzyme cleaves Ac-Phe-Lys-Arg-Pro, at the Lys-Arg bond, and that this substrate is not hydrolyzed by tissue kallikreins such as horse urinary and porcine pancreatic kallikrein [5] .

The existence of a lower molecular weight derivative of plasma kallikrein was sugested by Movat et al. [6] . An enzymatic activity was isolated during the purification of plasma kallikrein [7] . Sampaio et al. [8] have shown that the incubation of plasma kallikrein with different proteolytic enzymes can generate lower molecular fragments. The light chain of plasma kallikrein was generated after mild reduction of the native enzyme, and was demonstrated to be active , at least upon synthetic substrates [9] .

The aim of this work is to compare the enzymatic properties of α-kallikrein, β-kallikrein and the active light chain.

Human plasma kallikrein, purified under the conditions of a described procedure [10] , is usually α-kallikrein, and upon incubation at room temperature is transformed into β-kallikrein; the actual concentration of both forms was measured by NPGB active site titration [11] . Kallikrein chains were separated by the procedure described by van der Graaf [2] , and isolated by affinity chromatography on soybean-trypsin inhibitor-Sepharose. Identification of α- and β-kallikrein and light-chain, was performed, with reduced and non reduced samples, on SDS-polyacrilamide gel electrophoresis [12] .

Specific p-nitroanilide peptides [13] were a kind from Dr. Luis Juliano (Departamento de Biofisica, Escola Paulista de Medicina). The incubations with kallikrein were performed in 0.1 M tris-HCl, pH 8.0, 37°C in 200 uL-final volume, being the reactions interrupted after 2 to 20 minutes, depending on the substrate, by the addition of 15% (v/v) acetic acid. Kallikrein kinin releasing activity was followed on fresh human normal plasma as substrate, and the released kinin was estimated on isolated guinea-pig ileum [14] . The hydrolysis of purified high-molecular weight kininogen, prepared by a described procedure [15] , was followed by SDS-polyacrylamide gel electrophoresis. Tosyl-arginine methyl ester (TAME) hydrolysis was followed in a pH-stat [10] .

RESULTS

The activity of all forms of kallikrein was measured on TAME, after active site titration, and the esterolytic activity was found to be higher for the light chain when compared to both α-kallikrein and β-kallikrein, being respectively 275, 72 and 101 umols TAME hydrolyzed per minute per mg enzyme.

The hydrolysis of p-nitroanilides of N-α-substituted dipeptides showed that Ac-Phe-Arg-pNA is a better substrate than Bz-Phe-Arg-pNA. The presence of a third amino-acid residue at position P3 (Pro or Gly) does not improve significantly the ability of the three enzyme forms to cleave those substrates (table 1). Light chain is always more efficient to cleave the anilide bond in those peptides, and the best substrate for this molecular species is H.D-Pro-Phe-Arg-pNA. The hydrolysis of Ac-Phe-Arg-pNA is not changed by the concomitant addition of free heavy chain to the incubates (table 2).

On the other hand, the kinin releasing activity, is present mostly in α-kallikrein; β-kallikrein activity towards high-molecular weight kininogen is 25% of that observed for α-kallikrein; light chain does not release bradykinin from kininogen, although all forms of enzyme can cleave high-molecular weight kininogen, as seen by product-analysis of these incubates performed by SDS-polyacrylamide gel electrophoresis (not shown).

DISCUSSION

The results indicate that the activity of light chain upon synthetic substrates is higher than for α- or β-kallikrein; in the case of dipeptides, the increased efficiency measured by kcat/Km ratio is due chiefly to a higher catalytic activity; in tripeptides there is also an important contribuition of Km, that is lower for light chain when compared to the other two enzyme forms. One possible explanation for this difference would be an easier diffusion of the substrate, in the absence

Table 1

HYDROLYSIS OF DI- AND TRIPEPTIDES BY KALLIKREIN FORMS

ENZYME	SUBSTRATE	Km (mM)	kcat (sec -1)	kcat/Km (mM x sec)-1
α-HuPK		0.90	71.30	79.22
β-HuPK	AcPhe-Arg-pNA	0.87	113.70	129.86
LC		0.83	179.90	216.75
α-HuPK		0.85	35.70	42.00
β-HuPK	BzPhe-Arg-pNA	1.17	55.50	47.44
LC		1.36	120.70	88.75
α-HuPK		0.52	29.10	55.96
β-HuPK	BzPro-Phe-Arg-pNA	1.97	62.20	31.57
LC		0.34	86.90	255.59
α-HuPK		1.68	117.82	380.06
β-HuPK	AcGly-Phe-Arg-pNA	1.54	178.20	15.71
LC		0.47	141.80	301.70
α-HuPK		0.31	117.82	380.06
β-HuPK	H.D-Pro-Phe-Arg-pNA	0.54	116.38	215.52
LC		0.21	329.74	1570.19

LC: Light chain

of the enzyme heavy chain. The association of free heavy and light chains is not spontaneous since no changes in the kinetic parameters were detected when heavy chain was added to light chain solutions.

Heavy chain is fundamental for the association of kallikrein to kininogen, and only one cleavage on heavy chain impairs the efficiency for bradykinin release; furthermore, the heavy chain does not seem to be necessary for unespecific cleavages of kininogen, as seen by SDS-electrophoresis (not shown) but only for bradykinin generation.

Table 2

HYDROLYSIS OF Ac-Phe-Arg-pNA BY KALLIKREIN
ISOLATED CHAINS

ENZYME	Km (mM)	kcat (sec -1)	kcat/Km (mM x sec)-1
LC	0.83	179.9	216.8
HC	n.d.	n.d.	n.d.
LC + HC	1.01	186.1	184.6

LC: Light chain;   HC: Heavy chain
n.d.: not detected

REFERENCES

1 - D.W. Chung, K. Fujikawa, B.A. McMullen, and E.W. Davie, Human plasma prekallikrein, a zymogen to a serine protease that contains four tandem repeats, <u>Biochemistry,</u> 25: 2410 (1986).

2 - F. van d. Graaf, G. Tans, B.N. Bouma and J.H. Griffin, Isolation and functional properties of the heavy and light chains of human plasma kallikrein, <u>J. Biol. Chem.</u>, 257: 14300 (1982).

3 - R.W. Colman, Y.T. Wachtfogel, U. Kucich, G. Weinbaum, S. Hahn, R.A. Pixley, C.F. Scott, A. Agostini, D. Burger and M. Schapira, Effect of cleavage of the heavy chain of human plasma kallikrein on its functional properties, <u>Blood</u>, 65: 311 (1985).

4 - D. Burger, W.D. Schleuning and M. Schapira, Human plasma prekallikrein. Immunoaffinity purification and activation to α- and β-kallikrein, <u>J. Biol. Chem.</u>, 261: 324 (1986).

5 - E. S. Prado, M. S. Araujo-Viel, M. A. Juliano, L. Juliano, R.C.R. Stella and C.A.M. Sampaio, Tetrapeptide substrates for the discrimination among kallikreins and other trypsin-like serine proteinases, <u>Biol. Chem. Hoppe Seyler</u>, 367: 199 (1986).

6 - H. Z. Movat, The plasma kallikrein-kinin system and its interrelationship with other components of blood, <u>Handb. Exp. Pharmacol.</u>, 25 (supp) :1 (1979).

7 - M.L. Oliva, D. Grisolia, M.U. Sampaio and C.A.M. Sampaio, Properties of highly purified human plasma kallikrein, <u>Agents</u> and <u>Actions</u>, 9: 52 (1982).

8 - C.A. M. Sampaio, S.Vidmar, A.Hamaguchi and M.U. Sampaio, Hydrolysis of plasma kallikreins by trypsin and plasmin and the formation of active fragments, in <u>Kinins IV</u>, part B, L.Greenbaum and H. Margolius, eds, Plenum Press, New York 105 (1986).

9 - F. van d. Graaf, J.A. Koedam, J.H. Griffin and B.N. Bouma, Interaction of human plasma kallikrein and its light chain with C1-inhibitor, <u>Biochemistry,</u> 22: 4860 (1983).

10- C. Sampaio, S. C. Wong and E. Shaw, Human plasma kallikrein. Purification and preliminary characterization, <u>Arch. Biochem. Biophys.</u>, 165: 133 (1974).

11- T. Chase Jr. and E. Shaw, Titration of trypsin, plasmin and thrombin with p-nitrophenyl p-guanidinobenzoate HCl, <u>Meth. Enzymol.</u>, 19:20 (1970).

12- U. K. Laemmli, Cleavage of structural proteins during the assembly of the head of bacteriophage T4, <u>Nature,</u> 227: 680 (1970).

13- M. A. Juliano and L. Juliano, Synthesis and kinetic parameters of hydrolysis by trypsin of some acyl-arginyl-p-nitroanilides and peptides containing arginyl-p-nitroanilide, <u>Brazilian J. Med. Biol. Res.</u>, 18: 435 (1985).

14- C.A.M. Sampaio, S.T. Nunes, M.G.N. Mazzacoratti and J.L. Prado, Inactivation of kinins by chymotrypsin, <u>Biochem. Pharmacol.</u>, 25: 2391 (1976).

15- B. Dittmann, A. Steger, R. Wimmer and H. Fritz, A convenient large-scale preparation of high-molecular weigh kininogen from human plasma, <u>Hoppe Seylers Z. Physiol. Chem.</u>, 362: 919 (1981).

PURIFICATION OF FACTOR XII FROM PORCINE PLASMA AND ITS ACTIVATION BY

PORCINE PLASMA KALLIKREIN

Kiyoshi Kato, Hiroshi Mashiko, Kyoichi Fujii, Kumiko Shiina,
Kenichi Miyamoto, Noriko Kohashi and Hidenobu Takahashi

Division of Chemistry of Hygiene, Meiji College of Pharmacy
1-35-23 Nozawa, Setagaya-ku, Tokyo 154, Japan

INTRODUCTION

Factor XII (F. XII) is a single polypeptide-chain glycoprotein that
circulates in plasma as a precursor form of a serine protease. It participates in the early or contact phase of blood coagulation, fibrinolysis and
kinin release when these reactions are initiated by surface activation. It
is revealed that the contact activation occurs on a negatively charged surfaces in the presence of high-molecular-weight (HMW) kininogen, F. XI and
plasma prekallikrein, using purified protein components of bovine or human
plasma (see reviews, Ref. 1-4). By this reaction, F. XII converts to activated F. XII (F. XIIa) which composed of two polypeptide-chains linked by a
disulfide bond. However, no report has appeared on the activation of porcine F. XII. To study the activation mechanism, we tried to isolate F. XII
from porcine plasma according to the purification method of F. XII from
human,[5] bovine,[6-7] rabbit,[8] or guinea pig[9] plasma, however, we usually
obtained F. XIIa. So, for the purification of F. XII, an improved method
to prevent completely the activation of F. XII during the isolation procedure is required. For this, the addition of large amounts of polybrene or
the addition of diisopropylfluorophosphate (DFP) at purification step was
necessary. This approach allowed us to purify F. XII from porcine plasma,
and we studied the activation of F. XII by purified porcine plasma
kallikrein.

MATERIALS AND METHODS

Materials

DEAE-Sephadex A-50, Q-Sepharose and S-Sepharose were purchased from
Pharmacia Fine Chemicals, Sweden. Synthetic fluorogenic substrates were
obtained from the Peptide Institute Inc., Japan. Rabbit brain cephalin, a
kit of standard protein markers (MW-SDS-200), soybean trypsin inhibitor
(SBTI, type I-S), sulfatide and ellagic acid were obtained from Sigma Chemical Co., U.S.A. Porcine plasma kallikrein was purified according to the
method of Ishihara et al.[10] The sources of other materials were as follows: DFP from Katayama Kagaku Kogyo Co., Ltd., Japan; Trasylol from Bayer,
West Germany; polybrene from Aldrich Chemical Co., Inc., U.S.A.; F. XII-
and F. XI-deficient plasmas and Fitzgerald plasma from George King Bio-
Medical, U.S.A.; and lima bean trypsin inhibitor (LBTI) from Worthington

Biochemical Corp., U.S.A. Fresh porcine blood containing sodium citrate
was collected in polyethylene bottles at a slaughterhouse, and was centrifuged at 3,000 rpm for 30 min at 20°C. The plasma was supplemented with
polybrene at a concentration of 0.5 g/liter, and stocked at -80°C until use.

Methods

Assay of F. XII

The assay of F. XII was carried out according to the method of Fujikawa
et al.,[6] using F. XII-deficient plasma. Activity was calculated from a
calibration curve where the log of F. XII concentration was plotted against
the log of the clotting time. One unit of activity is defined as the
amount of activity present in 1 ml of normal porcine plasma. For the assay
of F. XIIa, an equal volume of saline was added to the test tube instead of
the kaolin suspension. The amidase activity of F. XIIa was determined by
the method of Morita et al.,[11] using various synthetic fluorogenic substrates.

Protein Concentration

Protein concentrations were determined by measurements of the absorbance at 280 nm, assuming that an absorption value of 1.0 equals 1 mg/ml.

Electrophoresis

SDS-polyacrylamide gel disc electrophoresis was done according to the
method of Weber and Osborn.[12] The gels were stained with 0.25% Coomassie
brilliant blue R-250 and destained with a mixture of 7.5% acetic acid and
5% methanol. The molecular weight of F. XII was estimated from its relative mobility of 7.5% gel, in comparison with those of standard proteins
reduced with 2-mercaptoethanol.

RESULTS AND DISCUSSION

Purification of F. XII

All purification procedures were performed in a cold room at 4-5°C.
All of the columns and fraction tubes were silicon-coated before use.

Fresh or frozen porcine plasma was dialyzed against 20 liters of 0.02
M Tris-HCl buffer, pH 8.0, containing 0.02 M NaCl, overnight. After the
resulting precipitate was removed by centrifugation, polybrene (0.3 g/
liter) was added to the dialyzed fraction from 675 ml of plasma. And this
fraction was chromatographed on a DEAE-Sephadex A-50 column (7.5 x 48 cm)
equilibrated with 0.02 M Tris-HCl buffer, pH 8.0, containing 0.02 M NaCl.
The column was washed with 2 liters of the same buffer, then proteins were
eluted with a linear concentration gradient of NaCl from 0.02 M to 0.4 M
in 0.02 M Tris-HCl buffer, pH 8.0, containing polybrene (0.2 g/liter).
The elution was made with each 1 liter of 0.02 M and 0.08 M, followed with
0.08 M and 0.15 M, and finally with 0.15 M and 0.4 M NaCl. F. XII fractions
with clotting activity of F. XII-deficient plasma were pooled and dialyzed
against 20 liters of 0.02 M acetate buffer, pH 6.0, containing 0.08 M NaCl,
overnight. In the dialyzed solution, polybrene was added to obtain 0.2 g/
liter at a final concentration. After this solution was applied to a DEAE-
Sephadex A-50 column (5 x 45 cm) equilibrated with 0.02 M acetate buffer,
pH 6.0, containing 0.08 M NaCl, the column was washed with 600 ml of the
same buffer. And proteins were eluted by a salt gradient formed by 1 liter
of 0.08 M NaCl in 0.02 M acetate buffer (pH 6.0) and 1 liter of 0.25 M NaCl
in 0.02 M acetate buffer (pH 6.0). Both solutions also contained polybrene

Table 1. Purification of Porcine Factor XII

Purification step	Total protein (mg)	Total activity (units)	Specific activity (units/mg)
Plasma (675 ml)	54,000	675	0.01
1st DEAE-Sephadex A-50	4,460	338	0.08
2nd DEAE-Sephadex A-50	1,570	259	0.17
Q-Sepharose	918	237	0.26
S-Sepharose (F. XII-1)	8.5	175	20.59
(F. XII-2)	2.3	45	19.57

(0.2 g/liter). F. XII fractions were pooled and dialyzed against 20 liters of 0.02 M acetate buffer, pH 6.0, containing 0.02 M NaCl, overnight. In the dialyzed solution, 1 ml of 0.1 M DFP was added and polybrene was also added to obtain 0.2 g/liter at a final concentration. After this solution was applied to a Q-Sepharose column (3 x 21 cm) equilibrated with 0.02 M acetate buffer, pH 6.0, containing 0.02 M NaCl, the column was washed with 450 ml of the same buffer. And proteins were eluted by a salt gradient formed by 500 ml of 0.02 M NaCl in 0.02 M acetate buffer (pH 6.0) and 500 ml of 0.4 M NaCl in 0.02 M acetate buffer (pH 6.0). Both solutions also contained polybrene (0.1 g/liter). F. XII fractions were pooled and dia-lyzed against 10 liters of 0.02 M acetate buffer, pH 6.0, containing 0.2 M NaCl for 2 hr. In the dialyzed solution, polybrene was added to obtain 0.2 g/liter at a final concentration. After this solution was applied to an S-Sepharose column (3 x 20 cm) equilibrated with 0.02 M acetate buffer, pH 6.0, containing 0.2 M NaCl, the column was washed with 600 ml of the same buffer. Then proteins were eluted by a salt gradient formed by 500 ml of 0.2 M NaCl in 0.02 M acetate buffer (pH 6.0) and 500 ml of 0.5 M NaCl in 0.02 M acetate buffer (pH 6.0). Both solutions also contained polybrene (0.2 g/liter). Two protein peaks appeared on this chromatogram, however, F. XII activity was in parallel with the elution profile of the two protein peaks. F. XII contained in the faster eluted fraction was named F. XII-1, and F. XII contained in the slower eluted fraction was named F. XII-2. They also have the same migration on SDS-polyacrylamide gel electrophoresis.

A summary of the purification of F. XII is shown in Table 1. About 8.5 mg of F. XII-1 and 2.3 mg of F. XII-2 were obtained from 675 ml of por-cine plasma. The increase of specific activity was about 2,000-2,100-fold, and the specific activity of the final preparation was nearly 20 units/mg of protein of each preparation.

Polybrene, which prevents the surface binding of F. XII on the nega-tively charged materials such as kaolin, glass or ellagic acid, was added to the buffers throughout the entire procedure. Protease inhibitor, DFP, was also added to the solution during the purification procedure for pro-tection of activation of F. XII by plasma kallikrein or plasmin. [13]

Purity

The purity of both final preparations (F. XII-1 and -2) was examined by SDS-polyacrylamide gel disc electrophoresis in the presence or absence of 2-mercaptoethanol. These preparations gave a single band on the elec-trophoresis before or after reduction with 2-mercaptoethanol. These re-sults suggest that these porcine F. XIIs consist of a single polypeptide

chain. In the absence of kaolin, the coagulation time of F. XII-deficient
plasma was almost the same as that of saline as a control. Therefore,
these preparations contained no detectable F. XIIa. Furthermore, these
preparations did not contain other coagulation factors such as F. XI or
HMW kininogen, because these preparations did not shorten the abnormal
clotting time of F. XI-deficient plasma or Fitzgerald plasma. For study
the contamination of plasma kallikrein or prekallikrein in these preparations, they were dialyzed against 1 liter of 0.05 M Tris-HCl buffer, pH
8.0, for 1 hr at 4°C to remove polybrene in these preparations. When the
clotting time of F. XII-deficient plasma was measured using each of dialyzed preparations in the presence or absence of kaolin, both preparations
had the ability to correct the abnormal clotting time of the plasma in the
presence of kaolin, but not in the absence of kaolin. After each of dialyzed preparations was allowed to stand for 3 days at 4°C, the assay was
carried out under the same condition as described above. F. XII-2 had the
ability to correct the abnormal clotting time of the plasma in the presence
of kaolin, but not in the absence of kaolin, however, F. XII-1 had the
ability to correct the abnormal clotting time of the plasma in the presence
or absence of kaolin. This result indicates that F. XII-1 converts to F.
XIIa under the condition, and the activation of F. XII-1 is due to induce
by kallikrein or prekallikrein in this preparation or to occur by autoactivation. The datailed studies will be required in near future.

Determination of Molecular Weight

For the determination of the molecular weight of F. XII-2, standard
proteins were simultaneously subjected to SDS-polyacrylamide gel disc electrophoresis. And the calibration curve was obtained from the relative electrophoretic mobilities of protein markers. By comparison with the relative
mobilities of protein markers, the molecular weight of purified F. XII was
estimated to be about 90,000.

Properties of Porcine F. XIIa

Before the study of the activation of F. XII by plasma kallikrein, we
investigated the properties of purified porcine F. XIIa obtained from the
fraction which was spontaneously activated during the purification procedure
as described above. At first, the substrate specificity of F. XIIa on
various synthetic fluorogenic substrates was investigated. The enzyme
potently hydrolyzed tert-butoxycarbonyl (Boc)-Val-Pro-Arg-4-methylcoumaryl-
7-amide (MCA) and Boc-Glu(OBzl)-Gly-Arg-MCA among these substrates used.
On the other hand, bovine F. XIIa also potently hydrolyzed Boc-Glu(OBzl)-
Gly-Arg-MCA, however, the enzyme weakly hydrolyzed Boc-Val-Pro-Arg-MCA. [14]
Furthermore, the activity of porcine F. XIIa was completely inhibited by
the addition of SBTI, LBTI and DFP, however, the activity of human or bovine
F. XIIa was inhibited by the addition of DFP and LBTI, but not by the
addition of SBTI. [5,14] These results indicate that F. XIIa is a serine
protease and activates prekallikrein to kallikrein, but the properties of
porcine F. XIIa differ from the properties of human or bovine F. XIIa.

Activation of Porcine F. XII by Porcine Plasma Kallikrein

To study the activation of F. XII by plasma kallikrein, F. XII-2 was
used, and the amount of F. XIIa induced by kallikrein was determined by the
measurement of amidase activity using Boc-Glu(OBzl)-Gly-Arg-MCA. At first,
we investigated the effects of foreign surfaces on the activation of F. XII
by plasma kallikrein. From this experiment, most effective foreign surfaces
on the activation was sulfatide among other materials such as ellagic acid,
dextran sulfate and kaolin used. Then, time course of activation of F. XII
by plasma kallikrein in the presence or absence of sulfatide is investi-

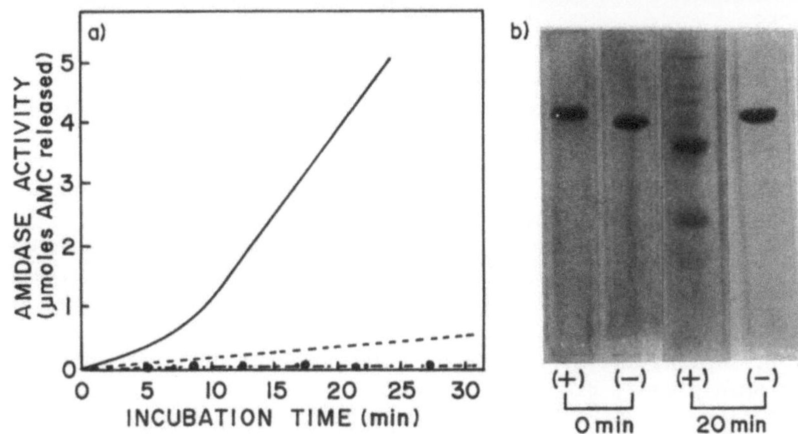

Fig. 1a. Time course of activation of F. XII by plasma kallikrein in the
presence or absence of sulfatide. Porcine F. XII-2 (2.6 µg),
sulfatide (37.5 µg), Boc-Glu(OBzl)-Gly-Arg-MCA and porcine plasma
kallikrein (0.054 µg) were used. The amount of 7-amino-4-methyl-
coumarin (AMC) liberated was measured by the method of Morita et
al. [11] ——, F. XII + plasma kallikrein + sulfatide; ----, F. XII
+ plasma kallikrein;—·●--, F. XII + sulfatide.

Fig. 1b. SDS-polyacrylamide gel electrophoresis of the incubated mixture of
F. XII and plasma kallikrein. After 11.2 µg of F. XII-2 was incubated with 0.01 µg of porcine plasma kallikrein for 20 min in the
presence of sulfatide, the incubated mixture was subjected to SDS-
polyacrylamide gel electrophoresis in the presence (+) or absence
(-) of 2-mercaptoethanol.

gated (Fig. 1a). From this result, plasma kallikrein rapidly activated F.
XII in the presence of sulfatide, and the activation rate of F. XII by the
kallikrein increased 20 times faster than that of F. XII by the kallikrein
in the absence of sulfatide. Moreover, F. XII was not activated by the
addition of sulfatide in the absence of plasma kallikrein. This result
suggests that the autoactivation of F. XII does not occur, even though suitable amount of sulfatide is present in the solution of F. XII. To study
the activation mechanism of F. XII by the kallikrein, the 20 min-incubated
mixture was subjected to SDS-polyacrylamide gel disc electrophoresis before
or after reduction with 2-mercaptoethanol (Fig. 1b). Before reduction of
the incubated mixture, the band of the incubated mixture showed almost the
same mobility as the original band (0 min-incubated mixture), however, the
incubated mixture gave new two bands showing a faster mobility than the
original band in the presence of 2-mercaptoethanol. These results indicate
that plasma kallikrein cleaves a single peptide bond on the disulfide-
bridged polypeptide-chain of the precursor molecule, and F. XIIa thus
induced is composed of two polypeptide-chains linked by a disulfide bond.
This activation mechanism of porcine F. XII by porcine plasma kallikrein is
almost the same as that of human or bovine F. XII by plasma kallikrein. [15-17]

It is shown that further fragmentation of human F. XIIa molecule occurs
on the prolonged incubation with plasma kallikrein. [4,5,15] This reaction
did not occur in the case of bovine. [16,17] Now, detailed studies of the
fragmentation of porcine F. XII by porcine plasma kallikrein are in
progress, and the results will be reported in the near future.

REFERENCES

1. H. Kato, Initiation mechanism of intrinsic blood coagulation: Activation of Factor XII and role of high-molecular-weight kininogen, Seikagaku (in Japanese) 52:1173 (1980).

2. R. L. Heimark, K. Kurachi, K. Fujikawa, and E. W. Davie, Surface activation of coagulation, fibrinolysis, and kinin formation, Nature 286:456 (1980).

3. B. N. Bouma, and J. H. Griffin, Initiation mechanism: The contact activation system in plasma, In: "New Comprehensive Biochemistry", Vol. 13, R. F. A. Zwaal, and H. C. Hemker, ed., Elsevier, New York (1986).

4. A. P. Kaplan, and M. Silverberg, The coagulation-kinin pathway of human plasma, Blood 70:1 (1987).

5. K. Fujikawa, and E. W. Davie, Human factor XII (Hageman factor), In: "Methods in Enzymology", Vol. 80, L. Lorand, ed., Academic Press, New York (1981).

6. K. Fujikawa, K. A. Walsh, and E. W. Davie, Isolation and characterization of bovine factor XII (Hageman factor), Biochemistry 16:2270 (1977).

7. T. Sugo, N. Ikari, H. Kato, S. Iwanaga, and S. Fujii, Functional sites of bovine high molecular weight kininogen as a cofactor in kaolin-mediated activation of factor XII (Hageman factor), Biochemistry 19:3215 (1980).

8. C. G. Cochrane, and K. D. Wuepper, The first component of the kinin-forming system in human and rabbit plasma. Its relationship to clotting factor XII (Hageman factor), J. Exp. Med. 134:986 (1971).

9. T. Yamamoto, and C. G. Cochrane, Guinea pig Hageman factor as a vascular permeability enhancement factor, Am. J. Pathol. 105:164 (1981).

10. F. Ishihara, H. Mashiko, and H. Takahashi, Evidence for the presence of two kininogens in porcine plasma and the isolation of high-molecular-weight kininogen, Chem. Pharm. Bull. 34:4694 (1986).

11. T. Morita, H. Kato, S. Iwanaga, K. Takada, T. Kimura, and S. Sakakibara, New fluorogenic substrates for α-thrombin, factor Xa, kallikreins, and urokinase, J. Biochem. 82:1495 (1977).

12. K. Weber, and M. Osborn, The reliability of molecular weight determination by dodecyl sulfate-polyacrylamide gel electrophoresis, J. Biol. Chem. 244:4406 (1969).

13. A. P. Kaplan, and K. F. Austen, A prealbumin activator of prekallikrein. II. Derivation of activators of prekallikrein from active Hageman factor by digestion with plasmin, J. Exp. Med. 133:696 (1971).

14. T. Sugo, Y. Ohno, T. Shimada, H. Kato, and S. Iwanaga, Mechanism of surface-mediated activation of bovine factor XII and prekallikrein, In: "Advances in Experimental Medicine and Biology", Vol. 156A, H. Fritz, N. Back, G. Dietze, and G. L. Haberland, ed., Plenum Press, New York (1983).

15. S. D. Revak, C. G. Cochrane, and J. H. Griffin, The binding and cleavage characteristics of human Hageman factor during contact activation. A comparison of normal plasma with plasmas deficient in factor XI, prekallikrein, or high molecular weight kininogen, J. Clin. Invest. 59:1167 (1977).

16. K. Fujikawa, R. L. Heimark, K. Kurachi, and E. W. Davie, Activation of bovine factor XII (Hageman factor) by plasma kallikrein, Biochemistry 19:1322 (1980).

17. T. Sugo, A. Hamaguchi, T. Shimada, H. Kato, and S. Iwanaga, Mechanism of surface-mediated activation of bovine factor XII and plasma prekallikrein, J. Biochem. 92:689 (1982).

STUDY ON THE IN VITRO ASSAY METHOD FOR EVALUATING THE INHIBITORY EFFECT OF VARIOUS SUBSTANCES ON THE PRODUCTION OF PLASMA KALLIKREIN

Katsumi Nishikawa, Hitoshi Kawakubo, Kenji Matsumoto,
Hisashi Yago, Yoshio Toyomaki and Seishi Suehiro

Institute of Bio-Active Science, Nippon Zoki Pharmaceutical
Co. Ltd., Yashiro-cho, Hyogo 673-14, Japan

SUMMARY

The assay method based on the principle of kallikrein-kinin cascade
was established for evaluating the inhibitory effects of various
substances on the production of plasma kallikrein. In this _in vitro_
assay, it was found that indomethacin, ketoprofen, ibuprofen and an
extract obtained from inflamed rabbit skin inoculated with vaccinia virus
(NSP) had the inhibitory effect on the production of plasma kallikrein.
Kinins generated in the reaction mixture were measured by RIA. It was
shown that the generation of kinins was also inhibited by these
substances. From these results, it is hoped that this assay method may be
useful for screening the substances which inhibited the production of
kinin.

INTRODUCTION

The assay methods for measurement of plasma prekallikrein by the
complete conversion of prekallikrein to kallikrein had been reported[1-7].
However, the assay method for evaluating the effects of various substances
on the kallikrein-kinin system has not been reported. Therefore, the _in
vitro_ assay system for evaluating the inhibitory effects of substances on
the production of plasma kallikrein was tried to be established and
evaluated.

MATERIALS AND METHODS

Chemicals

Synthetic substrate S-2302 (D-Pro-Phe-Arg-p-nitroanilide) was
purchased from Kabi Vitrum. Lima bean trypsin inhibitor (LBTI, Sigma
Co.), kaolin (acid washed, American standard, Fisher Scientific Co.),
bradykinin (BK), lys-bradykinin (Lys-BK) and met-lys-bradykinin (Met-Lys-
BK, Peptide Inst., Osaka) were used. Sep-pak® column was purchased from
Waters-Millipore Co. For the separation of kinins, Nucleosil $5C_{18}$ column
(guard column, 4.6mmI.D.×50mm; separation column, 4.6mmI.D.×250mm, Nagel
Co.) was used. Aminopyrine, aspirin, indomethacin, ketoprofen, ibuprofen,
pentazocine, morphine and an extract obtained from inflamed rabbit skin

inoculated with vaccinia virus (NSP) were the substances which were
investigated in this study.

Human Plasma

Nine ml of whole blood was collected from healthy human subjects and
immediately transferred to a plastic tube containing 1ml of 130mM sodium
citrate. The tube was centrifuged 1700×g for 10min. at 4°C. Plasma was
diluted by saline and used as soon as possible.

The Assay Method

Plasma kallikrein activity was evoked by the addition of kaolin
suspension to a reaction mixture and 0°C. LBTI was added in order to
terminate the reaction. Kallikrein activity in the reaction mixture was
measured by using synthetic substrate S-2302.

Extraction of Kinins from the Reaction Mixture

Acetonitrile was added to the reaction mixture in order to
deproteinize as well as to free kinins from kaolin. After centrifugation
followed by filtration of supernatant, the filtrate was dried under
reduced pressure. The residue was dissolved in appropriate solvent, and
applied to Sep-pak C_{18} cartridge column[8-9]. The fraction between 15% and
50% of aqueous acetonitrile was collected and dried again. The final
residue in buffer was measured for kinins by RIA[10].

RESULTS

The Optimal Conditions of the Assay

The optimal conditions of this assay were as follows; The
concentration of sodium chloride and kaolin were 100mM and 1.25mg/ml
respectively. The reaction time was determined to be 20min. LBTI above
5mg/ml of the final concentration completely inhibited the generation of
kallikrein activity when used before the initiation of the reaction.
Taking the safety margin into consideration, 15mg/ml of the final
concentration of LBTI was chosen. At this concentration, it inhibited the
further increase of kallikrein activity without affecting kallikrein
activity itself. The optimal pH of reaction was 8.0

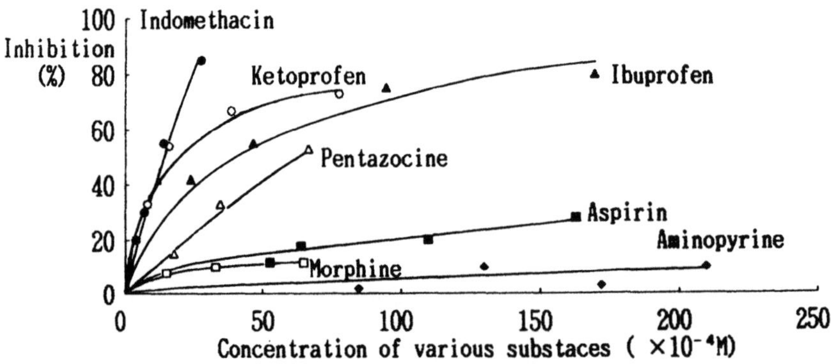

Fig: 1 Inhibitory effects of various substances on the production
of plasma kallikrein.

<u>The Inhibitory Effects of Various Substances on the Production of Plasma Kallikrein</u>

The inhibitory effects of various substances on the production of plasma kallikrein were determined by the method described (Fig. 1). Indomethacin, ketoprofen and ibuprofen showed the strong inhibitory effects on the production of plasma kallikrein dose-dependently in this assay system, but aspirin, morphine and aminopyrine didn't.

An extract obtained from inflamed rabbit skin inoculated with vaccinia virus, NSP, was also tested (Table 1). It was found that NSP also inhibited the production of plasma kallikrein dose-dependently.

<u>Inhibitory Effects of Various Substances on the Kinin Formation</u>

Inhibitory effects of various substances on the kinin formation were determined. Indomethacin, ketoprofen and NSP inhibited the formation of kinin strongly as well as the production of plasma kallikrein (Table 2 and 3). A good correlation was observed between inhibitory effect on the production of plasma kallikrein and the inhibition of the formation of kinins.

Table 1   Inhibitory effect of an extract obtained from inflamed rabbit skin inoculated with vaccinia virus (NSP) on the production of plasma kallikrein.

Concentration of NSP (μg/ml)	Inhibition (%)
25	26
50	45
100	83

Table 2   Inhibitory effects of indomethacin and ketoprofen on the formation of kinins.

Substances	Concentration ($\times 10^{-4}$M)	Inhibition (%)
Indomethacin	5	24
	10	38
	25	87
Ketoprofen	20	44
	40	66
	80	89

Table 3   Inhibitory effect of an extract obtained from inflamed rabbit skin inoculated with vaccinia virus (NSP) on the formation of kinins.

Concentration of NSP (μg/ml)	Inhibition (%)
25	9
50	57
100	90

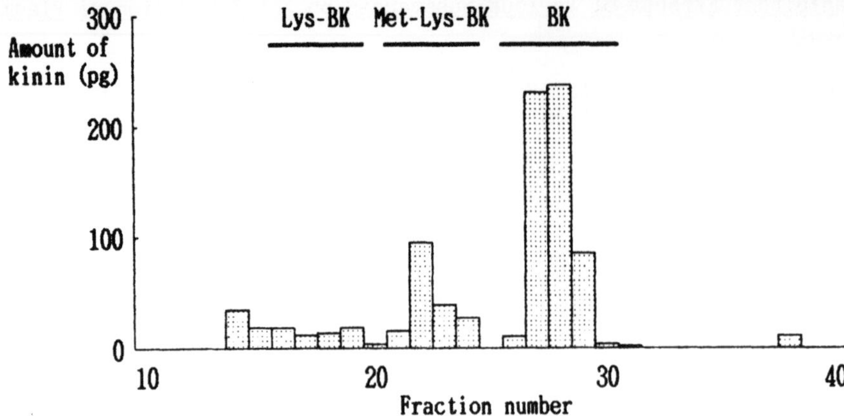

Fig. 2 Elution pattern of generated kinin by HPLC. Generated kinin
was separated on Nucleosil 5C$_{18}$ column using a mobile phase of
10% isopropylalcohol containing 0.1% TFA.

HPLC Fraction of Generated Kinins

The kinins generated in a control reaction mixture were fractionated
by HPLC and the species of kinins were investigated. Kinins were
separated by HPLC column into two peaks (Fig.2). From the elution pattern
of authentic kinins, one peak was found to be Met-Lys-BK and another BK.
It was found that both peaks were equally affected when the formation of
kinins was inhibited.

DISCUSSION

An _in vitro_ assay system in evaluating the inhibitory effects of
various substances on the production of plasma kallikrein was established
in this study. To determine the inhibitory effect, it was necessary to do
fixed time assay when kallikrein activity increased linearly. At the end
of the desired time, the further increase of kallikrein activity had to be
terminated.

It was found that indomethacin, ketoprofen, ibuprofen and NSP had the
inhibitory effects on the production of kallikrein in this assay. These
substances also inhibited the kinin formation in the reaction mixture.
From these results, it is suggested that these substances have some
effects on the kallikrein-kinin system. Furthermore, this assay method
may be useful for screening the substances which act on the kinin
formation.

It is of interest to note that kinins separated by HPLC were Met-Lys-
BK and BK. Met-Lys-BK has been known to be excreted in human urine, but
its formation in plasma level isn't well known. Recently, the release of
BK and Met-Lys-BK from purified low molecular weight kininogen with the
help of neutrophil elastase by plasma kallikrein was reported[11]. It may
be a mechanism of the formation of Met-Lys-BK found in the plasma.
Currently studies are underway in investigating in this respect.

REFERENCES

1. R. J. Mandle, R. W. Colman, and A. P. Kaplan, Identification of
   prekallikrein and high-molecular-weight kininogen as a complex in
   human plasma, _Proc. Natl. Acad. Sci._, 73,4179, (1976).
2. C. Kluft, Determination of prekallikrein in human plasma: optimal

conditions for activating prekallikrein, <u>J. Lab. Med.</u>, 91, 83, (1978).

3. T. Guido, and J. H. Griffin, Properties of sulfatides in factor-XII-dependent contact activation, <u>Blood</u>, 59, 69, (1982).

4. H. L. Meier, J. V. Pierce, R. W. Colman, and A. P. Kaplan, Activation and function of human hageman factor, <u>J. Clin. Invest.</u>, 60, 18, (1977).

5. S. Oh-ishi, and M. Katori, Fluorometric assay for plasma prekallikrein using peptidylmethyl coumarinyl amide as a substrate, <u>Thromb. Res.</u>, 14, 551, (1979).

6. M. Kato, Y. Nagano, T. Suzawa, S. Konishi, M. Fujimaki, and K. Fukutake, Methodological and clinical observation of chromogenic substrate for plasma prekallikrein and prekallikrein assay, <u>Blood & Vessel</u>, 10, 90, (1979).

7. M. Fujimaki, and M. Kato, Synthetic chromogenic substrates for determination of blood clotting and fibrinolytic factor, <u>J. Med. Enzymol.</u>, 3, 554, (1980).

8. A. Barlas, K. Sugio, and L. M. Greenbaum, Release of T-kinin and bradykinin in carrageenin induced inflammation in the rat, <u>FEBS letter</u>, 190, 268, (1985).

9. A. Barlas, H. Okamoto, and L. M. Greenbaum, T-kininogen - the major plasma kininogen in rat adjuvant arthritis, <u>Biochem. Biophys. Res. Comm.</u>, 129, 280, (1985).

10. M. Minami, H. Togashi, M. Sano, T. Endoh, H. Saito, F. Hashimoto, K. Fujita, H. Yasuda, Y. Kuriyamoto, and T. Nishino, Plasma bradykinin concentration in patients with essential hypertension, effort angina and other cardiac diseases, <u>Folia Pharmacol. Japon.</u>, 82, 159, (1983).

11. F. Sato, and S. Nagasawa, Release of kinins from human low molecular weight kininogen in cooperation with human plasma kallikrein and neutrophil elastase, <u>Seikagaku</u>, 59, 665, (1987).

A NEW ANALYTICAL SYSTEM FOR THE PROTEASES AND ANTIPROTEASES ASSESSMENT

Jean Boulanger[1], Pierre Ers[1], M-Violaine Lemaire[1],
Michel Notche[1], and Albert Adam[1,2]

[1]Laboratoire de Biologie clinique, C.H. Sainte Ode B-6970 Baconfoy and
[2]Faculté de Pharmacie, Université de Montréal, Montréal, Canada

INTRODUCTION

The classical coagulation analyses are performed either by using mechanical and optic principles for dectection the end-point of the reaction : the clot formation. However, the development of specific synthetic chromogenic substrates allows photometric assays for coagulation and fibrinolysis factors, independently of the concentration of fibrinogen and the presence of heparine. These photometric methods can be automated with a significant improvement of the standardization and the reproducibility. For such purposes, a new analytical system, the CHROMOTIMER has been developed by Behringwerk, Marburg, RFA. This is based on the measurement of the time necessary to attain a fixed increase in absorbance rather than an increase of absorbance as a classical spectrophotometer (1-3). The purpose of this work is to apply this new system to the enzymatic determination of prokallikrein (pKK), and two antiproteases : antithrombin III (AT III) and C1 esterase inhibitor C1IN). After an analytical study, we compare the obtained results in emergency medicine with those furnished by classical spectrophotometric methods.

MATERIAL AND METHODS

1. The chromotimer system

Description of the instrument

The BEHRING CHROMOTIMER consists of an analyzer: a four channel glass-fiber photometer (completely thermostated) and an Apple II GS computer with a printer.
The operator controls the system via the computer with a menu-software. The computer controls the analyzer and runs and evaluates tests specified by the user.

Measuring principle

In routine testing, activation of the coagulation cascade is produced by addition of aPT- or aPTT-type reagent, similar to the actual clotting methods. A coloured dye is then released by the activity of thrombin on a chromogenic substrate. The time required for the absorbance to increase by 0.10 (fixed A method) is measured at 405 nm.

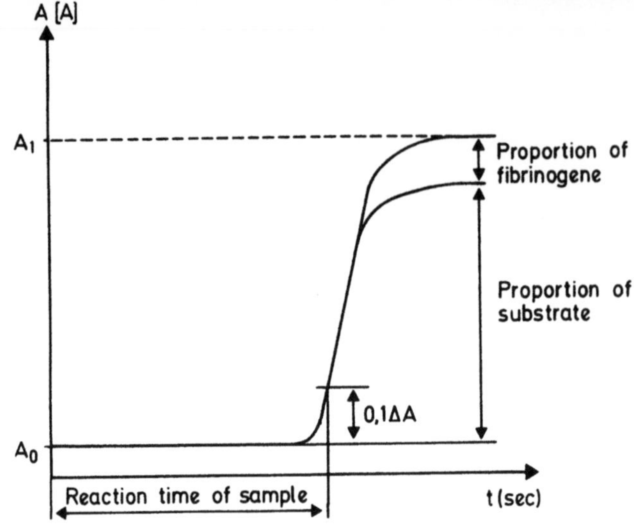

Fig. 1. Principle of coagulation measurements with the chromotimer system.

Test with a fixed time principle can also be performed on the Chromotimer.

2. Reagents : pKK, C1IN and AT III were quantified using chromogenic substrates purchased respectively by Kabi-Vitrum Stockolm, Sweden (Coa-set Prekallikrein) and by Behringwerke (Berichrom-C$_1$ inactivator and Berichrom-Antithrombin III).

3. Methods : Spectrophotometric methods used our an laboratory on HITACHI 705 (NAKA-WORKS JAPAN) have been adapted on the chromotimer system.

RESULTS

Protease and antiprotease activities are expressed as % of a pool of normal plasmas obtained from blood donors.

Table 1. Intrabatch precision (CV %) of the results obtained with the chromotimer system at 5 levels of activity.

Level	pKK	ATIII	C1IN
100 %	2.5	2.7	0.7
75	5.4	1.6	1.9
50	2.0	2.9	0.9
25	3.8	8.2	3.2
10	1.5	5.4	9.1

1. Precision and limit detection levels

The intrabatch reproducibility expressed by CV % has been calculated at five levels of activity (100 - 75 - 50 - 25 - 10 %). The results are shown in table 1. Although we found 2 CV values (AT III 25 %, C1IN 10 %) near 10 percent, in the majority of cases (n = 13), CV was lower or equal to 5 %.

For the 3 investigated parameters, we could measure a limit detection level $\leqslant$ 5 % of activity.

2. Correlation between the classic photometric and the chromotimer method

This correlation could be calculated by quantifying, pKK, AT III and C1IN, by both methods on 50 plasma samples obtained in acute pancreatitis, burned patients, septic shock and polytrauma. The results are shown in figure 2. For each quantified parameter the correlation is excellent, in fact the coeficient correlation equals respectively 0.98 for pKK (y = 1.05 x - 0.74), 0.92 for C1IN (y = 0.92 x + 6) and 0.97 for AT III (y = 0.98 x - 0.63).

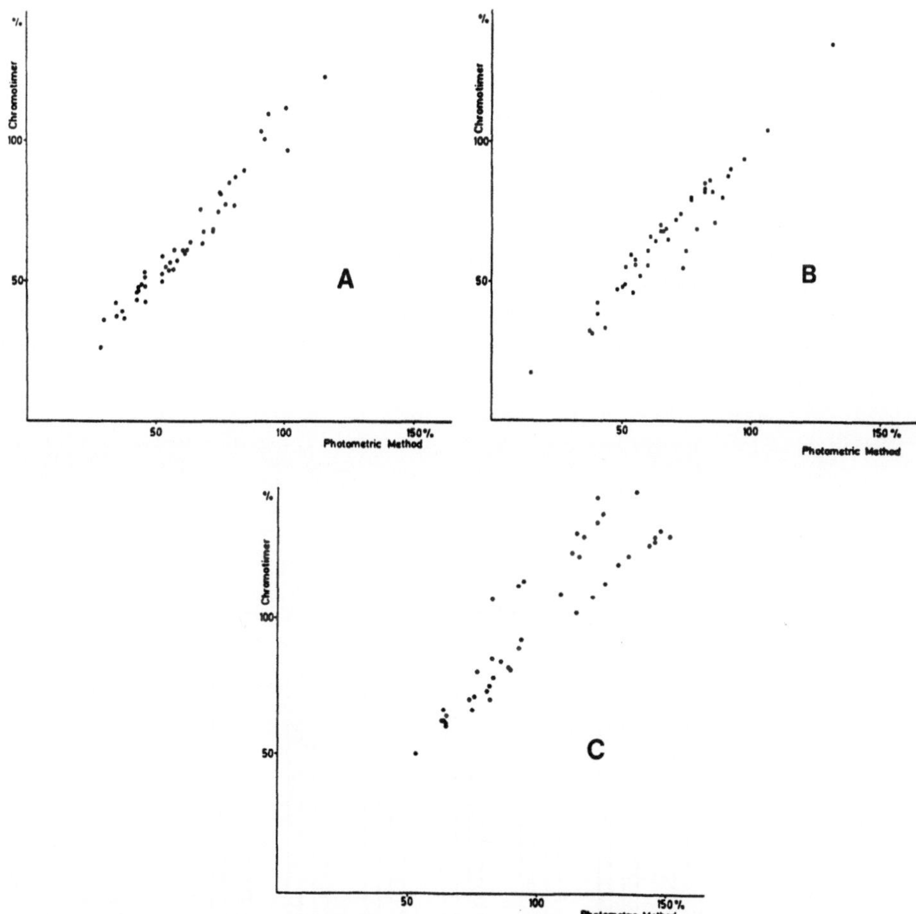

Fig. 2. Correlation of activities measured with the chromotimer system with those obtained with the classical photometric method A: prokallikrein, B: C1 esterase inhibitor, C: Antithrombin III.

3. Use of the chromotimer system in critical care medicine

In figure 3, we illustrate, the usefulness of the chromotimer system in the followup of the liver transplantation.

Before transplantation, plasma pKK and AT III are significantly reduced (40 % and 58 % of activity) although C1IN values are normal (80 - 120 % of activity). In the postoperative period, we can observe a progressively and parallel increase of pKK and AT III, until the second week of observation, although, C1IN activities remain unchanged since the first day after transplantation.

DISCUSSION

The activation of plasma pKK play a key role in the pathology of acute inflammatory processes. Therefore, the quantification of pKK and plasma antiproteases inhibiting active kallikrein (C1IN, AT III, and a2 macroglobulin) can be helpful in the diagnosis and the therapeutic monitoring of the intravascular coagulation, the septic shock and the acute respiratory distress syndrome. In fact, several authors have considered pKK activation as the primum movens of such acute complications often seen in intensive care medicine (4 - 5).
Altough enzymatic methods using chromogenic substrates are now available for the quantification of the chemistries considered here, they remain relatively unknown and unused in emergency and intensive care medicine. Actually, these methods are still considered as time consuming and unpracticable.
The chromotimer system fills up these gaps. In fact, it is particularly applicable to emergencies, performing individual tests in a short period of time.
Moreover the results obtained by this system are analytically reliable. They are reproducible and sensible allowing the early detection of the prokallikrein activation and the precise variation in time during the follow up. In clinical application, they correlate perfectly with those obtained with spectrophotometric methods.
From these results, we can conclude that the chromotimer opens a new area in the assessment of the protease-antiprotease system in critical care medicine.

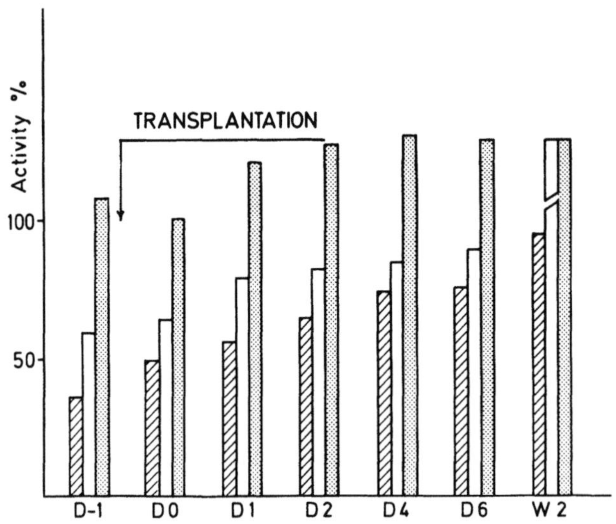

Fig. 3 Evolution of the enzyme activities of prokallikrein (▨), C1 esterase inhibitor (▒), and antithrombin III (▢), before and after liver transplantation.

REFERENCES

1. H. J. Kolde · Chromotime System. A new generation of coagulation analyses. <u>Behring Inst. Mitt.</u>, 78:176 (1985).
2. H. J. Kolde, F. Dati. Experience with a new photometric prothrombin time assay. <u>Haemostasis</u> 15:71 (1985).
3. F. Dati, U. Becker, A. Hissung, F. Keller. New perspectives in diagnosis of haemostasis disorders. Comptes rendus de la IV° Rencontre internationale de Biologie clinique. Biologie clinique en soins intensifs. <u>Ann. Biol. Clin.</u> (in press).
4. A. Kaplan, M. Silverberg. The coagulation-kinin pathway of human plasma. <u>Blood</u>, 1:1 (1987).
5. R.W. Colman. Surface-mediated defense reactions: the plasma contact activation sustem. <u>J. Clin. Invest.</u> 73:1249 (1984).

cDNA CLONING OF KININASE 1

Wolfgang Gebhard[+], Matthias Schube[+] and Manfred Eulitz

[+]Abteilung für Klinische Chemie und Klinische Biochemie in
der Chirurgischen Klinik, Universität München, München, FRG
and Institut für Hämatologie der GSF, Abteilung für Immu-
nologie, München, FRG

INTRODUCTION

Kininase 1 (carboxypeptidase N, anaphylatoxin inactivator, arginine
carboxypeptidase, EC 3.4.17.3) cleaves C terminal basic amino acids of
kinins and other peptides (1–3). The enzyme exists in plasma as a tetra-
meric complex of Mr about 280,000 (4,5) comprising two large carbohydrate containing subunits of Mr about 83,000 and two active subunits of
Mr about 48,000 (6,7). Isolated small subunits are as active as the intact enzyme (6).

PURIFICATION OF KININASE 1

Kininase 1 was isolated from plasma using ion exchange chromatography and arginine-Sepharose affinity chromatography according to a reliable and efficient scheme (6) with the expected yield. Peptidase activity
was determined using furylacryloylalanyl-L-lysine (8).

In SDS–PAGE no contaminants could be detected after Western blotting
and silver staining (fig. 1). As expected, the carbohydrate free small
subunits are stained more intensively. The large subunits are represented
by a double band. Wether this is due to a different carbohydrate content
or the existence of isoforms remains to be proven. Long-term storage at
-20°C leaves the small subunit unaffected. The large subunits become
smaller, but the double band pattern remains. The degradation is probably
due to the presence of trace amounts of proteases, e.g. plasmin.

cDNA CLONING

Polyclonal antibodies generated in rabbits preferentially detect the
small subunit of kininase 1. We used the antibodies to screen a human liver cDNA expression library in lambda gt11 (kindly provided by Dr. S.L.C.
Woo, ref.9), but without success concerning the small subunit.

We therefore isolated the small subunit of purified kininase 1 by
linear gradient (10–18%) SDS-PAGE and electroelution of the protein from
the stained, excised gel. After determination of the N-terminal amino-
acid sequence (fig. 2) a unique 59–mer oligonucleotide probe was deduced
according to the rules of Lahte (10).

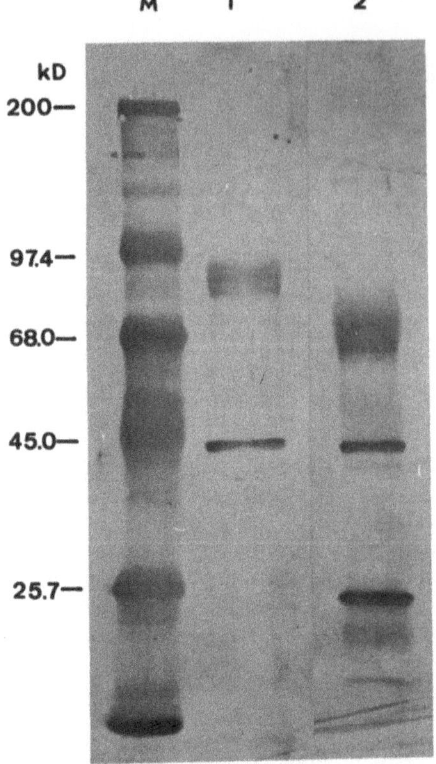

Fig. 1. Subunits of isolated kininase 1 after SDS–PAGE, Western blotting
and silver staining. M: Marker; lane 1: freshly prepared material;
lane 2: after 17 months at -20°C.

```
        V  T  F  R  H  H  R  Y  D  D  L  V  R  T  L  Y  K  V  Q  N

     GTGACCTTCCGGCATCATCGGTATGATGACCTGGTGCGGACCCTGTACAAGGTGCAGAA
            *  *  *  *  *        *  *        *              *
     GTGACCTTTCGCCACCACCGCTATGATGATCTTGTGCGGACGCTGTACAAGGTGCAAAA
```

Fig. 2. First line: N–terminal amino acid sequence of the isolated small
subunit; second line: the nucleic acid probe derived from the
amino acid sequence; third line: the obtained cDNA sequence;
stars mark mismatches.

                    10   20   30   40   50   60
      GTGAGGGAGGAGAGATGAGTGGCTATTCCAGAACGACATAAAGAATTTCCAGCCTTGGAC

                    70   80   90   100   110   120
      GGACAGCTGGGAACGTCTTCCAATTTGGACTGGTGTTTACAAGCGGGAAGCTAGGTGGAC

                   130   140   150   160   170   180
      CTTGGATTTTGGCGGGTGAAGAGGCTAGGTTGTTTAAGGAGGTGGGGAGCGTTTCAGTGG

                   190   200   210   220   230   240
      CTCTCTTTGAAAAAGCCCAGCAAGATGTCAGACCTGCTCTCAGTCTTCCTCCACCTCCTC
                                       M   S   D   L   L   S   V   F   L   H   L   L

                   250   260   270   280   290   300
      CTTCTCTTCAAGTTGGTTGCCCCGGTGACCTTTCGCCACCACCGCTATGATGATCTTGTG
        L   L   F   K   L   V   A   P   V   T   F   R   H   H   R   Y   D   D   L   V

                   310   320
      CGGACGCTGTACAAGGTGCAAAAC
        R   T   L   Y   K   V   Q   N

      Fig. 3. N-terminal amino-acid sequence of kininase 1 derived from its
              cDNA. The signal peptide cleavage site is marked by a triangle.
              In frame stop codons in the 5'untranslated regions are under-
              lined.

      A total of 60 000 plaques were screened using the oligolabeled probe
(4 x10^7 cpm/ g) and the same cDNA library as before. One plaque hybrid-
ized sufficiently.

ANALYSIS OF KININASE 1 cDNA

      The isolated phage-DNA contains a cDNA-insert of about 1.7 kbp. Af-
ter subcloning in plasmid pTZ18R we sequenced the double stranded DNA
from both ends. From the analysis of both cDNA ends we know that the
clone represents a full length cDNA. The 3'end of the cDNA contains the
noncanonical polyadenylation sequence AATACA and, in the right distance,
the polyadenylation site followed by a poly(A)-tract of 15 bp. The 5'part
of the cDNA sequence is shown in fig. 3.

      The sequence contains within an unusually long 5'non-coding region
two in-frame stop codons. Therefore, the expression of a fusion protein
is impossible. This is the reason why we were unable to detect any full-
length cDNA clone with anti-kininase 1 antibodies.

      After a signal sequence the derived amino-acid sequence matches com-
pletely the predetermined N-terminal amino-acid sequence. There are only
9 mismatches in the 59-mer oligonucleotide used as the probe (fig. 2).

      The full-length cDNA of kininase 1 now opens the possibility to stu-
dy its hereditary diseases and the role as well as the possible therapeutical application of this enzyme in inflammation.

REFERENCES

1. E. G. Erdös, Kininases, in: "Handbook of Experimental Pharmacology," Vol. XXV Suppl., pp 427-487, E. G. Erdös, ed., Springer-Verlag, Heidelberg (1979).
2. V. A. Bokisch and H. J. Müller-Eberhard, Anaphylatoxin inactivator of human plasma: its isolation and characterization as a carboxypeptidase, J. Clin. Invest. 49: 2427-2436 (1970).
3. N. C. Corbin, T. E. Hugli, and H. J. Müller-Eberhard, Serum carboxypeptidase B: a spectrophotometric assay using protamine as substrate, Anal. Biochem. 73: 41-51 (1976).
4. G. Oshima, J. Kato, and E. G. Erdös, Subunits of human plasma carboxypeptidase N (kininase 1, anaphylatoxin inactivator), Biochim. Biophys. Acta 365: 344-348 (1974).
5. G. Oshima, J. Kato, and E. G. Erdös, Plasma carboxypeptidase N, subunits and characteristics, Arch. Biochem. Biophys. 170: 132-138 (1975).
6. Y. Levin, R. A. Skidgel, and E. G. Erdös, Isolation and characterization of the subunits of human plasma carboxypeptidase N (kininase 1), Proc. Natl. Acad. Sci. USA 79: 4618-4622 (1982).
7. T. H. Plummer and M. Y. Hurwitz, Human plasma carboxypeptidase N, isolation and characterization, J. Biol. Chem. 253: 3907-3912 (1978).
8. R. A. Skidgel and E. G. Erdös, Carboxypeptidase N (arginine carboxypeptidase), in: "Methods of Enzymatic Analysis," 3rd. ed., Vol. V, Enzymes 3, pp 60-72, H. U. Bergmeyer, ed., Verlag Chemie, Weinheim (1984).
9. S. C. M. Kwok, F. D. Ledley, A. G. DiLella, K. J. H. Robson, and S. L. C. Woo, Nucleotide sequence of a full length complementary DNA clone and amino acid sequence of human phenylalanine hydroxylase, Biochemistry 24: 556-561 (1985).
10. R. Lahte, Synthetic oligonucleotide probes deduced from amino acid sequence data, theoretical and practical considerations, J. Mol. Biol. 183: 1-12 (1985).

CYSTEINE PROTEASE INHIBITORS WITH S-(3-NITRO-2-PYRIDINESULFENYL)-CYSTEINE

RESIDUE IN AFFINITY ANALOGS OF PEPTIDE SUBSTRATES

Rei Matsueda, Hideaki Umeyama*, Eiki Kominami**, and
Nobuhiko Katunuma**

New Lead Research Laboratories, Sankyo, Co., Ltd.
Shinagawa-ku, Tokyo 140, Japan
 *School of Pharmaceutical Sciences, Kitasato University
  Minato-ku, Tokyo 108, Japan
**Institute for Enzyme Research, The University of Tokushima
  Tokushima,770, Japan

INTRODUCTION

The recently shown 3-nitro-2-pyridinesulfenyl (Npys) halides[1] react
readily and smoothly with free thiol functions to afford S-Npys derivatives. N-t-butyloxycarbonyl-S-(3-nitro-2-pyridinesulfenyl)-cysteine (Boc-
Cys(Npys)-OH) can be prepared from Boc-Cys(SH)-OH with Npys halides or
by conversion of conventional S-protecting groups such as benzyl, t-butyl,
acetoamidomethyl, and trityl into S-Npys with Npys halides[2].

An important feature of S-Npys is the ability of a peptide containing S-Npys-cysteine residue to react selectively with free thiol of
another cysteine containing peptide to afford an unsymmetrical disulfide
bond as depicted in Fig. 1.

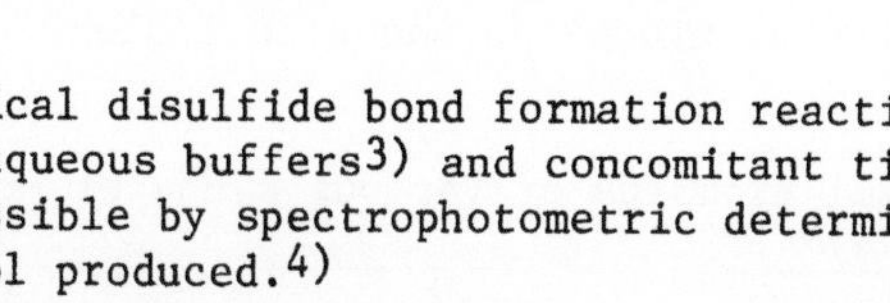

Fig. 1   Unsymmetrical Disulfide Bond Formation Between the S-Npys
         Residue and the Free Thiol Residue

This unsymmetrical disulfide bond formation reaction takes place over
a wide pH range in aqueous buffers[3] and concomitant titration of sulfhydryl groups is possible by spectrophotometric determination of the 3-
nitro-2-pyridinethiol produced.[4]

Boc-Cys(Npys)-OH can be used directly in solid phase synthesis of
Cys(Npys)-containing peptides since the S-Npys group is stable toward trifluoroacetic acid and HF. The S-Npys group can be used to advantage in
syntheses of peptides with unsymmetrical disulfide bond and it was successfully applied to the syntheses of human fibrin model peptides[3], α-human
atrial natriuretic peptides[5], and cyclic analogs of substance P[6].

This reaction is also effective for modification of thiol enzyme.
The modification and concomitant inactivation of the catalytic subunit of

bovine heart cAMP-dependent protein kinase were attained by specific
analogs of peptide substrates with Cys(Npys) residue.[4]

This principle has been further investigated to synthesize inhibitors
toward cysteine proteases.

SYNTHESES OF CYSTEINE PROTEASE INHIBITORS

Cathepsin B is an intracellular proteolytic enzyme which belongs to
the group of closely related thiol proteinase including cathepsin H and L.
The physiological role of this enzyme is thought to be that of the
degradation of tissue proteins within the lysosomes and has been postulated to be involved in proteolytic processing of protein and hormone
precursors.[7]   Design and syntheses of cathepsin B inhibitors have been
attempted by using the recently shown three-dimensional structure of rat
liver cathepsin B.[8]

1. Transition State Analog

It has been proposed that the 3S-hydroxyl of internal statine residue
in pepstatin is an analog of the transition-state or tetrahedral-inter-
mediate for the enzyme reaction of hydrolysis.[9]   One of the authors has
shown that statine (Sta) containing peptides are effective as renin inhibitors.[10]

H-Arg-Arg-Sta-Phe-OH was designed and prepared based on this approach.
The inhibitory potencies of this peptide are rather weak as shown in
Table 1.

Table 1. Inhibitory Potencies of H-Arg-Arg-Sta-Phe-OH

Compound	Inhibition % at 250 µM		
	Cathepsin B	Cathepsin L	Cathepsin H
H-Arg-Arg-Sta-Phe-OH	4.5	34.5	23.7

The weak inhibitory potencies of the peptide may due to the difference
of dependence on substrate specificity: renin is an angiotensinogen
specific enzyme but the cathepsin B, H, L and papain degrade various kinds
of peptides as substrates. Further investigation on statine position and
peptide chain may be necessary to have higher potency analogs by this
approach.

2. Affinity Labeling Approach

The proteases may be classified into 4 categories according to their
activities and functional groups as shown in Table 2.

Table 2. Examples of Various Kinds of Proteases

Serine Proteases	Thiol Proteases	Acid Proteases	Metalloproteases
Trypsin	Papain	Pepsin	Carboxypeptidase A
Chymotrypsin	Cathepsin B	Renin	Angiotensin-Converting Enzyme
	Calpain		

The serine proteases have reactive serine residues, the acid proteases and metalloproteases have catalytically important carboxylates, and
the cysteine proteases have reactive cysteine residues.

Many peptide chloromethyl ketones were designed as potential enzyme
inhibitors. However, there are potential problems with using these
inhibitors as drugs since the chloromethyl ketone indiscriminately
alkylate non-target enzymes. To overcome this problem, an affinity
labeling approach was considered to be effective if an inhibitor can
selectively modify the functional group of the target enzyme. An
approach of affinity labeling of active sites of enzymes is depicted in
Fig. 2.

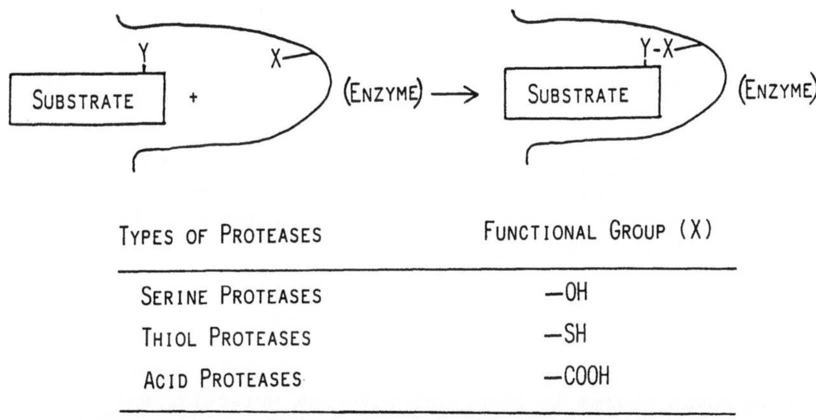

Types of Proteases	Functional Group (X)
Serine Proteases	—OH
Thiol Proteases	—SH
Acid Proteases	—COOH

Y SHOULD REACT SELECTIVELY WITH THE X OF THE TARGET ENZYME.

Fig. 2 Affinity Labeling of Active Sites of Enzymes

In this approach, the functional group Y which is bound to substrate or substrate-like peptide should selectively react with the functional group X of the target enzyme to form a covalent bond and inactivate
the enzyme. For example, Y of a cysteine protease inhibitors should react
selectively with the SH group of cysteine proteases and should not react
with the OH group of serine proteases or the COOH group of acid proteases.
A principle of selective labeling of cysteine proteases by the use
of the S-Npys group is depicted in Fig. 3.

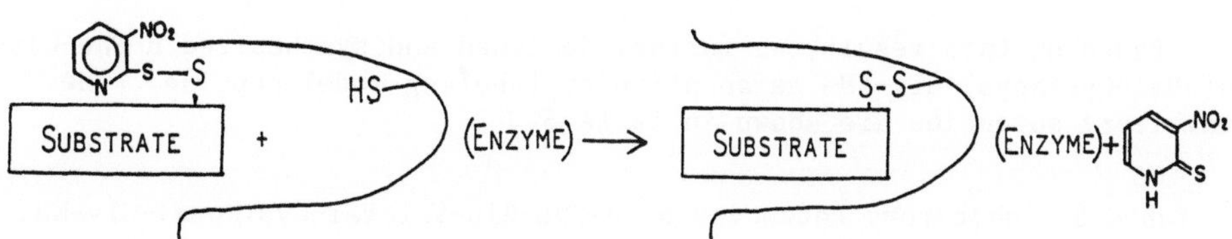

Fig. 3 Principle of Selective Labeling of Cysteine Proteases by the
        Use of the S-Npys Group

Some of the inhibitors designed by this approach for cathepsin B
and their inhibitory potencies are shown in Table 3.

Table 3 Design and Syntheses of Cysteine Protease Inhibitors

Compounds		Inhibitory Potencies*		
		Cathepsin B	Cathepsin H	Papain
H-Arg-Ser-Cys(Npys)-OH	200 μM	3.2%	26.0%	20.0%
H-Arg-Arg-Cys(Npys)-OH	200 μM (IC$_{50}$ 1.8x10^{-3}M)	55.8%	51.1%	41.1%
H-Arg-Arg-Cys(Npys)-Phe-OH	IC$_{50}$	5.5x10^{-4}M	——	——
Ac-Ala-Arg-Arg-Cys(Npys)-Phe-OH	IC$_{50}$	1.0x10^{-4}M	2.5x10^{-4}M	9x10^{-5}M
Ac-Phe-Arg-Arg-Cys(Npys)-Phe-OH	IC$_{50}$	5.0x10^{-5}M	1.2x10^{-4}M	1.9x10^{-4}M

*Inhibitory potencies were assayed by using Z-Phe-Arg-MCA for cathepsin B
and papain and Arg-MCA for cathepsin H as substrates in the presence of
0.01 M cysteine which partially decomposes inhibitors. Net inhibitory
potencies are higher than the observed.

3. Design of Inhibitors from Kininogen Sequence

Ohkubo et al. recently reported that the cysteine protease inhibitor
(α_2 TPI) in human plasma is identical with low molecular weight kininogen
and they have the conservative common amino acid sequence of Gln-Val-Val-
Ala-Gly.[11] Okada et al. also showed recently that benzyloxycarbonyl-
Gln-Val-Val-Ala-Gly-OMe weakly inhibits papain activity.[12]
We synthesized Ac-Ala-Gln-Val-Val-Ala-Gly-NH$_2$ and tested inhibitory
potency against cathepsin B, H and papain. The results are shown in Table
4.

Table 4 Inhibitory Potencies of Ac-Ala-Gln-Val-Val-Ala-Gly-NH$_2$ against
Cysteine Proteases

Compound	Inhibitory Potencies, IC$_{50}$		
	Cathepsin B	Cathepsin H	Papain
Ac-Ala-Gln-Val-Val-Ala-Gly-NH$_2$	1x10^{-4}M	1.7x10^{-4}M	9x10^{-5}M

Based on this result, we further designed and synthesized H-Phe-Gln-
Val-Val-Cys(Npys)-Gly-NH$_2$ as an affinity labeling model peptide. The
inhibitory potencies are shown in Table 5.

Table 5 Inhibitory Potencies of H-Phe-Gln-Val-Val-Cys(Npys)-Gly-NH$_2$

Compound	Inhibitory Potencies, IC$_{50}$		
	Cathepsin B	Cathepsin H	Papain
H-Phe-Gln-Val-Val-Cys(Npys)-Gly-NH$_2$	2x10^{-5}M	9x10^{-5}M	4x10^{-5}M

MATERIALS AND METHOD

Peptides were prepared by solid phase synthesis. Details of the syntheses will be published elsewhere.

Inhibitors were assayed with N-Benzyloxycarbonyl-L-phenylalanyl-L-arginine 4-methyl-cumaryl-7-amide for cathepsin B, L and papain and L-arginine 4-methyl-cumaryl-7-amide for cathepsin H as substrates by the method of Barret.[13] The enzyme 50 μℓ (0.1 μg/ml) was preincubated with the inhibitor 0.41 ml (0.4 M Na-acetate buffer, pH 5.5, containing 4 mM EDTA) for 3 min. at 37°C. Reaction was initiated by the addition of substrate in Na-acetate buffer, 0.25 ml and the mixture was incubated at 37°C for 6 min. The reaction was stopped by adding 1 ml of 0.1 M Na-chloroacetate buffer, pH 4.3 and 0.5 ml of water. The liberated 7-amino-4-methyl-cumarin was assayed by using exitation at 370 nm with emission wave length at 460 nm.

DISCUSSION

Table 3 shows the inhibitory potencies of inhibitors against cathepsin B, H and papain. Substitution of Phe residue for both N and C-terminal residues improved inhibitory potencies. IC_{50} of Ac-Phe-Arg-Arg-Cys(Npys)-Phe-OH was 5×10^{-5}M but a net potency may be higher than this value since assays were carried out in the presence of 0.01 M cysteine which partially decomposes inhibitors.

It is assumed that the Arg-Arg part of the inhibitor binds ionically to Asp(67) and Glu(241) and N-terminal Phe binds to Tyr(73) and C-terminal Phe binds to Tyr(173), Leu(179) and Trp(219) of the recently shown rat liver cathepsin B model.[8] Thus, Cys(Npys) residue of the inhibitor may be able to react with Cys(29) and inactivate the enzyme.

The affinity labeling approach by the use of the S-Npys group is effective for the design and syntheses of cystein protease inhibitors, because it is rather easy to design from their substrates and can make cysteine protease specific inhibitors which do not modify serine proteases or acid proteases. Further application of this approach to other thiol enzymes and modification of receptors with cysteine residue are under investigation.

Inhibitors with the S-Npys group may be of use to investigators studying the roles of cysteine proteases and of clinical value in the treatment of certain proteases-associated diseases.

REFERENCES

1. R. Matsueda and K. Aiba, Chem. Lett., 951 (1978).
2. R. Matsueda, T. Kimura, E.T. Kaiser, and G.R. Matsueda, Chem. Lett., 737 (1981).
   R. Matsueda, S. Higashida, R.J. Ridge, and G.R. Matsueda, Chem. Lett., 921 (1982).
   Boc-Cys(Npys)-OH as well as Npys-amino acids are commercially available from Kokusan Chemical Works, Ltd., 3-9 Nihonbashi-Honcho, Chuo-ku, Tokyo, 103 Japan.
3. M.S. Bernatowicz, R. Matsueda, and G.R. Matsueda, Int. J. Peptide Protein Res., 28, 107 (1986).
4. H.N. Bramson, N. Thomas, R. Matsueda, N.C. Nelson, S.S. Taylor, and E.T. Kaiser, J. Biol. Chem., 257, 10575 (1982).
5. N. Chino, K. Yoshizawa-Kumagaye, Y. Noda, T.X. Watanabe, T. Kimura, and S. Sakakibara, Biochem. Biophys. Res. Commun., 141, 665 (1986).
6. O. Ploux, G. Chassaing, and A. Marquet, Int. J. Peptide Protein Res., 29, 162 (1987).

7. S. Ansorge, H. Kirschke, and K. Freidrick, Acta Biol. Med. Ger.,
    36, 1723 (1977).
    P.S. Quinn and J.D. Judah, Biochem. J., 172, 301 (1978).
    K. Docherty, R.J. Carroll, and D.F. Steiner, Proc. Natl. Acad.
    Sci. U.S.A., 79, 4613 (1982).
8. K. Akahane and H. Umeyama, Enzyme, 36, 141 (1986).
9. J. Marcincszyn, J.A. Hartsuck, and J. Tang, J. Biol. Chem., 251,
    7088 (1976).
10. R. Matsueda, Y. Yabe, H. Kogen, S. Higashida, H. Koike, Y. Iijima,
    T. Kokubu, K. Hiwada, E. Murakami, and Y. Imamura, Chem. Lett.,
    1041 (1985).
11. I. Ohkubo, K. Kurachi, T. Takasawa, and M. Sasaki, Biochemistry,
    23, 5691 (1984).
12. Y. Okada, N. Teno, N. Itoh, and H. Okamoto, Chem. Pharm. Bull.,
    33, 5149 (1985).
    N. Teno, S. Tsuboi, Y. Okada, N. Itoh, and H. Okamoto, Int. J.
    Peptide Protein Res., 30, 93 (1987).
13. A.J. Barrett and H. Kirschke, in Methods in Enzymology (L. Lorand
    ed.), Vol. 80, Part C, pp. 553, Academic Press, New York (1981).

STUDIES ON NEW SYNTHETIC INHIBITORS OF KALLIKREINS AND CHYMOTRYPSIN

T. Yokoyama, N. Yokoo, F. Sato, K. Ikegaya, E. Hattori,
K. Watanabe, J. Kirihara, M. Nagakura, and S. Fujii(*)

Tokyo Research Laboratories, Kowa Co., Ltd., Higashimurayama
Tokyo 189, Japan. (*) The Osaka Foundation for Promotion of
Fundamental Medical Research, Otsu, Shiga 520-01, Japan

INTRODUCTION

We have previously reported strong, reversible, and specific inhibitory
effects of 1,2,3,4-tetrahydro-α-naphthoate, α-naphthylacetate, and mono- and
di-substituted indoleacetate derivatives on chymotrypsin(Fujii et al.,1984).
Moreover, we also reported strong, reversible inhibitory effects of
various ω-guanidino acid esters, and p-guanidinobenzoate derivatives on
trypsin, plasmin, plasma kallikrein, thrombin, C1r, and C1 esterase(Muramatu
et al., 1971, 1972, and 1972; Tamura et al., 1977; Fujii et al., 1981).
Among the various inhibitors examined, p-guanidinobenzoate derivatives were
more inhibitory than ω-guanidino acid esters. On the other hand, Markwardt
and coworkers (1972), and Kanaoka and coworkers(Tanizawa et al., 1977),
reported the inhibitory effect of aromatic amidino compounds on trypsin and
thrombin.
This paper describes the strong inhibitory effects of several p-amidinophenylester derivatives on kallikreins, chymotrypsin, trypsin, thrombin,
plasmin, tissue plasminogen activator(TPA), urokinase, factor Xa, and
elastase. Studies on the mechanism of enzyme inhibition of these compounds
are also described. Furthermore, the promoting effect of above inhibitors
on the intestinal absorption of tissue kallikrein are also examined.

MATERIALS AND METHODS

Enzymes
Porcine tissue kallikrein was purchased from Roman Industries Co.,
Ltd., Tokyo, Japan; bovine α-chymotrypsin and trypsin were purchased from
Böhringer Mannheim Co., Ltd., West Germany; and human thrombin, bovine
factor Xa, and porcine elastase were purchased from Sigma Chemical Company,
St. Louis, MO, USA. Porcine plasma kallikrein, human urokinase, and TPA
were from Tokyo Research Laboratories, Kowa Co., Ltd., Tokyo, Japan. Human
plasmin was from Green Cross Co., Osaka, Japan. Each enzyme was dissolved in
0.1M Tris-HCl buffer, pH 8.0, containing 10mM $CaCl_2$ in the case of trypsin.

Substrates and Inhibitors
S1, Pro-Phe-Arg-MCA(4-methylcoumaryl-7-amide); S2, Z(carbobenzoxy)-Phe-
Arg-MCA; S3, Suc(succinyl)-Ala-Ala-Pro-Phe-MCA; S4, Boc(t-butyloxycarbonyl)-
Phe-Ser-Arg-MCA; S5, Boc-Val-Pro-Arg-MCA; S6, Boc-Val-Leu-Lys-MCA; S7, Glt-
(glutaryl)-Gly-Arg-MCA; S8, Boc-Ile-Glu-Gly-Arg-MCA; and S9, Suc-Ala-Pro-
Ala-MCA were purchased from the Foundation for Protein Research, Minoh,
Osaka, Japan. Soybean trypsin inhibitor(SBTI) was also purchased from

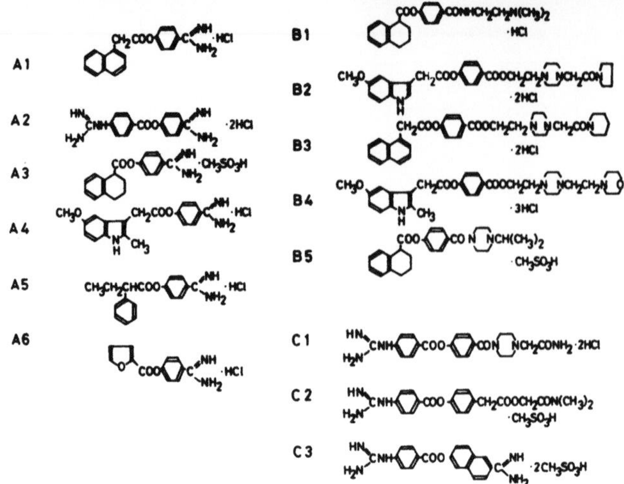

Fig. 1. Structural formulae of A1, A2, A3, A4, A5, A6, B1, B2, B3, B4, B5, C1, C2, and C3.

Sigma, and aprotinin was obtained from Bayer, West Germany.

4-Amidinophenyl naphthyl-1-acetate hydrochloride(A-1); 4-amidinophenyl 4-guanidinobenzoate dihydrochloride(A-2); 4-amidinophenyl 1,2,3,4-tetrahydro-1-naphthoate methanesulfonate(A-3); 4-amidinophenyl 5-methoxy-2-methylindole-3-acetate hydrochloride(A-4); 4-amidinophenyl 2-phenylbutylate hydrochloride(A-5); 4-amidinophenyl furan-2-carboxylate hydrochloride(A-6); 4-[2-(dimethylamino)ethylaminocarbonyl]phenyl 1,2,3,4-tetrahydro-1-naphthoate hydrochloride(B-1); 4-[(2-[4-(pyrrolidinocarbonylmethyl)-piperazino]-ethyl)oxycarbonyl]phenyl 5-methoxyindole-3-acetate dihydrochloride(B-2); 4-(2-[4-(piperidinocarbonylmethylpiperazino)ethyl]oxycarbonyl)phenyl 1-naphthylacetate dihydrochloride(B-3); 4-([2-(4-[2-morpholinoethyl]piperazino)ethyl]oxycarbonyl)phenyl 5-methoxy-2-methylindole-3-acetate trihydrochloride(B-4); 4-(4-isopropylpiperazinocarbonyl)phenyl 1,2,3,4-tetrahydro-1-naphthoate methanesulfonate(B-5, FK-448); 4[4-(carbamoylmethyl)piperazinocarbonyl]phenyl 4-guanidinobenzoate dihydrochloride(C-1, KF-526); N,N-dimethylcarbamoylmethyl 4-(4-guanidinobenzoyloxy)phenylacetate methanesulfonate(C-2, FOY-305); and 6-amidino-2-naphthyl 4-guanidinobenzoate dimethanesulfonate(C-3, FUT-175) were synthetized from each component carboxylic acid and p-substituted phenol by methods of thionylchloride or dicyclohexylcarbodiimide in pyridine. The structural formulae of these compounds are shown in Fig. 1.

Experiments on inhibition of various enzymes

The rate of hydrolysis for each of the following was determined as described by Iwanaga and coworkers (1979) at a substrate concentration of 0.1mM: S1 by tissue kallikrein; S2 by plasma kallikrein; S3 by chymotrypsin; S4 by trypsin or TPA; S5 by thrombin; S6 by plasmin; S7 by urokinase; S8 by factor Xa; and S9 by elastase.

For measurement of inhibitoroy effects, mixtures of enzyme solution and inhibitor were preincubated at 37°C for 5min and then residual enzyme activity was determined as the hydrolytic activity of an appropriate substrate mentioned above. <u>Km</u> values and <u>Ki</u> values were determined from Lineweaver-Burk plots of the results(Lineweaver et al., 1934).

Experiments on the residual ester determination in reactions of chymotrypsin or trypsin with inhibitors

The residual ester determination was examined in reactions of chymotrypsin or trypsin with some esteric inhibitors by Hestrin's method (1949), modified by Roberts(1958).

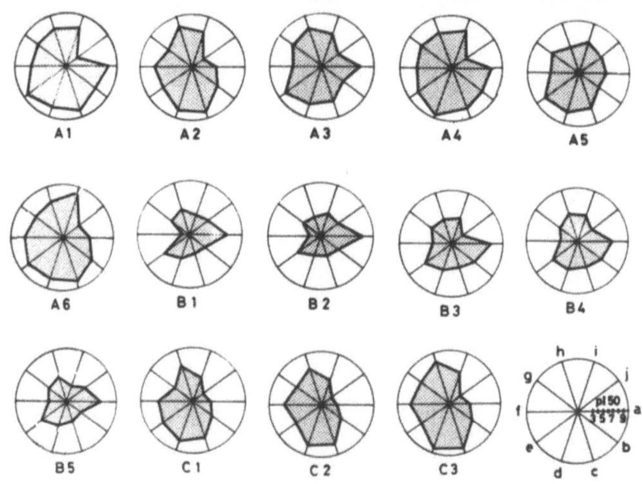

Fig. 2. Radar scope of IC50 values of inhibitor with respect to ten enzymes (a, chymotrypsin; b, tissue kallikrein; c, plasma kallikrein; d, trypsin; e, thrombin; f, plasmin: g, TPA; h, urokinase; i, factor Xa; and j, elastase).

Table I. $\underline{Ki}$ values for above enzymes. Data are indicated as $-\log[\underline{Ki}]$ (M).

Enzyme/Inhibitor

	A1	A2	A3	A4	A5	A6	B1	B2	B3	B4	B5	C1	C2	C3
(a)	8.54	4.85	7.60	7.92	5.68	5.62	7.43	8.15	7.43	7.07	7.12	3.80		4.27
(b)	7.28	6.39	5.09	7.00	5.07	7.42						5.62	4.85	6.82
(c)	9.25	8.38	7.00	8.14	7.29	9.36						8.38	8.38	9.15
(d)	8.85	8.60	7.80	9.07	7.85	8.77						8.70	8.64	9.20
(e)	9.52	6.85	8.54	8.68	8.30	8.89						7.37	6.20	6.96
(f)	6.85	7.01	5.43	6.82	5.72	7.60						7.96	8.30	8.96
(g)	6.80	6.01	7.14	7.31	6.60	6.92						4.24	4.82	6.92
(h)	8.06	8.37	7.89	7.59	7.08	7.07						7.28	7.36	8.20
(i)	8.03	7.11	6.68	7.68	7.80	6.77						4.96	5.21	6.31
(j)			3.85	3.15	5.38	4.12								

<u>Experiments on intestinal absorption of tissue kallikrein in rats and rabbits</u>

Rats were anesthetized with pentobarbital(60mg/kg, intraperitoneally), and a front midline incision was made to expose the viscera. A hypodermic needle attached to a syringe containing the test solution was then carefully inserted into the lumen of the jejunum 2cm under the pylorus. Tissue kallikrein(10,000U/kg) was dissolved in saline with or without 20mg/kg of the inhibitor, and injected at 2ml/kg. For measurement of plasma Pro-Phe-Arg-MCA hydrolytic activity, samples of 0.2 ml of blood were drawn from cannulated femoral artery of rats before, 0.25, 0.5, 1, 1.5, and 2 hr after medication as a citrated blood(0.38%), and were centrifuged at 3000rpm for 10min. Its plasma Pro-Phe-Arg-MCA hydrolytic activity was checked whether being inhibited by 100µg/ml SBTI(as an inhibitor of plasma kallikrein) or by 100KIU/ml aprotinin(as an inhibitor of both kallikreins).

The plasma concentration of tissue kallikrein was indicated as mU/ml, which was calculated as above mentioned. The basal enzyme activity in plasma was subtracted from the data.

In the case of rabbit, the catheter for administration of the sample directly into intestine had been implanted 2 or 3 weeks before use. The test solution was administered through the tube, and the blood was drawn (until 180min) and examined similarly as in the case of rats.

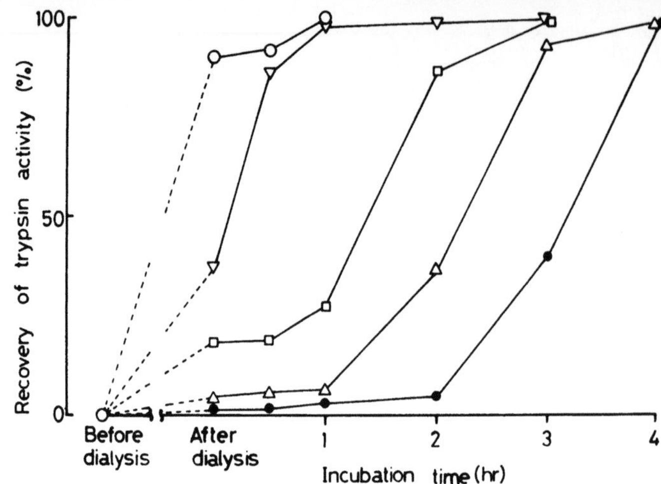

Fig. 3. Effect of dialysis and incubation on amidolysis of inhibitor-treated trypsin. A mixture of the enzyme(20μg/ml) and inhibitor(1mM) in 0.1M Tris-HCl buffer, pH 8.0 containing 1mM $CaCl_2$, was incubated at 37°C for 5min and then dialyzed against the same buffer overnight at 4°C. The dialysate was incubated at 37°C for the indicated periods and then the amidase activity of the enzyme was determined by incubating the mixture at 37°C for 10min after addition of 0.1mM Boc-Phe-Ser-Arg-MCA as substrate: o—o ;with A1, △—△;with A2, ▽—▽ ;with A3, □—□ :with A4, and ●—● :with C1.

Table 2. Residual inhibitor concentration determined by Hestrin-Roberts' method. Each inhibitor(2mM) was incubated with various amounts of trypsin or chymotrypsin in 0.1M Tris-HCl buffer, pH 8.0 containing 10mM $CaCl_2$ in the case of trypsin at 37°C for 30min, and then the residual ester was determined.

Enzyme (mM)	Inhibitor with trypsin							Inhibitor with chymotrypsin						
	A1	A2	A3	A5	A6	B5	C1	A1	A2	A3	A5	A6	B5	C1
1	1	61	63	0	7	73	84	0	13	47	5	34	48	32
1/2	2	78	76	4	7	84	92	18	17	76	22	40	74	18
1/4	15	99	97	71	17	88	100	48	22	84	50	39	92	17
1/8	56			91	60	95		69	16	90	74	51	99	21
1/16	82			100	86			80	20	98	88	77		28
1/32	100				97			87	50		95	85		67
1/64								95	75			93		87
1/128									85			94		
1/256									95					

RESULTS AND DISCUSSION

The effects of p-amidinophenylester derivatives(A1 to A6) on the amidolysis with peptidyl-MCA of various enzymes were examined, comparing those of B1 to B5 and C1 to C3, and the concentration for 50% inhibition are shown in Fig. 2 as radar scopes.

We have previously reported (Fujii et al., 1984) that some tetrahydro-α-naphthoate, α-naphthylacetate, and indoleacetate derivatives were strong and specific inhibitors of chyomotrypsin, and their inhibitory activities were almost the same as that of the bacterial inhibitor chymostatin. As shown in Fig. 2, p-amidinophenylester derivatives which comprise aromatic carboxylic acid residues as mentioned above, are strongly inhibitory to both

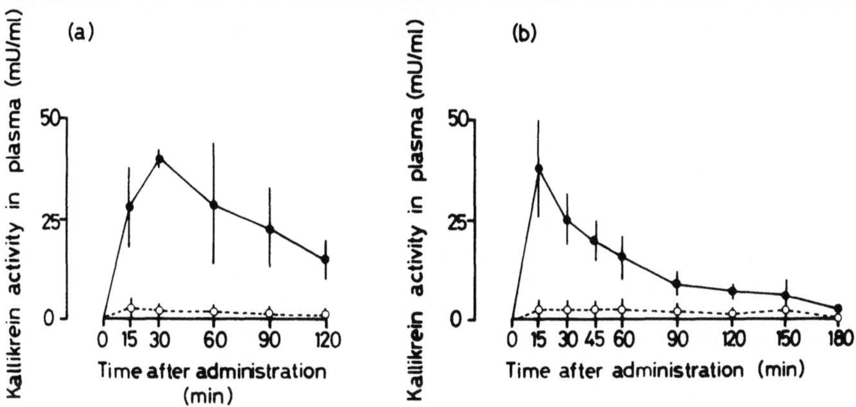

Fig. 4. Intestinal absorption of kallikrein. Tissue kallikrein 10,000U/kg
was administered without(O⋯O) or with(●—●) 20mg/kg of B5 to rats(a) and
rabbits(b), intraduodenally. The ordinate shows the change of kallikrein
activity in plasma(mU/ml, mean values ± S. E., n=4, respectively) and the
abscissa indicates the time after administration(min).

chymotrypsin and trypsin-like enzymes. On the other hand, A2 is strongly
inhibitory only to trypsin-like enzymes as well as C1 to C3.

Next determined were the $\underline{Ki}$ values of these inhibtors on the amidolysis
with the peptidyl-MCA substrates. Table I shows that the $\underline{Ki}$ values of these
compounds for tissue kallikrein were in the range of 0.01 to 1μM, and those
for plasma kallikrein were 0.1 to 10nm. These compounds are all competitive
inhibitors except A5 for thrombin and C3 for trypsin — are non-competitive.

The $\underline{Km}$ values of the substrates for the enzymes were in the range of
0.01 to 0.1mM as reported earlier. The fairly small $\underline{Ki}$ values of these
compounds with respect to enzymes seem due, in large part, to acylation of
the enzyme, because they are hydrolyzable by the enzyme during incubation as
indicated in Table II. These inhibitors are all reactivatable with respect
to both of the enzymes shown.

The several compounds described above were reversible and hydrolysable
inhibitors of these enzymes. For example, as shown in Fig. 3, A1 was mostly
removed from the inhibited enzyme by dialysis and it was completely removed
by incubating the inhibited enzyme at 37°C for 2hr. On the other hand, A2,
A3, A4, and C3 were partly removed from the inhibited enzyme by dialysis,
but after that, they were completely removed by incubating the inhibited
enzymes at 37°C, for 4hr at most. Except for A2, other amidinophenyl
derivatives were rather more easily removed from the inhibited enzyme than
those of p-guanidinobenzoate such as C1. This result is not inconsistent
with the results of Kanaoka and coworkers(Tanizawa et al., 1977) in which
they reported that amidinophenylesters were "Inverse-substrates" for
trypsin-like enzymes, and therefore, these compounds were rather easily
removed from the enzyme. The inhibition of these amidinophenylesters tested
in this study is rather temporary; however, they are still strongly
inhibitory to these enzymes, because their acyl-intermediate with trypsin
are somewhat more stable than those of Kanaoka and coworkers. The compounds
used in the present work may be useful as a tool for making a temporary
inhibited enzyme such as an acylated enzyme — especially when a
trypsin-like enzyme is used in the reaction.

It is interesting that, except A2, these aromatic carboxylates of
amidinophenol are strongly inhibitory to both chymotrypsin and trypsin-like
enzymes, and they are reactivatable for both enzymes. It is also of
interest that such simple esters could inhibit the enzyme activities that
are known to possess restricted substrate specificity, especially in the
cases of thrombin, plasmin, TPA, urokinase, factor Xa, and kallikreins.

Fig. 4A shows the effect of chymotrypsin specific inhibitor(B5) on the
intestinal absorption of tissue kallikrein in rats. In the presence of B5,
the increase in plasma Pro-Phe-Arg-MCA hydrolytic activity level was
observed. The basal Pro-Phe-Arg-MCA hydrolytic activity in plasma was
mostly inhibited by adding 100μg/ml SBTI, and the increased activity after
administration was only inhibited by adding 100U/ml aprotinin. Therefore,
it seems that the increased plasma Pro-Phe-Arg-MCA hydrolytic activity may
be caused by absorbed kallikrein.

In the case of rabbit, as shown in Fig. 4B, the combined administration
of tissue kallikrein and B5 also produced the aprotinin sensitive and SBTI
insensitive increase in plasma Pro-Phe-Arg-MCA hydrolytic activity.
Therefore, like the case of insulin(Fujii et al., 1985), kallikrein could be
absorbed from intestine only in combining with chymotrypsin specific
inhibitor(B5). The increase in plasma could not be observed when kallikrein
was combined with A or C type inhibitors(data are not shown).

REFERENCES

Fujii, S. and Hitomi, Y., 1981, New synthetic inhibitors of C1r̄, C1 esterase
    thrombin, plasmin, kallikrein, and trypsin. Biochim. Biophys. Acta, 661,
    342-345.

Fujii, S., Yokoyama, T., Ikegaya, K., and Yokoo, N., 1984, New synthetic
    inhibitors of chymotrypsin. J. Biochem., 95, 319-322.

Fujii, S., Yokoyama, T., Ikegaya, K., Sato, F., and Yokoo, N., 1985,
    Promoting effect of the new chymotrypsin inhibitor FK-448 on the
    intestinal absorption of insulin in rats and dogs. J. Pharm. Pharmacol.,
    37, 545-549.

Hestrin, S., 1949, The reaction of acetylcholine and other carboxylic acid
    derivatives with hydroxylamine, and its analytical application. J. Biol.
    Chem., 180, 249-261.

Iwanaga, S., Morita, T., Kato, H., Harada, T., Adachi, N., Sugo, T.,
    Maruyama, I., Takada, K., Kimura, T., and Sakakibara, S., 1979,
    Fluorogenic peptide substrates for proteases in blood coagulation,
    kallikrein-kinin and fibrinolysis systems. Adv. Exp. Med. Biol., 120A,
    147-163.

Markwardt, F., Wagner, G., Walsmann, P., Horn, H., and Stürzbecher, J.,
    1972, Inhibition of trypsin and thrombin by amidinophenol esters of
    aromatic carboxylic acids. Acta Biol. Med. Germ., 28, K19-K25.

Muramatu, M. and Fujii, S., 1971, Inhibitory effects of ω-amino acid esters
    on trypsin, plasmin, plsma kallikrein, and thrombin. Biochim. Biophys.
    Acta, 242, 203-208.

Muramatu, M. and Fujii, S., 1972, Inhibitory effects of ω-guanidino acid
    esters on trypsin, plasmin, plasma kallikrein, and thrombin. Biochim.
    Biophys. Acta, 268, 221-224.

Muramatu, M., Shiraishi, S., and Fujii, S., 1972, Inhibitory effects of
    ω-amino and ω-guanidino acid esters on the first component of human
    complement. Biochim. Biophys. Acta, 285, 224-234.

Roberts, P. S., 1958, Measurement of the rate of plasmin action on synthetic
    substrates. J. Biol. Chem., 232, 285-291.

Tamura, Y., Hirado, M., Okamura, K., Minato, Y., and Fujii, S., 1977,
    Synthetic inhibitors of trypsin, plasmin, kallikrein thrombin, C1r, and C1
    esterase. Biochim. Biophys. Acta, 484, 417-422.

Tanizawa, K., Kasaba, Y., and Kanaoka, Y., 1977, "Inverse substrates" for
    trypsin. Efficient enzymatic hydrolysis of certain esters with a cationic
    center in the leaving group. J. Amer. Chem. Soc., 99, 4485-4488.

INHIBITION OF HUMAN AND RAT TISSUE KALLIKREINS BY PEPTIDE ANALOG

ANTAGONISTS OF BRADYKININ

Jocelyn Spragg, Raymond J. Vavrek*, and John M.
Stewart*

Harvard Medical School and Brigham and Women's
Hospital, Boston MA 02115; and *University of
Colorado Health Sciences Center, Denver CO 80252

SUMMARY

Three representative bradykinin receptor antagonists have
been examined for their capacity to inhibit purified human and
rat urinary kallikreins. In an amidolytic assay, the K_i values
for the inhibition of human urinary kallikrein were 0.5, 0.3,
and 2.5 µM for B4307(DArg-Arg-Pro-Hyp-Gly-Thi-Ser-DPhe-Thi-Arg),
B4308 (Lys-Lys-Arg-Hyp-Hyp-Gly-Thi-Ser-DPhe-Thi-Arg) and B3852
(Arg-Pro-Hyp-Gly-Phe-Ser-DPhe-Phe-Arg), respectively. B4308 and
B3852 inhibited rat urinary kallikrein with K_i's of 1.0 and 5.5
µM, respectively. B4308 (0.4 to 1.6 µM) also inhibited the
kininogenase activity of human urinary kallikrein on human low
molecular weight kininogen in a dose-dependent fashion. These
bradykinin receptor antagonists may inhibit the kallikrein-kinin
system both by blocking the binding of kinins to B2 receptors
and by inhibiting the cleavage of kinins from kininogens.

INTRODUCTION

The plasma and tissue (glandular) kallikrein-kinin systems
not only generate kinins but appear to have additional,
kinin-independent functions determined by the action of
kallikreins on alternative substrates. Plasma kallikrein
activates coagulation factor XII[1], while the family of tissue
kallikreins may be involved with prorenin activation[2] or with
the activation of peptide prohormones such as proinsulin[3], high
molecular weight atrial natriuretic peptide[4], and intermediates
in pro-opiomelanocortin metabolism[5]. Apolipoprotein B-100 is
cleaved by both types of kallikrein[6]. Identification of the
relevant in vivo functions of tissue kallikreins will require
the use of specific kallikrein inhibitors[7-10] and kinin receptor
antagonists[11-13].

Specific substrate sequence analog inhibitors of tissue
kallikreins have some of the features of bradykinin B2 receptor

antagonists, including a bulky D-amino acid at position P3 and a preference for L-arginine over L-lysine at position P1[7,8,11]. This observation has led to an examination of the capacity of bradykinin analog receptor antagonists to inhibit also the enzymatic activity of tissue kallikreins[14].

MATERIALS AND METHODS

Bradykinin sequence analog antagonists[11] (Table 1) were used to inhibit purified human urinary kallikrein (specific activity: 0.5 to 4 mg kinin/min/mg enzyme protein)[8] in a kinetic assay with 10 or 35 μM substrate (Kabi, S-2266) at pH 9.0 and 37°C[15]. Similar assays were performed with 10 and 25 μM substrate and rat urinary kallikrein (specific activity: 0.2 to 1.0 mg kinin/min/mg enzyme protein) prepared by published procedures[16] and generously provided by Dr. Manfred Maier, Vienna, Austria. The release of p-nitroaniline in the presence or absence of 0.2 to 20 μM antagonist was monitored for 10 minutes at 405 nM, and the linear change in optical density/minute was converted to nmoles of p-nitroaniline generated/min/ml. Data were evaluated by linear regression analysis and Dixon plots[17].

Inhibition of the kininogenase activity of human urinary kallikrein on purified human low molecular weight kininogen[18] was examined on the estrous rat uterus[19] standardized with 0.05 to 0.50 ng of synthetic bradykinin (Bachem). B4308 was added to mixtures of kallikrein (20 ng) and kininogen (400 ng) either at the beginning of a 5-minute incubation period at 37°C, or immediately before the incubation mixture was added to the bioassay.

RESULTS AND DISCUSSION

The three kinin receptor antagonists inhibited the amido-lytic activity of human and rat urinary kallikreins in a dose-

Table 1. The structure of sequence analog antagonists of brady-kinin tested as tissue kallikrein inhibitors. The stucture of bradykinin (BK) is shown for comparison.

	P11	P10	P9	P8	P7	P6	P5	P4	P3	P2	P1
BK			Arg	Pro	Pro	Gly	Phe	Ser	Pro	Phe	Arg
B4307[a]		DArg	Arg	Pro	Hyp	Gly	Thi	Ser	DPhe	Thi	Arg
B4308	Lys	Lys	Arg	Hyp	Hyp	Gly	Thi	Ser	DPhe	Thi	Arg
B3852			Arg	Pro	Hyp	Gly	Phe	Ser	DPhe	Phe	Arg

[a]Hyp = L-4-hydroxyproline; Thi = beta-(2-thienyl)-L-alanine

Table 2. The inhibition of the amidolytic activity of human
         urinary kallikrein (HUK) and rat urinary kallikrein
         (RUK) by sequence analog antagonists of bradykinin[a].

Antagonist	K_i for HUK (μM)	K_i for RUK (μM)
B4307	0.5	--
B4308	0.3	1.0
B3852	2.5	5.5

[a]From Spragg et al (14) with permission of the publishers.

dependent fashion and Dixon plots of the data obtained indicated
that the inhibition was competitive[14]. The K_i values obtained
for these representative receptor antagonists are in the micro-
molar range and the two analogs containing the beta-
(2-thienyl)-L-alanine residues in the P2 and P5 positions appear
to be one half to one log more potent in this assay than the
similar analog which contains the native phenylalanine residue
in positions P2 and P5 and lacks any additional N-terminal
residues (Tables 1 and 2). B4307 and B4308 also appear to be
approximately one order of magnitude more potent than B3852 in
their capacity to inhibit the binding of radiolabelled bradykinin to bovine uterine myometrium[20] (Charles E. Odya, personal
communication).

The capacity of B3852 to inhibit kininogenase activity was
tested on human urinary kallikrein, which lacks direct oxytoxic
activity[21]. Kinin antagonist (0.4 to 1.6 μM) added at the
beginning of the incubation of kallikrein and kininogen yielded
a dose-dependent reduction of contractile activity in the rat
uterus assay that was 3 to 8 times greater than that seen when
the antagonist was added after the incubation period and just
before the sample was added to the bioassay bath. While further
studies are required in systems that are not sensitive to the
multiple effects of these antagonists, these results suggest
that kinin receptor antagonists block both the amidolytic and
kininogenase activities of tissue kallikreins. If these
antagonists are also shown to inhibit the action of tissue
kallikreins on alternative substrates[2-5], these effects may influence the interpretation of data obtained with these
inhibitors _in vivo_ or in isolated organ experiments.

ACKNOWLEDGEMENTS

This study was supported in part by grants
AI-23401, HL- 35949, and HL-26284 from the National Institutes
of Health. The authors thank Marilyn Pontone and Robert Wolff
for technical assistance.

REFERENCES

1. C. G. Cochrane, S. D. Revak, B. S. Aiken, and K. D. Wuepper, The structural characteristics and activation of Hageman factor, in:"Inflammation: Mechanisms and Control," I. H. Lepow and P. A. Ward, eds., Academic Press, New York (1972).

2. J. E. Sealey, S. A. Atlas, J. H. Laragh, N. B. Oza, and J. W. Ryan, Human urinary kallikrein converts inactive renin to active renin and is a possible physiologic activator of renin. Nature, 275:144 (1978).

3. O. ole-MoiYoi, D. C. Seldin, J. Spragg, G. S. Pinkus, and K.F. Austen, Sequential cleavage of proinsulin by human pancreatic kallikrein and a human pancreatic kininase. Proc. Natl. Acad. Sci.(USA), 76:3612 (1979).

4. M. G. Currie, D. M. Geller, J. Chao, H. S. Margolius, and P. Needleman, Kallikrein activation of a high molecular weight atrial peptide. Biochem. Biophys. Res. Comm.,120:461 (1984).

5. E. S. Prado, L. Prado de Carvalho, M. S. Araujo-Viel, N. Ling, and J. Rossier, A met-enkephalin-containing peptide, BAM 22P, as a novel substrate for glandular kallikrein. Biochem. Biophys.Res. Comm., 112:366 (1983).

6. A. D. Cardin, K. R. Witt, J. Chao, H. S. Margolius, V. H. Donaldson, and R. L. Jackson, Degradation of apolipoprotein B-100 of human plasma low density lipoproteins by tissue and plasma kallikreins. J. Biol. Chem., 259:8522 (1984).

7. H. Okunishi, J. Burton, and J. Spragg, Specificity of substrate analogue tissue kallikrein inhibitors. Hypertension, 7:I-72 (1985).

8. H. Okunishi, J. Spragg, and J. Burton, The design of substrate analogue tissue kallikrein inhibitors. Hypertension, 8:I-114 (1986).

9. H. Okunishi, J. Spragg, and J. Burton, In vivo assay of specific kallikrein inhibitors. Agents and Actions, in press.

10. H. Okunishi, J. Spragg, J. Burton, and N. Toda, In vivo inhibition of tissue kallikreins by kininogen sequence analogue peptides.This volume.

11. R. J. Vavrek and J. M. Stewart, Competitive antagonists of bradykinin. Peptides, 6:161 (1985).

12. A. Benetos, H. Gavras, J. M. Stewart, R. J. Vavrek, S. Hatinoglou, and I. Gavras, Vasodepressor role of endogenous bradykinin assessed by a bradykinin antagonist. Hypertension, 8:971 (1986).

13. A. Benetos, I. Gavras, and H. Gavras, Hypertensive effect of a bradykinin antagonist in normotensive rats. Hypertension 8: 1089 (1986).

14. J. Spragg, R. J. Vavrek, and J. M. Stewart, The inhibition of glandular kallikrein by peptide analog antagonists of bradykinin. Peptides, in press (1988).

15. E. Amundsen, J. Putter, P. Friberger, M. Knos, M. Larsbraten, and G. Claeson, Methods for the determination of glandular kallikrein by means of a chromogenic tripeptide assay. Adv. Exp. Med. Biol., 120A:83 (1978).

16. M. Maier, E. Polivka, and B. R. Binder, Application of hydrophobic interaction chromatography for purification of pig urinary kallikrein - characterization of the enzyme and its antibody. Z. Physiol. Chem., 362:883 (1981).

17. M. Dixon and E. C. Webb, "The Enzymes," Academic Press, New York (1979).

18. M. Maier, K. F. Austen, and J. Spragg, Purification of single-chain human low molecular weight kininogen and demonstration of its cleavage by human urinary kallikrein. <u>Anal.Biochem.</u>, 134:336 (1983).

19. R. P. Orange and K. F. Austen, The biological assay of slow reacting substances - SRS-A, bradykinin, prostaglandins <u>in</u>: "Methods in Immunology and Immunochemistry, vol V," C. A. Williams and M. W. Chase, eds., Academic Press, New York (1976).

20. M. J. Fredrick, R. J. Vavrek, J. M. Stewart, and C. E. Odya, Further studies of myometrial bradykinin receptor-like binding. <u>Biochem. Pharmacol.</u>, 33:2887 (1984).

21. J. Chao, J. Buse, K. Shimamoto, and H. H. Margolius, Kalli-krein-induced uterine contraction independent of kinin formation. <u>Proc. Natl. Acad. Sci. (USA)</u>, 78:6154 (1981).

CHANGES OF T-KININOGEN LEVELS IN PLASMA AND LIVER DURING

DEVELOPMENT OF RATS

Izumi Hayashi, Atsushi Kusunoki, Yoshinao Nagashima,
Masahiko Hayashi and Sachiko Oh-ishi

Department of Pharmacology, School of Pharmaceutical
Sciences, Kitasato University, 5-9-1 Shirokane
Minatoku, Tokyo 108, Japan

SUMMARY

T-kininogen levels of plasma and liver were measured in rats
during development by RIA.   We found that higher levels of T-kininogen in plasma and liver of neonates and of the mother rats at around
term.   The plasma level of mature male rats was as low as 1/5 to 1/2
of that of mature femal rats. T-kininogen levels in male and female
rats increased after treatment with estradiol, indicating that sex
hormones may regulate the physiological level of T-kininogen in rats.

INTRODUCTION

T-kininogen is known to increase after inflammatory stimuli[1-2],
and it is considered as one of the acute phase reactants in rats[3].
Darcy reported that alpha-globulin in rats plasma increased after
turpentine injection, surgery, bearing tumor, and the delivery[4-5]. In
this communication we report T-kininogen levels in plasma and liver of
rats during development as well as their sexual differences.

MATERIALS AND METHOD

<u>Animals:</u> Brown Norway Katholiek rats were bred and kept in an
experimental animal room as previously described[6].   Mature Wistar
rats of both sexes were purchased (Charles-River Japan, Atsugi and
Shizuoka Experimental Animal Center, Hamamatsu) and bred as above.
Blood and liver samples were prepared as previously described[7].

<u>Assay</u> <u>of</u> <u>T-kininogen</u> <u>and</u> <u>protein:</u> T-kininogen levels in plasma and
liver were measured by radioimmunoassay as previously reported[3].
Protein content of samples was measured by the method of Lowry[8].

<u>Agents</u> <u>used:</u> Estradiol dipropionate (Teikokuzoki, Tokyo) and
testosterone propionate (Mochida Pharm. Co., Tokyo) were injected into
5-week old Wistar rats of both sexes, one every 3 days, in a doses of
0.5 mg and 1 mg per rat per day simultaneously. Sesame oil (Japanese
Pharmacopeia standard) was injected into control rats as the vehicle.

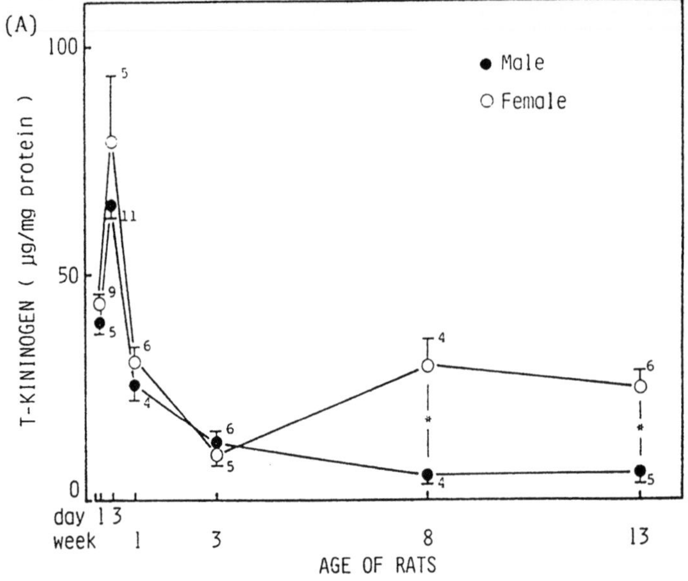

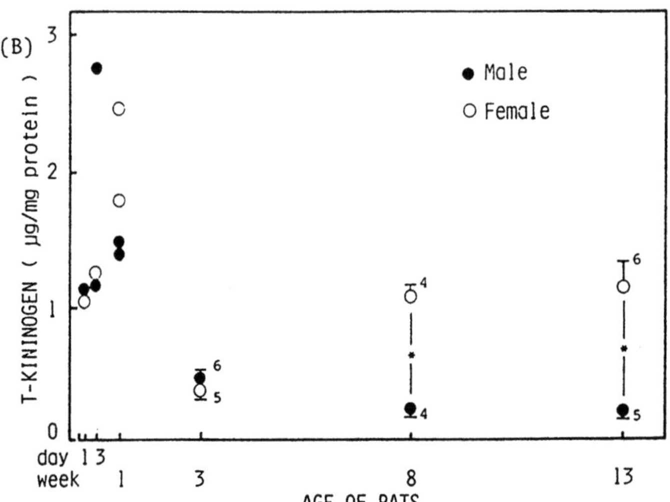

Fig. 1.   T-kininogen contents in plasma (A) and liver microsomal fraction (B) of male and female B/N-Katholiek rats during development.

T-kininogen was assayed by RIA and the levels were expressed as the values per mg protein. * indicates the value is statistically different between male and female at 5% level of significance. Figures by the circles indicate the numbers of rats used.

RESULT

T-kininogen levels of plasma and liver of Brown Norway Katholiek rats were measured by RIA during development and illustrated in Fig. 1A and B.   In male rats plasma and liver levels higher at 1 and 3 days after birth and then decreased with ages to the lowest level of

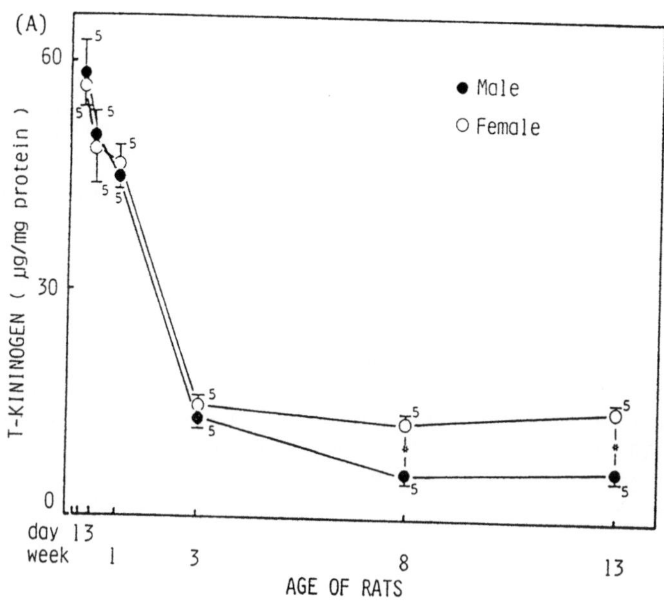

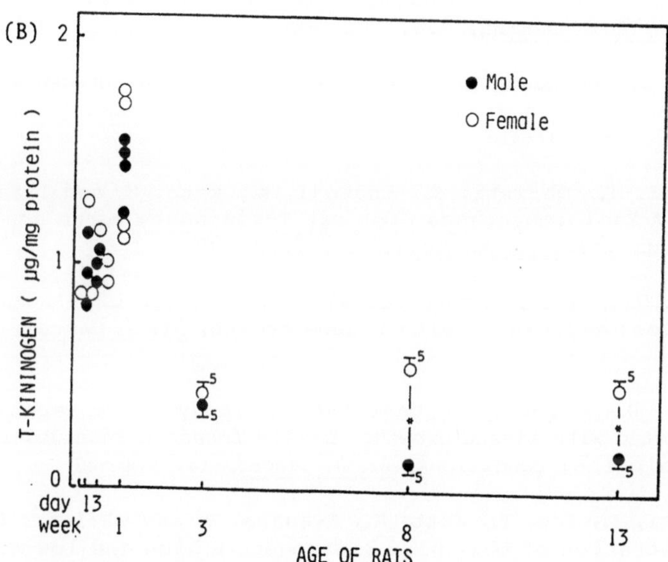

Fig. 2. T-kininogen contents in plasma (A) and liver microsomal fraction (B) of male and female Wistar rats during development. Figures and marked are the same as those in Fig. 1.

13 weeks old. Although in female rats the levels at 1 day to 3 weeks old were similar to those of male rats, the levels at 5 weeks old were not decreased, but about 2-3 times higher than those of male rats.

The similar observation was seen in Wistar strain as shown in Fig. 2A and B.   Furthermore the plasma levels of T-kininogen in mother rats around term were 2-4-fold higher than that of mature female rats. These results indicate that there may be hormonal regulation on the plasma level of T-kininogen.

Therefore we studied the effect of estradiol, and testosterone on the T-kininogen level.   Pretreatment with estradiol dipropionate increased T-kininogen level of male rats about 2-3 fold of that of control, and also increased the level of female rats about 1.5-fold. However pretreatment with testosterone propionate decreased the female level about 0.7-fold , and no effect on the male level.   Taken together all these results we conclude that sexual hormones may regulate physiological level of T-kininogen in rats.   The reason why T-kininogen level in neonate was higher is not known. Darcy mentioned that the increased level of globulin in mother rats might cause the higher level seen in neonates[3]. Further study is necessary for clarification.

REFERENCES

1. Barlas, A., Okamoto,H. and Greenbaum, L.M., 1985, T-kininogen - The major plasma kininogen in rat adjuvant arthritis, Biochem. Biophys. Res. Commun., 129, 280-286

2. Damas, J. and Adam, A., 1985, The relationship between kininogens and kallikreins in deficient Brown Norway rat plasma, Mol. Physiol., 8, 307-316

3. Hayashi, I., Oh-ishi, S., Enjyoji, K., Kato, H. and Iwanaga, S., 1986, A Radioimmunoassay for rat T-kininogen as an acute phase reactant, Chem. Pharm. Bull., 34, 3502-3505

4. Darcy, D.A., 1957, Immunological demonstration of a substance in rat blood associated with tissue growth, Br. J. Cancer, 11, 137-147

5. Darcy, D.A., 1960, A Quantitative study of a serum protein associated with tissue growth. Levels found in rats under various physiological conditions, Br. J. Cancer, 14, 524-533

6. Hayashi, I., Ino, T., Kato, H., Iwanaga, S. and Oh-ishi, S., 1984, Demonstration of the third kininogen in high and low molecular weight kininogens-deficient Brown Norway Katholiek rat, Thrombosis Res., 36, 509-516

7. Oh-ishi, S., Hayashi, I., Kusunoki, A., Nagashima, Y., Hayashi, M., Yamaki, K., Utsunomiya, I., and Yamasu, A., 1988, Developmental and sexual differences in T-kininogen levels in rat plasma and liver, Biochem. Biophys. Res. Commun., (in press)

8. Lowry, O.H., Rosebrough, N.J., Farr, A.L. and Randall, R.J.,1951, Protein measurement with the folin phenol reagent, J. Biol. Chem., 193, 265-275

LEUKOCYTE-INDUCED REGULATION OF HEPATIC PRODUCTION

OF T-KININOGEN

Norio Itoh, Katsutoshi Yayama and Hiroshi Okamoto

Department of Pharmacology
Faculty of Pharmaceutical Sciences
Kobe-Gakuin University
Ikawadani-cho, Nishi-ku, Kobe 673, Japan

INTRODUCTION

T-kininogen is a major plasma kininogen in rat[1], characterized as a protein precursor of biologically active peptide T-kinin[2]. Plasma concentration of T-kininogen as well as hepatic level of T-kininogen mRNA increases 10-20 fold after the induction of acute inflammation[1,3], indicating that the protein is an acute-phase reactant in rats. T-kininogen has also been identified to be a cysteine-proteinase inhibitor in rat plasma[4]. Recently, we have demonstrated that macrophages prepared from the site of inflammation have the ability to enhance secretion of T-kininogen from rat hepatocytes in primary culture[5], indicating that, similarly with other acute-phase reactants, acute-phase response of T-kininogen is mediated by a macrophage-derived factor, monokine.

Macrophage-derived proteins, interleukin-1 (IL-1) and hepatocyte-stimulating factor (HSF), have recently been identified to be mediators which directly act on hepatocytes to stimulate the production of several acute phase reactants[6]. Hepatic synthesis of cysteine-proteinase inhibitor, presumably corresponding to T-kininogen, has also been reported to be stimulated by HSF[6].

During the course of experiments to better understand the underlying mechanisms for the induction of T-kininogen, we found that leukocytes, which were stimulated in vitro for prolonged periods by lipopolysaccharide (LPS), suppressed hepatic production of T-kininogen. The evidence presented here strongly suggest a presence of the negative control system for hepatic production of acute-phase reactant.

MATERIALS AND METHODS

Animals and Materials

Male Fisher-344 rats, weighing 100-150 g, (Shizuoka Laboratory Animal Center, Hamamatsu, Japan) were used. The following materials were obtained commercial sources: LPS (Staphylococcus typhosa 0901; Difco, Detroit, Mich); fetal calf serum (M.A. Bioproducts, Walkersville, Md); Millicell-HA inserts (Millipore Products Division, Bedford, Ma); collagenase (Wako Chemicals, Osaka, Japan).

T-kininogen was determined by radioimmunoassay using [^{125}I]labeled T-kininogen and rabbit anti-T-kininogen serum as described previously[7].

Preparation of Macrophage-enriched or Macrophage-deprived Cells

A single cell suspension of spleen cells was prepared from rats. Macrophage-enriched cells were prepared from spleen cells by means of adherence to plastic dishes[8]. Macrophage-deprived cells were prepared by passing spleen cells through a Sephadex G-10 column[9].

Coculture of Hepatocytes with Spleen Cells

Spleen cells were cultured in William's E medium supplemented with insulin (10^{-7} M), gentamycin (50 μg/ml), dexamethasone (10^{-7} M) and fetal calf serum (5%) (modified WE medium) in the presence of LPS (5 μg/ml) for different times, washed and then resuspended in modified WE medium. Rat hepatocytes, which were prepared as described previously[5], were cultured in the modified WE medium for 48 hr, the medium was changed to 2 ml of fresh modified WE medium, and then 30-mm Millicell-HA insert with membrane filter of 0.45 μm pore size was placed into each culture dish of hepatocytes. One-milliliter suspension of spleen cells (2×10^{2} - 2×10^{4}/ml) was added to the interior of each Millicell-HA insert. By this technique, hepatocytes and spleen cells could be cultured in the same medium across a membrane filter. Following the culture for 48 hr, the amount of T-kininogen secreted from hepatocytes into culture medium was assayed.

RESULTS

Induction of Suppressive Leukocytes on Hepatic Production of T-kininogen by a Prolonged Stimulation with LPS

Leukocytes from several sources, such as peritoneal exudate cells, Kupffer cells and peripheral blood monocytes, have been used to determine their factors which stimulate hepatic production of acute-phase reactants. In the present study, we used rat spleen to prepare leukocytes. Our initial objective was to determine whether the period of LPS-exposure affects on the stimulatory activity of leukocytes on hepatic production of T-kininogen. Spleen cells were prepared from normal F-344 rats, stimulated _in vitro_ for different periods by LPS and then cocultured with hepatocytes prepared from F344 rats. As shown in Fig.1, spleen cells stimulated for 8 hr caused a significant enhancement of T-kininogen secretion from hepatocytes. However, 2-hr stimulation no longer enhanced T-kininogen secretion. Surprisingly, 48-hr stimulation caused a significant reduction of T-kininogen secretion. Only 200 spleen cells exhibited 50% reduction (Fig. 1). These results suggest that LPS-stimulated leukocytes initially secrete a factor stimulating hepatic production of T-kininogen and subsequently secrete another factor inhibiting T-kininogen production.

Identification of Suppressive Leukocytes on Hepatic Production of T-kininogen

In order to identify leukocyte which may be responsible for secreting an inhibitory factor on hepatic production of T-kininogen, LPS-stimulated spleen cells were separated into two fractions, i.e., the macrophage-enriched and the macrophage-deprived cells. These fractions of leukocytes were then cocultured with hepatocytes to assess which fraction of leukocytes is responsible for producing an inhibitory factor. As shown in Fig.

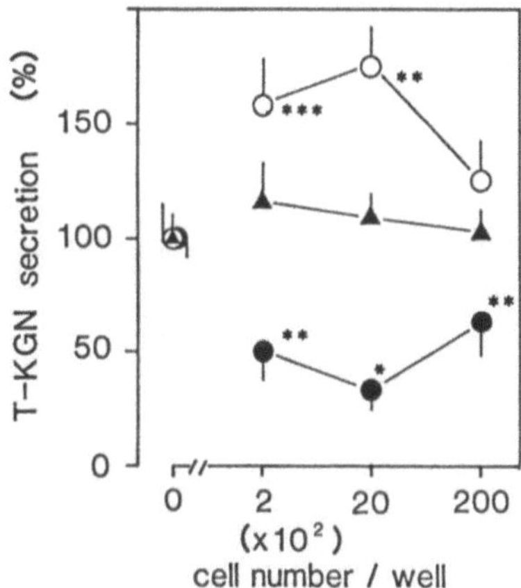

Fig. 1. Time-dependent induction of stimulatory and suppresive leukocytes on hepatic production of T-kininogen. Rat spleen cells were cultured in the presence of LPS (5 µg/ml) for 2 hr (▲), 8 hr (o) or 48 hr (●), and the cells in the number shown in the figure were cocultured with rat hepatocytes for 48 hr. T-kininogen secretion from hepatocytes were exprssed as % of those from hepatocytes cultured alone. Significantly different from basal secretion (*p<0.05, **p<0.01, ***p<0.001; n=6).

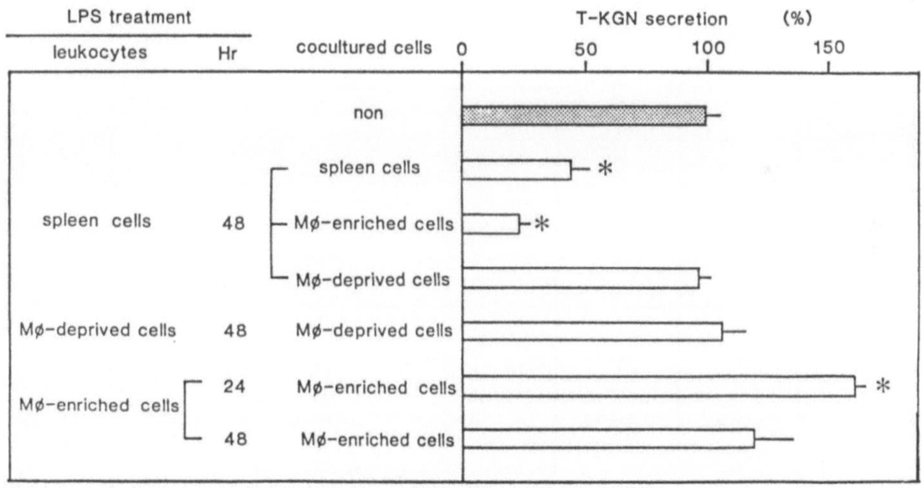

Fig. 2. Effect of LPS-stimulated leukocytes on hepatic production of T-kininogen. Spleen cells, macrophage-deprived cells and macrophage-enriched cells were stimulated with LPS for the periods shown in the figure. Spleen cells were then separated into macrophage-enriched or macrophage-depreived cells after LPS-stimulation, as described in the text. These cells were cocultured with hepatocytes for 48 hr, and T-kininogen secreted into culture medium was measured. Significantly different from basal T-kininogen secretion (*p<0.001; n=6).

2, LPS-stimulated spleen cells for 48 hr suppressed T-kininogen secretion by 50% of control. The macrophage-enriched cells prepared from these LPS-stimulated spleen also exhibited a significant suppression of T-kininogen secretion. By removing macrophages from LPS-stimulated spleen cells, the suppressive effect was significantly reduced. These results indicate that macrophages are responsible for producing an inhibitory factor. We term here these macrophages as the suppressive macrophages.

In order to ascertain whether some leukocytes other than macrophages are involved in the induction of suppressive macrophages, spleen cells were first separated into macrophage-enriched or macrophage-deprived cells, and then these cells were stimulated with LPS for 48 hr and cocultured with hepatocytes. As shown in Fig. 2, neither fraction of cells affected on T-kininogen secretion from hepatocytes. These results indicate that some leukocytes other than macrophages are necessary in the induction phase of suppressive macrophages. In contrast, macrophage-enriched cells, which were stimulated in the absence ofother leukocytes for 24 hr by LPS, exhibited an enhancement on T-kininogen secretion from hepatocytes. Therefore, macrophages, which produce a stimulatory factor on T-kininogen production, are inducible in the absence of other leukocytes.

Possible Contribution of Prostaglandin (PG) in the Induction of Suppressive Macrophage

Several evidence has implicated that PGs, especially E_1 and E_2, act as inhibitors for the immune system[10], such as on the production of lym-

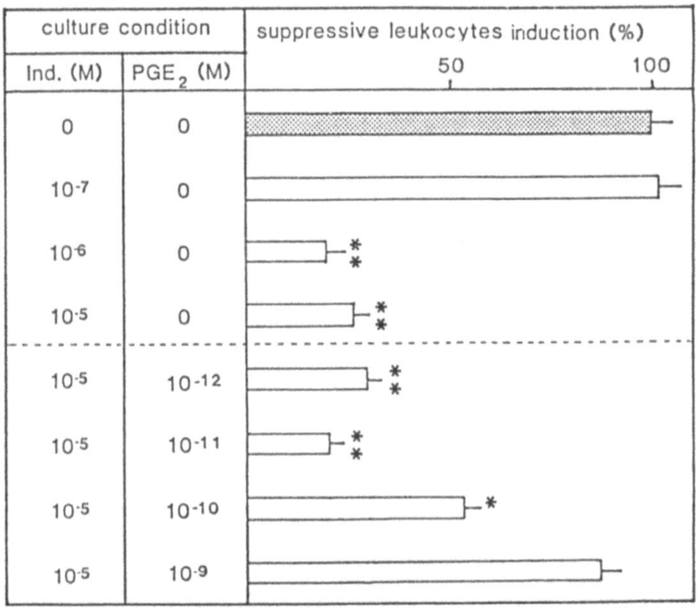

culture condition		suppressive leukocytes induction (%)
Ind. (M)	PGE_2 (M)	
0	0	▨
10^{-7}	0	
10^{-6}	0	**
10^{-5}	0	**
10^{-5}	10^{-12}	**
10^{-5}	10^{-11}	**
10^{-5}	10^{-10}	*
10^{-5}	10^{-9}	

Fig. 3. Effects of indomethacin and PGE_2 on the induction of suppressive leukocytes. Spleen cells were stimulated with LPS for 48 hr in the presence of indomethacin or indomethacin plus PGE_2 at different concentrations shown in the figure, and then these cells were cocultured with hepatocytes. Inhibition by these cells on T-kininogen secretion was measured and represented as the induction of suppressive leukocytes. Data were expressed as % of the induction of suppressive leukocytes in the absence of indomethacin or PGE_2; *p<0.01, **p<0.001 (n=6).

phokines, the mitogen-induced DNA synthesis of T-cell, the induction of killer T-cell, the antibody production and the induction of natural killer cell. Thus, PGs have been considered to be important factors regulating immune responses. In addition, the most obvious role for PGs in the immune response is as mediators of inflammation. These evidence made us expect some contribution of PGs in the induction phase of suppressive macrophages. Spleen cells were stimulated _in vitro_ for 48 hr by LPS in the presence or absence of several concentrations of indomethacin or a combination of indomethacin and PGE_2. Then, spleen cells were washed and co-cultured with hepatocytes. As shown in Fig. 3, addition of indomethacin at the concentrations more than 1×10^{-6} M during LPS- stimulation significantly inhibited the induction of suppressive macrophages. Under the presence of indomethacin (1×10^{-5} M) which was expected to inhibit endogenous PGs synthesis of spleen cells, PGE_2 was added at the concentrations from 1×10^{-12} to 1×10^{-9} M during LPS-stimulation. As shown in Fig. 3, the induction of suppressive macrophages, which was inhibited under the presence of indomethacin, again appeared by the addition of PGE_2 in a concentration-dependent manner. Indomethacin-induced inhibition of the induction of suppressive leukocytes was completely abolished by 1 nM of PGE_2.

DISCUSSION

T-kininogen[2] has been identified in rat plasma to be a protein precursor of kinin[2], an endogenous inhibitor for cysteine-proteinase[4] and an acute-phase reactant[1,3]. However, its function in the inflammatory condition is still obscure.

Several investigators have demonstrated that monokines, which may be produced and secreted from the 'activated' macrophages at the site of inflammation, directly act on hepatocytes to stimulate the synthesis of acute-phase reactants[6]. Like other known acute-phase reactants, hepatic production of T-kininogen (or cysteine-proteinase inhibitor) has been known to be stimulated by a factor secreted from the 'activated' macrophages[6].

In addition to this stimulatory system by leukocytes, we found for the first time the presence of an inhibitory system by leukocytes on hepatic production of acute-phase reactant, T-kininogen. The inhibitory system by leukocytes were characterized as followed: first, it was induced in leukocytes by a prolonged exposure of stimulus ; second, an inhibitory factor for hepatic production of T-kininogen was secreted from macrophages, and therefore the effector cell is macrophage; third, leukocytes other than macrophages were needed in the induction phase of suppressive macrophages; forth, the induction phase was blocked by indomethacin, and the blockade was abolished by PGE_2, indicating a key role of PGE_2 in the induction phase of suppressive macrophages. In contrast, macrophages, which secrete a stimulatory factor for T-kininogen production, could be induced in the absence of other leukocytes. These evidence suggest that, at the site of inflammation, inflammatory stimuli may initially cause direct activativation of macrophages to secrete a stimulatory factor and, subsequently, induce suppressive macrophages in the process of cell to cell interation between macrophages and other leukocytes. PGs may play an important role in the induction phase of macrophages.

We already observed that implantation of suppressive leukocytes, which were induced _in vitro_ in spleen cells by LPS-stimulation, into the peritoneal cavities of normal rats caused a significant reduction of plasma T-kininogen level (data not shown), indicating that suppressive leukocytes are effective on hepatic production of T-kininogen not only _in_

<u>vitro</u> but also <u>in vivo.</u> By a single injection of LPS into rats, plasma T-kininogen level increases until 48 hr and thereafter turns to decrease. These evidence may indicate that, in the process of acute inflammation, the initial stimulation of T-kininogen production by a stimulatory factor are followed by a suppression of its production. Thus, hepatic production of T-kininogen seems to be closely controlled in the process of inflammation. Significance of this inhibitory system in other acute-phase reactants are investigating in our laboratory.

REFERENCES

1. A. Barlas, H. Okamoto, and L. M. Greenbaum, T-kininogen - The major plasma kininogen in rat adjuvant arthritis, <u>Biochem. Biophys. Res. Commun.</u> 129: 280 (1985).
2. H. Okamoto and L. M. Greenbaum, Isolation and structure of T-kinin, <u>Biochem. Biophys. Res. Commun.</u> 112: 701 (1983).
3. R. Kageyama, N. Kitamura, H. Ohkubo, and S. Nakanishi, <u>J. Biol. Chem.</u> 260: 12060 (1985).
4. T. Sueyoshi, K. Enjyoji, T. Shimada, H. Kato, S. Iwanaga, Y. Bando, E. Kominami, and N. Katunuma, A new function of kininogens as thiol-proteinase inhibitors, <u>FEBS Letters</u> 182: 193 (1985).
5. N. Itoh, T. Toyohama, H. Okamoto, H. Kawano, T. Mayumi, and T. Hama, Involvement of inflammatory leukocytes in hepatic induction of T-kininogen in rat, <u>Inflammation</u> 11: 345 (1987)
6. H. Baumann, V. Onorato, J. Gauldie, and G. P. Jahreis, Distinct sets of acute phase plasma proteins are stimulated by separate human hepato-cyte-stimulating factors and monokines in rat hepatoma cells, <u>J. Biol. Chem.</u> 262: 9756 (1987).
7. H. Okamoto, N. Itoh, and M. Uwani, Identification of T-kininogen in rat urine, <u>Biochem. Pharmac.</u> 36: 2979 (1987).
8. D. E. Mosier, A requirement for two cell types for antibody formation in vitro, <u>Science</u>, 158: 1573 (1967).
9. A. L. Y. Iris and I. M. Robert, Separation of mouse spleen cells by passage through column of Sephadex G-10, <u>J. Immunol. Methods,</u> 5: 239 (1974).
10. J. S. Goodwin and D. R. Webb, Regulation of the immune responses by prostaglandins, <u>Clin. Immunol. Immunopathol.</u> 15: 106 (1980)

IDENTIFICATION OF THIOL-ACTIVATED T-KININOGENASES

IN THE RAT AND MOUSE SUBMANDIBULAR GLANDS

A. Barlas, X. Gao and L.M. Greenbaum

Department of Pharmacology and Toxicology and
School of Graduate Studies
Medical College of Georgia
Augusta, GA. 30912, USA

SUMMARY

T-kininogen is a unique protein(s) which is directed for synthesis
following inflammation such as that caused by adjuvant arthritis and
carrageenin. The properties of the protein include thiol-protease inhibition
and the potential to act as a substrate to release Ile-Ser-bradykinin
(T-kinin). During the inflammatory response, free T-kinin is found in the
blood and inflammatory fluids indicating that T-kininogenase (T-kgnase)
enzymes exist that release T-kinin and perhaps related T-kinins involved in
inflammation. We report here that T-kininogenases have been found in the rat
and mouse submandibular glands and in rat peritoneal white cells. The pH
optimum is about 8.0. The enzymes must be thiol-activated. Thus, the rat has
the complete T-kgnase-T-kinin system. Since T-kininogen is a member of the
superfamily of cysteine protease inhibitors, members of the superfamily may
be directed for synthesis in inflammatory diseases including ascites in
other species including humans.

INTRODUCTION

Studies in our laboratory led to the discovery of T-kininogen I & II
and T-kinin (1,2). We also demonstrated that T-kininogens, but not
K-kininogens (kallikrein substrates) are acute phase proteins in the rat
which increases in peripheral blood some 7-10 fold in adjuvant arthritis (3).
This was confirmed by the demonstration by Furuto et al that mRNAs of
T-kininogen I & II are synthesized following an inflammatory response (4).
Since T-kininogens were found to be similar in structure to 1 cysteine
protease inhibitors, it has been claimed that thiol inhibition is the sole
property of T-kininogens (5). In the current communication, we review and
relate our recent findings that T-kgnases are present in the rat and mouse
submandibular glands and white cells which demonstrate the completeness of
the T-kgnase - T-kininogen system in the rat and that the role of T-kininogen is to release T-kinin as well as serving as a thiol protease inhibitor.

Table 1. Increases in Free T-Kinin and T-Kininogen Levels in Rats Treated With Carrageenin

KGEN	DAY 0	DAY 1
Plasma	ug/ml	ug/ml
T-KGN	280	2,072
H-KGN	45	56
L-KGN	54	54
Inflammatory fluid		
T-KGN	–	448
H-KGN	–	3
L-KGN	–	45

KININ	DAY 0	DAY 1
Blood	ng/ml	ng/ml
T-kinin	0.05	0.26
Bradykinin	0.04	0.16
Inflammatory fluid		
T-kinin	–	0.34
Bradykinin	–	0.13

Table 2. Tissue Content of T-Kgnase

TISSUE	UNITS/DTT	UNITS/NO DTT
Rat Submandibular Gland	75	18
Mouse Submandibular Gland	56	28
Guinea Pig Submandibular Gland	1	1

DTT (Dithiothreitol) concentration was 10^{-3}M. One unit of enzyme liberates 1 ng of T-kinin in 30 minutes (7). The following rat tissues showed negligible activity: liver, lung, heart, kidney, pancreas and spleen.

RESULTS

Table 1 demonstrates that <u>free</u> T-kinin increases in the blood and is present in inflammatory fluid of the rat that has been injected a day before with 4ml of a 2% carrageenin solution into a rat with a dorsum air pouch. The increase in free T-kinin is accompanied by the acute phase response of an increase in T-kininogen, but not H or L kininogens.

Table 2 demonstrates that a thiol- activated T-kgnase is found in the submandibular gland of the rat and the mouse, but not the guinea pig. The products of the rat enzyme acting on a pure T-kininogen substrate is T-kinin and an unknown kinin.

In addition to the rat submandibular gland, a thiol-activated T-kgnase has been identified in white cells. Thus the T-kgnase-T-kininogen system of the rat is established. T-kininogen acts as a substrate for endogenous and pathological T-kgnases which promote the release of T-kinin and account for the presence of T-kinin in blood and inflammatory fluids of the rat following an inflammatory challenge. It should be noted that Cathepsin D also releases T-kinin (6).

The T-kgnase-T-kininogen system may be representative of genetically related thiol protease inhibitors synthesized in response to injury in humans and other species and which promote healing. The mechanisms by which it is signalled to be synthesized may be of importance in the understanding of the inflammatory response in humans and other species. A full report has been published (7).

REFERENCES

1. H. Okamoto and L.M. Greenbaum, Isolation and Structure of T-kinin, Biochem. Biophys. Res. Commun, 112: 707-708 (1983).

2. H. Okamoto and L.M. Greenbaum, Kininogen Substrates for Trypsin and Cathepsin D in Human, Rabbit & Rat Plasmas, Life Sci, 32: 2007-2013, (1983).

3. A. Barlas, H. Okamoto, and L.M. Greenbaum, T-kininogen - The Major Plasma Kininogen in Rat Adjuvant Arthritis, Biochem, Biophys. Res Commun, 129: 280-286, (1985).

4. S. Furuto-Kato, A. Matsumoto, N. Kitamura and S. Nakanishi, Primary Structures of the mRNAs Encoding the Rat Precursors for Bradykinin and T-kinin, J. Biol. Chem, 260, 12054 (1985).

5. M. Moreau, N. Gutman, A. EL Moujahed, F. Esnard, and F. Gauthier, Relationship Between Cysteine-Proteinase-Inhibitory Function of Rat T-kininogen and the Release of Immunoreactive Kinin Upon Trypsin Treatment, Eur. J. Biochem, 159: 341-346, (1986).

6. H. Okamoto and L.M. Greenbaum, Isolation and Properties of Two Rat Plasma T-kininogens, ADV. in EXPERIMENTAL MED, 198, 69, "Kinins IV" eds. L.M. Greenbaum and H. Margolius, Plenum Press, N.Y. (1986).

7. A. Barlas, X. Gao and L.M. Greenbaum, Isolation of a Thiol-activated T-kininogenase from the Rat Submandibular Gland. FEBS Lett., 218, 266 (1987).

SEX DIMORPHISM AND ESTROGEN REGULATION OF KININOGENS IN RAT SERUM,
ADRENAL GLAND AND KIDNEY

Julie Chao, Steven Chao, William Xiong, Limei Chen,
Christopher Swain and Lee Chao

Departments of Pharmacology and Biochemistry
Medical University of South Carolina, Charleston, SC, USA

The present studies demonstrate sex dimorphism of kininogen content
in rat serum and various tissues. Kininogen levels were determined by
measuring the levels of released kinin after treatment with trypsin. In
perfused female adrenal gland and kidney, kininogen content was 10.2-
and 5.3-fold higher than that in corresponding male tissues. Ovariectomy resulted in a 5- to 10-fold reduction of kininogen levels in these
tissues, and estradiol treatment of the ovariectomized rats restored
renal kininogen content to the level of female sham-ovariectomized rats.
In female rats, serum kininogen levels are 5-fold higher than those of
males. Western blot analysis of serum proteins on a 2-dimensional
polyacrylamide gel using a kinin-directed kininogen monoclonal antibody
revealed that in female rats the levels of several 68,000 dalton kininogens varying in charge were higher than those in male rats. The
results indicate that a sex difference exists with regard to kininogens
in rat serum and tissues and that kininogen levels are regulated by
estrogen. The impact of hormone-regulated kininogens on cardiovascular
function awaits further study.

INTRODUCTION

Kininogens are the biosynthetic precursors of vasoactive kinins
(1). Kinins have a broad spectrum of biological activities including
effects on the cardiovascular system, smooth muscle contraction, ion
transport, prostaglandin synthesis, cell proliferation, capillary
permeability, pain production, and inflammation (1). Kininogens are
distributed in mammalian plasma and liver. Three forms of kininogen
have been identified as high molecular weight (HMW) kininogen, low
molecular weight (LMW) kininogen (2), and a T-kininogen which has been
found so far only in rat plasma (3,4).

Recently a novel function of the intact kininogen molecule unrelated to kinin release has been discovered. The kininogens were
demonstrated to be potent inhibitors of cysteine proteinases and an
acute phase protein of the rat (4-7). Kininogens are thus multi-func-
tional proteins which serve not only as the precursors of vasoactive
kinins and as inhibitors of cysteine proteinases, but also as a major
acute phase protein. To further analyze the structure, regulation and
function of kininogen, we have recently produced monoclonal antibodies
against the bradykinin moiety of kininogen (8). These antibodies were

used to identify kininogen distribution by Western blotting and immunohistochemical localization. The present studies show that a major sex
difference in kininogen levels exists in rat serum, adrenal gland, and
kidney and that kininogen levels are regulated by sex hormones in these
tissues.

EXPERIMENTAL PROCEDURES

Determination of Kininogen Levels

Aliquots (0.2 ml, ~6-7 mg protein/ml) of tissue extracts were added
to 0.6 ml of 0.02 M Tris-HCl, pH 8.0, and boiled for 30 min to eliminate
kininase activity. Aliquots (100 µl) of the supernatants were collected
after centrifugation for 5 min with a Microfuge. TPCK-trypsin (40 µg)
(Sigma Chemical Co., St. Louis, MO, USA) in 0.3 ml of 0.02 M Tris HCl,
pH 8.0, was added to each aliquot for releasing kinin moiety from
kininogens. The samples were then incubated at $37^{\circ}C$ for 30 min. The
reaction was stopped by boiling for 10 min, and aliquots were used in a
kinin radioimmunoassay (9) utilizing rabbit antiserum against ^{125}I-
labelled tyrosyl-bradykinin. Kininogen levels were expressed as kinin
equivalent/mg protein.

Hormonal Treatment and Tissue Preparation

Sprague-Dawley (200-250 g) ovariectomized female rats and the
sham-operated controls were used in groups of six animals each. Three
weeks after surgery performed by the supplier, rats began to receive
subcutaneous injections of estradiol benzoate (30 µg/kg body weight)
suspended in sesame oil or sesame oil alone every 48 h for 2 weeks.
After the treatments, kidney and adrenal gland tissues were prepared
from the perfused animals as previously described (10).

Western Blot Analyses of Serum Proteins on Two-dimensional Gels

Two dimensional gel electrophoresis was performed according to
O'Farrell (11). Rat serum (10 µl) was initially separated in the 1st
dimensional focusing system (pH 4-6) of the tube gel (10 cm x 2 mm).
Second dimensional electrophoresis was performed on a 7.5-15% linear
gradient polyacrylamide gel containing 0.1% SDS. The proteins were
either stained with Coomassie brilliant blue or transferred to nitrocellulose for Western blot analysis. The blot was incubated for 2 h at
room temperature with affinity-purified ^{125}I-labelled kinin directed
kininogen monoclonal antibody (5 x 10^5 cpm/ml) (1D$_{10}$) and for another 2
h at $37^{\circ}C$ in a buffer containing 0.15 M NaCl, 0.005 M EDTA, 0.05 M
Tris-HCl (pH 7.4), 3% BSA, and 0.05% Nonidet P-40. The blots were
washed, and kininogen binding was displayed visually by autoradiography.

RESULTS

Sex Difference of Kininogen and Kallikrein Levels in the Male and Female Rat Kidney and Adrenal Gland

Kininogen levels were measured by a kinin radioimmunoassay and
expressed as trypsin-generated kinin equivalents per mg protein. Figure
1 shows a major sex difference of kininogen content in rat kidney and
adrenal gland. The contents of immunoreactive kininogen in kidney and
adrenal gland of female rats are 5.3- and 10.2-fold higher, respectively, than that of male rats. However, there is no significant sex
difference of tissue kallikrein content in the adrenal gland. In the
female rat kidney, tissue kallikrein level is only ~ 1.6-fold higher
than that in the male ones (data not shown).

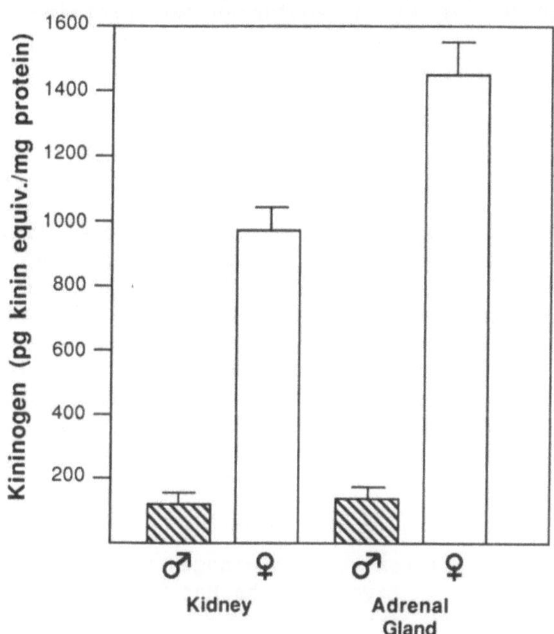

Figure 1. Sex difference of kininogen levels in kidney and adrenal gland of male and female rats. Values shown are mean ± S.E.M. of five animals.

Hormonal Effect on Kininogen Levels in the Rat Kidney

Figure 2 shows the effect of estradiol on kininogen content in the rat kidney. Ovariectomy of female rats results in a 5.3-fold decrease in kininogen content in the kidney from 969.0 ± 81.90 to 181.64 ± 56.97 ng kinin equivalent/mg protein (n=5). Kininogen levels in the kidney of ovariectomized female rats are similar to those of normal male rats

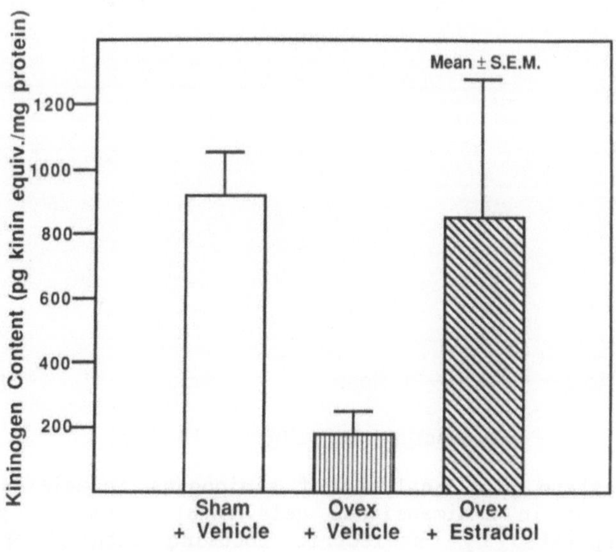

Figure 2. Effect of estradiol on kininogen content in ovariectomized (Ovex) female rat kidneys. Values shown are mean ± S.E.M. of five animals.

(114.45 ± 40.38 ng kinin equivalent/ml protein, n=5). Estradiol replacement in ovariectomized females restored renal kininogen content to a level not significantly different from that of sham ovariectomized rats (Figure 2).

Quantitative and Qualitative Difference of Serum Kininogens in Male vs Female Rats Analyzed by Radioimmunoassays and Western Blotting

Table 1 shows a comparison of immunoreactive kininogen and kallikrein levels in male and female rat serum. Kininogen concentrations in male and female rat serum are 1.55 ± 0.10 and 7.83 ± 1.01 µg kinin equivalent/ml (n=5), respectively. The results show that kininogen levels in the serum are ~ 5-fold higher in the female rat. However, rat serum tissue kallikrein levels are 60% higher in males than in female rat serum. These results indicate that a differential regulation of kininogen and kallikrein levels in the serum and tissues by sex hormones exists.

Table 1

Sex Differences of Kininogen and Kallikrein
Levels in the Rat Serum

Sex	Source	Kininogen (µg kinin equiv./ml)	Kallikrein (ng/ml)
♂	Serum	1.55 ± 0.10	334.72 ± 24.55
♀	Serum	7.83 ± 1.01	250.6 ± 17.7

Figure 3 shows Western blot analyses of kininogens in male and female rat serum. Serum samples were run in 2-dimensional gels. Total

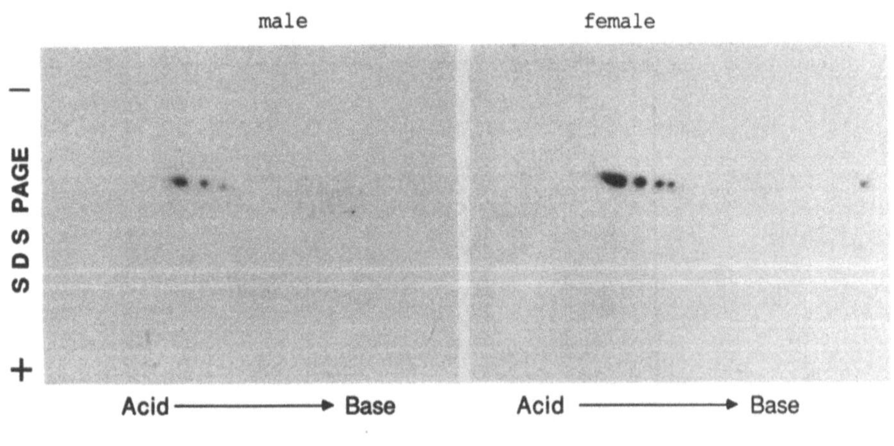

Figure 3. Western blot analysis of kininogens in male and female rat serum in 2-dimensional gels. Rat serum (10 µl) was first separated by isoelectric focusing with pH 4-6 system in 1st-dimension and then by 2nd-dimensional SDS-polyacrylamide gel electrophoresis.

serum proteins were first separated by isoelectric focusing in a pH 4-6 1st-dimensional system and then by 2nd-dimensional SDS-polyacrylamide gel electrophoresis. After electrophoretic transfer of proteins onto nitrocellulose, kininogens were identified by their ability to bind to a ^{125}I-labelled kinin-directed kininogen monoclonal antibody. Several 68,000 dalton kininogens can be identified in the 2-D gel shown below. In comparison with levels in male serum, female serum has greater amounts of kininogens which are similar in molecular weight but different in isoelectric points (Figure 3).

DISCUSSION

The present studies show sex dimorphism of kininogen content in rat kidney, adrenal gland and serum. In females, kininogen concentrations are several-fold higher than those in males. Ovariectomy of female rats results in a reduction of kininogen to levels similar to those of male rats, and estradiol treatment restores kininogen content to that of sham-ovariectomized female rats. Kininogen levels were measured in the perfused tissues by a kinin radioimmunoassay following trypsin treatment of the extracts and were expressed as kinin equivalents per mg protein in tissues or per ml of serum. In our recent studies, using a newly established direct radioimmunoassay for measuring rat kininogen, we also demonstrated a difference in immunoreactive kininogen between male and female rats (Chao et al., unpublished results). Previous works revealed that there is a difference in plasma kininogen levels between male and female rats and that this difference might be related to sex hormones (13). Several studies have reported the possible roles which plasma kininogen may play in oestrous cycle, pregnancy, parturition and puer- perium of rats, goats as well as in the human menstrual cycle (14-18). We measured kininogen levels by a kinin radioimmunoassay, which is ~ 100 fold more sensitive than bioassay methods used by other investigators. This method may partially account for the greater difference in rat serum kininogen levels between sexes in comparison with previous work. Furthermore, this paper is the first demonstration of the existence of immunoreactive kininogen in the rat kidney and adrenal gland and of the regulation of kininogen levels in these tissues by estradiol.

Analysis of Western blots from a 2-dimensional gel using our kinin-directed kininogen monoclonal antibody reveals that, in female serum, the concentrations of several kininogens, similar in molecular weights but different in isoelectric points, are higher than in male serum. Since the reported molecular weights of rat LMW kininogen and T-kininogens are similar, ~ 68,000 dalton, the varying charges of these kininogens may reflect either a difference in carbohydrate content or a small number of amino acid substitutions. HPLC analyses of the types of rat kininogen found by measuring kinins released after trypsin treatment showed that the levels of three types of immunoreactive kinins are higher in female rats than in males. The results suggest that low molecular weight kininogen, T-kininogen, and other proteins containing kinin moiety are expressed at higher levels in female rats.

The liver is the major site of synthesis of kininogens and several other acute-phase proteins of inflammation. Since serum contains high levels of kininogen, the possibility that kininogens detected in the perfused kidney or adrenal gland originate from serum cannot be elim- inated. However, human renal kininogen has been localized immunohisto- chemically in the distal tubules of the kidney (12). Dot blot analysis using a kinin oligonucleotide probe showed that kininogen mRNA was present in rat kidney (Chao et al, unpublished results). The studies also showed that renal kininogen levels are regulated by estrogen.

Whether kininogen gene expression in kidney, liver and other tissues is also regulated by estrogen remains to be determined.

Since the ovary is an important part of a very complex endocrine system and bears multifunctional characteristics, ovariectomy not only decreases the level of estradiol but also causes a lot of changes in the homeostasis of organisms. Consequently, other factors may also contribute to the regulation of kininogen during this process, such as progesteron.

It is interesting to note that angiotensinogen, a precursor of the vasoconstrictor, angiotensin II, is an acute phase protein and is also regulated by sex hormones. Angiotensinogen has been found to be an acute-phase protein in man (19), and its mRNA in rat liver increased rapidly following acute inflammation (20). Estradiol treatment of the rat resulted in a 50% increase in angiotensinogen levels (21), and these levels are higher during pregnancy and in women taking oral contraceptives (22). Therefore, we have found numerous parallels between the regulation of kininogen and angiotensionogen, despite the active form of the former causing vasodilatation and the latter causing vasoconstriction. Collectively, the above results suggest that kininogen may play some novel roles in various physiological and pathological conditions during normal pregnancy, toxemia of pregnancy, hypertension, hyperthyroidism and Cushings disease, all of which are closely related to the renin-angiotensin-aldosterone system. It is important to elucidate the relationship of kininogen with other hormones and metabolites such as progesterone and angiotensinogen.

REFERENCES

1. M. Schachter, Kallikreins (kininogens) - a group of serine protease with bioregulatory actions, Pharmacol. Rev. 31, 1-17 (1980).

2. H. Kato, S. Nagasawa, and S. Iwanaga, S., HMW and LMW kininogens. Methods Enzymol. 80, 172-198 (1981).

3. H. Okamoto, and L.M. Greenbaum, Biochem. Biophys. Res. Commun. 112, 701-708 (1983).

4. A. Barlas, H. Okanoto, L.M. Greenbaum, T-kininogen - The major plasma kininogen in rat adjuvant arthritis. Biochem Biophys. Res. Commun. 112: 701-708 (1985).

5. I. Ohkubo, K. Kurachi, T. Takasawa, H. Shiokawa, and M. Sasaki, Isolation of a human cDNA for α_2-thiol proteinase inhibitor and its identity with low molecular weight kininogen. Biochemistry 23, 5691-5697 (1984).

6. T. Sueyoshi, K. Enjyoji, T. Shimada, H. Kato, S. Iwanaga, Y. Bando, E. Kominami, and N. Katunuma, A new function of kininogens as thiol-proteinase inhibitors: inhibition of papain and cathepsins B,H and L by bovine, rat and human plasma kininogens. Febs. Lett. 182, 193-195 (1985).

7. W. Muller-Esterl, H. Fritz, W. Machleidt, A. Ritonja, J. Brzin, M. Kotnik, V. Turk, J. Kellermann, and F. Lottspeich, Human plasma kininogens are identical with α-cysteine proteinase inhibitors. Febs. Lett. 182, 310-314 (1985).

8.   J. Chao, D.M. Tillman, and J. Chao, Isolation and characterization of a target-directed monoclonal antibody to kininogens. Fed. Proc. 45, 1916 (1986).

9.   K. Shimamoto, T. Ando, T. Nakao, S. Tanaka, M. Sakuma, and M. Miyahara, A sensitive radioimmunoassay method for urinary kinin in man. J. Lab. Clin. Med. 91: 721-   (1978).

10. J. Chao, L. Chao, C. Swain, J. Tsai, and H.S. Margolius, Tissue kallikrein in rat brain and pituitary: Regional distribution and estrogen induction in the anterior pituitary. Endocrinology 120(2), 475-482 (1987).

11. P.H. O'Farrell, High resolution two-dimensional electrophoresis of proteins. J. Biol. Chem. 250, 4007-4021 (1975).

12. D. Proud, M.I. Perkins, J.V. Pierce, N. Yates, P.F. Highet, Herring, M. Mangkornkanok/Mark, R. Bahu, F. Carone, and J.J. Pisano, Characterization and localization of human renal kininogen. J. Biol. Chem. 256, 10634-10639 (1981).

13. J.T. McCormick and J. Senior, The effect of sex hormones on plasma kininogen levels in the rat. Arch. Int. Pharmacodyn. 210, 221-231 (1974).

14. J.T. McCormick and J. Senior, Plasma kinin and kininogen levels in the female rat during the oestrous cycle, pregnancy, parturition and the puerperium. Br. J. Pharmac. 50, 237-241 (1974).

15. C. Smith and A.M. Perks, The kinin system and ovulation changes in plasma kininogens and in kinin-forming enzymes in the ovaries and blood of rats with 4 day oestrous cycles. Can. J. Physiol. Vol 61. 736-742 (1983).

16. M. McDonald and A.M. Perks, Plasma bradykininogen and reproductive cycles: studies during the oestrous cycle and pregnancy in the rat, and in the human menstrual cycle. Can. J. Zool. Vol. 54, 941-947 (1975).

17. S.P. Prasad, V. Raviprakash, M. Sabir and N.K. Bhattacharyya, Changes in blood histamine and bradykininogen levels during different periods of the oestrous cycle in goats. J. Reprod. Fent. 42, 229-232 (1975).

18. L.L. Espey, D.H. Miller, and H.S. Margolius, Ovarian increase in kinin-generating capacity in PMSG/hCG-primed immature rat. Am. J. Physiol. 251, E362-E365 (1975).

19. A.H. Nielsen and F. Knudsen, Angiotensinogen is an acute-phase protein in man. Scand. J. Clin. Lab. Invest. 47, 175-178 (1987).

20. R. Kageyama, H. Ohkubo and S. Nakanishi, Induction of rat liver angiotensinogen mRNA following acute inflammation. Biochemical and Biophysical Research Communications Vol. 129 No. 3, 826-832 (1985).

21. V.J. Dzau and H.C. Hermann, Hormonal control of angiotensinogen production. Life Sciences Vol 30, 577-584 (1982).

22. O.M. Helmer and W.E. Judson, Influence of high renin substrate levels on renin-angiotensin system in pregnancy. Am. J. Obst. & Gynec. Vol. 99, No. 1, 9-17 (1967).

MONOCLONAL ANTIBODIES AGAINST THE COMPLEX BETWEEN HMW KININOGEN AND

CALPAIN I

Iwao Ohkubo, Shigeki Higashiyama and Makoto Sasaki

Department of Biochemistry, Nagoya City University Medical
School, Mizuho-ku, Nagoya 467, Japan

INTRODUCTION

High and low molecular weight kininogens (HMW and LMW kininogens)
are specific inhibitors towards thiol proteinases including cathepsins
(B, H, L), calpains (I, II), ficin and papain[1,2]. Recently, we reported[3]
that both kininogens are capable of forming instantly the complex with
calpains I and II in the presence of calcium ion. It is easily
speculated that both kininogens capture the thiol proteinases derived
from the damaged tissues and blood cells in pathological conditions such
as inflammation, immunological reaction, and cancer. However, little is
known about the vicissitude _in vivo_ of the complexes formed between
kininogens and thiol proteinases.

In this paper, as the first step to know the vicissitude of the
complexes _in vivo_, we report the attempt to prepare the monoclonal
antibodies recognizing the complex between HMW kininogen and calpain I,
and to establish an assay system for detection of the complex.

MATERIALS AND METHODS

Purification of HMW and LMW kininogens from human plasma

HMW kininogen was purified from fresh human plasma by DEAE-Sephadex
and Zinc-chelate Sepharose column chromatographies[4]. LMW kininogen was
also purified from fresh human plasma by a procedure employing DEAE-
Sephadex, DEAE-Sephacel, Red Sepharose, HA-Ultrogel and butyl-Toyopearl
(unpublished data).

Purification of calpains I and II

Calpain I from human erythrocytes[5] and calpain II from human liver
or kidney were purified by employing column chromatographies on DEAE-
cellulose, Ultrogel AcA 34, Blue Sepharose and DEAE Bio-Gel A.

Complex formation between kininogens and calpains

In order to form complexes between kininogens and calpains, a
reaction mixture containing kininogen and calpain was incubated for 10
min at 30°C in a kininogen to calpain molar ratio of 1:1 in 20 mM borate

buffer, pH 8.0, containing 5 mM $CaCl_2$ (N complex). Further, to form cross-linked complex (CL complex), the reaction mixture was added to 1 mM disuccinimidyl suberate[6], and it was incubated for an additional 30 min at room temperature. To confirm the complex formation, the reaction mixture was subjected to SDS polyacrylamide slab gel electrophoresis.

Cell fusion and antibody production

BALB/c mice were injected subcutaneously at weekly intervals with 10 µg of cross-linked complex between HMW kininogen and calpain I emulsified in Freund's complete adjuvant. Four days prior to fusion, the donor mice were injected intravenously with 10 µg of the complex in saline solution. Spleen cells of the mice were harvested, and fused with NS-1 mouse myeloma cells in the presence of 50% polyethylene glycol 1500[7]. Positive hybridoma cells surviving in HAT medium were identified by enzyme-linked immunosorbent assay (ELISA). The hybridoma cells then were subcloned by limiting dilution in HT (hypoxanthine-thymidine) medium, expanded and grown for 3 ~ 4 days in DMEM containing 1% Nutridoma SP by inoculation of 1×10^7 cells.

Screening of antibodies against complex by ELISA

Wells of 96-well microtiter plates were coated with 100 µl of CL-complex (5 µg/ml) in 20 mM Tris-HCl, pH 7.5, for 2 h at room temperature. The wells were washed three times with TBS-Tween buffer and blocked with 1% BSA in the same buffer for 1 h at room temperature. The wells were washed three times with TBS-Tween buffer, and 50 µl of hybridoma supernatant and 50 µl of TBS-TPB buffer were added to the wells and the plate was left for 2 h at room temperature. The wells were then washed three times with TBS-Tween buffer and 100 µl of peroxidase conjugated goat anti-mouse Igs (IgA, IgG and IgM), which were diluted 10^4-fold in TBS-TPB buffer, was added to the wells. The plate was left for 2 h at room temperature. The wells were washed three times with TBS-Tween buffer, and 100 µl of o-phenylenediamine (0.4 mg/ml) containing 1.82 mM H_2O_2 in 0.1 M citrate phosphate buffer, pH 5.0, was added to the wells in the dark. The enzymatic reaction was stopped after 10 min by the addition of 50 µl of 2 N H_2SO_4. The amount of peroxidase product in each well was estimated spectrophotometrically at 492 nm[8].

For competitive inhibition assay, 50 µl of competitor protein solution (0.1 ~ 500 µg/ml) and 50 µl of antibody solution (2 µg/ml) were added to the wells coated with antigen (CL complex or N complex). The plates were incubated for 4 h at room temperature. The following steps were performed as described above.

RESULTS AND DISCUSSION

Complex formation of HMW kininogen with calpain I was performed according to the method described in Materials and Methods, and analyzed by disc gel electrophoresis in the absence of SDS. As shown in Fig. 1, in a HMW kininogen to calpain I molar ratio of 1:1, complex formation was clearly observed, but the complex was easily dissociated by 20 mM EGTA. This suggests that the complex is linked with noncovalent bond(s).

In order to avoid dissociation of complex when the complex is immunized to animal(s), the complex of HMW kininogen and calpain I was cross-linked with disuccinimidyl suberate. As shown in Fig. 2 (lane B), the cross-linked complex was migrated with very slow mobility.

Several fusions of spleen cells from mice immunized with cross-linked complex of HMW kininogen and calpain I to NS-1 mouse myeloma

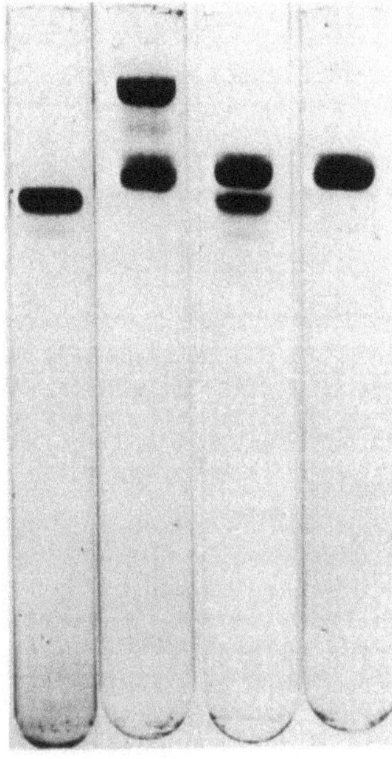

Fig. 1 Complex formation between HMW kininogen and calpain I in the
presence of 5 mM $CaCl_2$, and its dissociation by 20 mM EGTA.
A: calpain I, B: HMW kininogen·calpain I mixture (1:1) in the
presence of 5 mM $CaCl_2$, C: HMW kininogen·calpain I mixture with
20 mM EGTA, D: HMW kininogen.

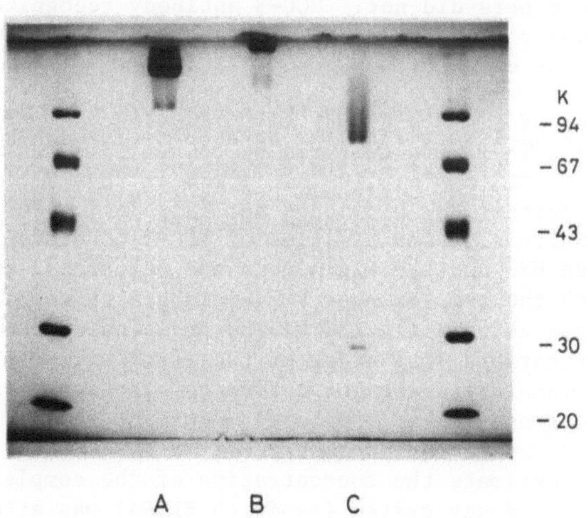

Fig. 2 SDS-polyacrylamide slab gel electrophoresis of HMW kininogen,
calpain I and cross-linked complex.
A: HMW kininogen, B: cross-linked complex, C: calpain I.

Table 1

Monoclonal antibodies to HMW KG - calpain I complex

Monoclonal antibodies	CL complex[b]	Calpain I	HMW KG[c]	N complex[d]	Subclass	Light chain subtype
HCC 1	0.53[a]	0	0	0	Ig M	κ
HCC 2	0.25	0	0	0	Ig M	κ
HCC 3	0.77	0.01	0	0.45	Ig M	κ
HCC 4	0.30	0	0	0.14	Ig M	κ
HCC 5	0.14	0.02	0	0	Ig M	κ
control	0	0	0	0		

a) Figures indicate absorbance at 492 nm. Antigens were bound to the microtiter plates at a concentration of 500 ng/100 μl/well (CL complex and N complex) or 250 ng/100 μl/well (Calpain I and HMW KG) overnight at 4°C. Antibodies were used as culture media containing 10% FCS. Optical density was measured at 15 min after the addition of substrate.
b) CL complex, cross-linked complex.
c) HMW KG, high molecular weight kininogen.
d) N complex, non-linked complex.

cells gave five hybridomas (HCC-1 ~ 5). These five hybridomas were subcloned further by limiting dilution. Large quantities of monoclonal antibodies were purified from DMEM containing 1% Nutridoma-SP with these hybridomas by ammonium sulfate precipitation at 50% saturation followed by chromatography on a Sephacryl S-300 column.

The class of immunoglobulin from each clone was determined by ELISA by using specific antisera to each mouse immunoglobulin class. The anti cross-linked HMW kininogen·calpain I complex antibodies obtained were found to be only IgM, and all five antibodies had κ light chains (Table 1).

Among these five monoclonal antibodies, both HCC-3 and -4 antibodies recognized noncross-linked HMW kininogen·calpain I complex (N complex), but others did not. HCC-3 antibody recognized the complex (N complex) stronger than HCC-4 did. Consequently, the monoclonal antibody, HCC-3 was used for subsequent studies.

Reactivities of HCC-3 antibody to CL complex, N complex, HMW kininogen and calpain I were analyzed by competitive inhibition assay. HCC-3 reacted with CL complex 150-fold stronger than N complex, while it reacted with neither HMW kininogen nor calpain I. Further, in the experiment of analysis of reactivities of HCC-3 to cross-linked complexes between HMW and LMW kininogens and calpains I and II, HCC-3 also reacted with the complexes of HMW kininogen·calpain I; and in turn with HMW kininogen·calpain II, LMW kininogen·calpain I and LMW kininogen· calpain II. Furthermore, the order of the reactivities of HCC-3 to noncross-linked complexes (see above four combinations) was similar to that of HCC-3 to cross-linked complexes (data not shown).

In order to estimate the concentration of the complex in the plasma, establishment of an assay system (sandwich ELISA) was attempted by using HCC-3. For this assay system, affinity purified anti calpain I IgG (polyclonal antibody) was used as a solid-phase antibody, and biotinylated HCC-3 as the first antibody and peroxidase conjugated avidin instead of the second antibody used in routine ELISA were employed (Fig. 3). Standard curves of cross-linked and noncross-linked HMW kininogen·calpain I complexes were shown in Fig. 4. It was possible

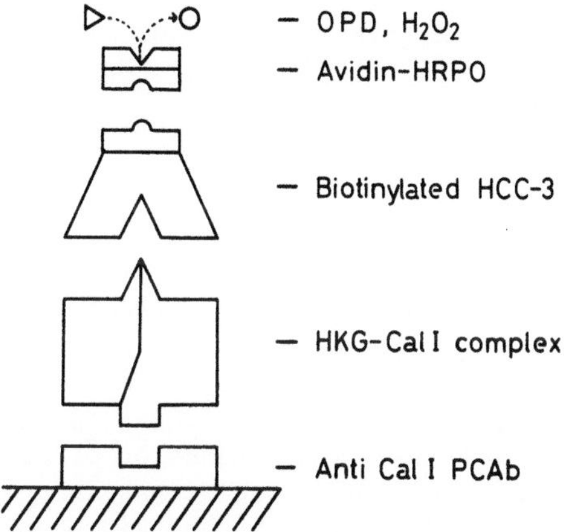

Fig. 3 Scheme of assay for HMW kininogen·calpain I complex.

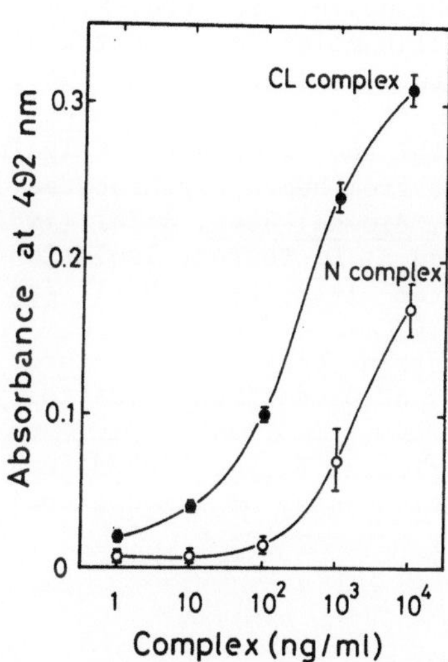

Fig. 4 Standard curves for determination of HMW kininogen·calpain I
complex level.
CL complex: cross-linked HMW kininogen·calpain I complex
N complex: noncross-linked HMW kininogen·calpain I complex

to estimate the amounts of the complexes up to 1 ng/ml (for CL complex)
and 100 ng/ml (for N complex), respectively. By using the standard
curves, the quantitative estimation of N complex level was practically
applied for normal plasma. Since the level of N complex in normal
plasma (n=5) was less than 100 ng/ml, a more sensitive assay method to
detect trace amounts of the complex must be established. Obviously, the
establishment of the assay system using monoclonal antibodies to the
complex(es) will be useful for the clinical applications, namely, the
qualitative and quantitative investigations of kininogens, calpains and
their complexes in various pathological states such as tissue
inflammation and cancer.

REFERENCES

1. M. Sasaki, K. Taniguchi, K. Suzuki and K. Imahori, Human plasma α_1-
   and α_2-thiol proteinase inhibitors strongly inhibit Ca-activated
   neutral protease from muscle, Biochem. Biophys. Res. Commun., 110:
   256 (1983).
2. T. Sueyoshi, K. Enjoji, T. Shimada, H. Kato, S. Iwanaga, Y. Bando, E.
   Kominami and N. Katunuma, A new function of kininogens as thiol-
   proteinase inhibitors: Inhibition of papain and cathepsins B, H
   and L by bovine, rat and human plasma kininogens, FEBS Lett., 182:
   193 (1985).
3. H. Ishiguro, S. Higashiyama, C. Namikawa, M. Kunimatsu, E. Takano, K.
   Tanaka, I. Ohkubo, T. Murachi and M. Sasaki, Interaction of human
   calpains I and II with high molecular weight and low molecular
   weight kininogens and their heavy chain: Mechanism of interaction
   and the role of divalent cations, Biochemistry, 26:2863 (1987).
4. S. Higashiyama, I. Ohkubo, H. Ishiguro, M. Kunimatsu, K. Sawaki and
   M. Sasaki, Human high molecular weight kininogen as a thiol
   proteinase inhibitor: Presence of the entire inhibition capacity
   in the native form of heavy chain, Biochemistry, 25:1669 (1986).
5. M. Hatanaka, T. Kikuchi and T. Murachi, Calpain I, a low Ca^{2+}-
   requiring protease from human erythrocytes: Purification and
   subunit structure, Biomed. Res., 4:381 (1983).
6. I. Sen, H. G. Bull and R. L. Soffer, Isolation of an angiotensin II-
   binding protein from liver, Proc. Natl. Acad. Sci. USA, 81:1679
   (1984).
7. G. Köhler and C. Milstein, Continuous cultures of fused cells
   secreting antibody of predefined specificity, Nature (London),
   256:495 (1975).
8. E. Engvall and P. Perlmann, Enzyme-linked immunosorbent assay
   (ELISA), Quantitative assay of immunoglobulin G, Immunochemistry,
   8:871 (1971).

KININ-CONTAINING KININOGEN IS PRESENT IN HUMAN SEMINAL PLASMA

Edwin Fink*, Wolf-Bernhard Schill** and Werner Miska**

Abteilung für Klinische Chemie und Klinische Biochemie in der
Chirurgischen Klinik Innenstadt* and Dermatologische Klinik und
Poliklinik** der Universität München

INTRODUCTION

It has been shown recently that human seminal plasma contains the components of tissue kallikrein-kinin systems: tissue kallikrein, kininases
and kininogens. Both tissue kallikrein and kininases are present in seminal
plasma in enzymatically active forms (1-3); kininogens, however, have been
demonstrated by immunological methods (2,4) which did not allow to distinguish between kinin-containing and kinin-free kininogen.

It was the aim of the present study to elucidate whether kininogen of
seminal plasma contains the kinin moiety and, hence, can react as an active
component of the tissue kallikrein kinin system.

METHODS

The ejaculates investigated were either from healthy donors or from
men attending the andrological service. The semen was obtained by masturba-
tion after 3-5 days of sexual abstinence.

In order to block proteolytic enzymes including tissue kallikrein and
kininases semen samples were mixed with an equal volume of 123 mM NaCl, 5 mM
KCl, 37 mM Tris/HCl, 90 mM EDTA, 9 mM 1,10-phenanthroline, 10 mM 4-chloro-
mercuribenzoic acid, 20 mg/l aprotinin, 3 mM phenylmethylsulfonyl fluoride,
ph 8.0. After 5 min centrifugation at 10 000 g the supernatant seminal plasma
was removed and stored at -20 °C.

The seminal plasma samples were analyzed by measuring the kinin contents of ethanolic extracts of each sample both with and without trypsin
treatment. In this way total kinin (= free + releasable kinin) and free
kinin were determined, the difference representing the kinin-containing
kininogen. For the determination of free kinin 0.05 ml of seminal plasma
were mixed with 0.5 ml 100 % ethanol and incubated for 10 min at 70 °C.
After 10 min centrifugation at 10 000 g the supernatant was transferred to
a second tube and evaporated to dryness. For determination of total kinin
0.09 ml seminal plasma were mixed with 0.01 ml 0.27 M HCl, after 15 min at
37 °C 0.01 ml of 0.25 M NaOH, 0.15 ml 0.3 M Tris/HCl, pH 7.8, and 0.01 ml
of a solution of bovine trypsin, 10 mg/ml in 2.5 mM HCl, were added. After
30 min at 37 oC 1.0 ml 100 % ethanol was added and proceeded as described

above. The kinin contained in the dry residues was measured by a radioimmunoassay as previously described (3).

The time course of kinin release was investigated by incubating ejaculate at 25 and 37 $^{\circ}$C. At certain time intervals aliquots were removed,
mixed with an equal volume of the inhibitor containing buffer (cf. above)
and analyzed as described.

RESULTS AND DISCUSSION

Kininogen Contents of Seminal Plasma

In earlier studies we had not been able to detect free or releasable
kinin in samples of human seminal plasma. However, these samples had been
obtained after all routine determinations of semen parameters had been performed and without taking any precautions to prevent kinin release and degradation. Since seminal plasma contains enzymatically active tissue kallikrein and also kininases (1-3) one has to expect that during normal treatment of the samples for routine analysis any kinin present in kininogens
will be released and free kinin will be degraded.

Therefore, in the present study the seminal plasma samples were mixed
with a buffer containing inhibitors for tissue kallikrein, kininases and
other proteinases either immediately after ejaculation or – in the case of
patient specimen – after liquefaction (i. e. 0.5–1 h after ejaculation). A
total number of 11 samples has been analyzed (Tables 1 and 2).

In all samples kinin could be released by treatment with typsin (Tables 1 and 2). Free kinin was present in all samples to which the inhibitor
buffer had been added immediately after ejaculation (Table 2) and, though
at a lower concentration, in most samples to which the inhibitors had been
added with a time-lag (Table 1).

Table 1. Kinin Contents of Semen Samples to which Inhibitor
          Buffer was Added 0.5–1.0 h after Ejaculation.

Sample Nr.	Free Kinin pmole/ml	Total Kinin pmole/ml	Releasable Kinin pmole/ml
1	1.2	7.6	6.4
2	1.6	5.8	4.2
3	0.9	6.7	5.8
4	0.5	8.3	7.8
5	0	1.6	1.6
6	0	9.1	9.1
7	1.3	4.4	3.1
Mean value	0.8	6.2	5.4
± SEM	0.24	1.0	1.0

Table 2. Kinin Contents of Semen Samples to which Inhibitor
          Buffer was Added Immediately after Ejaculation.

Sample Nr.	Free Kinin pmole/ml	Total Kinin pmole/ml	Releasable Kinin pmole/ml
8	3.4	8.8	5.4
9	0.9	5.0	4.1
10	2.9	4.8	1.9
11	5.2	8.5	3.3
Mean value	3.1	6.8	3.7
± SEM	0.9	1.1	0.7

The free kinin present even if the inhibitor mixture was added immediately after ejaculation may represent either kinin release within the
male tract prior to ejaculation or after ejaculation during the time elaps-
ing until all kininogenase activity is blocked by the added inhibitors. The
latter explanation seems less probable with regard to the relatively slow
kinin release in ejaculates (Fig. 1).

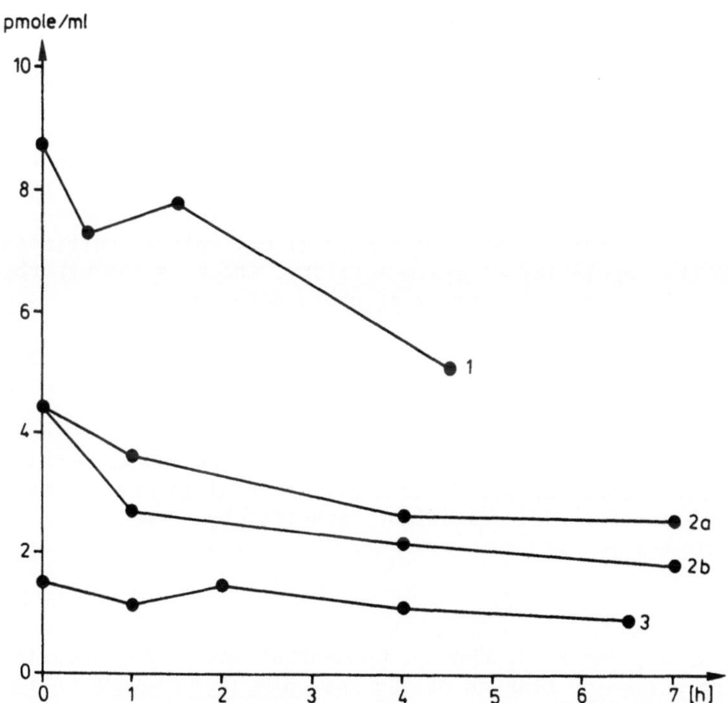

Fig. 1 Time course of the decrease of kinin-containing ki-
        ninogen in seminal plasma. Three semen samples with
        different kininogen levels obtained between 0.5 and
        1 h after ejaculation were incubated at 25 $^{\circ}$C (curves
        1, 2a and 3) and at 37 $^{\circ}$C (curve 2b) and the releas-
        able kinin determined after certain time intervalls.

The concentrations of total kinin are of the same order of magnitude
as but still clearly lower than the concentrations of 11.5–38.2 pmole/ml
reported by Schill et al (4) for total immunoreactive kininogen which represents the sum of kinin-free and kinin-containing kininogens. However,
because of the low number of investigated samples in both studies, any
discussion of this difference would be meaningful only if both parameters
were measured in the same samples. Unfortunately, the direct enzyme immunoassay for total kininogen was not available during our studies.

Studies on the Rate of Kinin Release

The time course of kinin release was followed by incubating whole
ejaculates at 25 or 37 ^{o}C and determining free and total kinin in the seminal plasma at certain time intervals. These studies revealed that kinin is
liberated at a rather low rate both at 25 and 37 ^{o}C (Fig. 1). Compared to
the kallikrein activity the kininase activity is obviously high since no
free kinin was detectable in the incubated samples. The low rate of kinin
liberation is easily understandable since both tissue kallikrein (3) and
the substrate kininogen are present in semen in low concentrations. In addition, one has to assume that the kallikrein activity is continuously reduced by complex formation with the slow reacting α_1-proteinase inhibitor
which is also present in seminal plasma (4).

CONCLUSIONS

It has been demonstrated for the first time that kinin-containing kininogen is present in human seminal plasma. Thus, all components necessary
for a functional kallikrein-kinin system are present in human semen in a
biologically active form.

In ejaculates kinin is released continuously at a low rate for at
least several hours. Because of concomitant degradation of the released
kinin the actual kinin concentration in ejaculate is very low but maintained for several hours. The low kinin level may well be sufficient to
take part in the regulating of sperm motility, which is the hypothetical
role of the kallikrein-kinin system of human semen.

ACKNOWLEDGMENT

This work was supported by the Deutsche Forschungsgemeinschaft, Sonderforschungsbereich 207, B2, B3. We are very grateful to Mrs. G. Godec and
Mrs. C. Hirschauer for their excellent technical assistance.

REFERENCES

1. Cushman, D. W., and H. S. Cheung, Concentrations of angiotensin-
   converting enzyme in tissues of the rat. Biochim. Biophys. Acta (Amst.)
   250:261–265, (1971).

2. Palm, S., and H. Fritz, Components of the kallikrein-kinin-system
   in human midcycle cervical mucus and seminal plasma. In: "Kallikrein",
   G. L. Haberland, J. W. Rohen, C. Schirren and P. Huber, Eds., Schattauer
   Verlag, Stuttgart, pp. 17–21, (1975).

3. Fink, E., W.-B. Schill, F. Fiedler, F. Krassnigg, R. Geiger, and K. Shimamoto, Tissue kallikrein of human seminal plasma is secreted by the
   prostate gland. Biol. Chem. Hoppe-Seyler 366:917–924, (1985).

4. Schill, W.-B., F. Krassnigg, W. Müller-Esterl, and E. Fink, Quantitative determination of different proteins in normal and pathological semen. Protides Biol. Fluids, Proc. Colloq. 32:293-297, (1985).

4. Schill, W.-B., F. Krassnigg, W. Müller-Esterl, and E. Fink, Quantitative determination of different proteins in normal and pathological semen. Protides Biol. Fluids, Proc. Colloq. 32:293-297, (1985).

STUDIES OF THE CLEAVAGE OF HUMAN HIGH MOLECULAR WEIGHT KININOGEN
BY PURIFIED PLASMA AND TISSUE KALLIKREINS, AND UPON CONTACT
ACTIVATION OF PLASMA

Sesha Reddigari and Allen P. Kaplan

Division of Allergy, Rheumatology, and Clinical Immunology
Department of Medicine, SUNY-Stony Brook, HSC
Stony Brook, New York 11794-8161

INTRODUCTION

Activation of the Hageman factor dependent pathways in human plasma
leads to cleavage of HMW-Kininogen (HMWK) at LYS-ARG and ARG-SER bonds
with release of the vasoactive peptide bradykinin[1]. This leaves two chains
that are disulfide linked which are separable upon reduction[2]. The N-
terminal chain has been shown to be a cysteine-protease inhibitor while the
C-terminal chain is a coagulation cofactor[2,3-7]. This latter activity is
dependent upon binding to initiating surfaces and interaction with PK and
factor XI[8,9]. Prior studies have demonstrated that those two chains have
similar molecular weights; in some studies indistinguishable on SDS gels[7,10,11]
and in others, appearing as a heavy chain of 62,000 daltons (N-
terminal chain) and a light chain of 56,000 daltons (C-terminal chain)[12-14]
. The latter is subsequently cleaved to 45,000[2,5]. Factor XIa has
also been shown to be capable of cleaving the light chain so as to destroy
its coagulant activity[15]. We have prepared monoclonal antibodies to the
heavy and light chain of HMWK and in this study, have used an anti-LC
monoclonal to assess the chain size and evolution upon kallikrein activation of purified HMWK and activation of NHP and plasma congenitally deficient in contact factors. Further we have assessed the LC coagulant activity of these plasmas with increasing time of incubation with kaolin and
dextran sulfate and demonstrate that proteolysis of the LC in plasma is not
a significant control mechanism. Finally we demonstrate the potential use
of immunoblotting for quantitative assessment of HMWK cleavage.

<u>Monoclonal Antibodies</u>: Monoclonal antibodies (MAbs) to the HMWK light
and heavy chains were prepared by the method of Lipsich et al[16]. Anti-
LC MAbs were produced by immunizing the mice with native HMWK. Anti-HC
MAbs were made by immunizing the mice with purified reduced and alkylated
HC which was a gift from Dr. Werner Muller-Esterl (Univ. Munich, Munich,
W. Germany). Ascites fluids were prepared by intraperitoneal injection
of 2-3 x 10[6] cells of active subcloned hybridoma cells into pristane-
treated Balb/c female mice (retired breeders).

Antibody isotyping was done by ELISA techniques using a commercial
isotyping kit (from Southern Biotechnology Associates, Birmingham, Ala).
Antibodies were purified by 40% ammonium sulfate precipitation followed
by ion-exchange chromatography on DE-52 (Whatman) in 10mM Tris-HCl

(pH 8.0) and eluted with a 0-0.3 M NaCl gradient in the same buffer.
Peak fractions containing anti-LC activity were pooled, concentrated to
3.0 mg/ml, and stored at -70°C.

<u>Activation of Plasma with Kaolin and Dextran Sulfate</u>: NHP or plasmas de-
ficient in Factor XII, PK or Factor XI were activated with 2 mg/ml kaolin
(stock 20 mg/ml in PBS) at 37°C[15] with frequent agitation. Aliquots were
withdrawn at indicated time points and either diluted 1-10 into TBS and
added to the coagulation assay mixture or added to SDS-PAGE sample buffer
and heat-denatured immediately. Activation of plasma with dextran sulfate
(mol. wt. 500,000) was performed at 4°C as described by Van der Graaf et
al.[17] at a final concentration of 12.5ug/ml. Samples at various time
points were taken for immunoblotting and determination of HMWK coagulant
activity as described earlier.

<u>Enzyme Linked Immunosorbant Assay (ELISA)</u>: ELISA's were performed by
standard procedures with 96-well microtiter plate (Dynatech, Immulon-2).
Wells were coated with 20 or 40 ng of antigen in 0.05M sodium carbonate
buffer (pH 9.6) by incubation at 4°C overnight. Blocking was for 30 min
at 37°C with 3% BSA in PBS. Wells were then incubated with various dilutions of primary antibody in PBS containing 0.05%-Tween-20 for 2 hrs
followed by a 2 hr incubation with the secondary antibody, [goat anti-
mouse IgG (gamma chain) conjugated to alkaline phosphatase, Jackson Im-
munoresearch] at a dilution suggested by the manufacturer. After washing, p-nitrophenylphosphate (1 mg/ml) in 10% diethanolamine-HCl buffer
(pH 9.6) was added to the wells and the absorbance read at 405 nm on a
Dynatech ELISA reader.

<u>Immunoblotting</u>: Proteins were electroblotted from gels onto nitrocellu-
lose sheets (0.2u, BA83, Schleicher and Schuell) according to Towbin
et al[18]. Following transfer, the nitrocellulose membrane was treated
with 3% BSA in PBS-Tween at room temperature for 1 hour to block the unbound sites. The membrane was then treated with a 1:1000 dilution of
primary antibody at room temperature for 2 hrs, rinsed and then treated
with goat anti-mouse IgG (gamma chain) - alkaline phosphatase conjugate
in PBS-Tween at a dilution suggested by the manufacturer for 2 hrs at
room temperature. The final wash was done in PBS-Tween containing 0.5M
NaCl for 1 hr at 37°C. The bands were developed in substrate mixture
containing 5-bromo-4-chrlorindoxyl phosphate and nitroblue tetrazoleum
in Tris-HCl buffer (pH 9.5)[19].

RESULTS

<u>Immunoblotting of HMWK after Digestion with Plasma Kallikrein</u>: A time
course of digestion of HMWK by purified plasma kallikrein was performed
and subjected to SDS-PAGE under reducing and nonreducing conditions
(Fig. 1). The slab gel was then immunoblotted with anti-LC MAb. As can
be seen in Fig. 1, under non-reducing conditions, the antibody recognized
major bands of native HMWK at 120 Kd and 103 Kd. A minor band is seen at
about 116 Kd. With increasing time of digestion the 120 Kd material was
converted to bands seen at 103 Kd and 96 Kd.

Upon reduction bands were seen at zero time, at 116 Kd, 100 Kd,
85 Kd, 62 Kd,and 49 Kd indicating that HMWK used in these experiments
was partially cleaved although these cleavage products were not that apparent in coomassie blue stained gels at zero time (Fig. 1). The 116 Kd,
100 Kd and 85 Kd bands were very quickly digested and as digestion proceeded, the 62 Kd band became more intense (Fig. 1, 10 min.) and then
appeared to decrease in intensity while the band seen at 49 Kd
progressively increased (Fig. 1).

NHP and Factor XI-deficient plasmas were activated with dextran sulfate. Aliquots immediately before and 5, 10, and 30 minutes after the addition of dextran sulfate were immunoblotted. The results shown in Fig. 2 indicate that in NHP, HMWK was cleaved almost completely within five minutes and the two LC forms could be seen at 62 Kd and 49 Kd, respectively. At ten minutes, the 62 Kd form was fainter and the 49 Kd form was more intense. by thirty minutes, all the 62 Kd form was converted to the lower form. In Factor XI-deficient plasma the cleavage was minimal at five minutes but thereafter it was similar to NHP. When plasma deficient in prekallikrein is similarly examined the rate of disappearance of native HMWK is slow relative to normal or factor XI deficient plasma and some uncleaved HMWK can still be seen after 2 hrs. The 62 Kd form of LC remains prominent and conversion to 49 Kd is minimal even after ninety minutes of incubation. There was no apparent cleavage of HMWK in factor XII deficient plasma.

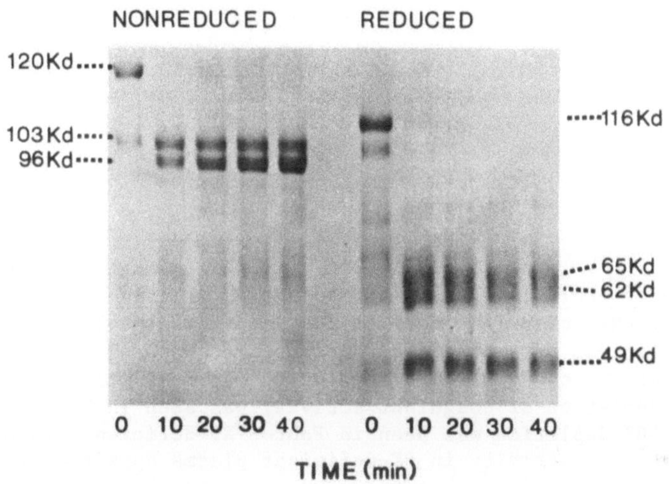

Figure 1. HMWK digestion with plasma kallikrein. HMWK was incubated with plasma kallikrein at 1% wt/wt of enzyme/substrate. Samples at indicated time points were electrophoresed under reducing and non-reducing conditions and immunoblotted with anti LC Mab.

It can be seen from Fig. 1 that the cleavage pattern of HMW kininogen in non reduced gels can be followed by immunoblotting. Further, if the total kininogen content of plasma is known, the ratio of the stained binding intensity at 105,000 plus 95,000 divided by the staining intensity at 120,000 gives the fraction cleaved. Fig. 2 demonstrates that these binds can be assessed in whole plasma as well as with purified components. In Fig. 3 is shown a dose response curve obtained by immunoblotting increasing quantities of NHP (in duplicate) and the average values for each quantity plotted against staining intensity. The linearity of values obtained for uncleaved HMWK (Fig 3) as well as for cleaved HMWK (not shown) suggest that our method for immunoblotting and quantitation of stained bands can be applied to plasma samples with varying degrees of activation. The calculated value for cleaved HMWK allows one to estimate the theoretical quantity of liberated bradykinin.

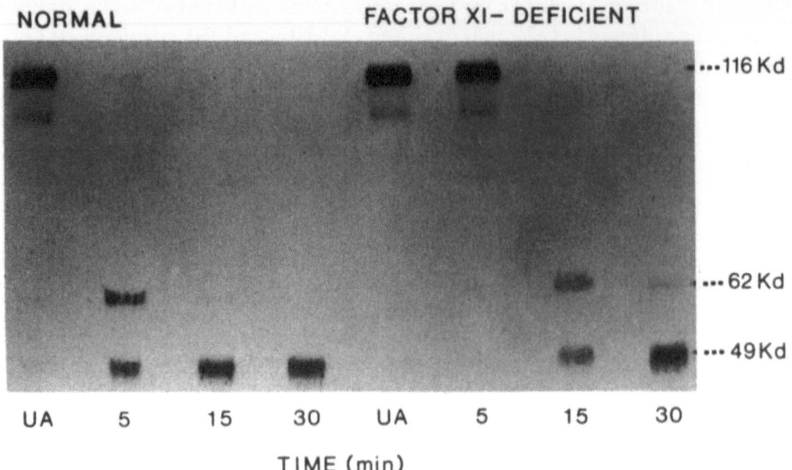

Figure 2.   Immunoblot of unactivated (UA) or dextran sulfate activated NHP and Factor XI-deficient plasma. Plasma samples were activated for indicated times with dextran sulfate.

<u>Time Course of Depletion of HMWK Coagulant Activity</u>: A time course of depletion of HMWK coagulant activity during the first 30 min of activation by kaolin was next assessed. Aliquots of each sample were diluted, added to HMWK deficient plasma and clotted for residual HMWK. Approximately 30% depletion of coagulant activity was seen in NHP by 30 min while only 18% depletion was seen in Factor XI-deficient plasma. Depletion of coagulant activity in PK-deficient plasma appeared slower during the initial twenty minutes but was very close to the other two plasmas by 30 minutes. When NHP was activated with dextran sulfate for 24 hours, its HMWK coagulant activity decreased by 60% whereas in similarly treated Factor XI-deficient plasma, the decrease was 40% (Table I).

Table 1.   HMWK-Dependent Coagulant Activity in Dextran sulfate Activated Plasma

Plasma	HMWK-Dependent Activity (units/ml)	
	Unactivated	24 hr Activation
NHP	1.4 (100%)	0.55 (39.3%)
Factor XI Deficient	0.95 (100%)	0.58 (61%)

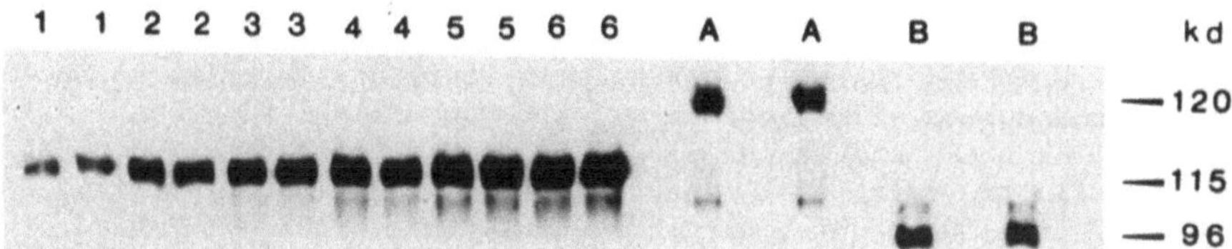

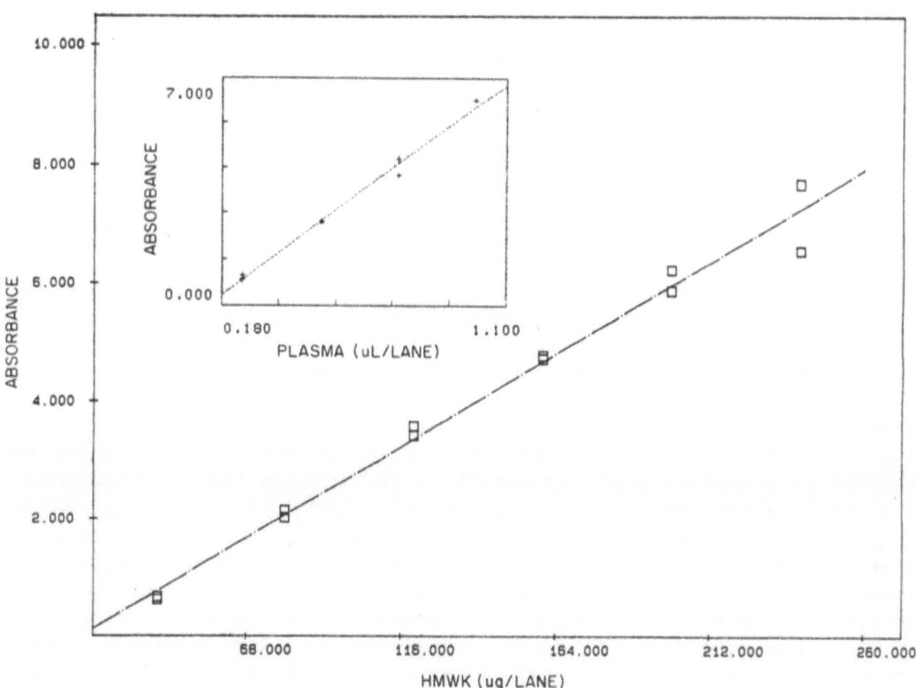

Figure 3. Upper panel shows immunoblotting pattern of six doses of HMW-Kininogen each of which is immunoblotted in duplicate. A and B represent 2ul of plasma that is either native (A) or fully activated (B) to show the difference in mobility and the comparable staining intensity. Below is shown the dose response of absorbance/ug HMWK and the inset shows the same analysis of dilutions of plasma.

DISCUSSION

It is known that when purified HMWK is cleaved by purified plasma kallikrein, two initial cleavages result in bradykinin release and formation of a two chain form of HMWK in which one chain is susceptible to further proteolysis. Some reports indicate that reduction of kinin-free HMWK yields chains of equal size (65 Kd) on SDS gel electrophoresis[7,10,11]. Others find a LC of 56,000 distinguishable from the heavy chain, which then undergoes further digestion[12-14]. We considered the possibility that LCs of 62-65,000, 56,000, and 46-49,000 form sequentially and that conversion of the 62-65,000 form to the 56,000 form might be exceedingly rapid and therefore variable in different experiments in different laboratories. Immunoblotting, with an anti-LC monoclonal allows one to follow this pattern in gels without superimposed HC. Our data indicate only two forms of LC when we assess digestion of purified HMWK by kallikrein. The 62 Kd band can be converted to the 49 Kd band progressively[13] and the rate is proportional to the enzyme concentration. We also confirm the relative inability of tissue kallikrein to convert the 62 Kd LC to 46-49 Kd during the digestion times utilized in our experiments. Further slow conversion can be seen but requires many hours of digestion[11]. Berretini et al[20] have also utilized anti-LC and anti-HC monoclonals to demonstrate cleavage of HMWK. They reported similar cleavage products when assessed non-reduced but upon reduction the LC forms could not be clearly delineated on their immunoblots.

Although kallikrein is clearly the primary enzyme required for the generation of bradykinin, other enzymes also can cleave HMWK. These include Factor XIIa[21], Factor XIa[15], and plasmin[22]. The pattern of digestion of HMWK by Factor XIIa is similar to that seen with kallikrein, but the rate of cleavage is considerably slower. Factor XIa, however, has a different cleavage pattern and results in formation of a LC of 45,000 (the same as that formed by kallikrein and XIIa) and a larger chain of 75,000 daltons. Further cleavage of the latter protein resulted in formation of a HC of 65,000, a 10,000 dalton peptide and bradykinin. The 45,000 dalton species, responsible for the coagulant activity is further digested into smaller peptides resulting in complete loss of coagulant activity[15]. This led to the suggestion that Factor XIa might be responsible for the depletion of LC coagulant activity in plasma following the initiation of clotting. When NHP was activated with dextran sulfate, the same two LC forms were observed, although almost all the 62 Kd form was converted to 49 Kd within ten minutes which remained stable. Factor XII deficient plasma did not activate. PK deficient plasma showed a marked diminution in rate of activation as well as no conversion of the 62 Kd LC to the 49 Kd LC. These are each kallikrein dependent processes thus those cleavages seen are due to interaction of factor XIIa[21] or perhaps Factor XIa with HMWK.

The decrease in coagulant activity observed for NHP or factor XI deficient plasma with prolonged incubation with either kaolin or dextran sulfate was relatively small, the maximum of 60% loss occurred after a 24 hr. incubation with dextran sulfate (Table I). Thus although Factor XI has been reported to function as a control protein which inactivates HMWK, considering that a level of HMWK of 15% is sufficient to normalize coagulation in kininogen deficient plasma[23] and any error inherent in our clotting assay would not change our data from 70% residual activity to less than 15%, the data presented here indicate that proteolytic inactivation of the LC or HMWK by Factor XIa or other enzymes is too slow to be an important control mechanism.

Frankly, we have adapted immunoblotting using an anti light chain monoclonal antibody for quantitation of the cleavage of HMW-kininogen in human plasma. Such an assay is dependent upon the linearity of band quantitation (Fig. 3) for native and cleaved HMW kininogen and proportionality between the loss of native material and gain of bands representing the cleavage product. We hope to combine such an assay with methods for determination of enzyme inhibitor complexes[24,25], radioimmunoassay of bradykinin[26], and assessment of kinin degradation products as a profile of the status of the intrinsic coagulatin-kinin system that can be applied to a wide variety of disorders.

REFERENCES

1. J.V. Pierce, M.E.Webster. Purification and some properties of the two different kallidinogens, in "Hypotensive Peptides", Erdos, E.G., Back, N., Sicuteri, F. (eds) Springer, New YOrk, (1966).

2. R.E. Thompson, R. Mandle, Jr., A.P. Kaplan. Characterization of human high molecular weight kininogen. Procoagulant activity associated with the light chain of kinin-free high molecular weight kininogen. J. Exp. Med. 147:488 (1978).

3. T. Sueyoshi, K. Enjyoji, T. Shimada, H. Kato, S. Iwanaga, Y. Bando, E. Kominami, N.L. Katunuma. A function of kininogens as thiol-proteinase inhibitors: inhibition of papain and cathepsins B, H, & L by bovine, rat, and human plasma kininogens. FEBS Letters 182:193 (1985).

4. W. Muller-Esterl, H. Fritz, I.W. Machleidt, A. Ritonja, J. Brzin, M. Kotnik, V. Turk, J. Kellermann, F. Lottspeich. Human plasma kininogens are identical with α_2-cysteine protease inhibitors. Evidence from immunological, enzymological, and sequence data. FEBS Lett 182:310 (1985).

5. D.M. Keribiriou, J.H. Griffin: High molecular weight kininogen. Studies of structure-function relationships and of proteolysis of the molecule occurring during contact activation of plasma. J. Biol Chem. 254:12020 (1979)

6. R.E. Thompson, R. Mandle Jr., A.P. Kaplan. Studies of the binding of prekallikrein and factor XI to high molecular weight kininogen and its light chain. Proc. Natl Acad Sci USA, 76:4862 (1979).

7. P.E. Bock, J.D. Shore. Protein-protein interactions in contact activation of blood coagulation. Characterization of a fluorescein-labeled human high molecular weight kininogen light chain as a probe. J Biol Chem 258:15079 (1983).

8. R. Mandle Jr., R.W. Coleman, A.P. Kaplan. Identification of prekallikrein and HMW-kininogen as a circulating complex in human plasma. Proc Natl Acad Sci USA 73:4174 (1976).

9. R.E. Thompson, R. Mandle Jr., A.P. Kaplan. Association of Factor XI and high molecular weight kininogen in human plasma. J. Clin Invest 60:1376 (1977).

10. S. Schiffman, C. Mannhalter, D. Tynerk. Human high molecular weight kininogen. Effects of cleavage by kallikrein on protein structure and procoagulant activity. J. Biol Chem. 255:6433 (1980).

11. M. Maier, K.F. Austen, J. Spragg. characterization of the procoagulant chain derived from high molecular weight kininogen (Fitzgerald factor) by tissue kallikrein. Blood 62:457 (1983).

12. T. Nakayasa, S. Nagasawa. Studies on human kininogen I. Isolation, characterization and cleavage by plasma kallikrein of high molecular weight (HMW) kininogen. J. Biochem 85:249 (1979).

13. K. Mori, S. Nagasawa.: Studies on human high molecular weight (HMW) kininogen II. Structural change of HMW-kininogen by the action of human plasma kallikrein II. J. Biochem 84:1465 (1981).

14. C.F. Scott, L.D. Silver, M. Schapira, R.W. Colman. Cleavage of human high molecular weight kininogen markedly enhances its coagulant activity. Evidence that this molecule exists as a procofactor. J. Clin Invest 73:954 (1984).

15. S.F. Scott, L.D. Silver, A.D. Purdon, R.W. Colman. Cleavage of human high molecular weight kininogen by Factor XIa in vitro. Effect on structure and function. J. Biol. Chem. 260:10856 (1985).

16. L.A. Lipsich, A.J. Lewis, J.S. Brugge. Isolation of monoclonal antibodies that recognize the transforming proteins of avian sarcoma viruses. J. Virology 48:352 (1983).

17. F. Van Der Graaf, F.J.A. Keus, R.A.A. Vlooswijk, B.N. Bouma. The contact activation mechanism in human plasma: Activation induced by dextran sulfate. Blood 59:1225, (1982).

18. H. Towbin, T. Staehelin, J. Gordon. Electrophoretic transfer of proteins from polyacrylamide gels to nitrocellulose sheets. Proc Natl Acad Sci. USA 76:4350 (1979).

19. M.S. Blake, K.H. Johnston, G.J. Russel-Jones, E.C. Gotschlich. A rapid, sensitive method for detection of alkaline phosphatase-conjugated anti-antibody on Western blots. Anal Biochem 136:175 (1984).

20. M. Berrettini, B. Laemmle, T. White, M. Jo Heeb, H.P. Schwartz, B. Zuraw, J. Curd, J. Griffin. Detection of in vitro and in vivo cleavage of high molecular weight kininogen in human plasma by immunoblotting with monoclonal antibodies. Blood 68:455 (1986).

21. R.C. Wiggins. Kinin release from high molecular weight kininogen by the action of Hageman factor in the absence of kallikrein. J. Biol Chem 258:8963 (1983).

22. F.M. Habal, c.E. Burrowes, H.Z. Movat. Generation of kinin by plasma kallikrein and plasmin and the effect of α_1-antitrypsin and anti-thrombin III on kininogenases. In "Advances in Experimental Medicine and Biology" Vol 70 – Kinins Pharmacodynamics and Biological Roles ed F. Sicuteri, N. Back, and G.L. Haberland, Plenum Press, N.Y. (1975).

23. R.W. Colman, A. Bagdasarian, R.C. Talamo, C.F. Scott, M. Seavey, J.A. Guimaraes, J.V. Pierce, A.P. Kaplan. Williams trait in human kininogen deficiency with diminished levels of plasminogen activator and prekallikrein associated with abnormalities of the Hageman factor dependent pathways. J Clin Invest 56:1650 (1975).

RADIOIMMUNOASSAY OF KININS AND ITS APPLICATION TO PURIFICATION OF

KININOGENS

Toshiyuki Yasui and Takao Saruta

Department of Internal Medicine, Keio University
35 Shinanomachi, Shinjuku, Tokyo 160 Japan

INTRODUCTION

Bradykinin, which decreases vascular resistence and increases
sodium diuresis, is considered to play an important role in pathogenesis
of hypertension. Kininogens, either precursors of kinins or thiol
proteinase inhibitor[1], can be supposed to participate in pathogenesis of
hypertension. Recent progress in technology of molecular biology enabled
us to manifest the mechanism of biosynthesis of kininogens[2,3]. However,
in review of the literatures, physiological contribution of kininogens
to pathogenesis of hypertension has not yet been fully elucidated. We
consider specific quantitation for both substances such as immunoassay
is essential to reveal patho-physiological role of kininogens in
hypertension. Although immunoassay for human kininogens has been already
reported[9,10,11], the assay has not yet been popular means to investigate
the pathophysiology of hypertension.
In the present study, we developed radioimmunoassay for kinins and
attempted to apply the radioimmunoassay to purification of high
molecular weight kininogen. Furthermore, we attempted to solve the
problem on the extraction of kinins from blood, which has been a matter
of debate for a long time.

MATERIALS AND METHODS

CHEMICALS

Bradykinin, lys-bradykinin and met-lys-bradykinin were purchased
from Peptide Institutes. Des-arg[1]-bradykinin, des-arg[9]-bradykinin and
des-phe[8]-arg[9]-bradykinin were purchased from Bachem. Crystalized bovine
serum albumin was of Sigma. Aprotinin and gabexate mesilate was generous
gift from Bayer Pharmaceutical and Ono Phramceutical, respectively.
DEAE-cellulose, SP-Toyopearl (polyvinyl based matrix) and epoxy-
activated-Sepharose were products of Whatman, Tosoh, Pharmacia,
respectively. Chelating agarose affinity media was made by coupling of
epoxy-activated Sepharose with imino-diacetic acid. Octadecyl silica
cartridge column (Sepak C_{18}) was of Waters Associates. Radio-iodinated
tyr[8]-bradykinin was purchased from New England Nuclear Research
Products. All other reagents were of reagent grade.

ANTI-BRADYKININ-ANTISERA

According to the metohod of Shimamoto et al.[4], 25 mg of bradykinin
was conjugated with 50mg of crystalized bovine serum albumin in the
presence of water-soluble carbo-diimide. Three New Zealand White rabbits
were immunized by the multiple injection of 25ug of the conjugate in
emulsion with Freund's adjuvant (per one rabbit) every two weeks for one
month and after then every four weeks for five month. Characterization
of the raised antisera was done by radioimmunoassay described below.

RADIOIMMUNOASSAY

Incubation buffer and incubation time was optimized by a few
attempts as described in the results. One reaction tube was composed of
$100\mu l$ of appropriately diluted sample, $200\mu l$ of diluted antisera and
$200\mu l$ of buffer containing radio-labeled bradykinin. According to the
results as follows, incubation time for the routine assay was decided as
twenty hours. Antibody bound peptide was separated by dextran-chracoal
method and radioactivity of the sedimented dextran-charcoal adsorbing
free radio-labeled bradykinin was counted by gamma counter (ISOFLEX) of
50% counting efficiency. As far as the study on the sensitvity and
characteriation of antisera, gel-filtration of the purchased radio-
labeled bradykinin was performed, based on the method of Alhenc-Gelas et
al.[6]

EXTRACTION OF KININS FROM SAMPLED BLOOD

Prior to the experiment on extraction of the peptides, elution
condition was determined by reverse phase high performance liquid
chromatography using octadecyl silica column. Blood was corrected from
ante-cubital vein into syringe containing inhibitor solution composed of
10mg/dl of gabaxate mesiltate, 50U/ml of aprotinine, 10mM of EDTA-2Na
and 5mg/dl of benzamidine in normal saline. Portion of the inhibitor
solution in sample was 20% by volume. Sampled blood was transfered into
ice-cooled plastic tube and plasma was separated by centrifuge(2000xg)
for five minutes at $4^{o}C$ and applied to octadecyl silica cartridge column
(Sepak C_{18}). After washing the cartridge with 10ml of 5% acetic acid,
objective peptides were eluted with 2ml of 100% methanol into the
siliconized glass tube. Methanol was evaporated by forced air blow into
tube on the heating block of $40^{o}C$ and the dried residue was redissolved
with RIA buffer and subsequently assayed by the radioimmunoassay.

RESULTS

RADIOIMMUNOASSAY

Optimal pH for the assay was proved to be 7.1 by an experiment on pH
dependency and consequently we took 0.1M of sodium-phosphate buffer
containing 0.002M o-phenanthroline, 0.002M EDTA, 50000U/1 of aprotinin
and 1mg/ml of lysozyme as assay buffer. Incubation time for routine
assay was decided to be 20hrs, as indicated in Figure 1.
Antisera which would deserve to perform radioimmunoassay were
obtained from two different rabbits. Raised antisera were estimated for
their titer by capability of binding radiolabeled bradykinin. Buffer for
the tentative assay was same as that of Reis et al.[5] As shown in Figure
2., two different antisera (aB2 and aB3) at a final dilution of 10^{4}
folds both bound 50% of total radio-labeled bradykinin. The more
antisera were diluted, the less radio-labeled bradykinin were bound. No
obvious difference was observed between two different antisera. Among
two different antisera, aB3 was selected to pursue susequent
experiments.

Standard curve for bradykinin by this radioimmunoassay was demonstrated as Figure 3. Eight pg/tube of bradykinin was capable of displacing 50% of total radio-labeled bradykinin. Thus the assay can be regarded to detect 30pg/ml of bradykinin. Lys-bradykinin displaced radio-labeled bradykinin as much as equal amount of bradykinin, whereas met-lys-bradykinin displaced 80% of radio-labeled bradykinin which would be displaced by same amount of bradykinin. These results indicate that the antiserum crossreacts with met-lys-bradykinin and lys-bradykinin by 80% and 100% respectively. Crossreactivity with vasoactive peptides such as angiotensin I, angiotensin II and arginine-vasopressin could not be found. However, little cross-reactivity with bradykinin-related peptides such as des-arg^1-bradykinin and des-arg^9-bradykinin was observed (Table 1).

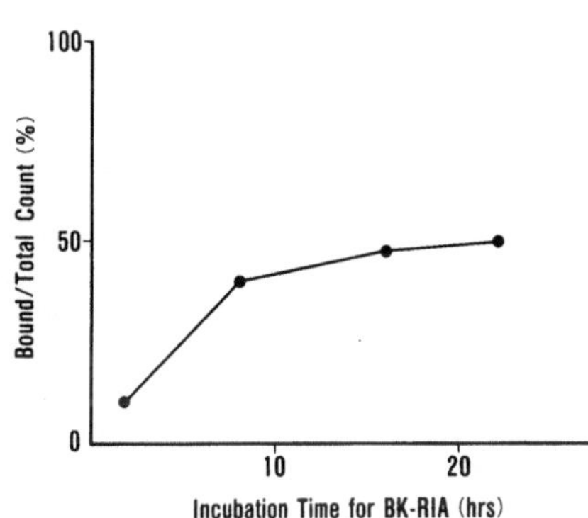

Fig. 1 Time dependency of antigen-antibody reaction. Dilution of anti-serum was 10^4 folds (aB3).

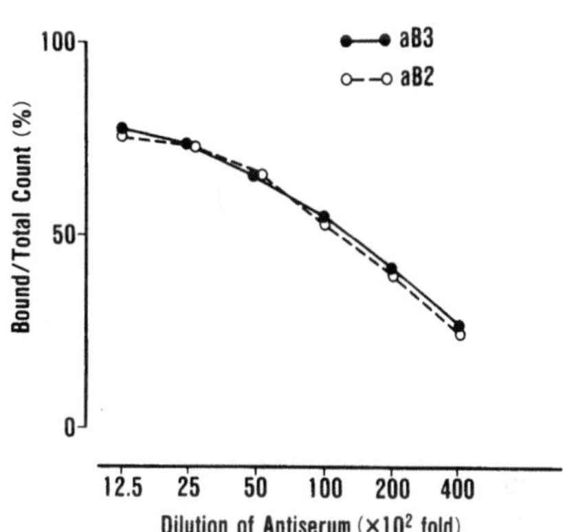

Fig. 2 Capability of antisera to bind ^{125}I-tyr^8-bradykinin.

TABLE 1

CROSS-REACTIVITY OF VARIOUS PEPTIDES WITH ANTI-BRADYKININ ANTISERUM aB3.

BRADYKININ	100 %
des-arg$_9^1$-BRADYKININ	0.5 %
des-arg$_8^9$-BRADYKININ	0.5 %
des-phe^8-arg^9-BRADYKININ	<0.1 %
ANGIOTENSIN I	<0.1 %
ANGIOTENSIN II	<0.1 %
ARGININE VASOPRESSIN	<0.1 %

EXTRACTION OF KININS FROM BLOOD

High performance liquid chromatography revealed that bradykinin could be thoroughly eluted from octadecyl silica column between 20% of methanol in water and 50% of methanol in water. Loss of the peptide during the procedure was as little as to be ignored. It was also confirmed that wash with 5% acetic acid and evaporation at 40°C by air blowing did not affect the recovery rate. Figure 5. indicates the result of extraction of kinins from blood. Within 15 minutes after sampling at 4°C, exogenously added bradykinin recovered almost 100% and concentration of endogenous kinins derived of 2ml of plasma was almost undetectable level. At 25°C, even treated within 15 minutes, neither

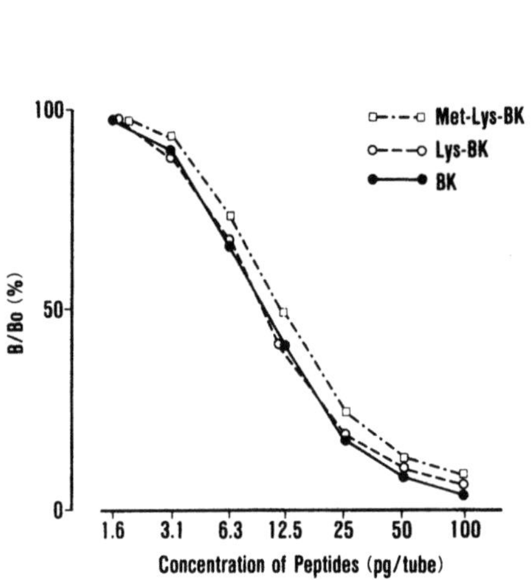

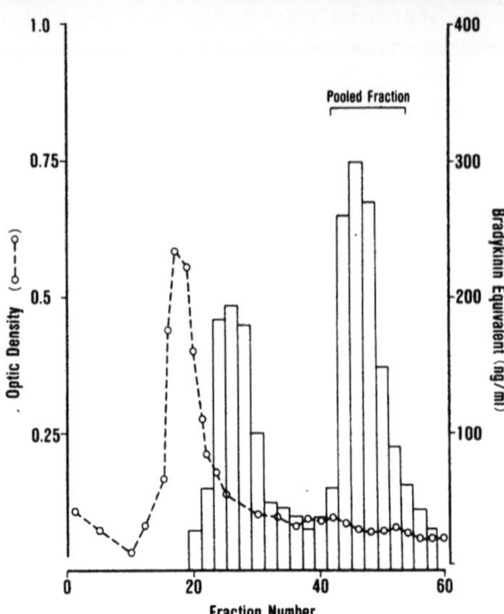

Fig. 3 Standard curve of the radio-immunoassay for bradykinin and related peptides. Antiserum(aB3) was diluted by 2×10^4 folds (final dilution).

Fig. 4 Elution profile from SP Toyopearl cation exchange chromatography. Flow rate was 12.5 ml/hr and volume of each fraction was 5ml. Linear gradient was performed between 0.075M NaCl and 1.2M NaCl in sodium acetate buffer (pH 5.3).

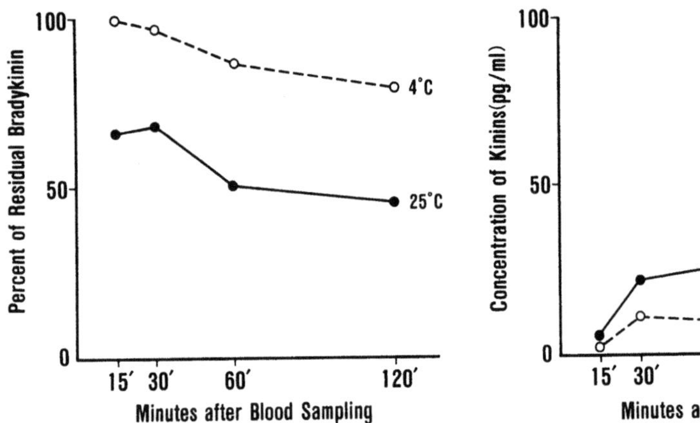

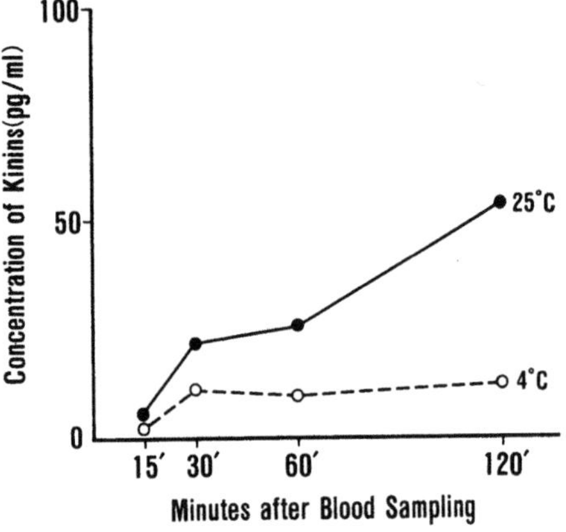

Fig. 5 Left figure indicates natural degradation of exogenously added bradykinin (10ng) into sampling syringe. Right figure indicates spontaneous generation of kinins after blood sampling. Incubations were stopped by transfering the samples onto Sepak C_{18} cartridge and immediate wash with 5% acetic acid.

spontaneous degradation nor spontaneous generation could be avoided. This result indicate that reproducible extraction of kinins from biological fluid might be expected by this procedure.

First step of the purification was anion exchange chromatography described by Hayashi et al.[7] Volume of the starting material was 150ml and column size was 5x18cm. After confirming that expected fractions whose chloride ion concentration exceeded 200mM can be hydrolyzed by exogenously added trypsin to release kinins, the fractions were pooled, concentrated by ultrafiltration with Amicon YM-10 membrane and succeessively applied to cation exchange chromatography (SP Toyopearl; 2.5x10cm) based on the report of Kerbiriou et al.[8] Gradient elution from the cation exchange chromatography was done by increasing the concentration of sodium chloride. Elution profile of cation exchange chromatography was indicated in Figure 4. Active fractions were obtained with buffer whose concentration of NaCl was around 350mM and 800mM. Copper-chelating chromatography was necessary to eliminate contaminating protein. After extensive washing with starting buffer, active fractions were acquired by the elution with the buffer containing 10mM of EDTA.

DISCUSSION

As far as vasoactive peptides and commercially available bradykinin-derived peptides were tested, no remarkable crossrectivity was observed. This result is similar to that of previous investigation[6]. The result that lys-bradykinin crossreacted 100% with anti-bradykinin antiserum and contrarily des-phe^8-arg^9-bradykinin lost antigenicitity with that antiserum implicate that carboxy terminal was major determinant site of the antigenicity. With respects to the property of kininase II which would hydrolyze dipeptide from carboxy terminal of the peptide, the radioimmunoassay seems highly valuable means to estimate specifically the enzyme from aspect of its function, whereas direct radio-immunoassay[12] is a tool to quantitate the enzyme as a protein.

A lot of investigation on the extraction of bradykinin from blood have been reported and the method has been for a long time a matter of dispute. Octadecyl silica cartridge column is widely used to efficiently extract the substance of small molecule such as peptides, nucleotides, lipids, steroids and so on. However, a few reports on the extraction of bradykinin from bilogical materials with octadecyl silica cartridge column can be seen and we attempted to obtain more reproducible method for the extraction of bradykinin in biological materials, using newly developed material. Blood sampling has been also a problem because spontaneous generation of kinins from plasma kininogens and spontaneous degradation of endogeneous kinins can occur. Recently, gabexate mesilate, protease inhibitor of wide spectrum such as plasma kallikrein, plasmin, trypsin and thrombin has been developed and we employed the inhibitor to solve the problem. Although innate bradykinin from 2ml of plasma was near undetectable level, increase of plasma as much as 10ml and increase in sensitivity with puirified tracer described in methods would solve the problem. Elution with 100% methanol did not affect performance of radioimmunoassay owing to other substances than kinins but was more efficient and time-saving than 50% methanol.

Pathogenesis of hypertension has been investigated from various aspects. Although role of vasodepressor kallikrein-kinin system in the pathogenesis of hypertension has been long investigated, pathophysiology of kininogens, particularly circulating ones, has not yet been fully elucidated. Purified kininogen is indispensable to acquire immunological tool, which will enable us to evaluate the protein more specifically and let us know its patho-physiological role in hypertension.

REFERENCES

1. Ohkubo I., Kurachi K., Takasawa T., Shiokawa H. and Sasaki M. Isolatioon of a Human cDNA for α_2-Thiol Proteinase Inhibitor and Its Identity with Low Molecular Weight Kininogen. (1984) <u>Biochemistry</u> 23,5691-5697.

2. Nawa H., Kitamura N., Hirose T., Asai M., Inayama S. and Nakanishi S. Primary structure of bovine liver low molecular weight kininogen precursors and their two mRNAs. (1983) <u>Proc. Natl. Acad. Sci.</u> 80,99-94.

3. Kitamura N., Takagaki Y., Furuto S., Tanaka T., Nawa H. and Nakanishi S. A single gene for bovine high molecular weight and low molecular weight kininogens. (1983) <u>Nature</u> 305,545-549.

4. Shimamoto K., Ando T., Nakao T., Tanaka S., Sakuma M. and Miyahara M. A sensitve radioimmunoassay method for urinary kinins in man. (1978) <u>J. Lab. Clin. Med.</u> 91,721-728.

5. Reis M. L., Alhenc-Gelas F., Alhenc-Gelas M., Allegrini J., Kerbiriou-Nabias D., Corvol P. and Menard J. Rat high-molecular weight kininogen: purification, production of antibodies and demonstration of lack of immunoreactive kininogen in a strain of Brown Norway rats. (1985) <u>Biochim. Biophys. Acta</u> 831,106-113.

6. Alhen-Gelas F., Marchetti J., Allegrini J., Corvol P. and Menard J. Measurement of Urinary Kallikrein Activity. Species Differences in Kinin Production. (1981) <u>Biochim. Biophy. Acta</u> 677,477-488.

7. Hayashi I., Kato H., Iwanaga S. and Ohishi S. Rat High-molecular-weight Kininogen. (1985) <u>J. Biol. Chem.</u> 260,6115-6123.

8. Kerbiriou D. M. and Griffin J. H. Human High Molecular Weight Kininogen. (1979) <u>J. Biol. Chem.</u> 254,12020-12027.

9. Proud D., Pierce J. V. and Pisano J. J. Radioimmunoassay of human high molecular weight kininogen in normal and deficient plasmas. (1980) <u>J. Lab. Clin. Med.</u> 95,563-574.

10. Kerbiriou-Nabias D. M., Garcia F. O. and Larrieu M. Radioimmunoassay of human high and low molecular weight kininogens in plasmas and platelets. (1984) <u>Br. J. Haematol.</u> 56, 273-286.

11. Muller-Esterl W., Rauth G., Lottspeich F., Kellermann J. and Henschen A. Limited Proteolysis of human low-molecular-mass kininogen by tissue kallikrein. (1985) <u>Eur. J. Biochem.</u> 149,15-22.

12. Yasui T., Alhenc-Gelas F., Corvol P. and Menard J. Characterization of angiotensin I converting enzyme in amniotic fluid. (1985) <u>J. Lab. Clin. Med.</u> 104,141-151.

MEASUREMENT OF des -Phe^8-Arg^9-BRADYKININ BY ENZYME-IMMUNO-

ASSAY --- A USEFUL PARAMETER OF PLASMA KININ RELEASE

Masataka Majima, Akinori Ueno, *Noriyuki
Sunahara and Makoto Katori

Department of Pharmacology, Kitasato University
School of Medicine, Sagamihara, Kanagawa 228
*Dainippon Pharmaceut. Co., Osaka, Japan

INTRODUCTION

Detection of free bradykinin (BK) in the inflammatory
exudate is the conclusive evidence of the involvement of
plasma kallikrein-kinin system in the inflammatory process.
Thus, we have developed an enzyme-immunoassay of BK[1].
However, it is difficult to detect free BK itself, because
kinins are rapidly degraded in vivo by kininases. It is
well known that kininase I inactivates bradykinin to des-
Arg^9-bradykinin (des-9-BK), and that kininase II does it to
des-Phe^8-Arg^9-bradykinin (des-8,9-BK).

This paper describes that des-8,9-BK could be detected
as a major transient metabolite after in vitro incubation of
BK with the inflammatory exudate or plasma and could be
taken as a parameter of the plasma kinin release in the
inflammatory exudate in vivo.

MATERIALS AND METHODS

Sprague-Dawley strain male SPF rats (8-10 weeks old)
were used. For degradation study of BK, rat plasma or human
plasma was used as sources of kininases. Blood was
collected through the carotid artery of rats or the ante-
cubital vein of human male volunteers into a plastic tubes
containing 1/10 volume of 3.8% of sodium citrate. The
exudate of rat pleurisy, which was induced by injection of
histamine (0.5 mg/0.5 ml) into the right pleural cavity of
rats, was also used as a source of kininases. The exudate
or plasma was diluted to the same concentrations to get an
adequate speed of the degradation of BK on high performance
liquid chromatoraphy (HPLC). BK (40 nmol) was incubated
with the diluted exudate or plasma (0.45 ml, 4 mg
protein/ml) at 37°C up to 60 min, and then the reaction was
stopped by addition of 10% trichloroacetic acid (TCA, 0.45
ml). The degradation products in the incubation mixture
were separated and measured by reversed-phase HPLC
(Trirotar, JASCO, Tokyo). When the standard mixture of the

peptides was applied to this HPLC system, pentapeptide (Arg-Pro-Pro-Gly-Phe), heptapeptide (des-8,9-BK), BK and octapeptide (des-9-BK) were eluted at 18 min, 21 min, 30 min and 38 min, respectively.

D,L-2-mercaptomethyl-3-guanidinoethylthiopropanoic acid (10 μM)[2] and captopril (33 μM) were used as a kininase I inhibitor and a kininase II inhibitor, respectively. 1,10-Phenanthroline (1 mM) was also used as an inhibitor of both kininases. These inhibitors were preincubated with the exudate or plasma for 5 min before addition of BK.

For an enzyme-immunoassay of des-8,9-BK, β-D-galactosidase, which was conjugated to N-terminal of des-8,9-BK, was used as a labeling enzyme. The first antibody against des-8,9-BK was produced from rabbits immunized with the conjugate of des-8,9-BK with albumin. The cross reactivities of the antibody against BK, Lys-BK, Met-Lys-BK, and T-kinin are very low (under 0.1%). The antigen-antibody reaction was performed for 1 hr at 37°C. The separation of the bound fraction from free was carried using the insoluble second antibodies against rabbit IgG obtained from goats. After centrifugation, the enzyme activities in the precipitate were measured with a synthetic substrate (2-nitrophenyl-B-D-galactopyranoside). The details in this method can be seen in other paper in this volume (Sunahara et al). When the samples were measured by both this enzyme-immunoassay and HPLC, the values determined by this enzyme-immunoassay correlated with those by HPLC. An enzyme-immunoassay of BK (Markit-A, Dainippon Pharmaceutical Co, Osaka)[3] was also used.

Kaolin was added to plasma of rats (10 mg/ml). The incubation was made at 37°C. At a given time, an aliquot (1 ml) was transferred to a tube, containing 0.2 ml of 10% TCA to stop the reaction. Des-8,9-BK and BK produced in the reaction mixture were determined by its own enzyme-immunoassay.

In order to test the validity of the detection of des-8,9-BK in the inflammatory exudate, a pleurisy was produced by injection of 0.1 ml of 2% lamda-carrageenin into the right pleural cavity of rats. After exsanguination at a given time until 24 hr, 5 ml of ethanol was injected into the pleural cavity for prevention of further degradation to smaller peptides. The fluid in the pleural cavity was harvested and centrifuged. The supernatant was evaporated under the reduced pressure. After the residue was washed with small amount of diethylether to remove the lipid, it was dissolved with an assay buffer of the enzyme-immunoassay of BK or des-8,9-BK.

RESULTS AND DISCUSSION

After the in vitro incubation of BK with plasma of rats, three peaks of the degradation products of BK were detected besides BK on the HPLC chromatogram. When each peak on the chromatogram was collected and analyzed by amino acid analysis, these were identified as pentapeptide (Arg-

Pro-Pro-Gly-Phe), heptapeptide (des-8,9-BK) and octapeptide (des-9-BK), respectively. The same three peaks were able to be detected on the chromatogram of the samples after incubation of BK with the exudate of histamine-induced pleurisy of rats or human plasma.

The time course of the degradation of BK by rat plasma revealed that the production of des-8,9-BK was two fold faster than that of des-9-BK at 10 min of the incubation and then the amounts of BK pentapeptide exceeded other two metabolites at 60 min. The sum of all three metabolites and the residual BK during the 60 min incubation period was not different from the original amount of BK added, so that further degradation from the BK pentapeptide to smaller fragments might be slow in this condition. The incubation of BK with rat exudate resulted in the same result, indicating that a major kininase in rat plasma or the exudate was kininase II, an angiotensin converting enzyme.

On the contrary, incubation of human plasma with BK in vitro disclosed that a major degradation product was des-9-BK, followed by des-8,9-BK up to 60 min.

Selective inhibitors of kininase I or II revealed that the degradation of BK was enzymatic (Fig. 1). The pre-incubation of rat plasma with a kininase I inhibitor, D,L-2-

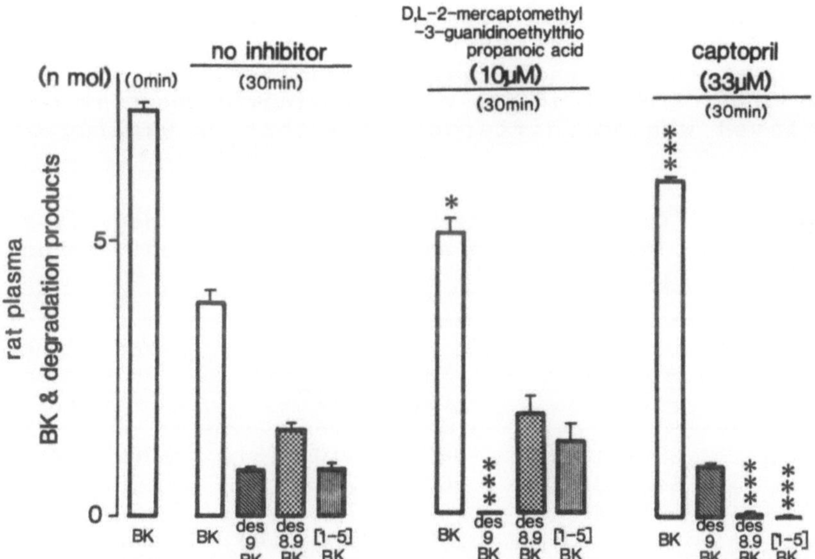

Fig. 1 Inhibition of bradykinin degradation in rat plasma by kininase inhibitor.

Each value indicates the mean (+SEM) of three or four experiments. Values of BK and its metabolites in each panel of the inhibitors were compared individually with those without addition of inhibitors (left panel). *: p<0.05, ***: p<0.001.

mercaptomethyl-3-guanidinoethylthiopropanoic acid (10 µM),
caused the complete inhibition of des-9-BK production,
whereas the des-8,9-BK formation and pentapeptide production
were not reduced. On the contrary, a kininase II inhibitor,
captopril (33 µM), inhibited the production of des-8,9-BK
and pentapeptide without a change of des-9-BK generation.
1,10-Phenanthroline (1 mM), an inhibitor for both kininase I
and II, inhibited the generation of all products. The
incubation of des-9-BK with plasma yielded pentapeptide of
BK and the degradation was inhibited by captopril (data not
shown). From these results, it can be concluded that
kininase II was not only a major kininase in rat plasma, but
also it may be involved in the degradation to pentapeptide.

The same results were obtained, using the exudate of
the histamine-induced pleurisy. When protein concentration
of the exudate for incubation was adjusted to the same as
that of plasma, the degradation rate of BK by the exudate
was not different from that by plasma, indicating that
kininases in the exudate of histamine-induced pleurisy may
be derived from plasma.

When Kaolin was added to plasma of rats in vitro,
factor XII and prekallikrein may be activated and BK was
generated at a peak of 4 min after addition of kaolin. The
BK levels declined with time and des-8,9-BK peaked at 6 min.
The total amount of des-8,9-BK under the curve was larger
than that of BK. Thus, des-8,9-BK could be used as a better
and a long-lasting parameter for kinin generation.

In carrageenin-induced pleurisy, the involvement of
plasma kallikrein-kinin system was predicted by the consumption of both prekallikrein and high molecular weight
kininogen in the inflammatory exudate[4]. In the present
experiment, free BK in the pleural exudate was measured, but
the level was not different from that in washing of the

Table 1. Changes of the BK levels and the des-8,9-BK
levels in the exudate of carrageenin-induced
pleurisy

Time after carrageenin	BK[a]		des-8,9-BK[a]
	(-)	captopril[b]	(-)
45 min	68 ± 18 (4)	3800 ± 1100 (3)	1000 ± 210 (4)[c]
1.5 hr	64 ± 36 (4)	5600 ± 2000 (4)	560 ± 170 (4)
3 hr	63 ± 48 (3)	1800 ± 180 (3)	680 ± 140 (3)
5 hr		1600 ± 170 (4)	470 ± 160 (6)
7 hr			530 ± 170 (3)
9 hr			400 ± 80 (4)
14 hr			340 ± 30 (7)
19 hr			410 ± 70 (3)
24 hr			370 ± 40 (3)

a: The levels were expressed as pg/rat.
b: Captopril (10 mg/kg, i.p.) was administered 30 min before
carrageenin.
c: Values indicates mean ± SEM (number of experiments).

pleural cavity of normal rats. However, as shown in Table
1, the pretreatment of rats with captopril (10 mg/kg, intraperitoneally, 30 min before carrageenin injection) allowed
to detect a large amount of BK in the exudate (1600-3800
pg/rat). The amount was over 30-80 times larger than that
of untreated rats.

On the other hand, as shown in Table 1, des-8,9-BK was
able to be detected in the entire course of the pleurisy
without any pretreatment with captopril, although des-8,9-BK
was not present in washing of the pleural cavity of normal
rats. These result indicated that, in rat carrageenin-
induced pleurisy, kininase II was a major kininase for the
degradation of BK. In the histamine-induced pleurisy, des-
8,9-BK was not detected, indicating that plasma prekallikrein was not activated in this model. From the above
results, it can be verified that plasma kallikrein-kinin
system was activated in the inflammatory site.

ACKNOWLEDGMENTS

We wish to give cordial thanks to Dr. T. Miyata and
Prof. S. Iwanaga (Kyushu University) for the determination
of the amino acid sequences of the degradation products of
BK and Mrs. C. Shima and Mrs. M. Takagi for their technical
assistances.

REFERENCES

1.   Ueno, A., Oh-ishi, S., Kitagawa, T. & Katori, M.
     Enzyme immunoassay of bradykinin using β-D-
     galactosidase as a labeling enzyme. Biochem.
     Pharmacol., 30: 1659-1664, 1981.

2.   Plummer, T. H. & Ryan, T. J. A potent mercapto bi-
     product analogue inhibitor for human carboxy-
     peptidase N. Biochem. Biophys. Res. Comm., 98: 448-
     454, 1981.

3.   Uchida, Y., Majima, M. & Katori, M. A method of
     determination of human plasma HMW and LMW kininogen
     levels by bradykinin enzyme immunoassay. Pharmacol.
     Res. Comm., 18: 831-846, 1986.

4.   Uchida, Y., Tanaka, K., Harada, Y., Ueno, A. & Katori,
     M. Activation of plasma kallikrein-kinin system and
     its significant role in pleural fluid accumulation
     of rat carrageenin-induced pleurisy. Inflammation,
     7: 121-131, 1983.

CHARACTERIZATION OF AN SH-PROTEINASE INHIBITOR FROM Bothrops jararaca

PLASMA

A.M. Chudzinski*, M.L.V. Oliva, M.U., Sampaio and C.A.M. Sampaio

Departamento de Bioquimica, Escola Paulista de Medicina
Caixa Postal 20372, 04034 S. Paulo, SP, Brazil
*Instituto Butantan

INTRODUCTION

Kininogens are the kinin carriers and natural substrates for plasma and tissue kallikrein. Most of known mammalian plasmas contain at least two types of kininogen, high and low molecular weight[1]. Kininogens share the N-terminus located heavy chains and the consecutive kinin moiety, but differ in the structural properties of the C-terminus located light chains [1]. Only light chain of high molecular weight kininogen accomodates plasma prokallikrein binding site, distal to bradykinin and near the C-terminus of kininogen[2]. Mammalian kininogens are now also known as the main plasma SH-proteinase inhibitors, and both high and low molecular weight kininogen exhibit this property, assigned to the heavy chain of the molecule [3,4,5,6,7].

Studies on the presence of kininogen in snake plasma have been approached by the estimation of released kinin , upon incubation with kininogenases. With regard to the kinin yielding property, snake plasma has been reported as either a kininogen missing plasma[8] or, alternatively, the absence of detectable amounts of kinin has been attributed to rapid and potent inactivation of released kinin by kininases[9].

The aim of this work is to study the presence of a kininogen-type protein with SH-proteinase inhibitor activity, in Bothrops jararaca plasma, a poisonous Brazilian snake.

MATERIAL AND METHODS

Papain was from Boehringer; bromelain, bovine trypsin, phenylmethylsulfonylfluoride (PMSF), L-trans-epoxysuccinyl-leuccylamido (4-guanidino) butane (E-64), DL-dithiothreitol (DTT), were from Sigma; bovine thrombin was from Roche; human plasma kallikrein was purified by a described procedure[10]. DEAE-Sephadex A 50 was a Pharmacia product; CM-papain-Sepharose was prepared by a described procedure[11]. Tosyl-arginine methyl ester (TAME) was from Merck, and the chromogenic substrate acetyl-phenylalanine-arginine-p-nitroanilide (Ac-Phe-Arg-pNA) was a kind gift of Dr. L. Juliano, Departamento de Biofisica, Escola Paulista de Medicina. Polybrene was from EGA-Chemie and Nembutal was from Abbott.

Snake plasma from male and female B. jararaca, with 250 g average weight, was used. Snakes were subcutaneously anesthesized with 5 mg/ml saline sodium Nembutal (30 mg/kg). Approximatelly 20 min later, being the snakes deeply anesthesized, they were extensively bled through a 5 cm ventrally made longitudinal incision, near the heart, that exposed the aorta artery. Blood (10 to 13 ml) was withdrawn in plastic syringes containing 1 mL mixture composed of 2.5% glucose, 0.1 mM EDTA, 100 mg/L polybrene, 1 mM PMSF, in 0.15 M NaCl. Collected blood was transferred to plastic centrifuge tubes, and kept in ice-bath until being centrifuged at 2,000 x g, 4°C, for 15 min. Plasma separated into plastic tubes was immediately frozen and kept at -70°C up to its use.

CM-papain-Sepharose [8] was preliminarily used as a single step purification. Resin (2 mL) was equilibrated with 0.1 M tris-HCl buffer, pH 7.0. Following sample (10 mL plasma diluted to 20 mL with equilibrium buffer) application, the resin was extensively washed with the same buffer, until the absorbance at 280 nm (A 280) was lower than 0.05. Elution of bound material was carried out with 0.5 M KCl-HCl buffer, pH 2.0, in 2.0 mL fractions, and immediately neutralized with 60 ul 1.0 M tris-HCl, pH 8.0 buffer. Protein elution was spectrophotometrically monitored at A 280 and fractions active upon papain were pooled for further characterization.

An ion-exchange chromatography on DEAE- Sephadex A 50 was initially used, as a second procedure. Column (22 x 1.5 cm) was equilibrated with 0.05 M tris-HCl, pH 8.0 buffer, containing 1 mM EDTA, 1 mM PMSF, 100 mg/L polybrene, 0.01 % tymerosal and 0.03 M NaCl. Following sample application (10 mL plasma diluted to 20 ml with equilibrium buffer), at 4°C, column was extensively washed with equilibrium buffer until A 280 was lower than 0.05, and subsequently with increasing NaCl concentration (0.08; 0.12; 0.20 and 0.50 M) in the same buffer system. Protein elution was followed by A 280 and peak-fractions were pooled for activity assay upon papain. Active pools were dialyzed against 0.015 M NaCl. The most active pool was lyophilized and dissolved in a volume of 0.1M tris-HCl, pH 7.0 buffer equivalent to approximately 1/10 of the original pooled volume.

DEAE-Sephadex A 50 chromatographed material was rechromatographed on CM-papain-Sepharose, under the conditions described above, except that 1.0 mL fractions were collected. Active fractions were pooled, for further characterization.

Papain and bromelain activities were measured by the hydrolysis of Ac-Phe-Arg-pNA, as described previously[12,13].Papain inhibition rate was followed by the incubation of the inhibitor with 0.12 ug activated papain, in 1.0 mL final volume of 10 mM sodium phosphate buffer, pH 6.8 containing 1 mM EDTA and 2 mM DTT, at 37 C, and at different intervals 2 mM (final) Ac-Phe-Arg-pNA was added. Spectrophotometric recordings at 405 nm were performed for 10 min, following substrate addition. Actual concentration of papain and bromelain were determined by titration with E-64 reagent [13]. One inhibitor unit was defined as the amount of protein which inhibits 1.0 mg papain.

Polyacrylamide gel eletrophoresis was performed on 5-15% or 10-20% gradient slab gels, under the conditions described by Laemmli[16], and stained with Coomassie Blue or silver nitrate [14] Protein concentration is expressed as absorbance at A 280 nm.

Assay of biological activity: on isolated guinea-pig preparation, bathed with 10 mL Tyrode solution, and standardized with synthetic bradykinin, variable amounts of the purified snake plasma inhibitor were assayed in the presence of 50 ug trypsin. Bradykinin elicited contractions

were recorded for 1 min, and contractions elicited by trypsin direct
incubation were recorded for about 3 min [15].

RESULTS

The protein purified on CM-papain Sepharose, as single step, appears
on SDS-polyacrylamide gel (5-15%) with apparent molecular weight 100,000
(unreduced). The protein purified by the two-step chromatographic
procedures, DEAE-Sephadex A 50 and CM-papain-Sepharose, is seen as a major
58,000 molecular weight protein, on SDS-polyacrylamide gel (10-20%),
either reduced or unreduced.

Trypsin incubates of both protein forms release a biologically
active material, when assayed upon the isolated guinea-pig ileum
preparation (figure 1), resembling kinin formation from mammalian
kininogen incubated under the same conditions (not shown).

The dissociation constant of inhibition was calculated from the
inhibition curves, by hydrolysis of Ac-Phe-Arg-pNA, and an example of
inhibition of papain and bromelain by the low molecular weight inhibitor,
is shown in the figure 2. Ki values were respectively of the order of
10-7 M for the 100,000 molecular weight preparation and 10-9 M for the
58,000 molecular weight preparation. For bromelain, apparent Ki values
were of the order of 10-6 M for both preparations.

Serine proteinases, bovine trypsin, bovine thrombin and human plasma
kallikrein activity upon TAME was not inhibited (not shown).

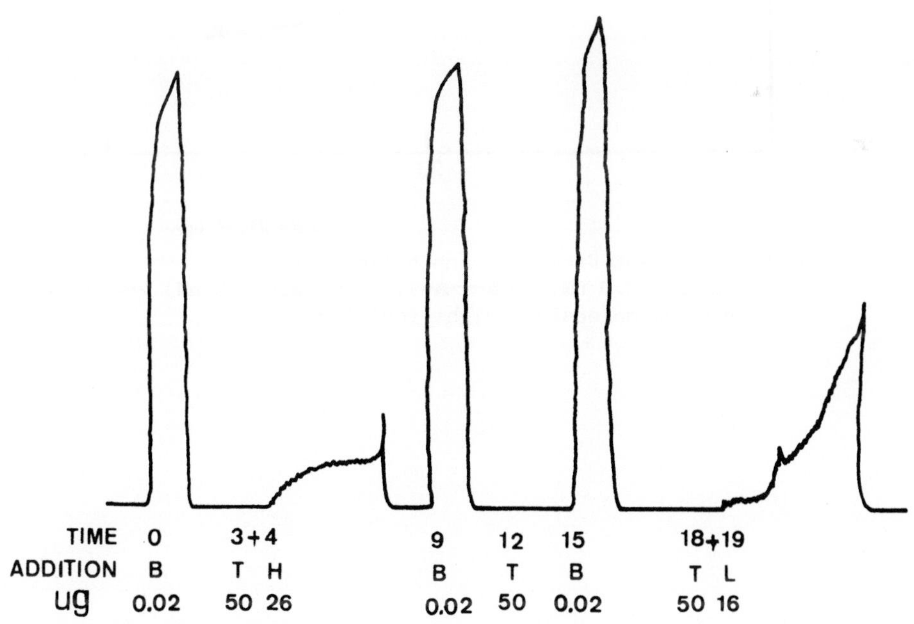

Figure 1. Kinin like release from the purified thiol-proteinase inhibitors
from B. jararaca plasma.
Bradykinin (B); Trypsin (T); 100.000-inhibitor (H);
58,000-inhibitor (L).

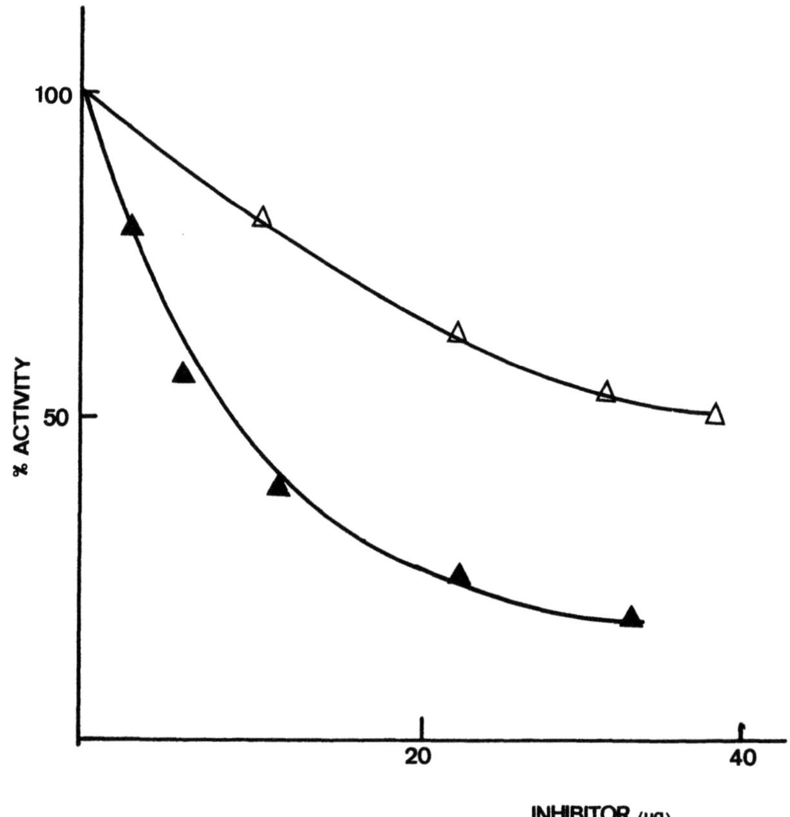

Figure 2. Papain and Bromelain inhibition curve.
Papain (6.0 nM) (—▲——▲—); Bromelain (15 nM) (—△—△—)
and low molecular weight inhibitor.

Ten minute pre-incubation of inhibitors, at different temperatures between 0° and 100 °C, showed that the inhibitory ability on papain enzyme activity is fully kept up to 50 °C; and time course experiments showed that maximal papain inhibition by B. jararaca plasma inhibitor is very rapidly attained (not shown).

DISCUSSION

B. jararaca plasma was shown to contain SH-proteinase inhibitor activity. Its preliminary characterization, based upon affinity chromatography on CM-papain-Sepharose, resulted in active protein forms, with molecular weights approximately 58,000 and 100,000. Isolated proteins were able to inhibit both SH-proteinases studied, papain and bromelain.

The release of a biologically active material, from the isolated protein incubated with trypsin, has not been detected with snake whole plasma although low activity was released from the purified thiol-proteinase inhibitors. The presence of these inhibitors in snake plasma, with general molecular characteristics of the mammalian kininogen, is an indication that the same type of protein is being expressed in snakes, although it has a low detectable content of kinin-like activity. It maybe that the peptide is linked through peptide bonds not susceptible to usual kinin-releasing enzymes, or the released peptide is not pharmacologically as active as bradykinin, on biological preparations as the isolated guinea pig ileum.

REFERENCES

1 - H. Kato, S. Nagasawa and S. Iwanaga, HMW and LMW kininogens, Methods Enzymol., 80: 172 (1981).
2 - J.F. Taiti and K. Fujikawa, Identification of the binding site for plasma prekallikrein in human high molecular weight kininogen, J.Biol. Chem., 261: 15396 (1986).
3 - I. Ohkubo, K. Kurachi, T. Takasawa, H, Shiokawa and M. Sasaki, Isolation of a human cDNA for α-2 thiol proteinase inhibitor and its identity with low molecular weight kininogen, Biochemistry, 23: 5691 (1984).
4 - T. Sueyoshi, K. Enjyoji, T. Shimada, H. Kato, S. Iwanaga, Y. Bando, E. Kominami and N. Katunuma, A new function of kininogens as thiol-proteinase inhibitors: inhibition of papain and cathipsins B, H and L by bovine rat and human plasma kininogens, FEBS Letters, 182: 193 (1985).
5 - T. Cole, A.S. Inglis, C.M. Roxburgh, G.J. Howlett and G. Schreiber, Major acute phase α-1-protein of the rat is homologous to bovine kininogen and contains the sequence for bradykinin: its synthesis is regulates at the mRNA level, FEBS Letters, 182: 57 (1985).
6 - W. Muller-Esterl, H. Fritz, W. Machleidt, A. Ritonja, J. Brzin, M. Kotnik, V. Turk, J. Kellermann and F. Lottspeich with α-cysteine proteinase inhibitors. Evidence from immunological, enzymological and sequence data, FEBS Letters, 182: 310 (1985).
7 - A.J. Barret, The cystatins: a diverse superfamily of cysteine peptidase inhibitors, Biomed. Biochim. Acta, 45: 1363 (1986).
8 - A.A.C. Lavras, M. Fichman, E. Hiraichi, M.A. Boucault, T. Tobo, P. Schmuziger,. L. Nahas and Z.P. Picarelli, Deficiency of kallikrein-kinin system and presence of potent kininase activity in the plasma of Bothrops jararaca (Serpentes, Crotalinae), Ciencia Cult., 31: 168 (1979).

9 - A.A.C. Lavras, M. Fichman, E. Hiraichi, T. Todo and M.A. Boucault; The kininases of Bothrops jararaca plasma, <u>Acta Physiol. Latinoam.</u>,30: 269 (1980).

10- M.L. Oliva, M.U. Sampaio and C.A.M. Sampaio, Properties of highly purified human plasma kallikrein, <u>Agents Actions</u>, 9: 52 (1982).

11- A. Anastasi, M.A. Brown, A.A. Khembhavi, M.J.H. Nicklin, C.A. Sayers, D.C. Sunter and A.J. Barret, Cystatin,a protein inhibitor of cysteine proteinases, <u>Biochem. J.</u>, 211: 129 (1983).

12- M.L.V. Oliva, M.U. Sampaio and C.A.M. Sampaio, Serine and SH-proteinase inhibitor from Enterolobium contortisiliquum beans, Purification and preliminary characterization, <u>Braz. J. Med. Biol.</u>, 20: 780 (1987).

13- S. Zucker, D.J. Butler, M.J.H. Nicklin and J.S. Barret, The proteolytic activities of chymopapain, papain, and papaya proteinase III, <u>Biochim. Biophy. Acta</u>, 828: 204 (1985).

14- J.H. Morrissey, Silver stain of protein polyacrilamide gels: a modified procedure with enhanced uniform sensitivy, <u>Anal. Biochem.</u>, 117: 307 (1981).

15- C.A.M. Sampaio, S.T. Nunes, M.G.N. Mazzacoratti and J.L. Prado, Inactivation of kinins by chymotrypsin, <u>Biochem. Pharmacol.</u>, 25: 2391 (1976).

16- U.K. Laemmli, Cleavage of structural proteins during the assembly of the head of bacteriophage T4, <u>Nature</u>, 227: 680 (970).

A SENSITIVE METHOD FOR DIFFERENTIAL DETERMINATION OF KININASE I, II AND

NEUTRAL ENDOPEPTIDASE (NEP) IN HUMAN URINE

Hitoko Ogata, Nobuyuki Ura, Kazuaki Shimamoto, Toru Sakakibara,
Toshiaki Ando, Takatoshi Nishimiya, Motoya Nakagawa,
Shuzaburo Fukuyama, Atsushi Masuda, Yasukazu Yamaguchi,
Takashi Ise, Shigeyuki Saito, Mamoru Shiiki, Kikuya Uno and
Osamu Iimura

The Second Department of Internal Medicine, Sapporo Medical
College, S-1 W-16, Sapporo, Japan

SUMMARY

In order to clarify the significance of NEP in human renal kallikrein-
kinin system, an assay system was developed for the simultaneous determination of kininase I, II and NEP activities in human. Each kininase activity
was determined by measuring the hydrolysis of bradykinin in the presence of
specific inhibitors of kininase I (2-mercaptomethyl-3-guanidinoethylthiopro-
panoic acid), kininase II (captopril) and NEP (phosphoramidon) in 8 normal
subjects. The effects of the different assay buffers on kininase activities
were also investigated by using a phosphate buffer. Total kininase, kininase
I, II and NEP activities were 499 ± 65 ng/min/ml (mean$\pm$S.E.), 55 ± 8, 141 ± 21 and
299 ± 42, respectively in our method using a tris buffer, while a phosphate
buffer brought about activities of 358 ± 43, 45 ± 5, 156 ± 21 and 135 ± 25 ng/min/ml.
The relative contributions of kininase I, II and NEP to total kininase activity were 11, 29 and 59% in our assay system, while they were 13, 44 and 35%
when a phosphate buffer was used. From these results it was suggested that
1) phosphate may inhibit urinary NEP activity, so that a tris buffer should
be used as the incubation buffer, 2) NEP is the major component of human
urinary kininases, and 3) NEP may play an important role in the renal kallikrein-kinin system.

INTRODUCTION

The renal kallikrein-kinin system has been implicated in the regulation
of water and sodium excretion as well as in the pathophysiology of some
forms of hypertension (1-4). Although in some studies the urinary kinins
were measured, for the most part kallikrein excretion was the only component
of the system determined (3,5-7). It was assumed to reflect the changes in
the intrarenal concentration of kinins. However, kinins are rapidly metabolized by enzymes, collectively called kininases, and both renal tissue and
urine contain such kininases. Thus, the intrarenal concentration of kinins
may depend on both the production and destruction systems of this peptide.
The best known kininases are kininase I or carboxypeptidase N-type
enzyme which cleaves the C-terminal arginine, and kininase II, also known

as angiotensin I converting enzyme. Recently, a new kininase, neutral endopeptidase (NEP; enkephalinase A) (9) was found in rat urine, in which NEP
was responsible for 68% of the total kininase activity (13). In the present
study, to clarify the significance of NEP in human renal kallikrein-kinin
system, an assay system was developed for the simultaneous determination
of kininase I, II and NEP activities in human urine by modifying the method
for each kininase activity in rat urine.

MATERIALS AND METHODS

     Twenty-four hour urine samples were collected from 8 normal subjects,
and were desalted on a Sephadex G-25 fine column containing 0.1M tris buffer
(pH 7.2).   Thirty μl of a desalted urine sample and 50 μl of 0.1M tris
buffer (pH 7.2) were mixed in polypropylene tubes, and preincubated for 15
minutes at 37°C. Prewarmed 1.25 μg of synthetic bradykinin in 20 μl assay
buffer was added to each tube to initiate the reaction. The mixture was
incubated for 40-80 minutes at 37°C. The reaction was terminated by the
addition of 300 μl of an assay buffer containing 30mM EDTA and 3mM 1,10-
phenanthroline. For the assessment of the contribution of each enzyme to
the total kininase activity, the following specific inhibitors were added
to the incubation mixture prior to preincubation; 10 μM 2-mercaptomethyl-
3-guanidinoethylthiopropanoic acid (MGTA) to inhibit urinary kininase I;
10 μM captopril to inhibit kininase II ; and 1 μM phosphoramidon to inhibit
NEP. The amount of kinin in the reaction mixture was determined by RIA (8).
     Total urinary kininase activity was calculated from the difference in
the amount of kinin in the inhibited (EDTA + 1,10-phenanthroline) and uninhibited reaction tubes. Thus, combination of EDTA and 1,10-phenanthroline
inhibited the total kininase activity. Kininase I, II or NEP activity was

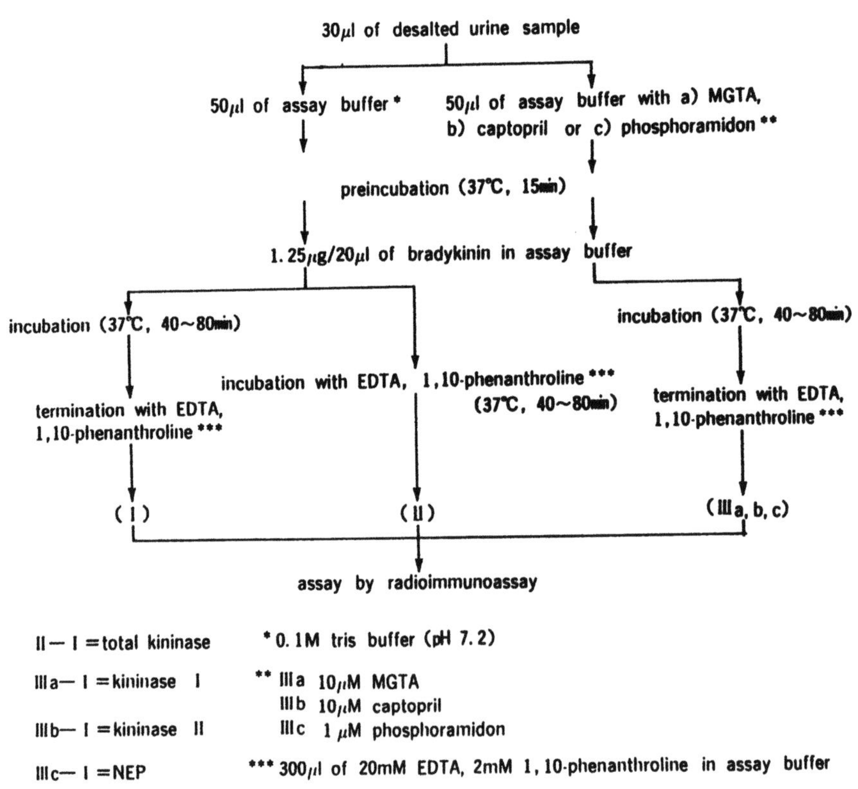

Fig. 1. Assay procedure for human urinary total kininase, kininase I,
         kininase II and NEP determination.

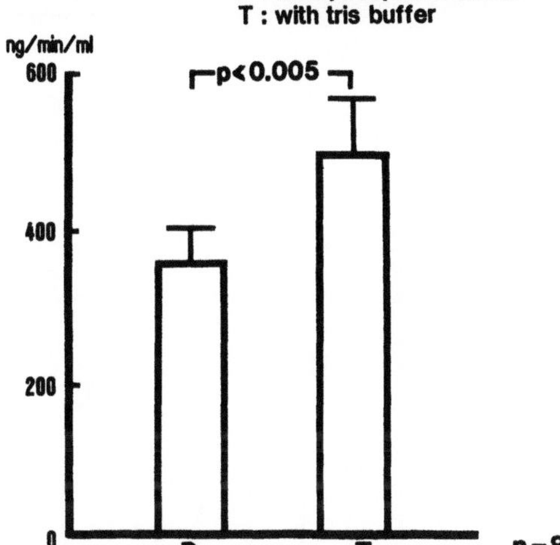

Fig. 2. Effects of tris or phosphate buffer on urinary total kininase
activity in normotensives.

calculated by subtracting the value found in the tubes containing MGTA,
captotril or phosphoramidon from the amount of bradykinin inactivated in the
absence of inhibitors at set time intervals. This procedure is shown in
Fig. 1. Additionaly, the effects of the different assay buffers on kininase
activities were investigated by comparing both the tris buffer and the
phosphate buffer.

RESULTS

Total kininase activity was 499 ± 65 ng/min/ml (mean$\pm$S.E.) in our method,
while it was 358 ± 48 ng/min/ml (mean$\pm$S.E.) when a phosphate buffer was used

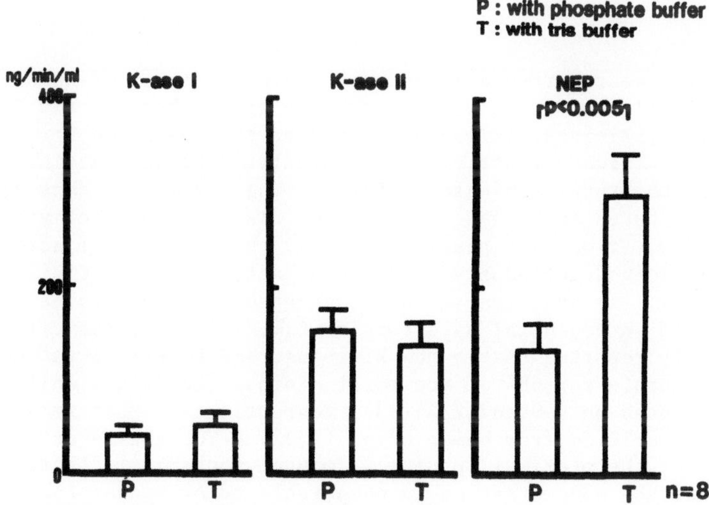

Fig. 3. Effects of tris or phosphate buffer on urinary kininase I, II
and NEP activities in normotensives.

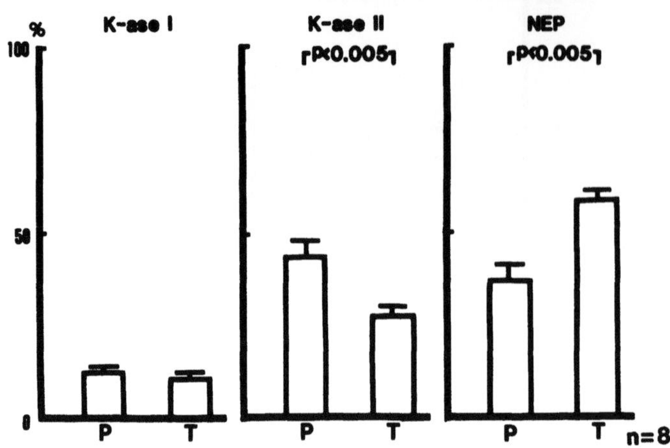

Fig. 4. Effects of tris or phosphate buffer on relative contributions of
kininase I, II and NEP to total kininase activity in normotensives.

instead of tris buffer (Fig. 2). Total kininase activity was significantly
inhibited by using a phosphate buffer. Kininase I, II and NEP activities
were 55+8, 141+21 and 299+42 ng/min/ml, respectively in our method, while
they were 45+5, 156+21 and 135+25 ng/min/ml by use of a phosphate buffer
(Fig. 3). Kininase I and II activities did not show any difference between
the two methods. But NEP activity was significantly lower in the case of the
phosphate buffer. The relative contributions of kininase I,II and NEP to
total kininase activity were 11.3+0.9, 28.5+2.0 and 59.2+2.1% in our assay
system, while they were 12.9+1.0, 44.0+3.6 and 37.1+3.4% in the method using
a phosphate buffer (Fig. 4). When a phosphate buffer was employed, the relative contribution of kininase II was elvaluated as a higher value and that of
NEP was significantly lower as compared to those obtained in our method.

DISCUSSION

     Previously, we reported a method for the measurement of human urinary
kininase I and II activities with bradykinin as a substrate (10,11). In this
previous method, kininase II was estimated as the inhibited activity with
captopril, and kininase I activity was calculated by subtracting kininase II
activity from the total kininase activity. The result was that kininase II
activity contributed more than half to the total kininase activity in human
urine. However, it was not possible to deny that kininase I activity measured by this method includes some kininase activity (or activities) other
than kininase I. In addition, it was suggested that non kininase II activity was elevated in essential hypertension (10,11). In these circumstances,
it was recently reported that a new kininase, NEP exists in rat urine, and
NEP was responsible for 68% of the total kininase activity, while kininase I
and II contributed only 9 and 23% (13), respectively. More recently, NEP
was partially purified from human urine (9,12). The enzyme originates from
brush border of the proximal tubules. Immunocytochemical electronmicroscopy
indicated that NEP concentration is comparable to or higher than that of
kininase II on the brush border of the human kidney. Thus, the possibility
was considered that NEP activity might exist to a significant degree in
human urine. The assay method for simultaneous determination of kininase I,
II and NEP activities in rat urine was modified for the measurement of each

kininase activity in human urine. The difference between the previously
reported method and the new method employed in this study is 1) using MGTA
as a kininase I inhibitor and phosphoramidon as a NEP inhibitor and 2) using
tris buffer as an incubation buffer. The results obtained in this study
revealed that NEP activity contributed more than half to total kininase activity in human urine as well as in rat urine. Total kininase activity and
NEP activity were significantly higher in the new method. This result suggested that phosphate may inhibit urinary NEP activity. Therefore, total
kininase activity in human urine may be inhibited when a phosphate buffer
was used because NEP activity contributed to more than half of that. Since
the sum of the relative contributions of kininase I, II and NEP was almost
100%, the possibility exists that no kininase other than kininase I, II and
NEP may be present in human urine as well as in rat urine. From these findings, it was suggested that NEP might play an important role in the regulation of renal kallikrein-kinin system. Therefore, the simultaneous determination of urinary kininase I, II and NEP activities with other components of
the kallikrein-kinin system should be considered to elucidate the pathophysiological role of renal kallikrein-kinin system in essential hypertension,
renal disease and others.

REFERENCES

1. R. K. Mayfield, H. S. Margolius, Renal Kallikrein-kinin System, Am. J.
      Nephrol., 3:145-155, (1983).
2. O. A. Carretero, A. G. Scicli, The renal kallikrein-kinin system, Am.
      J. Physiol., 238:F247-255, (1980).
3. H. S. Margolius, D. Horwiz, J. J. Pisano, H. R. Keiser, Relationship
      among urinary kallikrein, mineralocoticoids, and human hypertensive
      diseases, Fed. Proc., 35:203-206, (1976).
4. K. Shimamoto, T. Nakao, N. Ura, S. Tanaka, T. Ando, T. Nishimiya, T.
      Mita, M. Kondo, M. Nakagawa, O, Iimura, The role of the renal kalli-
      krein-kinin system in sodium metabolism in normal and low renin
      essential hypertension, Jpn. Cir. J., 47:1210-1215, (1983).
5. A. Lechi, G. Govi, G. Lechi, A. Corgani, E. Arocio, M. Zatti, L. A.
      Scuro, Urinary kallikrein excretion and plasma renin activity in
      patients with essential hypertension and primary aldosteronism,
      Clin. Sci. Mol. Med., 55:51-55, (1978).
6. S. B. Levy, J. J. Lilley, R. P. Frigon, R. A. Stone, Urinary kallikrein
      and plasma renin activity as determinants of renal blood flow,
      J. Clin. Jnvest., 60:129-138, (1977).
7. J. A. Mltas, S. B. Levy, R. Holle, R. P. Frigon, R. P. Stone, Urinary
      kallikrein activity in the hypertension of renal parenchymal disease,
      N. Engl. J. Med., 299:162-165, (1978).
8. K. Shimamoto, T. Ando, S. Tanaka, M. Sakuma, M. Miyahara, A sensitive
      radioimmunoassay method for urinary kinins in man, J. Lab. Clin. Med.
      91:721-728, (1978).
9. R. A. Skidgel, W. W. Sculz, L. T. Tam, E. G. Erdos, Human renal angio-
      tensin I converting enzyme and neutral endopeptidase, Kidney Int.,
      (suppl 20) 31:S45-S48, (1987).
10. A. Ogasawara, K. Shimamoto, Establishment of a Sensitive Method for
      Measurement of Urinary Kininase Activity and Its Clinical Application
      , The Sapporo Med. J., 53 (6):733-745, (1984).
11. N. Ura, K. Shimamoto, S. Tanaka, T. Nishimiya, T. Mita, M. Nakagawa,
      T. Maeda, Y. Yamaguchi, O. Iimura, Urinary Excretion of kininase I
      and kininase II Activities in essential Hypertension. A Sensitive
      and Simple Method for Its Kinin-Destroying capacity, J. Clin.
      Hypertens., 1:15-22, (1985).
12. J. T. Gafford, R. A. Skidgel, E. G. Erdos, L. B. Hersh, Human Kidney
      "Enkephalinase", a Neutral Metalloendopeptidase That Cleaves Active
      Peptides, Biochemistry, 22:3265-3271, (1983).

13. N. Ura, O. A. Carretero, E. G. Erdos, Role of renal endopeptidase 24, 11 in kinin metabolism in vitro and in vivo, <u>Kidney Int.</u>, 32:507-513, (1987).

LOCALIZATION OF NEUTRAL ENDOPEPTIDASE IN THE KIDNEY DETERMINED BY

THE STOP-FLOW METHOD

Thoru Sakakibara, Nobuyuki Ura, Kazuaki Shimamoto, Hitoko
Ogata, Toshiaki Ando, Shuzaburo Fukuyama, Yasukazu Yamaguchi,
Atsushi Masuda, Yoshihiro Mori, Shigeyuki Saito, Takashi Ise,
Yasumoto Sasa, Kazuaki Yamauchi and Osamu Iimura

The 2nd. Dept. of Internal Med. Sapporo Med. Col. Chuo-ku
S1 W16, Sapporo, Japan

SUMMARY

Recently, the existence of neutral endopeptidase (NEP) as a new
kininase in the kidney has been reported. In this study, the localization
of NEP in the nephron was investigated and compared with other components of
the renal kallikrein-kinin (K-K) system by using a stop-flow method in dog
kidneys. The stop-flow method was performed according to the procedures
previously reported by Scicli et al and Malvin et al. Five mongrel dogs
(weighing 15-20 kg) were used in this study. Kininase I, II and NEP were
measured by the modified procedure of Ura et al. Kallikrein and kinin were
found in the distal tubules, and kininase I and II were observed in both
the distal and proximal tubules. NEP was localized mainly in the proximal
tubules. A small peak was also recognized in the distal tubules. From
these results, it was suggested that, not only kininase I and II but also
NEP existing in the proximal tubules may destroy kinin filtered from the
glomeruli, and these kininases existing in the distal tubules may play an
important role in connection with kinin producing enzymes on the regulation
of activity in the renal kallikrein-kinin system.

INTRODUCTION

Since neutral endopeptidase (NEP) is suggested to contain the major
activity of renal kininases (1), the possibility should be considered that
the NEP localizes in the distal tubules as well as kallikrein and regulates
the activity of renal kallikrein-kinin system through the kinin metabolism.
Immunofluorescence technique revealed the existence of NEP in the bursh
border of the proximal tubules in human kidney (2 and 3).   However,
no evidence has been reported as to whether NEP is localized in
the distal tubules or not. In this study, using a stop-flow technique, the
localization of NEP in nephron was investigated in dog kidney.

MATERIALS and METHODS

The stop-flow methods were performed according to the procedures
reported by Scicli et al (4 and 5) and Malvin et al (6). The mongrel dogs

(weighing 15-20 kg) were anesthetized with sodium pentobarbital (30 mg/kg) and ventilated artificially with a Harverd positive pressure pump. Catheters were inserted into the femoral artery and veins, and a Tygon catheter was also inserted into the ureter. The tip of it was placed close to the beginning of the pelvic space.

After catheterization, the initial dose of inulin (60 mg/kg) was injected intravenously. Constant infusion of 0.9% inulin in 0.9% saline (1 ml/min) and 15% mannitol in 5% glucose and 0.9% saline (10 ml/min) were drip infused simultaneously. Urine was permitted to flow freely until it reached a stable value of 3-6 ml/min. Two 1 ml free-flow urine samples were collected immediately before the ureter was clamped for 5 minutes, then the occulusion was released and 16 urine fractions of 1 ml each were collected. From each fraction, a 100 μl urine sample was transfered to other tubes containing 2 μl of a pepstatin solution in 13 N-hydrochlolic acid (10 μg/ml) immediately after the sampling to determine the urinary kinin (8). The residual urine samples without any pepstatin hydrochloride solution were used for the determination of sodium, potassium, inulin, glucose, kallikrein activity, kiniase I, kininase II and NEP content.

Glucose and inulin were measured by the hexokinase methods and anthrone methods (7), respectively. Urinary sodium and potassium were determined by the ion electrode methods. The excretion of kinin was measured by direct radioimmunoassay (8). Kallikrein activity was estimated as the kininogenase activity which reflects the kinin generating capacity from the purified bovine low molecular weight kininogen (9). Kininase I, II and NEP activities were measured as the kinin destroying capacity, employing a kinin direct RIA. All variables were corrected by the inulin concentrations.

RESULTS

The figures below represent the stop-flow patterns of a typical case. Fig. 1. shows the stop-flow patterns for sodium, potassium and glucose. Fractions 4-5 were identified as the distal tubules, because sodium and potassium levels of those fractions showed the lowest value of the former and the highest peak of the latter. Fractions 12-16 were identified as the proximal tubules, because the glucose levels were low in the stop-flow pattern.

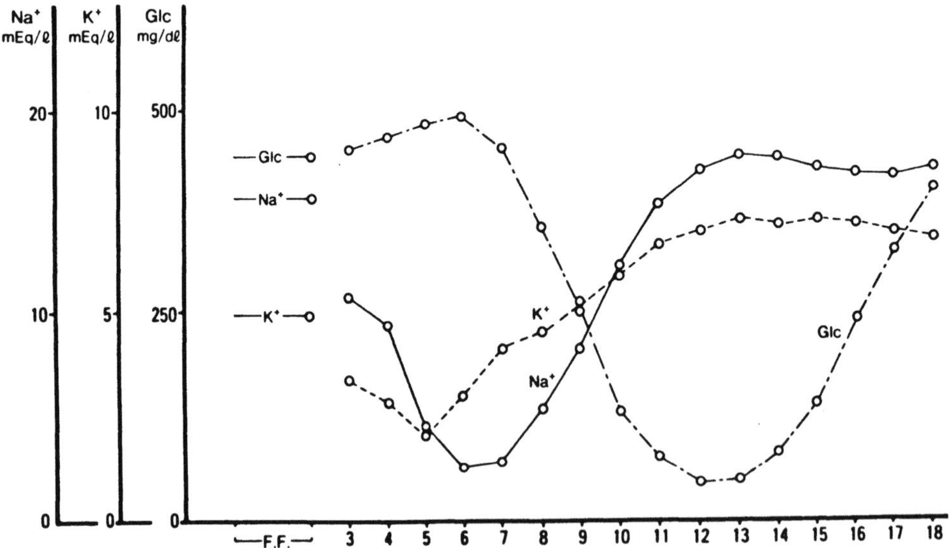

Fig. 1. Stop-flow patterns of sodium, pottasium and glucose in the dog (#1) kidney

The stop-flow patterns for kallikrein activity, kinin, kininase I, kininase II and NEP activities are shown in Fig. 2 and 3. Fig. 2 shows that the peak of kinin is observed at the fraction identical to the last part of the distal tubules and/or in the renal papilla. The peak of kallikrein activity is seen in the slightly more proximal part of the distal tubules.

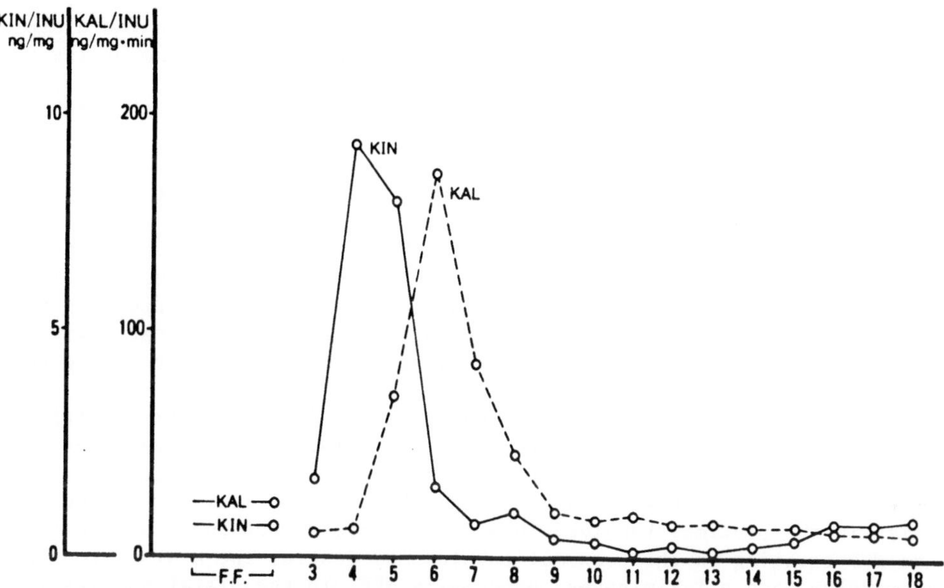

Fig. 2. Stop-flow patterns of KAL and KIN in the dog (#1) kidney

Fig. 3 shows that the peak of NEP activity exists in the distal and proximal tubules, although NEP activity in the distal part is rather small. It is the identical fraction to that of kinin.

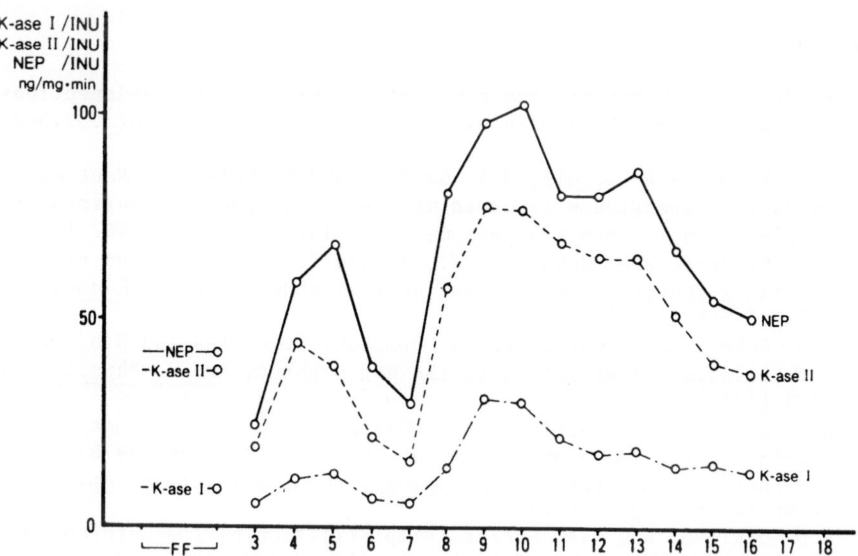

Fig. 3. Stop-flow patterns of K-ase I, II and NEP in the dog (#1) kidney

DISCUSSION

     Scicli et al reported by use of the stop-flow technique that renal
kallikrein-kinin system is located in the distal part of the nephron and
that the components are produced there. It has been reported that the
kallikrein-kinin system seems to regulate the renal blood flow and fluid-
sodium metabolism and that kallikrein-kinin system activity becomes deteri-
orated in those patients with hypertensive diseases.
     We already have reported that kininase I and II exist in the distal
part of the nephron, and that they take part in the regulation of the activity of the kallikrein-kinin system (10).
     However, it remains unknown whether NEP exists in the distal tubules
or not.
     As shown in the results of the stop-flow method in the dog kidney, it
was clarified that NEP localizes not only in the proximal but also in the
distal tubules, as well as kininase I and II.
     Kininase I and II in the proximal tubules are supposed to degenerate
kinin through the glomeruli. Since we recognized a great amount of NEP activity in the proximal part of the nephron, the same possibility can be
suggested in the case of NEP. In addition, NEP showed a greater activity
than kininase I or kininase II, approximately 40-55% activity of the total
kininase in all fractions.
     Moreover, a small peak of NEP was observed in the proximal portion of
the stop-flow pattern. Thus, from these results, it was proven that all
components of urinary kallikrein-kinin system including NEP localize in the
distal nephron, and that only kininases, kininase I, kininase II and NEP
exist in the proximal tubules. This data suggests that the kininase I, II
and NEP existing in the proximal tubules may destroy the kinin through the
glomerulus, and all kininases, especially NEP, in the distal tubules may
play an important role in the regulation of activity in the renal
kallikrein-kinin system.

ACKNOWLEDGMENT

     We wish to thank Miss K. Tanemura, Miss M. Mori, Miss R. Chiba and
Miss M. Toyooka for their technical assistance.

REFFERENCES

1. N. Ura, O.A. Carretero and E.G. Erdos, Role of renal endopeptidase 24
    11 in kinin metabolism in vitro and in vivo, Kidney Int.,32:507-513
    (1987)
2. E.G. Erdos, W.W. Schulz, J.T. Gafford and R. Defendin, Neutral
    metalloendopeptidase in Human male genital tract. Comparison to
    angiotensin I converting enzyme, Lab. Invest., 52:437-447 (1985)
3. R.A. Skidgel, W.W. Schulz, L.T. Tam and E.G. Erdos, Human renal angio-
    tensin I converting enzyme and neutral endopeptidase, Kidney Int.,
    31:545-548 (1987)
4. A.G. Scicli, O.A. Carretero, A. Hampton, P. Cortes and N.B. Oza, Site
    of kininogenase secretion in the dog nephron, Am. J. Physiol., 230:
    533 (1976)
5. A.G. Scicli, R. Gandorf and O.A. Carretero, Site of formation of
    kinins in the dog nephron, Am. J. Physiol., 234:F36 (1978)
6. R.L. Malvin, Hand book of physiology, renal physiology, Am. J. Soc.,
    Washington DC pp 119 (1973)
7. W.D. Davidson and M.A. Sacker, Simplification of the anthrone method
    for the determination of inulin in clearance studies, J. Lab. Clin.
    Med., 62:351 (1963)

8.   K. Shimamoto, T. Ando, T. Nakao, M. Sakuma and M. Miyahara, A sensi-
     tive radioimmunoassay method for urinary kinins in man, J. Lab. Clin.
     Med., 91:721-728 (1978)

9.   K. Shimamoto, S. Tanaka, T. Nakao, T. Ando, Y. Nakahashi, M. Sakuma and
     M. Miyahara, Measurement of urinary kallikrein activity by kinin radio-
     immunoassay, Jap. Circ. J., 43:147-152 (1979)

10. Y. Yamaguchi, K. Shimamoto, N. Ura, T. Nishimiya, M. Nakagawa, A.
     Masuda, T. Ando and O. Iimura, Localization of renal kallikrein-kinin
     system components in the dog kidney, Jap. J. Med., 25:9-12 (1986)

METABOLISM OF BRADYKININ BY MULTIPLE COEXISTING MEMBRANE-BOUND PEPTIDASES
IN LUNG: TECHNIQUES FOR INVESTIGATING THE ROLE OF EACH PEPTIDASE USING
SPECIFIC INHIBITORS

Arthur T. Orawski, Jean P. Susz, and William H. Simmons

Department of Biochemistry and Biophysics
Loyola University of Chicago Stritch School of Medicine
Maywood, Illinois 60153 USA

INTRODUCTION

The rapid metabolism of bradykinin (BK) during passage through the
pulmonary circulation is well documented[1-3]. Angiotensin converting enzyme
(ACE)[4], which is located on the plasma membrane of vascular endothelial
cells, has been implicated in this process[1-3]. However, there is evidence
that lung contains several additional membrane-bound peptidases which also
participate in the degradation of BK and/or its primary and secondary
metabolites[2,5-9].

The elucidation of a multi-enzyme metabolic pathway can present significant challenges. Indeed, we observed complex patterns of degradation of
BK by several enzyme preparations including: a) a detergent-solubilized
extract of membrane-bound peptidases from bovine lung[5], 2) bovine and rat
lung microsomes[6-8], 3) isolated perfused rat lung[2-3], and 4) rat brain
synaptic membranes[10]. The metabolites formed by each of these preparations
were separated by high performance liquid chromatography (HPLC). The large
number of peaks observed were subsequently identified by amino acid analysis,
end-group analysis, and comparison of retention times with synthetic peptide
standards. However, knowledge of the metabolites alone was not sufficient
to completely identify sites of cleavage in BK and its metabolites; nor was
this data sufficient to identify which enzymes were responsible for each
cleavage, or to establish precursor-product relationships among the metabolites. These problems were addressed by determining how various specific
peptidase inhibitors altered the HPLC pattern of metabolite peaks.

When using peptidase inhibitors for this purpose, it is essential that
the inhibitors be highly specific, inhibiting only the enzyme of interest.
For many of the inhibitors which we used, adequate information on inhibitor
specificity was not available. It was therefore necessary to determine this
specificity by developing inhibitor profiles for the various peptidases
present in lung.

As reported in this paper, we first identified membrane-bound peptidases present in a detergent-solubilized extract of bovine lung[5] using
specific model substrates. These substrates were then used to determine,
or confirm, key properties of the enzymes and to develop inhibitor profiles.
Comparative date were then obtained for a rat lung detergent extract and
for bovine and rate lung microsomes which contain the membrane-bound forms

of the peptidases. From this information, the most specific inhibitor for
each enzyme was chosen for studying of the role of each peptidase in BK
metabolism. A summary of the BK catabolic pathways which we elucidated for
several lung tissue preparations is also presented below.

METHODS

Enzyme Preparation and Assays

    Bovine lungs were obtained frozen from Pel-Freez while rat lungs
(Sprague-Dawley) were used fresh following decapitation. The "detergent
extracts" were prepared as described earlier[5]. Briefly, 0.25% sodium deoxycholate was used to extract membrane-bound peptidases from saline-washed,
delipidated acetone powder of bovine or rat lung. Microsomes from bovine
and rat lung were prepared from a 1:3 (w/v) homogenate of lung tissue in 0.1
M potassium phosphate, pH 7.4. Successive centrifugations were carried out
at 600 and 3300 x g (10 min), 10,000 x g (20 min), and 149,000 x g (50 min).
The final microsome-containing pellet was resuspended in 0.1 M potassium
phosphate, pH 6.8, and stored at either 4° for immediate use, or at -20° C.

    Most assays were performed at 37°C in 50 mM imidazole-HCl at pH 6.8.
In some cases (including all assays of microsomal preparations), 50 mM
potassium phosphate buffer, pH 6.8, was used as indicated in the text.
Assays for specific enzymes are described below. Degradation of BK was
monitored by HPLC as described earlier[5].

Inhibitors

    K_i values and additional kinetic parameters associated with mixed-type
inhibition were determined by the methods described by Segal[11]. In order
to evaluate the specificity of an inhibitor, the concentration of inhibitor
which produced nearly complete inhibition of the known target peptidase(s)
was determined. This concentration, which is indicated in Table 1, was then
used to determine whether the inhibitor was also able to affect the activities of the other peptidases present. In these assays, the concentration
of the peptidase substrates was always at the substrate K_m value.

RESULTS

    Several known membrane-bound peptidases were detected in the detergent
extract of bovine lung. Some of the more prominent of these are indicated
in Table 1 along with their sensitivities to various inhibitors.

    1. Aminopeptidase A (AP A) (glutamyl aminopeptidase) (EC 3.4.11.7)[4].
AP A was detected in the detergent extract of bovine lung using α-L-gluta-
myl-2-naphthylamide (Glu-2-NA) in the presence of 1.1 mM CaCl$_2$[4,12]. Calcium
was required for maximal activity. The K_m for Glu-2-NA was 0.14 mM. Amastatin was the best inhibitor of AP A activity with a K_i = 4.4 x 10^{-6} M
(competitive). Of the other agents in Table 1, only 1,10-phenanthroline
substantially blocked activity. Two inhibitors of aminopeptidase M (AP M),
puromycin and bestatin, had little or no effect on AP A. Discontinuities
in the kinetic curves for amastatin inhibition led to the conclusion that
Glu-2-NA is not an absolutely specific substrate for AP A. A second enzyme
in the mixture accounted for 15% of the Glu-2-NA cleavage and had a K_i for
amastatin of 5 x 10^{-8} M[13]. This second enzyme was presumably AP M (see
below).

    2. Aminopeptidase M (AP M) (microsomal alanyl aminopeptidase)
(EC 3.4.11.2)[4]. AP M was found in the detergent extract of bovine lung

Table 1. Specificity of Inhibitors Toward Solubilized Membrane-associated Peptidases from Bovine Lung[a]

Inhibitors (mM)	% Inhibition					
	Enzyme					
	AP A	AP M	AP P	DPP IV	EP 24.11	ACE
Bestatin (0.21)	12	89	1	1	0	8
Amastatin (0.17)	87	97	13	1	2	-3
Puromycin (0.30)	22	73	14	1	3	5
2-Mercaptoethanol (3.8)	0	23	90	17	2	13
DFP (1 hr preinc.) (2.0)	-5	0	3	98	4	15
Diprotin A (1.0)	13	14	8	98	5	9
Phosphoramidon (0.0004)	-1	-6	13	1	98	0
Thiorphan (0.0002)					96	72
(0.01)	0	0	-8	1		
(0.1)	0	4		4	100	99
Zincov (0.01)	6		13			
(0.05)	9	89		1	100	0
Captopril (0.001)	1	-1	0	-1	0	97
(1.0)	14	11		27		
o-Phenanthroline (0.5)	89	87	100	20		100

[a]Each enzyme was assayed using its specific substrate (see text) at a concentration equal to the Km value. Assays were at 37°C in 50 mM imidazole-HCl, pH 6.8, except for AP P which was in 50 mM potassium phosphate, pH 6.8. Abbreviations for inhibitors and enzymes are as indicated in the text. Levels of inhibition >70% are underlined.

using the substrate L-alanyl-2-naphthylamide (Ala-2-NA)[4,12] which had a K_m = 0.11 mM. An alternative substrate, L-arginyl-2-naphthylamide (Arg-2-NA), had a K_m = 0.10 mM. Both substrates gave identical inhibitory profiles for the enzyme. When used to assay an ion exchange chromatography run of the detergent extract, both substrates yielded superimposed peaks. The activity ratio of Ala-2-NA / Arg-2-NA was 2 when both substrates were assayed at K_m concentrations. The solubilized AP M activity in the detergent extract was stable upon freezing in phosphate buffer, but not in imidazole. Preincubation with 0.5% isopropanol completely inactivated AP M.

AP M was inhibited by amastatin, bestatin, and puromycin (Table 1). The best inhibitor was amastatin with a K_i = 4.7 x 10^{-8} M. Amastatin showed primarily competitive inhibition although detailed analysis suggested mixed-type with α = 10 and $\beta \neq 0^{11}$. Bestatin was a competitive inhibitor with a K_i = 1.0 x 10^{-6} M. Puromycin had a K_i = 8.4 x 10^{-6} M and exhibited mixed-type kinetics with α = 3.7, $\beta = 0^{11}$. Zincov was inhibitory only at relatively high concentration (5 x 10^{-5} M; but not at 10^{-7} M). One hour preincubation with 1,10-phenanthroline at different concentrations gave the following % inhibition: 87% at 1.7 mM, 69% at 0.3 mM, and 10% at 0.17 mM. The other agents in Table 1 had little or no effect on AP M activity. Only a higher concentration of 2-ME (19 mM) and p-chloromercuriphenylsulfonic acid (PCMPSA) (1 mM) significantly inhibited activity (90% and 56%, resp.).

3. Aminopeptidase P (AP P) (microsomal proline aminopeptidase) (EC 3.4.11.9)[4]. Several properties of solubilized AP P in the detergent

extract of bovine lung have been described previously[5]. AP P, which presumably releases N-terminal amino acids only when proline is in the penultimate position, was assayed in 50 mM potassium phosphate, pH 6.8, using Arg-Pro-Pro as substrate (K_m = 0.93 mM). Activity was quantitated following separation of Arg, Pro-Pro and substrate by HPLC[5]. The pH optimum for this substrate was 7.0. The release of glycine from Gly-Pro-Hyp in the presence of 10 mM $MnCl_2$ was also used to assay AP P[5] (using the standard imidazole buffer). $MnCl_2$, which had little effect on Arg-Pro-Pro cleavage, increased V_{max} for Gly-Pro-Hyp 10-fold over the range of 0-10 mM, but had no effect on K_m (0.34 mM). Evidence has been presented[5] that the AP P activity which hydrolyzes Arg-Pro-Pro and Gly-Pro-Hyp also cleaves the Arg^1-Pro^2 bond of BK. In addition, AP P was able to hydrolyze all N-terminal homologs of BK as well as Arg-Pro-Arg (0.43 times the rate of Arg-Pro-Pro, both at 1 mM) but not His-Pro-Phe or Ile-Pro-Ile (diprotin A).

Identical inhibitory profiles were obtained whether Arg-Pro-Pro, Gly-Pro-Hyp, or BK was used as a substrate for AP P. The results for Arg-Pro-Pro in Table 1 show that the best inhibitor of AP P activity was 2-mercaptoethanol (2-ME) which reduced activity 90% at 3.8 mM. AP P was partially, but maximally, inhibited 70% and 69% by the sulfhydryl group reagents, p-chloromercuribenzoate (PCMB) and PCMPSA, resp. Iodoacetic acid (1 mM) had no effect. The non-specific chelating agent, 1,10-phenanthroline, completely inhibited activity. MGTA (DL-2-mercaptomethyl-3-guanidino-ethylthiopropanoic acid) (1 mM) and citrate (25 mM) inhibited 54% and 60%, resp. None of the other agents in Table 1 significantly inhibited AP P.

4. Dipeptidyl Peptidase IV (DPP IV) (dipeptidylaminopeptidase IV) (EC 3.4.14.5)[4].

DPP IV specifically releases the N-terminal dipeptide from a substrate when the penultimate residue is proline (or alanine)[4]. DPP IV was detected in the bovine lung detergent extract using glycyl-prolyl-2-naphthylamide (Gly-Pro-2-NA) (K_m = 0.89 mM)[4,12]. Diisopropylphosphofluoridate (DFP) was a potent irreversible inhibitor of DPP IV. The second-order rate constant[14], $k_{obsd}/[DFP]$, was 11 $M^{-1}S^{-1}$ (using [DFP] at 1-4 x 10^{-5} M; 37°). The half-life for enzyme activity in the presence of 0.04 mM DFP was 27 min. The concentration of DFP used in the experiments shown in Table 1 (2 mM) inactivated DPP IV with a half-life of under 2 minutes.

Diprotin A (Ile-Pro-Ile) was a competitive inhibitor of DPP IV, having a K_i = 2.5 x 10^{-6} M. Other proline-containing tripeptides were also tested for their ability to inhibit cleavage of 0.5 mM substrate. The IC_{50} values were 1) diprotin A: 7 x 10^{-6} M; 2) Thr-Pro-Val: 4.0 x 10^{-5} M; 3) His-Pro-Phe: 1.5 x 10^{-4} M; 4) Ala-Pro-Gly: 2.0 x 10^{-4} M; 5) Arg-Pro-Arg: 6.0 x 10^{-4} M; 6) Arg-Pro-Pro: 1.0 x 10^{-3} M; 7) Gly-Pro-Hyp: no inhibition at 10^{-3} M. Some of the above tripeptides were shown by HPLC to be substrates for DPP IV and were cleaved in the following order (all peptides at 1 mM): His-Pro-Phe (rate comparable to Gly-Pro-2-NA) > Ala-Pro-Gly > Thr-Pro-Val > Arg-Pro-Arg (rate 13% of Gly-Pro-2-NA). Diprotin A and the two aminopeptidase P substrates, Arg-Pro-Pro and Gly-Pro-Hyp, were not cleaved.

None of the other agents in Table 1 significantly affected DPP IV activity. DPP IV was inhibited only 17% and 15% by 2-ME at 3.8 mM and 190 mM, resp., and was the only enzyme studied which was resistant to 2-ME at 190 mM. 1,10-Phenanthroline inhibited 20% and 50% at 0.5 mM and 5.9 mM, resp.

5. Endopeptidase 24.11 (EP 24.11) (neutral metalloendopeptidase, "enkephalinase", kidney microvillus proteinase) (EC 3.4.24.11)[15].

EP 24.11 specifically cleaves peptide substrates on the amino side of hydrophobic amino acids[16]. EP 24.11 activity was detected in detergent extracts of bovine lung using glutaryl-alanyl-alanyl-phenylalanyl-4-methoxy-2-naph-thylamide[16] (Glt-Ala-Ala-Phe-MNA) at the Km-concentration of 0.053 mM. A coupled assay was used in which the released Phe-MNA was hydrolyzed by endogenous AP M to give 4-methoxy-2-napthylamide which was then quantitated using the Garnet GBC method[12]. When testing inhibitors which blocked AP M and thus interferred with the coupled assay, HPLC was used to separate and quantitate the products.

Table 1 shows that the EP 24.11 activity in lung was inhibited by phosphoramidon. Inhibition was competitive with a K_i = 2.1 x 10^{-9} M. Zincov and thiorphan were also potent inhibitors with K_i's of 4 x 10^{-8} M and 4 x 10^{-9} M, resp. None of the other agents in Table 1, including captopril, were capable of inhibiting EP 24.11 activity. While 2-ME had no effect at 3.8 mM, it did reduce activity at the higher concentrations of 19 mM (44%) and 190 mM (98%). An alternative substrate for EP 24.11, succinyl-alanyl-alanyl-phenylalanyl-7-amino-4-methylcoumarin[17] (K_m = 0.046 mM), gave the same inhibitory profile as Glt-Ala-Ala-Phe-MNA.

HPLC anion exchange (Mono Q) chromatography of the detergent extracts from both bovine and rat lung gave single EP 24.11 activity peaks. The partially purified rat EP 24.11 had the same inhibitory profile as the bovine enzyme and, in addition, was shown to be unaffected by 0.001 mM teprotide but inhibited 88% by 10^{-8} M thiorphan.

6. Angiotensin Converting Enzyme (ACE) (peptidyl dipeptidase A, kininase II) (EC 3.4.15.1)[4]. ACE was detected using hippuryl-histidyl-leucine (Hip-His-Leu) at its K_m-concentration (0.27 mM) in the presense of 0.3 M NaCl[4] and following the release of His-Leu by HPLC. Chloride ion was stimulatory for this substrate as reported by others[4,18], increasing activity 8-fold under the conditions of the assay. Chloride had no effect on the cleavage of the Pro^7-Phe^8-bond of BK and was not included in assays of BK metabolism.

Table 1 shows that captopril completely inhibited ACE activity at 10^{-6} M (K_i = 1.4 x 10^{-9} M) (and probably at lower concentrations as well). When BK (at 0.5 mM) was used as a substrate instead of Hip-His-Leu (at 0.27 mM), 10^{-5} M captopril was required for complete inhibition. This difference can be explained by the fact that BK has a 2600-fold lower K_m than Hip-His-Leu and can therefore compete more successfully with captopril for the ACE active site[19]. Thiorphan (K_i = 8 x 10^{-8} M), as well as 1,10-phenanthroline (0.5 mM) and EDTA (1 mM), also completely inhibited ACE. Teprotide (nona-peptide inhibitor from B. jararaca) produced 95% inhibition at 10^{-6} M. None of the other agents in Table 1 significantly affected ACE activity. Phos-phoramidon had no effect on bovine lung ACE in either the detergent extract or in microsomes up to at least 10^{-5} M. However, in the case of rat lung, ACE activity in both the detergent extract and microsomes was partially inhibited by high concentrations of phosphoramidon: 8%, 10^{-8} M; 18%, 10^{-7} M; 31%, 10^{-6} M; 60%, 10^{-5}. The same inhibitory effect of phosphoramidon was also seen for rat lung ACE which had been partially purified by Mono Q anion exchange chromatography. 2-ME (3.8 mM) also exhibited different effects on ACE, depending on the preparation and species, with the maximal inhibition being 35% for ACE from bovine lung microsomes using Hip-His-Leu as substrate.

7. Other lung peptidases. The following peptidases, which are not shown in Table 1, were found to be present in one or more of the lung preparations used in these studies. Each peptidase was found to have some role in the degradation of BK or BK-metabolites in those preparations where it was found.

a. Dipeptidyl Peptidase I (DPP I) (Dipeptidylaminopeptidase I) (EC 3.4.14.1)[4]. The ability of the detergent extract from bovine lung to release Gly-Phe from Gly-Phe-2-NA (K_m = 0.13 mM) indicated the presence of a

DPP I-like enzyme[4,12]. In order to see activity, amastatin was required in
the assay to inhibit AP M which sequentially degrades the substrate as well
as the Gly-Phe product. The DPP I-like enzyme played a role in BK degradation by releasing Gly-Phe from BK metabolites (see below). Bovine lung
microsomes also contained the enzyme, but its contribution to the degradation of BK metabolites appeared to be small in comparison to other mechanisms leading to Gly-Phe release (see below).

       **b. Carboxypeptidase N-like (CP N) (Plasma Carboxypeptidase B)
(EC 3.4.17.3)[4]**. The detergent extracts of both bovine and rat lung, as well
as bovine and rat lung microsomes, contained an activity which contributed
in a minor way to the degradation of BK by releasing the C-terminal arginine
from BK. This CP N-like activity was completely inhibited by 1 mM MGTA.

       c. Dipeptidase (DP) (EC 3.4.13.-). We previously reported on a
dipeptidase (DP) from rat brain synaptosomes which could hydrolyze one of
the C-terminal metabolites of BK, Phe-Arg, as well as kyotorphin (Tyr-
Arg)[10,20]. A characteristic of DP is inhibition by bestatin but not by
amastatin. DP-like activity was observed in both bovine and rat lung
microsomes using an HPLC assay for Phe-Arg-cleavage. In addition, the
detergent extract of rat lung contained DP-activity which was inhibited 91%
by bestatin (0.12 mM) but 0% by amastatin (0.17 mM). On the other hand,
the extraction procedure apparently inactivated the DP activity of bovine
lung. The very low Phe-Arg-cleaving activity of this preparation could be
attributed to AP M since it was inhibited by amastatin and puromycin as well
as bestatin.

       d. Proline dipeptidase (P-DP) (prolidase) (EC 3.4.13.9)[4]. We
previously noted the presence of low levels of proline dipeptidase (P-DP)
activity in the detergent extract of bovine lung using the substrate
Arg-Pro[5]. This activity appeared to be responsible for the slow cleavage of
the dipeptide, Ser-Pro, which is an accumulated metabolite of BK produced by
other enzymes present in this preparation (see below). Although optimal
assay conditions for this enzyme were not used (e.g., + Mn^{+2}), bovine and
rat lung microsomes contained even less P-DP activity than the detergent
extract. This enzyme is known to co-purify with membrane-bound peptidases
and therefore may represent a cytosolic contaminant of the detergent solubilized bovine lung enzymes.

       e. Endopeptidase 24.15 (EC 3.4.24.15)[21]. An activity was
observed in bovine lung microsomes which could hydrolyze the Phe^5-Ser^6-bond
of BK. This activity was inhibited almost completely by 10^{-4} M N-[1-(R,S)-
carboxy-2-phenylethyl]-Ala-Ala-Phe-p-aminobenzoate (CPAAPA), suggesting the
activity was EP 24.15[21]. This enzyme was not observed in either the detergent extract of bovine lung, or in rat lung microsomes. However, EP 24.15
was the major enzyme responsible for BK degradation in rat brain synaptic
membranes[15]. In this latter preparation, phenelzine at 1 mM was also found
to cause nearly complete inhibition of EP 24.15.

       f. Peptidase activities which were not found. The dipeptide
metabolite, Pro-Pro, accumulated when BK was incubated with each of the
enzyme preparations. The fact that Pro-Pro was not cleaved indicated the
absence of prolyl dipeptidase (prolinase) (EC 3.4.13.8)[4]. Neither microsomal prolyl carboxypeptidase (carboxypeptidase P) (EC 3.4.17.-)[4] (substrate = Cbz-Pro-Ala) nor prolyl endopeptidase (EC 3.4.21.26) (Cbz-Gly-
Pro-2-NA) were observed in the detergent extract of bovine lung. The
cleavage of BK by the latter preparation was unaffected by the thiol
protease inhibitor, E-64, the acid protease inhibitor, pepstatin, and an
inhibitor of chymotrypsin-like proteases, chymostatin.

Several known membrane-bound peptidases were found in lung. Many of these have the potential to degrade BK and/or other biologically active peptides and may have a physiological role in the metabolism of circulating peptide hormones. In order to delineate the role of each enzyme in these processes, it is necessary to have available a series of enzyme-specific inhibitors. These inhibitors can then be used to demonstrate which enzyme is responsible for each of the specific peptide-bond cleavages in the substrate.

Towards this end, we determined inhibitor profiles for several peptidases as shown in Table 1. From this data, it was possible to select inhibitors which were specific for each enzyme. The results of this analysis are as follows:

<u>AP A</u>. Amastatin was the only agent tested which competitively inhibited AP A. While amastatin is not specific since it also inhibits AP M (but no other enzyme tested), it can still be used to identify AP A. If the release of an N-terminal amino acid (particularly Asp or Glu) from a peptide substrate is blocked by amastatin but not by bestatin, it is probably due to AP A rather than AP M. Furthermore, there is a concentration effect criterion since significant inhibition of AP M by amastatin can occur at 10^{-6}–10^{-8} M while inhibition of AP A requires 10^{-4}–10^{-6} M.

<u>AP M</u>. Bestatin is a selective inhibitor for AP M since it failed to inhibit all other enzymes in Table 1, including AP A, even at a concentration as high as 10^{-4} M. Only in the case of a dipeptide substrate is there possible ambiguity since a dipeptide could be a substrate for the bestatin-inhibited dipeptidase. However, if cleavage of such a dipeptide is also blocked by amastatin or puromycin, the enzyme responsible probably is AP M. In those cases where the concentration of AP A has been determined to be negligible, amastatin is preferred over bestatin as a routine inhibitor of AP M because of its 100-fold lower K_i.

<u>AP P</u>. 2-Mercaptoethanol (2-ME)is a selective inhibitor of AP P at 3.8 mM. At this concentration, 2-ME causes 90% inhibition of AP P, minimal inhibition of AP M, and no inhibition of the other enzymes in Table 1. However, a potent, specific active-site directed inhibitor must clearly be developed for AP P.

<u>DPP IV</u>. DPP IV is the only enzyme studied which can be completely and irreversibly inhibited by DFP. Diprotin A is also a selective inhibitor of DPP IV and is a competitive rather than covalent inhibitor. Diprotin A provides an attractive alternative to the use of toxic DFP and can be used more easily in physiological-type experiments such as the isolated perfused lung.

<u>EP 24.11</u>. Phosphoramidon is an effective, as well as selective, inhibitor of EP 24.11 in the 10^{-7}–10^{-8} M range. Above 10^{-7} M, partial inhibition of rat ACE, but not bovine ACE, also occurs. In the case of Zincov, the concentration range required to inhibit EP 24.11 overlaps that which inhibits AP M. Similarly, thiorphan blocks both ACE and EP 24.11. Therefore, Zincov and thiorphan are useful only in experiments designed to confirm the presence of EP 24.11. Retro-thiorphan, while not used in this study, has been reported to inhibit EP 24.11 but not ACE.

<u>ACE</u>. Captopril is selective for ACE. Thiorphan is not selective since it also inhibits EP 24.11. (It has been reported that captopril can inhibit prolidase with a K_i in the 10^{-5} M range[22].)

<u>Other Enzymes</u>. While other peptidases were not studied as systematically as those above in terms of sensitivity to inhibitors, some conclusions

can nevertheless be drawn. MGTA, which is a well-known inhibitor of carboxypeptidase N[4], also partially inhibits aminopeptidase P at 1 mM. Presumably, lower concentrations of MGTA would distinguish between these enzymes.
The very different primary substrate specificities of these enzymes should
not lead to confusion in any case.

    EP 24.15 is inhibited by CPAAPA[21]. In rat brain synaptic membranes
where EP 24.15-like activity is the major BK-degrading enzyme, CPAAPA
inhibited the cleavage of the Phe^5-Ser^6 bond in both BK and des-Arg^9-BK.
However, it had no apparent effect on cleavage of other bonds in BK or
BK-metabolites. These data suggest that at least among the synaptic
membrane peptidases studied, CPAAPA is specific for EP 24.15.

Determination of bradykinin metabolic pathways

    The pattern of bradykinin metabolism was determined for microsomes and
detergent extracts of bovine and rat lung, for the isolated perfused rat
lung, and for rat brain synaptic plasma membranes. Metabolites produced by
these preparations were separated by HPLC and identified. The effects of
the specific peptidase inhibitors discussed above on the HPLC pattern of
metabolites were determined. Conclusions were then drawn as to which peptide bonds in bradykinin were cleaved and which enzymes were responsible.
The details of these experiments will appear elsewhere. The following is
a summary of the results:

<u>Bovine lung microsomes[8]</u>:

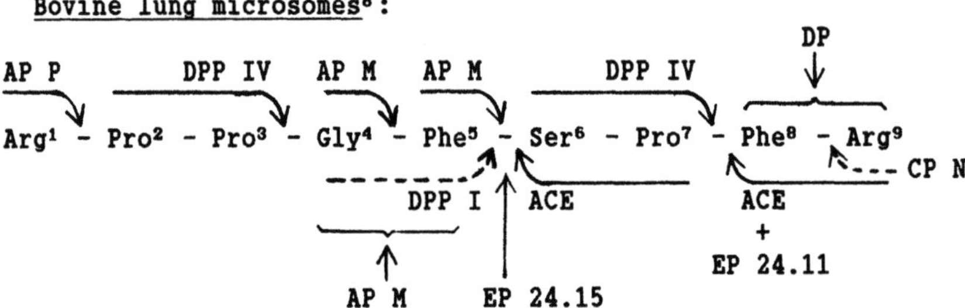

BK was degraded by bovine lung microsomes at several peptide bonds. The
N-terminal Arg was released by AP P (inhibited by 3.8 mM 2-ME). This was
followed by sequential release of Pro-Pro by DPP IV (inhibited by DFP and
diprotin A), Gly and Phe by AP M (inhibited by amastatin), and Ser-Pro and
Phe-Arg by DPP IV. EP 24.15 cleaved the internal Phe^5-Ser^6-bond in both BK
and BK_{1-8} (inhibited by CPAAPA). Both ACE and EP 24.11 released the C-terminal Phe-Arg dipeptide (partially inhibited by either captopril or phosphoramidon, completely inhibited by both when N-terminal degradation was
blocked). ACE further removed Ser-Pro. CP N had a minor role in releasing
the C-terminal Arg. The dipeptidase cleaved the Phe-Arg metabolite (inhibited by bestatin but not amastatin) while AP M slowly hydrolyzed Gly-Phe
(inhibited by amastatin). In terms of the initial cleavage of intact BK, it
was estimated that AP P, ACE, and EP 24.11 made about equal contributions,
while EP 24.15 acted at about one-half the rate of the others (using 0.5 mM
BK as substrate).

    <u>Detergent extract of bovine lung[5]</u>: ACE, EP 24.11, EP 25.15, CP N and
DP were relatively unimportant to BK degradation in this preparation compared to microsomes. This was probably due to poor extractability or
inactivation during the extraction procedure. The major mode of degradation
of BK in this case was sequential degradation from the N-terminus by AP P,
DPP IV and AP M (as outlined above for microsomes)[5]. AP P accounted for
over 90% of the cleavage of intact BK. Low levels of the DPP I-like enzyme
released Gly-Phe from BK_{4-9} while AP M slowly hydrolyzed both Gly-Phe and
Phe-Arg (in the absence of the dipeptidase).

Rat lung microsomes[1]: The mechanism of degradation of BK by rat lung microsomes was quite similar to that for bovine lung microsomes. The differences were that EP 24.15 was absent and both AP M and EP 24.11 activities were reduced in rat microsomes. The decreased AP M activity resulted in the accumulation of the Gly-Phe metabolite.   EP 24.11 was only about one-fourth as active as ACE in releasing the C-terminal Phe-Arg. Overall, the cleavage of intact BK at the C-terminus by ACE was somewhat faster than N-terminal hydrolysis by AP P.

Detergent extract of rat lung: The mechanism of BK degradation by this preparation was similar to the scheme shown above for bovine lung microsomes except that EP 24.11, EP 24.15 and CP N were not observed. Interestingly, rat ACE and dipeptidase survived the extraction procedure while the respective bovine enzymes did not. N-terminal cleavage by AP P and C-terminal cleavage by ACE occurred at about equal rates.

Isolated perfused rat lung[3]: When [^{3}H-2,3-Pro]BK was perfused through the isolated rat lung, the labelled substrate was degraded from both the N- and C-terminal ends. N-terminal cleavage was blocked by 2-ME and therefore was apparently due to AP P while C-terminal cleavage was blocked by captopril and was primarily due to ACE. The release of ^{3}H-Pro-Pro was blocked by diprotin A, indicating the involvement of DPP IV in the sequential degradation of bradykinin. Phosphoramidon had essentially no effect on BK degradation in the perfused lung. Thus, the results with the isolated perfused lung confirmed the in vitro results using rat lung microsomes.

Additional comments: The complicated BK degradation patterns discussed above are made even more complex by the observations that 1) AP P can cleave N-terminal fragments of BK more rapidly than BK itself, and 2) ACE can more readily hydrolyze fragments missing the N-terminal Arg-residue than BK itself. Thus, it would appear that simultaneous N- and C-terminal degradation can actually accelerate subsequent fragment degradation.

Our studies on BK degradation have essentially confirmed earlier elegant studies by Ryan and coworkers[2,23]. They demonstrated that the isolated perfused rat lung as well as cultured endothelial cells[23] can degrade BK at multiple sites giving rise to a variety of metabolites. We have been able to extend this work by identifying the peptidases responsible for the multi-step catabolism of BK. We have identified the specific cleavage sites in BK for each enzyme and have established precursor-product relationships among the metabolites. This work should provide the basis for subsequent experiments on the physiological role of lung peptidases other than ACE in the metabolism of circulating BK and other biologically active peptides.

ACKNOWLEDGEMENTS

This work was supported in part by U. S. Public Health Service grants AL28710, HL30970, and NS20252, and a Potts Estate grant from Loyola University of Chicago.

REFERENCES

1. S. H. Ferreira & Y. S. Bakhle, Inactivation of bradykinin and related peptides in lung, in: "Metabolic Functions of the Lung," Y. S. Bakhle and J. R. Vane, eds., pp 33-53, Marcel Dekker Inc, New York (1977).
2. J. W. Ryan, J. Roblero, & J. M. Stewart, Inactivation of bradykinin in rat lung, Adv. Exp. Med. Biol., 8:263-281 (1970).
3. M. Churchill, A. T. Orawski, P. N. AchutaMurthy, & W. H. Simmons,

Degradation of bradykinin by isolated perfused rat lung, <u>Fed. Proc. Fed. Am. Soc. Exp. Biol.</u>, 45:678 (1986) (Abstract).

4. J. K. McDonald & A. J. Barrett, "Mammalian Proteases: A Glossary and Bibliography, Vol. 2, Exopeptidases," Academic Press, London (1986).

5. A. T. Orawski, J. P. Susz, & W. H. Simmons, Aminopeptidase P from bovine lung: solubilization, properties, and potential role in bradykinin degradation, <u>Mol. Cell. Biochem.</u>, 75:123-132 (1987).

6. A. T. Orawski & W. H. Simmons, Differences in rat vs bovine lung peptidases involved in bradykinin degradation, <u>Fed. Proc. Fed. Am. Soc. Exp. Med.</u>, 46:1267 (1987) (Abstract).

7. A. T. Orawski, J. P. Susz, & W. H. Simmons, Degradation of bradykinin by rat lung microsomes, <u>in</u>: "Kinin '84 Savannah, International Congress Oct 21-25, 1984 Abstracts," pp. 102 (1984) (Abstract).

8. W. H. Simmons & A. T. Orawski, Degradation of bradykinin by bovine lung microsomes, <u>Fed. Proc. Fed. Am. Soc. Exp. Biol.</u>, 44:1243 (1985) (Abstract).

9. P. N. AchutaMurthy, A. T. Orawski, & W. H. Simmons, Partial purification and properties of aminopeptidase P from rat lung, <u>Fed. Proc. Fed. Am. Soc. Exp. Biol.</u>, 44:876 (1985) (Abstract).

10. A. T. Orawski & W. H. Simmons, Degradation of bradykinin by rat brain peptidases, <u>Soc. Neurosci. Abst.</u> 12 (Pt2): 1047 (1987) (Abstract).

11. I. H. Segal, "Enzyme Kinetics," John Wiley and Sons, New York (1975).

12. K. Felgenhauer & G. G. Glenner, The enzymatic hydrolysis of amino acid B-naphthylamides. II. Partial purification and properties of a particle-bound cobalt-activated rat kidney aminopeptidase, <u>J. Histochem. Cytochem.</u>, 14:401-413 (1966).

13. W. H. Simmons & A. T. Orawski, Aminopeptidase M (Ap<u>M</u>) & A (Ap<u>A</u>) and inhibition in bovine lung, <u>Fed. Proc. Fed. Am. Soc. Exp. Biol.</u>, 46:1267 (1987) (Abstract).

14. R. Kitz & I. B. Wilson, Esters of methane sulfonic acid as irreversible inhibitors of acetylcholinesterase, <u>J. Biol. Chem.</u>, 237:3245-3249 (1962).

15. A. J. Turner, Endopeptidase-24.11 and neuropeptide metabolism, <u>in</u>: "Neuropeptides and their peptidases," A. J. Turner, ed. pp. 183-201, VCH, New York (1987).

16. M. Orlowski & S. Wilk, Purification and specificity of a membrane-bound metalloendopeptidase from bovine pituitaries, <u>Biochemistry</u>, 20:4942-4950 (1981).

17. R. A. Mumford, A. W. Strauss, J. C. Powers, P. A. Pierzchala, N. Nishino, & M. Zimmerman, Purification of a membrane-bound metalloendopeptidase from procine kidney that degrades peptide hormones, <u>J.Biol. Chem.</u>, 255:2227-2230 (1980).

18. M. S. Rohrbach, E. B. Williams, Jr., & R. A. Rolstad, Purification and substrate specificity of bovine angiotensin-converting enzyme, <u>J. Biol. Chem.</u>, 256:225-230 (1981).

19. D. W. Cushman, H. S. Cheung, E. F. Sabo, B. Rubin, & M. A. Ondetti, Development of specific inhibitors of angiotensin I converting enzyme (kininase II), <u>Fed. Proc. Fed. Am Soc. Exp. Biol.</u>, 38:2778-2782 (1979).

20. A. T. Orawski & W. H. Simmons, Degradation of kyotorphin (Tyr-Arg) and other dipeptides by rat brain synaptosomal peptidases, <u>Fed. Proc. Fed. Am. Soc. Exp. Biol.</u>, 44:696 (1985) (Abstract).

21. M. Orlowski, C. Michaud, & C. J. Molineaux, Substrate-related potent inhibitors of brain metalloendopeptidase, <u>Biochemistry</u>, 27: 597-602 (1988).

22. V. Ganapathy, S. J. Pashley, R. A. Roesel, D. H. Pashley, & F. H. Leibach, Inhibition of rat and human prolidases by captopril, <u>Biochem. Pharm.</u>, 34:1287-1291 (1985).

23. J. W. Ryan, U. S. Ryan, A. Chung & G. H. Fischer, Metabolism of bradykinin by endothelial cells in culture, <u>Adv. Exp. Med. Biol.</u>, 156B: 775-781 (1983).

PURIFICATION OF ANGIOTENSIN-CONVERTING ENZYME FROM HUMAN INTESTINE

Makoto Hayakari, Ken-ichi Amano*, Hiroshi Izumi** and
Satoshi Murakami

Department of Legal Medicine and *Department of Bacteriology
Hirosaki University School of Medicine, Hirosaki, Aomori 036
and **Department of Physiology, Tohoku University School of
Dentisty, Sendai 980, Japan

Key words: purification, angiotensin-converting enzyme, human intestine

ABSTRACT

Angiotensin-converting enzyme (ACE) activity in the intestinal whole
homogenate was showed as three peaks on a column of Sephacryl S-300 HR gel
filteration. Over 90 % of total ACE activity was found in a soluble
fraction separated with an ultracentrifuge of the intestinal homogenate,
and the ACE activities were detected as two peaks on the same column. On
the other hand, two peaks of ACE activities were found in a membrane-bound
fraction of treated with trypsin on the Sephacryl column and confirmed with
the two peaks of the soluble fraction, while the fraction extracted with
Triton X-100 of the membrane-bound fraction showed only one peak as major
peak. All ACE peaks were inhibited by addition of EDTA or captopril and by
absence of chloride ion completely.

We purified one ACE from the soluble fraction by lisinopril-linked
Sepharose 6B affinity column chromatography and Cellulofine GCL-200 gel
filteration. This enzyme was a 1323-fold purification and its final
recovery was 25 %. The molecular weight of this enzyme (180,000) was
larger than that of ACE from human kidney (170,000), estimated by 7.5 %
SDS-PAGE. The Km value of the enzyme for HHL was 2.1 mM. The enzyme
activity was competitively inhibited by captopril.

INTRODUCTION

Angiotensin-converting enzyme (ACE, EC 3.4.15.1), which converts the
inactive decapeptide angiotensin I to vasoactive octapeptide angiotensin II
in the pulmonary circulation and also inactivates bradykinin (Yang et al.,
1970), is a widely occurring enzyme in animal organs (Cushman and Cheung,
1971) and human tissues (Lieber and Sastre, 1983; Sande et al., 1985a,
1985b), and were purified from human lung (Friedland et al., 1981), kidney
(Stewart et al., 1981; Takada, et al., 1981), blood plasma (Bull et al.,
1985), prostate (Yokoyama et al., 1980), testis (Lanzillo et al., 1985),
seminal plasma (Depierre et al.,1978), and urine (Kokubu et al., 1978).
Recently, orally active inhibitors of ACE have been shown to effectively
reduce blood pressure in essential hypertensive patient (Atkinson and

Robertson, 1979; Brunner et .al., 1981; Hodson et al., 1982) since these compounds inhibit the conversion of angiotensin I and the inactivation of bradykinin in the body.

It has been also reported that ACE from human lung can cleaves various peptides other than angiotensin I or bradykinin, releasing dipeptides from enkephaline, neurotensin, substance P, and Met-enkephalin-Arg-Phe, and tripeptides from des-Arg-bradykinin, substance P and lutenizing hormone releasing hormone (Erdos and Skidgel, 1986). This report suggested that this enzyme work as carboxypeptidase other than as ACE and play physiological roles other than the hypertension in human and animal.

In this report, we describe subcellular distribution, purification, and characterization of ACE in human small intestine which contains the high ACE activity.

METHODS

ACE assay. ACE activity was assayed spectrophotometically at 382 nm by using 5 mM hippuryl-histidyl-leucine (HHL) (Peptide Institute Inc. Osaka, Japan) dissolved in 100 mM sodium-borate buffer, pH 8.3, containing 0.8 M NaCl, at 37 C as previously described (Hayakari et al., 1984).

Enzyme purification. Human intestines were obtained from postmortem cases which were dead within 1 day prior to autopsy and stored at -85 C before use. The tissue was miced well with a standard kichen meat micer, then homogenized with a Polytron homogenizer in 5-fold volumes of 20 mM potassium phosphate buffer, pH 8.3 (buffer A), containing 1 mM phenylmethlsulfonyl fluoride (Nakarai Co Ltd., Tokyo, Japan) for 1 h at 4 C. The homogenate was filtered through two-layer cheese-cloth, and the filterate was centrifuged at 35,000 x g for 30 min. The obtained supernatant fraction was dialyzed against three changes of 10 1 of 20 mM potassium phosphate buffer, pH 8.3, containing of 0.3 M NaCl and 0.05 % Triton X-100 (buffer B) for 36 h. After centrifugation at 35,000 x g for 30 min, the supernatant was applied to a column of a Lisinopril-linked Sepharose 6B (4.2 x 40 cm) (Lanzillo et al., 1985) equilibrated with buffer B. The column was washed with 5 bed volumes of buffer B, ACE fraction was eluted with 500 ml of 5 M urea in buffer B. The fraction was dialyzed against 10 1 of 20 mM PB, pH 8.3, containing of 0.05 % Triton X-100 (buffer C) at 4 C over night twice and then concentrated with 20 % (by w/v) of polyethylene glycol (PEG) 6000 in buffer C. The concentrated material was applied to a column of Cellulofine GCL-2000 (2.2 x 100 cm; Seikagaku Kogyo, Co Ltd., Japan) equilibrated with buffer C. The active fraction was concentrated by 20 % of PEG-6000 to 2-3 ml and dialyzed against buffer C and used for the study of enzymic characterization. Protein concentrations were determined by using Bio-Rad Protein Assay Kit.

Sephacryl S-300 HR column chromatography. The tissue was homogenized and centrifuged at 35,000 x g as described above. The whole homogenate and 35,000 x g precipitate were treated with 1 % Triton X-100 for 1 h at 4 C or 10 mg trypsin/g protein for 1 h at 37 C and then centrifuged at 105,000 x g for 30 min at 4 C. After dialyzing against buffer C, the supernatant were applied to a column of Sephacryl S-300 HR equilibrated with buffer C. The soluble fraction of intestinal homogenate was applied to the column directly. The elution pattern was monitored by measuring of the ACE activity.

RESULTS AND DISCUSSION

Subcellular distribution of ACE. Several fractions which were isolated from the human intestine and treated with or without Triton X-100 and

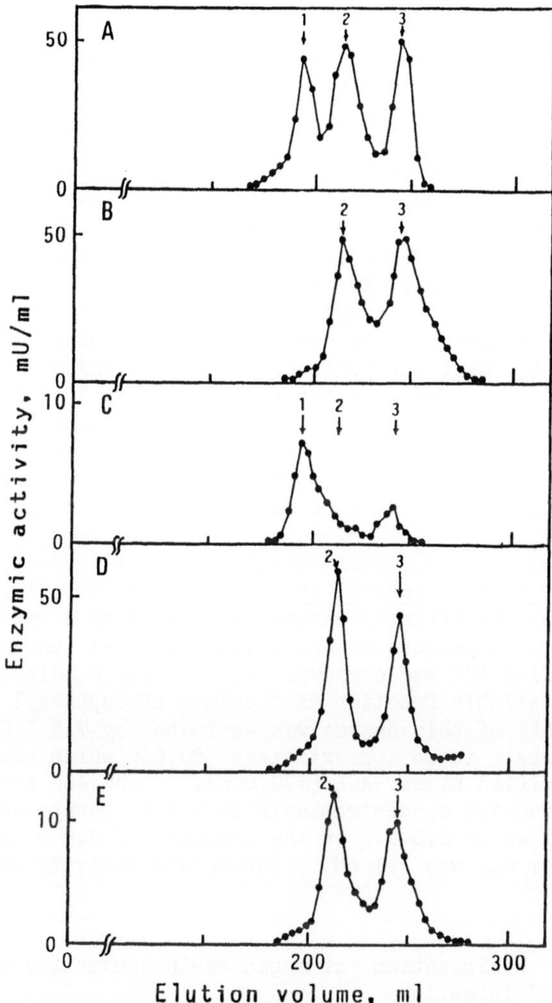

Fig. 1.   Sephacryl S-300HR gel chromatographic behaviour of angiotensin-converting enzyme. A, extract of intestinal whole homogenate with Triton X-100; B, soluble fraction of intestinal homogenate; C, extract of membrane-bound fraction with Triton X-100; D, extract of intestinal whole homogenate treated with trypsin; E, membrane-bound fraction treated with trypsin.

trypsin were analysed for the ACE profiles on the column of Sephacryl S-300 HR. The Triton X-100 extracted fraction (whole fraction) from the intestinal homogenate showed three ACE active peaks (Peaks 1, 2 and 3) on the column chromatogram (Fig. 1 A), while the soluble fraction of the homogenate without Triton X-100 trearment was detected only two active peaks (Peaks 2 and 3, Fig. 1B). The particulate fraction (membrane-bound fraction) extracted with Triton X-100 from the precipitate of the homogenate had one major peak which was same to Peak 1 in the whole fraction and two minor peaks which were same to Peaks 2 and 3 in the soluble fraction (Fig. 1C). These minor peaks of the membrane-bound fraction might be a contamination of the soluble fraction. After treatment of trypsin, Peak 1 in the whole and the membrane-bound fractions disappeared chromatographically, and Peaks 2 and 3 in both fractions significantly increased (Fig. 1 D and E). Furthermore, we checked whether the three peaks have characteristics as ACE or not. The ACE activities of all peaks were completely inhibited with the presences of EDTA and captopril, and also inhibited in the absence of chloride ion, indicating that the activities of three peaks originated in the ACE but not in other carboxypeptidases, because two inhibitors and one stimulator described above are specific for the ACE activity.

Thus, three forms (or isozymes) of the ACE were detected in the human intestine on the gel chromatogram, and it is clear that Peak 1 was distributed in the membrane portion and Peaks 2 and 3 were distributed in the soluble portion. Based on the fact that Peak 1 shifted to Peaks 2 and 3 by trypsin digestion, it is suggested that two soluble ACE are the products of membrane-bound ACE which were degraded by the endogenous proteolytic enzymes of the intestinal cells. However, it is unclear whether the two soluble ACE were derived from one membrane-bound ACE or from two.

    <u>Purification of intestinal ACE</u>. We tried to purify the ACE from the soluble fraction by affinity chromatography using a specific inhibitor, lisinopril-linked Sepharose 6B and Cellulofine gel chromatography (Table 1). The purified ACE was corresponded to a large molecular weight form, Peak 2, in the soluble fraction on a column of Sephacryl S-300 HR, and the molecular weight of this enzyme was estimated by 7.5 % SDS polyacryamide gel electrophoresis to be approximately 180,000 which was slightly larger than that of purified kidney ACE (170,000). The ACE activity was optimal at 0.8 M chloride-ion concentrationin in 0.1 M borate-sodium buffer, pH 8.3, and optimal at pH 8.0-8.5 in the presence of 0.8 M NaCl. The Km value of the enzyme for HHL was 2.1 mM. The enzyme activity was also completely

Table 1. Puripication of angiotensin-converting enzyme from human small intestine

Procedure	Total protein (mg)	Total activity (units)	Specific activity (units/mg)	Purification (-fold)	Yield (%)
Homogenate	7921	212.46	0.0268	1.0	100
25,000 g Supernatant	5621	186.59	0.0332	1.2	88
Affinity gel	2.81	63.50	22.629	931.6	30
Cellulofine GCL-2000	1.67	53.73	32.135	1323.0	25

inhibited by captopril.   These data for the ACE activity described above were corresponded with those of ACE from human kidney (Takada et al., 1981).

Thus, the enzyme obtained from human small intestine had the typical feature of ACE.   At this time, few reports have been published about the ACE of human intestine. Erdos and Skidgel (1987) reviewed that the intestinal ACE may be functioning by cleaveing a variety of peptides digested from proteins as dipeptidyl peptidase or tripeptidyl peptidase. Our obserbations of multiple forms in the human intstinal ACE point to the possibility that ACE works physiological roles, e.g., a digestive role in the human intestine.

REFERENCES

Atkinson, A.B. & Robertson, J.I.S., 1979, Captopril in the treatment of
        clinical hypertension and cardiac failure. Lancet, 2: 836.
Brunner, D.B., Desponds, G., Biollaz, J., Kellar, I., Ferber, F., Gavras,
        H., Brunner, H.R. & Schelling, J.L., 1981, Effect of a new
        angiotensin-converting enzyme inhibitor MK-421 and its lysine
        analogue on the components of the renin system in healthy subjects.
        Br. J. Clin. Pharmacol., 11: 461.
Bull, H.G., Thornberry, N.A. & Cordes, E.H., 1985, Purification of
        angiotensin-converting enzyme from rabbit lung and human plasma by
        affinity chromatography. J. Biol. Chem., 260: 2963.
Cushman, D.W. & Cheung, H.S., 1971, Concentration of angiotensin-converting
        enzyme in tissues of the rat. Biochim. Biophys. Acta, 250: 261.
Depierre, D., Bargetzi, J.P. & Roth, M., 1978, Dipeptidyl
        carboxypeptidase from human seminal plasma. Biochim. Biophys. Acta,
        523: 469.
Erdos, E.G. & Skidgel, R.A., 1986, The unusual substrate specificity and
        the distribution of human angiotensin I converting enzyme. Inter-
        Am. Soc. Proc. Suppl. I (Hypertension), 8: I-34.
Erdos, E.G. & Skidgel, R.A., 1987, The angiotensin-converting enzyme. Lab.
        Invest., 56: 345.
Friedland, J., Silverstein, E. & Drooker, M., 1981, Human lung angiotensin-
        converting enzyme: purification and antibody preparation. J. Clin.
        Invest., 67: 1151.
Hayakari, M., Seito, R., Furugori, A., Hashimoto, Y. & Murakami, S., 1984,
        An improved colorimetric assay of angiotensin-converting enzyme in
        serum. Clin. Chim. Acta, 144: 71.
Hodsman, G.P., Brown, J.J., Davies, D.L., Fraser, R., Lever, A.F., Morton,
        J.J., Murray, G.D. & Robertson, J.I.S., 1982, Converting enzyme
        inhibitor (MK421) in treatment of hypertension with renal artery
        stenosis. Br. Med. J., 285: 1697.
Kokubu, T., Kato, I., Nishimura, K., Hiwada, K. & Ueda, E., 1978,
        Angiotensin-convertine enzyme in human urine. Clin. Chim. Acta, 89:
        375.
Lanzillo, J.J., Stevens, J., Dasarathy, Y., Yostumoto, H. & Funburg, B.L.,
        1985, Angiotensin-converting enzyme from human tissues:
        Physilogical, catalytic, and immunological properties. J. Biol.
        Chem., 260: 14938.
Lieberman, J. & Sastre, A., 1983, Angiotensin-converting enzyme activity
        in postmortem human tissues. Lab. Invest., 48: 711.
Sande, M.V., Scharpe, S.L. & Neels, H.M., 1985a, Multiple forms of
        angiotensin-converting enzyme in human tissues and fluids. J. Clin.
        Chem. Clin. Biochem., 23: 381.
Sande, M.V., Schrpe, S.L. & Neel, H.M., 1985b, Distrbution of angiotensin-
        converting enzyme in human tissues. Clin. Chim. Acta, 147:255.

Stewart, T.A.m Weare, J.A. & Erdos, E.G., 1981, Purification and characterization of human converting enzyme (Kininase II). Peptides, 2: 145.

Takada, Y., Hiwada, K. & Kokubu, T., 1981, Isolation and characterization of angiotensin-converting enzyme from human kidney. J. Biochem., 90: 1309.

Yang, H.Y.T., Erdos, E.G. & Levin,Y., 1970, A dipeptidyl carboxypeptidase that converts angiotensin I and inactivates bradykinin. Biochim. Biophys. Acta, 241: 374.

Yokoyama, M., Hiwada, K., Kokubu, T., Takaha, M. & Takeuchi, M., 1980, Angiotensin-convertine enzyme in human prostate. Clin. Chim. Acta, 100: 253.

INVOLVEMENT OF ANGIOTENSIN-CONVERTING ENZYME (KININASE II) IN NEUROPEPTIDE METABOLISM

Hideyoshi Yokosawa, Yoshitaka Ohgaki, Mitsuo Satoh,
Yurika Fujii, Shogo Endo, and Shin-ichi Ishii

Department of Biochemistry
Faculty of Pharmaceutical Sciences, Hokkaido University
Sapporo 060, Japan

INTRODUCTION

All the components of the renin-angiotensin system have been
identified in the brain (Ganong, 1984). Angiotensin-converting enzyme
(ACE, EC 3.4.15.1) is a dipeptidyl carboxypeptidase which catalyzes the
generation of angiotensin II from angiotensin I (and also does the
degradation of bradykinin), releasing the C-terminal dipeptide. It is
unevenly distributed in the brain; whereas a positive correlation exists
between the contents of ACE and those of other components of the
renin-angiotensin system in some areas of the brain, such a correlation
cannot be found in other areas of the brain, such as substantia nigra.

The fact that the distribution of ACE does not correlate with that of
other components of the renin-angiotensin system but, inversely, correlates
with that of neuropeptides other than angiotensins in the latter regions of
the brain, together with the fact that the ACE activity is susceptible to
several neuropeptides, has led us to propose that ACE takes another role
than that for the renin-angiotensin system in such regions of the brain
(Yokosawa et al, 1983a).

This proposal was strengthened by our first discovery that ACE
purified from rat brain can hydrolyze substance P, which lacks a free
terminal carboxyl group (Yokosawa et al., 1983b). The result implys a new
feature of ACE: It also exhibits an endopeptidase activity. Successive
experiments with purified ACE preparations obtained from kidney and lung
(Skidgel et al., 1984; Cascieri et al., 1984; Yokosawa et al., 1985) and
also from brain (Strittmatter et al., 1985; Hooper and Turner, 1987) came
to almost the same conclusion. Furthermore, it has been demonstrated that
the enzyme shows an endopeptidase action toward luteinizing hormone-
releasing hormone (LH-RH), also lacking a free carboxyl terminus (Skidgel
and Erdos, 1985; Strittmatter et al, 1985; Hooper and Turner, 1987;
Yokosawa et al., 1987).

It is at present believed that several neuropeptides intracellularly
generated from their precursors act as neurotransmitters and/or
neuromodulators after secretion, and that their physiological activity is
terminated through enzymatic degradation at the synapse.

Could ACE in the brain function physiologically, in fact, on the metabolism of these neuropeptides ?

To answer this question, we used a homogenous cell line, the neuroblastoma cell, in tissue culture, as a possible model for the neuron, and investigated the effect of captopril on the degradation of several neuropeptides with its plasma membrane. In this study, we focused our attention on the degradation of three neuropeptides, substance P (Nicoll et all., 1980), LH-RH (Jan and Jan, 1983), and dynorphin (Herrera-Marschitz et al., 1986), all of which had been thought to function as neurotransmitters and/or neuromodulators and whose inactivation in the synaptic region had not been well elucidated. The presence of ACE in the plasma membrane of cultured neuroblastoma cells has been recently confirmed (Clemens et al., 1986).

MATERIALS AND METHODS

An established neuroblastoma cell line N-18 derived from mouse neuroblastoma C-1300 was used. The N-18 cells were cultured and collected as previously described (Endo et al., 1985). The plasma membrane of the neuroblastoma cells was prepared according to the method of Jones and Matus (1974).

Degradation of substance P (Endo et al, 1985), LH-RH (Yokosawa et al., 1987), and dynorphin (Satoh et al., 1986) with the membrane in the presence and absence of captopril and separation of their cleavage products by HPLC on a reversed-phase column of Nucleosil $5C_{18}$ (Marchery, Nagel, and Co.) were carried out as previously described. The cleavage products separated by HPLC were identified by determining their amino acid compositions on a Hitachi 835 amino acid analyzer. ACE was assayed by using hippuryl-His-Leu as a substrate (Yokosawa et al., 1983a).

Substance P, LH-RH, dynorphin(1-13), dynorphin(1-17), Leu-enkephalin, phosphoramidon, and hippuryl-His-Leu were purchased from the Peptide Institute, Osaka. Captopril was provided by Dr. A. Awaya of Mitsui Pharmaceuticals Inc., Tokyo. Leupeptin and bestatin were gifts from Dr. W. Tanaka of Nippon Kayaku Co., Tokyo.

RESULTS AND DISCUSSION

Degradation of substance P

Purified rat brain ACE hydrolyzed substance P (Arg-Pro-Lys-Pro-Gln-Gln-Phe-Phe-Gly-Leu-Met-NH_2)initially at the bond between Phe8 and Gly9 by an endopeptidase action, followed by successive release of dipeptide, Phe-Phe, by a dipeptidyl carboxypeptidase action (Yokosawa et al., 1983b). As a result, two fragments (9-11) and (7-8) accumulated as major cleavage products. Minor cleavage between the Phe7-Phe8 bond was also detected.

When substance P was submitted to the action of a plasma membrane preparation from neuroblastoma cells, HPLC pattern gave 11 newly formed peaks, among which that of fragment (9-11) was the highest (Endo et al., 1985). The appearance of almost all the peaks was completely inhibited with 0.1 mM EDTA. HPLC pattern in the presence of 0.1 mM captopril was almost identical to that in the absence of this inhibitor. Further quantitative analyses showed a little decrease (approximately twenty %) in the accumulation of fragment (9-11) and a disappearance of a small peak of Phe-Phe in the presence of the inhibitor. The similar results were obtained by measuring the decrease in the chromatographic peak area of substance P; the decrease was markedly inhibited with EDTA (97 %) but slightly inhibited with captopril (22%). Other inhibitors including p-chloromercuriphenylsulfonic acid (1 mM, 14 % inhibition), DFP (1 mM, 17 %), leupeptin (0.1 mM, 9 %), phosphoramidon (0.1 mM, 6 %), and bestatin (0.1 mM, 6 %) showed weak inhibitory effects. Thus, an EDTA-sensitive protease may play a major role in the degradation of substance P, while ACE makes a little contibution to its degradation.

Our attempt for identification of this putative EDTA-sensitive protease led to a finding of a novel rat brain substance P-degrading endopeptidase which hydrolyzed at the three sites between the Pro4-Gln5, the Gln5-Gln6, and the Gln6-Phe7 at the ratio of 2:2:3 (Endo, unpublished).

Degradation of LH-RH

Human kidney ACE has been reported to hydrolyze LH-RH (pGlu-His-Trp-Ser-Tyr-Gly-Leu-Arg-Pro-Gly-NH$_2$) initially at the two sites between the Trp3-Ser4 and the Leu7-Arg8 at a different ratio, dependent on NaCl concentration (Skidgel and Erdos, 1985). Our purified rat brain ACE also hydrolyzed LH-RH at least at 0.3 M NaCl and the generation of fragments (1-3) and (4-10) was detected (Yokosawa et al., 1987).

LH-RH was degraded also with the neuroblastoma cell membrane (Yokosawa et al., 1987). Although captopril exerted little effect on the decrease in the peak area of the initial peptide, LH-RH, on a HPLC chart, the appearance of several cleavage products was affected by the addition of captopril. These results imply that ACE may be involved in the secondary degradation of the products initially formed. Among 8 newly formed fragments, fragment (1-3) accumulated in the highest amount in the absence of captopril, while, in the presence of the inhibitor, the amount of fragment (1-5) was highest. Fragment (6-10) remained constant irrespective of the presence and the absence of captopril. These results suggest the generation of fragment (1-3) from fragment (1-5) by the dipeptidyl carboxypeptidase action of ACE.

This assumption was verified by the following two results. First, an inverse relationship was observed between the amount of fragment (1-5) and that of either fragment (1-3) or (4-5) as the concentration of captopril increased; the former increased, and the latter two fragments decreased. The formation of other fragments including fragment (6-10) was almost unaffected. Second, their inverse relationship was also observed in dependence on NaCl concentration; the formation of the latter two was stimulated approximately 3-fold by the presence of $>$0.1M NaCl, whereas that of the former was inhibited. Other fragment again remained constant.

Among the other inhibitors tested including DFP, phosphoramidon and bestatin, only p-chloromercuribenzoate (PCMB) completely inhibited the appearance of almost all the peaks. Thus, a PCMB-sensitive cysteine protease may be involved in the initial major cleavage at the Tyr5-Gly6. HPLC analyses showed the presence of minor peak of fragment (1-6) and its generation was also completely inhibited by PCMB but scarcely inhibited by the other inhibitors including captopril. It appears that ACE may not be involved in such initial cleavages that the putative cysteine protease is responsible for. However, further quantitative analyses indicated that the recovery of fragment (1-3) (60 % of LH-RH degraded) was higher than that of either fragment (4-5) (35 %) or (6-10) (47 %) and that a small peak of fragment (1-3) was detectable in the presence of PCMB. Therefore, it can be thought that ACE makes a minor contribution to the initial cleavage at the Trp3-Ser4.

The process for the degradation of LH-RH with the neuroblastoma cell membrane, disclosed by this study, was described in Fig. 1.

By HPLC on a Mono-Q column, we succeeded in separating the fragment (1-5)-generating enzyme from the fragment (1-6)-generating one in a cysteine protease-containing fraction which had been isolated from Brij 35-extract of the neuroblastoma cell membrane by p-mercuribenzoate (PMB)-Sepharose chromatography (Ohgaki, unpublished). ACE was recovered in the break-through fraction of PMB-Sepharose chromatography, further purified by HPLC on a Mono-Q column, and characterized.

Degradation of dynorphin

Many lines of evidence have been presented for the fact that the opiate activity of Leu-enkephain as well as of Met-enkephalin is terminated by the action of two peptidases, enkephalinase (endopeptidae-24.11, EC 3.4. 24.11) and an aminopeptidase (McKelvy and Blumberg, 1986). However, an inactivation mechanism in the neuron for dynorphin(1-17), an endogenous opioid peptide with the sequence Tyr-Gly-Gly-Phe-Leu-Arg-Arg-Ile-Arg-Pro-Lys-Leu-Lys-Trp-Asp-Asn-Gln, has not been well elucidated.

The neuroblastoma cell membrane degraded dynorphins (1-13) and (1-17), as well as Leu-enkephalin (Satoh et al., 1986). The degradation of dynorphins (1-13) and (1-17) detected by the decrease in the HPLC peak areas of the starting materials was inhibited by N-ethylmaleimide (NEM) (1 mM, 72 % and 81 % inhibition, respepctively) and slightly by DFP (1 mM, 15 % and 27 %). PCMB (1 mM, 75 % and 81 %) and p-aminobenzamidine (1 mM, 11 % and 21 %) also inhibited their degradation. Phosphoramidon (0.1 mM) and bestatin (1 mM) exhibited less inhibitory effects on the degradation of the two dynorphins (14 % and 15 % with the former inhibitor, and 3 % and 4 % with the latter, respectively) than on that of Leu-enkephalin (42 % with the former and 15 % with the latter). Inversely, NEM (5 %) and DFP (0 %) did less inhibitory effect on the degradation of Leu-enkephalin. These results with Leu-enkephalin fit well with the proposed involvement of enkephalinase and aminopeptidase, while those with dynorphins indicate the involvement of a cysteine protease and a serine protease.

Captopril showed little substantial effect on the decrease of all three peptides themselves, whereas it did a significant effect on the HPLC pattern of cleavage products generated from the two dynorphins. In the absence of captopril, 9 and 12 newly formed peaks were detected with dynorphins (1-13) and (1-17), respectively. Assignment of those fragments showed that they were derived by the cleavage around the three regions, the Phe4-Leu5-Arg6-Arg7, the Lys11-Leu12-Lys13 and the Asp15-Asn16 sequences. In the presence of the inhibitor, on the other hand, the two dynorphins gave 12 peaks, in either case, among which 5 and 3 peaks, respectively, appeared at the positions different from those of any ones detected in the absence. Almost all the peaks only detected in the presence of captopril were found to be N-terminal fragments such as (1-7), (1-6), (2-7), (2-6), and (1-8). Inversely, fragments arising from the N-terminal region such as (1-3), (1-5) and (2-5) disappeared. Furthermore, fragments (7-11), (8-11), (12-15), (13-15), and (14-15) decreased, accompanying with the increase of fragments (7-13), (8- 13), (12-17), (13-17), and (14-17). Generation of fragment (1-11) from dynorphin(1-13) was also inhibited. Thus, dynorphins seems to be degraded through the initial cleavage at the two regions around the Arg6-Arg7 and the Lys11-Leu12-Lys13 sequences by a cysteine protease, followed by the release of dipeptide by ACE. Additionally, ACE may be also resposible for the liberation of C-terminal dipeptide. The cleavage around the Arg6-Arg7 sequence may be most important from the viewpoint of dynorphin inactivation, because its cleavage results in a change of receptor specificity and a dramatic decrease of opiate activity.

The scheme for the degradation of dynorphin with the neuroblastoma cell membrane proposed from this study was shown in Fig. 2.

Recently, we succeeded in isolation of two types of cysteine proteases
functioning in degradation of dynorphin from Triton X-100-extract of the
neuroblastoma cell membrane. One cleaved dynorphin(1-17) at the Arg6-Arg7,
while the other did at the Lys11-Leu12 and the Leu12-Lys13. Trypsin-like
enzyme cleaving the Arg6-Arg7 bond and the Lys11-Leu12 bond was also
isolated (Satoh, unpublished).

Function of ACE

It has been established that a purified ACE exerts endopeptidase
action on substance P and LH-RH, both of which contain blocked C-terminal
amino acids. However, as demonstrated in this study, ACE present in the
plasma membrane of neuroblastoma cells scarcely attacks LH-RH directly by
its endopeptidase action. The ACE displays its dipeptidyl carboxypeptidase
action only after the peptide has been cleaved with other membrane
proteases. This situation may be explained by the reason that the latter
proteases, which have been characterized as cysteine proteases in this
study, can attack LH-RH more efficiently than ACE can. The similar
situation also takes place in the degradation of substance P. In this
case, an EDTA-sensitive endopeptidase may be involved in the initial
cleavage. Minor contribution of ACE to the initial cleavage of substance P
and LH-RH was, of course, demonstrated in this study. In the case of
dynorphin, ACE was again shown to contribute to the secondary cleavage of
the products initially formed. Although the release of C-terminal
dipeptide from the original peptide with ACE would occur, such a cleavage
may not result in important consequence from the viewpoint of inactivation
of dynorphin. In the case of dynorphin too, cysteine proteases were found
to play important roles as the first-attacking ones. In conclusion, we
propose that ACE may function as a role of "scavenger" rather than of
"trigger-pulling" enzyme in the neuropeptide metabolism in the synapse.

1. Major step

$$LH\text{-}RH(1\text{-}10) \xrightarrow{E1} \begin{array}{c} LH\text{-}RH(1\text{-}5) \\ + LH\text{-}RH(6\text{-}10) \end{array} \xrightarrow{ACE} \begin{array}{c} LH\text{-}RH(1\text{-}3) \\ + Ser\text{-}Tyr \end{array}$$

2. Minor step

$$LH\text{-}RH(1\text{-}10) \xrightarrow{E2} LH\text{-}RH(1\text{-}6) + LH\text{-}RH(7\text{-}10)$$

$$LH\text{-}RH(1\text{-}10) \xrightarrow{ACE} LH\text{-}RH(1\text{-}3) + LH\text{-}RH(4\text{-}10)$$

Fig. 1. Scheme for degradation of LH-RH with neuroblastoma cell membrane.
E1, fragment (1-5)-generating cysteine protease.
E2, fragment (1-6)-gerenating cysteine protease.

```
 1   2   3   4   5   6   7   8   9  10  11  12  13  14  15  16  17
Tyr-Gly-Gly-Phe-Leu-Arg-Arg-Ile-Arg-Pro-Lys-Leu-Lys-Trp-Asp-Asn-Gln
```

$$\begin{array}{l}
\quad\quad\quad\quad\quad\quad\quad\quad\quad\quad\quad\quad\quad ACE \\
I \quad \left\{ \begin{array}{l} Tyr\text{-}Gly\text{-}Gly\text{-}Phe\text{-}Leu\text{-}Arg\text{-}(Arg) \longrightarrow \\ (Arg)\text{-}Ile\text{-}Arg\text{-}Pro\text{-}Lys\text{-}(Leu)\text{-}(Lys) \longrightarrow \\ (Leu)\text{-}(Lys)\text{-}Trp\text{-}Asp\text{-}Asn\text{-}Gln \longrightarrow \end{array} \right. \\
II
\end{array}$$

<pre>
                                                         ACE
   I ⎧ Tyr-Gly-Gly-Phe-Leu-Arg-(Arg)   ------->
 ----->⎨ (Arg)-Ile-Arg-Pro-Lys-(Leu)-(Lys)   ------->
   II ⎩ (Leu)-(Lys)-Trp-Asp-Asn-Gln   ------->
                                                                  ACE
   ACE ⎧ Tyr-Gly-Gly-Phe-Leu-Arg-Arg-Ile-Arg-Pro-Lys-Leu-Lys-Trp-Asp ---->
 ------->⎨ Asn-Gln   ?
</pre>

Fig. 2. Scheme for degradation of dynorphin with neuroblastoma cell membrane
I, cysteine protease I; II, cysteine protease II.

REFERENCES

Cascieri, M. A., Bull, H. G., Mumford, R. A., Patchett, A. A., Thornberry, N. A., and Liang, T., 1984, Carboxyl-terminal tripeptidyl hydrolysis of substance P by purified rabbit lung angiotensin-converting enzyme and the potentiation of substance P activity in vivo by captopril and MK-422, Mol. Pharmacol., 25:287.

Clemens, D. L., Okamura, T., and Inagami, T., 1986, Subcellular localization of angiotensin-converting enzyme in cultured neuroblastoma cells, J. Neurochem., 47:1837.

Endo, S., Yokosawa, H., and Ishii, S., 1985, Degradation of substance P by the neuroblastoma cells and their membrane, Biochem. Biophys. Res. Commun., 129:694.

Ganong, W. F., 1984, The brain renin-angiotensin system, Ann. Rev. Physiol., 46:17.

Herrera-Marschitz, M., Christensson-Nylander, I., Sharp, T., Staines, W., Reid, M., Hokfelt, T., Terenius, L., and Ungerstedt, U., 1986, Striato-nigral dynorphin and substance P pathways in the rat. II. Functional analysis, Exp. Brain Res., 64:193.

Hooper, N. M., and Turner, A. J., 1987, Isolation of two differentially glycosylated forms of peptidyl-dipeptidase A· (angiotensin-converting enzyme) from pig brain: a re-evaluation of their role in neuropeptide metabolism, Biochem. J., 241:625.

Jan, Y. N., and Jan, L. Y., 1983, A LHRH-like peptidergic neurotransmitter capable of action at a 'distance' in autonomic ganglia, Trends Neurosci., 6:320.

Jones, D. H., and Matus, A. I., 1974, Isolation of synaptic plasma membrane from brain by combined flotation-sedimentation density gradient centrifugation, Biochim. Biophys. Acta, 356:276.

McKelvy, J. F., and Blumberg, S., 1986, Inactivation and metabolism of neuropeptides, Ann. Rev. Neurosci., 9:415.

Nicoll, R. A., Schenker, C., and Leeman, S. E., 1980, Substance P as a transmitter candidate, Ann. Rev. Neurosci., 3:227.

Satoh, M., Yokosawa, H., and Ishii, S., 1986, Degradation of dynorphin-(1-13) and dynorphin-(1-17) by the neuroblastoma cell membrane. Evidence for the involvement of a cysteine protease, Biochem. Biophys. Res. Commun., 140:335.

Skidgel, R. A., Engelbrecht, S., Johnson, A. R., and Erdos, E. G., 1984, Hydrolysis of substance P and neurotensin by converting enzyme and neutral endopeptidase, Peptides, 5:769.

Skidgel, R. A., and Erdos, E. G., 1985, Novel activity of human angiotensin I converting enzyme: Release of the NH_2- and COOH-terminal tri-peptides from the luteinizing hormone-releasing hormone, Proc. Natl. Acad. Sci. USA, 82:1025.

Strittmatter, S. M., Thiele, E. A., Kapiloff, M. S.. and Snyder, S. H., 1985, A rat brain isozyme of angiotensin-converting enzyme. Unique specificity for amidated peptide substrates, J. Biol. Chem., 260:9825.

Yokosawa, H., Ogura, Y., and Ishii, S., 1983a, Purification and inhibition by neuropeptides of angiotensin-converting enzyme from rat brain, J. Neurochem., 41:403.

Yokosawa, H., Endo, S., Ogura, Y., and Ishii, S., 1983b, A new feature of angiotensin-converting enzyme in the brain: hydrolysis of substance P, Biochem. Biophys. Res. Commun., 116:735.

Yokosawa, H., Endo, S., Ohgaki, Y., Maeyama. J., and Ishii, S., 1985, Hydrolysis of substance P and its analogs by angiotensin-converting enzyme from rat lung. Characterization of endopeptidase activity of the enzyme, J. Biochem., 98:1293.

Yokosawa, H., Fujii, Y., and Ishii, S., 1987, Degradation of luteinizing hormone-releasing hormone by neuroblastoma cells and their membrane: evidence for the involvement of a thiol protease and angiotensin-converting enzyme, J. Neurochem., 48:293.

DISTRIBUTION OF ANGIOTENSIN I CONVERTING ENZYME IN MALE REPRODUCTIVE SYSTEMS OF VARIOUS VERTEBRATES AND PROPERTIES OF THE GENITAL ENZYMES

Takamasa Yamaguchi, Masahiko Ikekita, Kazuyuki Kizuki and
Hiroshi Moriya

Department of Biochemistry, Science University of Tokyo
12 Ichigaya Funakawara-machi, Shinjuku-ku, 162 Tokyo, Japan

SUMMARY

The distribution of the angiotensin I converting enzyme (EC 3.4.15.1,
ACE) in male reproductive systems of various vertebrates including non-
mammalian species and properties of the genital ACEs were studied. In such
mammals as rat, dog and pig, it has been found that ACE activity is only
distributed in testis and epididymis (especially in the epididymal semen),
but not in accessory sex glands such as prostate, seminal vesicle and
coagulating gland. In the rat and dog, most of or all epididymal ACE has
been found to resemble testicular ACEs rather than pulmonary ACE in molecular weight. Besides the studies on mammals, it has been found that the
enzymes having characteristics of ACE are present in the genital systems of
such lower vertebrates as bird (domestic fowl) and fish (carp).

INTRODUCTION

It is known that a large amount of angiotensin I converting enzyme
(EC 3.4.15.1, dipeptidyl carboxypeptidase I, kininase II, ACE) is distributed
in the testes of many mammals.[1] Recently, it has been reported that the
ACEs in rabbit and rat testes are novel ACEs whose molecular weights
(100×10^3 by SDS-PAGE, 200×10^3 by Sephadex G-200 gel filtration) are lower than
those of the pulmonary ACEs (150×10^3 by SDS-PAGE, 290×10^3 by Sephadex G-200
gel filtration).[2,3,4] In the rabbit, it has been demonstrated that the testicular and the pulmonary ACEs are translated from the different m RNAs.[2,5]

In human, the sex glands other than testis have been reported to contain high molecular weight type ACE which resembles pulmonary ACE, although
the occurrence of a low molecular weight ACE has been confirmed in the testis.[6-8,15] These observations show difference in ACE of the testis and the
other sex glands. However, it seems undesirable to analogize the cases of
the other animals from these observations in humans, because of the difference in anatomical and functional features of genital systems among animal
species. In order to clarify the similarities and the dissimilarities in
ACE among sex glands and animal species, we examined the distribution of
ACE in male reproductive systems of various vertebrates including such non-
mammals as a bird (domestic fowl, *Gallus gallus domesticus*) and a fish
(carp, *Cyprinus carpio*) and characterized some of the genital ACEs.

MATERIALS AND METHODS

<u>Chemicals</u>. N$^\alpha$-hippryl-L-His-L-Leu-OH (HHL), angiotensins I and II, L-His-L-Leu and phosphoramidon were purchased from the Peptide Institute Inc. (Osaka, Japan). MK-422 was a kind gift from Nippon Merck Banyu Co. Ltd. (Tokyo, Japan). Other chemicals were of guaranteed reagent grade.

<u>Enzyme assay</u>. Enzyme activity of ACE was measured using 5 mM HHL as a substrate. Enzyme reaction was carried out for 30 min at 37°C in 0.1 M borate-bicarbonate buffer, pH 8.3, containing 0.8 M NaCl. The amount of hippuric acid enzymatically liberated from HHL was determined according to the spectrophotometric method of Cushman and Cheung.[10] One unit (U) of the enzyme was defined as the amount of enzyme that can hydrolyze 1 μmol HHL per minute under the conditions mentioned above.

<u>Preparation of tissue homogenate and collection of tissue fluid</u>. Each tissue was minced and suspended in four volumes of 10 mM Tris-HCl buffer, pH 8.0. The tissue suspension (except the case of carp testis) was homogenized for 5 min by Polytron homogenizer (Kinematica, Switzerland). After the homogenate was centrifuged for 10 min at 600 x g, the amount of HHL hydrolyzing activity of ACE in the supernatant was measured. In the case of carp testis, homogenization was carried out in the presence of 0.25 %(W/V) sodium deoxycholate and 5.5 %(W/V) streptomycin sulfate. After the homogenate was centrifuged for 1 h at 20 000 x g, enzyme activity in the supernatant was measured. Epididymal semen were collected from slit epididymal ducts of rat, dog and pig by micro pipette. The fluid in pig seminal vesicle was drained by syringe. Carp semen was obtained from the cloaca of conscious animal by pressing the abdomen.

<u>Enzyme preparations</u>. Rat testicular and pulmonary ACEs used in the gel filtration through a Sephadex G-200 column were purified according to the methods previously described.[3] Procedures of subcellular fractionation of rat epididymis and partial purifications of ACEs from each fraction have been previously reported in detail.[11]

<u>Angiotensin I converting activity</u>. Angiotensin I converting activity was examined by the Magunus method or thin layer chromatography analysis according to the methods previously reported.[3,11,12]

<u>Dipeptidyl carboxypeptidase activity toward HHL</u>. Site of action of the enzyme on HHL was analyzed by thin layer chromatography using silica gel plate (E. Merck. Darmstadt, West Germany) in the same manner as described previously.[12]

RESULTS

Distribution of ACE activity in male reproductive systems of rat, dog and pig

Results of the determination of ACE activity in each tissue homogenate and fluid are summarized in Table I. As shown in Table I, in rat, dog and pig, ACE activity was detected only in testis and epididymis. Only traces or no ACE activity was in accessory sex glands such as prostate, seminal vasicle and coagulating gland.

Properties of epididymal ACEs

Since a large amount of ACE was detected only in epididymis other than testis, properties of the epididymal ACEs of rat and dog were studied, particularly, the molecular weights.

Table I. Distribution of ACE Activity in Male Reproductive Systems of Rat, Dog and Pig

Animal Tissue, fluid		Enzyme activity* (U/g tissue or ml fluid)
RAT		
Testis	homogenate	10.36 ± 2.23 (n=5)**
Epididymis	homogenate	11.20 ± 1.17 (n=3)
	epididymal semen	7.39 (n=1)
Coagulating gland	homogenate	<0.050 (n=3)
Prostate	homogenate	not detectable (n=3)
Seminal vesicle	homogenate	
DOG		
Testis	homogenate	2.66 ± 0.66 (n=5)
Epididymis	homogenate	0.611 (n=1)
	epididymal semen	1.99 ± 0.29 (n=6)
Prostate	homogenate	not detectable (n=4)
PIG		
Testis	homogenate	7.88 ± 0.14 (n=4)
Epididymis	caput epididymal semen	9.22 ± 3.56 (n=3)
	corpus epididymal semen	18.63 ± 7.38 (n=9)
	cauda epididymal semen	40.31 ± 7.70 (n=14)
Prostate	homogenate	not detectable (n=4)
Seminal vesicle	fluid	not detectable (n=4)
Urethral muscle	homogenate	not detectable (n=4)

*; HHL hydrolyzing activity was measured in the absence or the presence of 1 µM MK-422. The value of enzyme activity of ACE was obtained by subtracting the value in the presence of MK-422 from the value in the absence of MK-422.

**; Mean ± S.D. of n times experiments.

Soluble and particulate fractions of rat epididymis were prepared from the homogenate by centrifugation (100 000 x g, 1 h). ACE activity was detected in both fractions, 55 and 42%, respectively. The soluble fraction and the solubilized materials obtained from the particulate fraction by the treatment with deoxycholate were separately fractionated by TEAE-cellulose chromatography. One ACE and Two ACEs (P-I and P-II with a peak area ratio of 1.4:1.0) were obtained from the soluble fraction and from the solubilized materials of the particulate, respectively.

The molecular weights of these three ACEs (soluble, P-I and P-II) were compared with those of rat testicular and pulmonary ACEs by gel filtration through a Sephadex G-200 column. Soluble ACE and P-I were found to have slightly lower molecular weights (170×10^3) than that of the testicular ACE (200×10^3), whereas P-II was found to have the same molecular weight as the pulmonary ACE (290×10^3).

The presence of three differnt forms of ACE were thus demonstrated in the rat epididymis. All these ACEs had angiotensin I converting activity (confirmed by Magnus method). They also had very similar enzymo-chemical properties with regard to activation by NaCl and sensitivities to ACE inhibitor MK-422 in spite of the structural difference.

Similar studies were made on the dog epididymal ACE. ACE was separately extracted from the homogenates of dog lung, testis and epididymis in

the presence of 0.25 %(W/V) sodium deoxycholate. Each ACE was then partially purified by ammonium sulfate fractionation and TEAE-cellulose chromatography. In the dog, multiple forms of ACE was not observed in the TEAE-
cellulose chromatography. Subsequently, molecular weights of the dog ACEs
were compared with each other by Sephadex G-200 gel filtration. Dog testicular ACE was found to have lower molecular weight (207×10^3) than dog
pulmonary ACE (290×10^3). The same was true in the rat. However, ACE in dog
epididymis was found to have the same molecular weight as testicular ACE.
The presence of high molecular weight type ACE was not observed in the dog
epididymis. It was confirmed by thin layer chromatography that these dog
ACEs had MK-422-sensitive angiotensin I converting activity.

<u>Distribution of ACE-like Peptidase in Male Reproductive Systems of Domestic</u>
<u>Fowl (*Gallus gallus domesticus*) and Carp (*Cyprinus carpio*)</u>

Besides studies on mammals, we searched for the enzyme having characteristics of ACE in male sex glands of lower vertebrates such as a domestic
fowl and a carp in order to clarify whether the presence of ACE is essential
to male reproductive function throughout the vertebrates.

First, the presence of hydrolyzing activity toward HHL was observed in
chicken testis (0.044±0.030 U/g tissue,n=6) and carp testis (0.230±0.090
U/g tissue,n=4). Next, some enzymo-chemical properties of the chicken and
carp testicular enzymes were studied after they were partially purified by
ammonium sulfate fractionation and TEAE-cellulose chromatography. It was

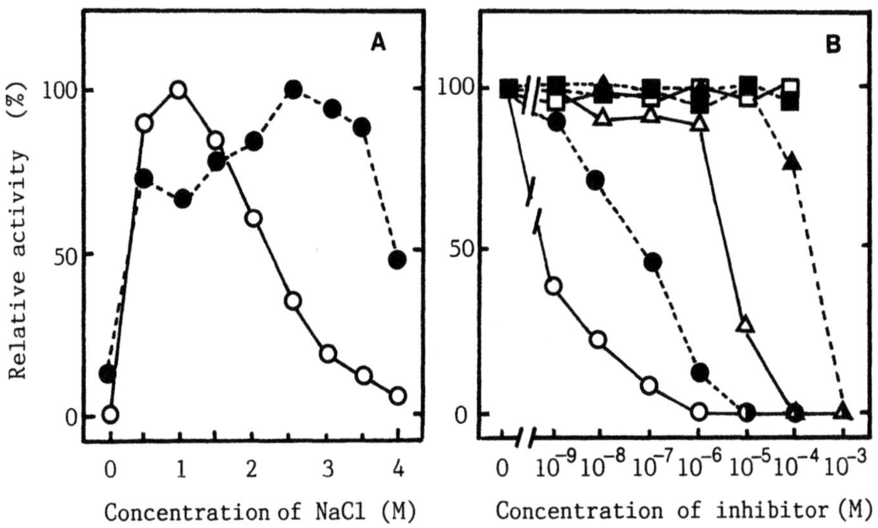

Fig. 1. Effects of NaCl, MK-422, EDTA and Phosphoramidon on the
Activities of the HHL Hydrolyzing Enzymes in Chicken and
Carp Testes.

A: HHL hydrolyzing activity of each enzyme (●,chicken;○,
carp) was measured in 0.1 M borate-bicarbonate buffer, pH
8.3, containing various concentrations of NaCl.

B: HHL hydrolyzing activity of each enzyme (closed symbols,
chicken; open symbols, carp) was measured in 0.1 M borate-
NaOH buffer, pH 8.3, containing 1.1 M NaCl and various concentrations of each inhibitor (circles, MK-422; triangles,
EDTA; squares, phosphoramidon).

demonstrated by thin layer chromatography that the chicken and carp testicular enzymes liberated the dipeptide His-Leu from the carboxyl terminus of HHL. As shown in Fig. 1-A, the HHL hydrolyzing activities of these enzymes were strongly activated by the addition of NaCl. The highest activities of the chicken and carp enzymes were observed in the presence of 1.0 M and 2.5 M NaCl, respectively. These properties of the chicken and carp testicular enzymes agreed well with those of mammalian ACEs previously reported.[13] Furthermore, as shown in Fig. 1-B, the HHL hydrolyzing activities of the chicken and carp enzymes were completely inhibited by typical ACE inhibitors such as EDTA (0.1-1.0 mM) and MK-422 (1-10 μM) but not by phosphoramidon (0.1 mM). From these observations, it was concluded that the HHL hydrolyzing enzymes in the chicken and carp testes could be classified in the same group as mammalian ACEs.

The presence of HHL hydrolyzing enzyme was detected also in the ejaculated semen of the carp. The carp seminal enzyme was also confirmed to be a NaCl-dependent and MK-422 sensitive dipeptidyl carboxypeptidase by thin layer chromatography.

DISCUSSION

In the present work it was established that ACE was only present in testis and epididymis, but not in accessory sex glands such as prostate, seminal vesicle and coagulating gland in the mammals such as rat, dog and pig. This observation differs from that in man where prostate and seminal vesicle were reported to contain more ACE than the testis and epididymis.[8,9] In man, the prostate is considered to be the major origin of ACE in the ejaculated semen. Contrary to this, we found that in the rat, dog and pig, the testis and epididymis were the only possible organs from which seminal ACE could be derived. Since a large amount of ACE was found in the epididymal semen of these animals (Table I), it is suggested that the ACE is discharged with epididymal spermatozoa.

The ACEs in the ejaculated semen of human and rabbit have been reported to be high molecular weight ACEs resembling the pulmonary ACEs.[14,15] These reports imply that certain sex glands produce this pulmonary type ACE. In man, the prostate has been shown to produce high concentrations of the ACE with the same molecular weight as that of the pulmonary or renal ACE.[7,8]

In the present work, the pulmonary type ACE was located in the particulate fraction of the rat epididymis. However, judging from ratio of the soluble to particulate ACE (55:42) and P-I-to-P-II ratio (7:5), the pulmonary type ACE was considered to account for only less than 20% of the total ACE in the epididymis. Most of the remaining epididymal ACE was considered to consist of soluble and insoluble ACEs with low molecular weight. Furthermore, in the dog, the pulmonary type ACE was not present in the epididymis, and all of the epididymal ACE was a low molecular weight ACE which was the same as that of the dog testicular ACE. Thus, in contrast to man, low molecular weight ACEs were predominantly distributed in the male reproductive systems in the rat and dog. From the overall results in mammals, it is strongly suggested that the synthesis and metabolism of ACE in male sex glands is remarkably different among animal species.

It was also demonstrated, for the first time, that ACE-like peptidases are distributed in the male reproductive systems of lower vertebrates such as a bird and a fish. It is generally accepted the mechanism of reproduction as well anatomical features are extremely diverse in different species. Nevertheless, the enzymes having characteristics of ACE are present in the

male reproductive organs of the different vertebrates which are phylo-
genetically far apart from each other. Therefore, ACE or ACE-like enzyme,
is assumed to be involved in reproductive processes in many vertebrates
in which the specific catalyzing function of these enzymes is required.
The physiological function of ACE in reproduction has not been clearly
understood even in mammals. However, our observations on ACEs in non-
mammalian vertebrates (the bird and fish) may help to clarify the significance of ACE in reproduction in vertebrates.

REFERENCES

1. D. W. Cushman and H. S. Cheung, Studies in vitro of angiotensin-
    converting enzyme of lung and other tissues, in: "Hypertension,"
    J. Genest and E. Koiw, eds., Springer-Varlag, Berlin (1972).
2. H. A. El-Dorry, H. G. Bull, K. Iwata, N. A. Thornberry, E. H. Cordes,
    and R. L. Soffer, Molecular and catalytic properties of rabbit tes-
    ticular dipeptidyl carboxypeptidase, J. Biol. Chem., 257:14128
    (1982).
3. T. Yamaguchi, M. Sekine, M. Ikekita, K. Kizuki, and H. Moriya,
    Enzymological properties of rat testicular angiotensin I-converting
    enzyme: comparison with rat pulmonary enzymes, Yakugaku Zasshi, 105:
    491 (1985).
4. P. A. Velletri, M. L. Billingsley, and W. Lovenberg, Thermal denatur-
    ation of rat pulmonary and testicular angiotensin-converting enzymes
    effects of chelators and $CoCl_2$, Biochim. Biophys. Acta, 893:71
    (1985).
5. H. A. El-Dorry, C. B. Pickett, J. S. MacGregor, and R. L. Soffer,
    Tissue-specific expression of m RNA for dipeptidyl carboxypeptidase
    isoenzymes, Proc. Natl. Acad. Sci. USA, 79:4295 (1982).
6. D. Depierre, J. P. Bargetzi and M. Roth, Dipeptidyl carboxypeptidase
    from human seminal plasma, Biochim. Biophys. Acta, 523:469 (1978).
7. M. Yokoyama, K. Hiwada, K. Kokubu, M. Takaha, and M. Takeuchi, Angio-
    tensin-converting enzyme in human prostate, Clin. Chim. Acta, 100:
    253 (1980).
8. E. G. Erdös, W. W. Schulz, J. T. Gafford, and R. Defendini, Neutral
    metalloendopeptidase in human male genital tract: comparison to
    angiotensin I-converting enzyme, Lab. Invest., 52:437 (1985).
9. M. E. van Sande, S. L. Scharpe, H. M. Neels, and K. O. van Camp,
    Distribution of angiotensin converting enzyme in human tissues,
    Clin. Chim. Acta, 147:255 (1985).
10. D. W. Cushman and H. S. Cheung, Spectrophotometric assay and properties
    of angiotensin-converting enzyme of rabbit, Biochem. Pharmacol.,
    20:1637 (1971).
11. T. Yamaguchi, H. Toyoda, M. Ikekita, K. Kizuki, and H. Moriya, Angio-
    tesnsin I converting enzymes in rat epididymis, Chem. Pharm. Bull.,
    34:418 (1986).
12. T. Yamaguchi, S. Kurihara, M. Ikekita. K. Kizuki, and H. Moriya, Angio-
    tensin I converting enzyme activity in the kidney of bullfrog (Rana
    catesbeiana), J. Pharmacobio-Dyn., 9:585 (1986).
13. E. G. Erdös, Kininases, in: "Hand. Exp. Pharm., Vol. XXV, Supple.,"
    E. G. Erdös ed., Springer-Verlag, Berlin (1979).
14. H. A. El-Dorry, J. S. MacGregor, and R. L. Soffer, Dipeptidyl carboxy-
    peptidase from seminal fluid resembles the pulmonary rather than the
    testicular isoenzyme, Biochem. Biophys. Res. Commun., 115:1096
    (1983).
15. J. J. Lanzillo, J. Stevens, Y. Dasarathy, H. Yotsumoto, and B. L.
    Fanburg, Angiotensin-converting enzyme from human tissues, J. Biol.
    Chem., 260:14938 (1985).

A NEW TYPE OF ULTRASENSITIVE BIOLUMINESCENCE ENZYME
SUBSTRATES FOR KININASES

Reinhard Geiger and Werner Miska[*]

Dept. Clin. Chem. Clin. Biochem. Surg. Clinic
and [*]Dermatol. Clinic Uni. Munich, D-8000 München
2, FRG.

INTRODUCTION

A number of chromogenic and fluorogenic substrates are
currently in use for the determination of kininases (1-4).
Relatively low amounts of enzymes (5) can be detected by these
methods, but highly sensitive enzyme tests, especially for the
measurement of small quantities of enzymes, e.g. in single
cells, are required.

More recently, highly sensitive bioluminescent and lumi-
nescent methods have become available for the determination of
ATP and many different analytes (6). Bioluminescence is a
natural phenomenon found in many lower forms of life. Naturally occuring bioluminescent systems differ with regard to the
structure and function of enzymes and cofactors, as well as in
the mechanism of the light emitting reactions (7 - 9).

The aim of this study was the development of a new type of
highly sensitive kininase substrates on the basis of firefly
luciferin (Photinus pyralis) derivatives. These new substrates

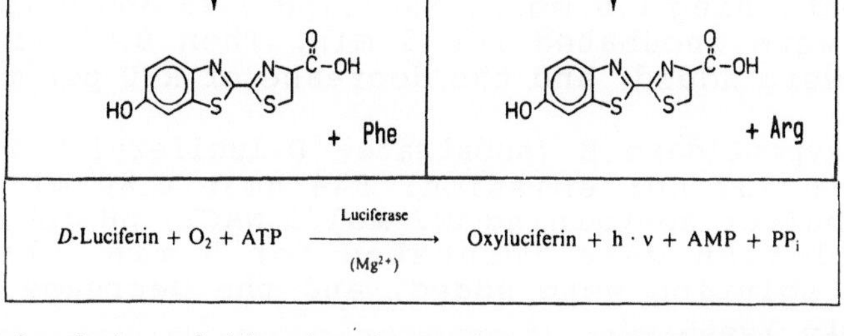

+ Phe

+ Arg

Luciferase

D-Luciferin + O_2 + ATP $\longrightarrow$ Oxyluciferin + h · v + AMP + PP_i

(Mg^{2+})

Fig. 1   Principle of the test systems. X, carboxypeptidases B
and N; E, carboxypeptidase A

can be used in enzymatic activity assays. The test principle
of these new substrates is the release of D-luciferin (Photinus pyralis) from D-luciferin derivatives by the action of
hydrolytic enzymes. D-Luciferin is the leaving group of the
substrate and can be easily quantified in a luminometric assay
(Fig. 1).

MATERIALS AND METHODS

Carboxypeptidases A (bovine pancreas; 50 U/mg) and B (bo-
vine pancreas; 175 U/mg) were purchased from Sigma, München,
FRG. Synthetic D-luciferin (Photinus pyralis) was a product of
Novabiochem AG, CH-4448 Läufelfingen, Switzerland. Luciferase
(Photinus pyralis; spec. act. 8 mU/mg) was a product of
Boehringer, Mannheim, FRG. ATP and NAD were purchased from
Merck, Darmstadt, FRG. Carboxypeptidase N (kininase I) was
kindly provided by W. Gebhard, München.

Synthesis and characterization of D-luciferin substrates
have been performed as described in ref. (9). D-luciferin
derivatives are commercially available by Novabiochem AG, CH-
4448 Läufelfingen, Switzerland.

<u>Luminometric assay (Determination of luciferin by lucifera</u>
<u>se</u>: Luciferin was measured luminometrically in a biolumino-
meter according to the following procedure (Biolumat, Fa.
Berthold Typ 9500 T, Wildbad, FRG; 25°C, volume: 0.5 ml,
(10)): 0.4 ml bioluminescence cocktail (30 mmol/l HEPES, 6.6
mmol/l $MgCl_2$, 0.66 mmol/l EDTA, 0.1 mmol/l DTT, 5 mmol/l ATP,
1 ug luciferase, pH 7.75) were preincubated at 25°C for 5 min
in a bioluminometer. Thereafter 0.1 ml luciferin solution
(standard or incubation mixtures of the tests (11)) were added
and light impulses were measured for 10 s.

<u>Determination of kinetic constants</u>: Michaelis-Menten con-
stant (K_m) were calculated according to Wilkinson (12) after
graphical inspection of the data in Lineweaver-Burk diagrams.
The assays were performed fluorimetrically as follows (test
volume: 0.5 ml; 37°C; substrate concentrations: 25, 50, 100,
250, 500, 750, 1000 umol/l).
Carboxypeptidase A (substrate: D-luciferyl-L-phenylalanine; excitation: 332 nm; emission: 543 nm): 0.40 ml 0.05
mol/l Tris/HCl buffer containing 3 g/l LiCl, pH 7.5 and 0.05
ml enzyme solution were incubated for 5 min. Then 0.05 ml
substrate solution was added, and the decrease of RFU per
minute were measured.
Carboxypeptidase N (substrate: D-luciferyl-L-N$^{\alpha}$-arginine;
excitation: 333 nm; emission: 544 nm): 0.40 ml 0.1 mol/l HEPES
buffer containing 0.5 mol/l NaCl, pH 7.75 and 0.05 ml enzyme
solution were incubated for 5 min. Then 0.05 ml substrate
solution were added, and the decrease of RFU per minute were
measured.
Carboxypeptidase B (substrate: D-luciferyl-L-N$^{\alpha}$-arginine;
excitation: 333 nm; emission: 544 nm): 0.40 ml 0.05 mol/l
Tris/HCl buffer containing 0.2 mol/l NaCl, pH 7.8 and 0.05 ml
enzyme solution were incubated for 5 min. Then 0.05 ml
substrate solution were added, and the decrease of RFU per
minute were measured.

Precisely quantified luciferin derivatives and luciferin
solutions were used as calibration standards for the fluorescence measurements.

k_{cat} values were calculated as described in (13).

<u>Enzymatic assay systems</u>: carboxypeptidase A (test volume:
0.5 ml; 37oC): 0.40 ml 0.05 mol/l Tris/HCl buffer containing 3
g/l LiCl, pH 7.5 and 0.05 ml substrate solution (40 mmol/l D-
luciferyl-L-phenylalanine in Tris/HCl buffer) were incubated
for 5 min. Then 0.05 ml enzyme solution was added and incubated for 30 min. Thereafter 0.1 ml of test solution was transfered to 0.4 ml bioluminescence cocktail and light impulses
were measured as described above.

Carboxypeptidase B (test volume: 0.5 ml; 37°C): 0.40 ml
0.05 mol/l Tris/HCl buffer containing 0.2 mol/l NaCl, pH 7.8
and 0.05 ml substrate solution (2 mmol/l D-luciferyl-L-N$^{\alpha}$-
arginine in Tris buffer) were incubated for 5 min. Then 0.05
ml enzyme solution were added and incubated for 30 min.
Thereafter 0.1 ml of test solution was transfered to 0.4 ml
bioluminescence cocktail and light impulses were measured as
described above.

Carboxypeptidase N (test volume: 0.5 ml; 37°C): 0.40 ml
0.1 mol/l HEPES buffer containing 0.5 mol/l NaCl, pH 7.75 and
0.05 ml substrate solution (0.5 mmol/l D-luciferyl-L-N$^{\alpha}$-argi-
nine in HEPES buffer) were incubated for 5 min. Then 0.05 ml
enzyme solution were added and incubated for 30 min.
Thereafter 0.1 ml of test solution was transfered to 0.4 ml
bioluminescence cocktail and light impulses were measured as
described above.

RESULTS AND DISCUSSION

Enzyme substrates withD-luciferin (Photinus pyralis) as a
leaving group have been developed for carboxypeptidases A, B
and N (Fig. 2). D-luciferyl-L-phenylalanine and D-luciferyl-L-
N$^{\alpha}$-arginine were synthesized via luciferin-N-hydroxysuccinimide. Luciferin-N-hydroxysuccinimide was prepared from luciferin and N-hydroxysuccinimide in the presence of N,N'-dicyclo-
hexylcarbodiimide and D-luciferyl-L-phenylalanine was obtained
in high yield (63%). Synthesis of D-luciferyl-L-N$^{\alpha}$-arginine is
more difficult to perform because of the presence of a reactive guanido group. Using slightly acid conditions (pH 6), D-
luciferyl-L-N$^{\alpha}$-arginine could be obtained in good yield (37%).

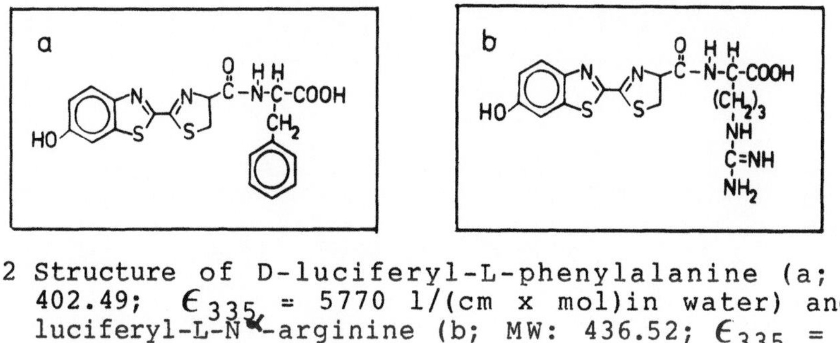

Fig. 2 Structure of D-luciferyl-L-phenylalanine (a; MW:
402.49; ϵ_{335} = 5770 l/(cm x mol)in water) and D-
luciferyl-L-N$^{\alpha}$-arginine (b; MW: 436.52; ϵ_{335} = 5710
l/(cm x mol) in water).

All synthetized luciferin derivatives were purified by high performance liquid chromatography (9). Because of the high sensitivity of the luminometric assay (9) in which traces of luciferin would interfere, all preparations of luciferin derivatives had to be absolutely free of luciferin. This was verified by thin layer chromatography (two systems), by several HPLC systems, and by the luminometric assay itself.

Identity of all luciferin derivatives was assessed by ultra violet and fluorescence spectroscopy, and by mass spectrometry. Amino acid analysis was used to determine the content of phenylalanine and arginine in D-luciferyl-L-phenylalanine and D-luciferyl-L-N$^\alpha$-arginine. D-luciferyl-L-phenylalanine had a phenylalanine content of 37.9% (calcd.: 38.4%). For D-luciferyl-L-N$^\alpha$-arginine, an arginine content of 38.7% (calcd.: 39.7%) was determined.

Furthermore, quantitative luciferin determinations after complete enzymatic hydrolysis were performed by the luminometric assay and by fluorescence measurements. The amount of luciferin found by both methods was close to the calculated values. In all these tests satisfactory results were obtained. The quantum yields of fluorescence of the derivatives relative to native D-luciferin was as follows (D-luciferin = 100): D-luciferyl-L-phenylalanine = 105; D-luciferyl-L-N$^\alpha$-arginine = 113.
m/z values found by FAB mass spectrometry for luciferin derivatives indicated the expected luciferin compounds.

Before use of the synthesized luciferin substrates in enzymatic tests the following questions had to be answered: 1) can different amounts of D-luciferin be quantified in the luminometric assay ?, 2) are the derivatives themselves substrates for luciferase ?; is a light emitting reaction induced ?, 3) are the derivatives inhibitors of luciferase ?; are the luminometric assays disturbed by these compounds ?, 4) can the derivatives be cleaved by enzymes ?, and 5) is D-luciferin released ?
As to the first question luciferin can easily be quantitated. As shown in Fig. 3 there is a linear relation between light output and used luciferin concentrations.

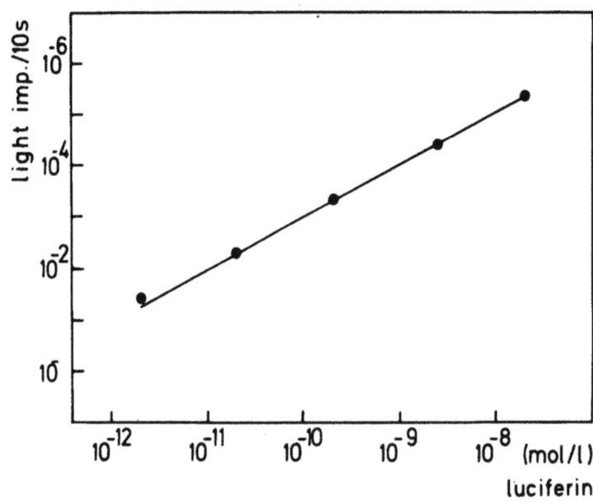

Fig. 3   Determination of D-luciferin in the luminometric assay (concentrations in test: 5 mmol/l ATP,1 µg luciferase). For details see Materials and Methods.

Enzymatic studies clearly demonstrate that luciferin derivatives applied in the luminometric assay up to 1 mmol/l cause
no light emission. In other words, the luciferin derivatives
are not substrates for firefly luciferase and are free of
luciferin.

Depending on the concentrations of luciferin derivatives
added to the luminometric assay (9), luciferin derivatives can
inhibit the light emitting reaction. To prevent this inter-
ference, which is essential for the sensitivity of the detection systems of the immunoassays, concentrations of luciferin
derivatives were later used in the detection systems which did
not interfere in the luminometric assay.

The most important point was whether the luciferin derivatives can be cleaved by kininases and whether luminometri
cally active luciferin is indeed released by these reactions.
As can be seen from the data in Table 1, which have been obtained by following the hydrolytic reactions by the luminometric assay, luciferin derivatives can be cleaved by appro-
priated enzymes. D-Luciferyl-L-phenylalanine was a substrate
for carboxypeptidase A. Formation of D-luciferin-L-N$^\alpha$-arginine
lead to a substrate for carboxypeptidase B and N. The Michae-

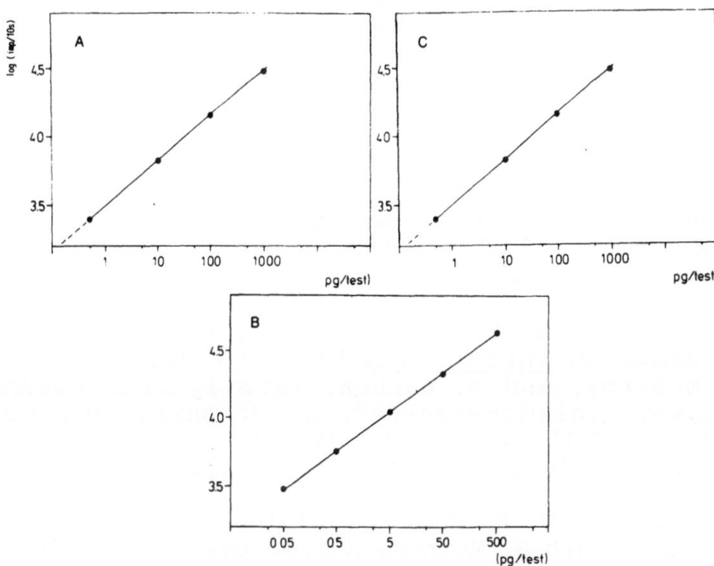

Fig. 4 Detection limits of D-luciferin derivatives in
the enzymatic test system. A, carboxypeptidase A, B
carboxypeptidase N and C, carboxypeptidase B.

Table 1 Kinetic data for carboxypeptidases and D-luciferin
substrates.

Enzyme	D-luciferin derivative	K_m (mol/l)	k_{cat} (1/s)	k_{cat}/K_m (l·mmol^{-1}·s^{-1})
Carboxypeptidase A	D-luciferyl-L-phenylalanine	3.5×10^{-3}	7.7[*]	2.2
Carboxypeptidase B	D-luciferyl-L-N$^\alpha$-arginine	2.0×10^{-4}	7.0[*]	35
Carboxypeptidase N	D-luciferyl-L-N$^\alpha$-arginine	0.5×10^{-4}	11.8[**]	236

[*]protein concentration was given by the manufactures;[**] protein concentration was determined
according to Bradford (13) using carboxypeptidase B as standard.

lis-Menten constants determined for the luciferin substrates
and the respective enzymes were in a range typical for other
substrates of these enzymes (Table 1). The detection limits of
the tests are between 50 fg and 500 fg per test for carboxypeptidases (Fig. 4). The results demonstrate that the sensitivity of the bioluminescence substrates are decades lower than
found with the usual substrates (5)and can be convieniently
used for ultra sensitive enzymatic acitivity test.

ACKNOWLEDGEMENT

We wish to thank Prof. Dr. H. Fritz for his support during the
work. We are indebted to Dr. F. Kovac, University Ljubljana,
Institut of Chemistry for FAB mass spectrometry studies and
for elementary analysis.

REFERENCES

1 H. U. Bergmeyer, Enzymes 3: Peptidases, Proteinases and
  Their Inhibitors, Methods of Enzymatic Analysis Vol 5,
  Verlag Chemie, Weinheim, FRG (1984).
2 L. Lorand, Proteolytic Enzymes, Methods of Enzymology 80,
  Academic Press, New York, USA (1981).
3 M. F. Scully and V. V. Kakkar, Chromogenic peptide
  substrates, chemistry and clinical usage, Churchill Living-
  stone, Edinburgh (1979).
4 T. H. Plummer, jr., and M. T. Kimmel, An improved spectrophotometric assay for human plasma carboxypeptidase N,
  Anal. Biochem. 108, 348 - 353 (1980).
5 R. E. Smith, E. R. Bissell, A. R. Mitchell, and   K. W.
  Pearson, Direct photometric or fluorometric assay of proteinases using substrates containing 7-amino-4-trifluoro-
  methylcoumarin, Thromb. Res. 17, 393 - 402 (1980).
6 W. D. McElroy, and M. DeLuca, firefly luminescence, in:
  "Chemi-and Bioluminescence", J. G. Burr, ed., pp. 387 -
  400, Marcel Dekker, New York (1985).
7 M. DeLuca, Bioluminescence and Chemiluminescence, Methods
  of Enzymology 57 (1978).
8 M. DeLuca, and W. D. McElroy, Bioluminescence and Chemiluminescence, Part B, Methods Enzymology 133 (1986).
9 W. Miska, and R. Geiger, Synthesis and characterization of
  luciferin derivatives for use in bioluminescence enhanced
  enzyme immunoassays. New ultrasensitive detection systems
  for enzyme immunoassays, I., J. Clin. Chem. Clin. Biochem.,
  25, 23 - 30 (1987).
10 A. Lundin, A. Rickardsson, and A. Thore, Continuous monitoring of ATP-converting reactions by purified firefly luciferase, Anal. Biochem. 75, 611 - 620 (1976).
11 R. Geiger, and W. Miska, Bioluminescence enhanced enzyme
   immunoassays. New ultrasensitive detection systems for
   enzyme immunoassays, II. , J. Clin. Chem. Clin. Biochem.,
   25, 31 - 38 (1987).
12 G. H. Wilkinson, Statistical estimations in enzyme kinetics, Biochem. J. 80, 324 - 332 (1961).
13 M. M. Bradford, A rapid and sensitive method for the quali-
   tation of microgram quantities of protein utilizing the
   principle of protein-dye binding, Anal. Biochem. 72, 307 -
   314 (1976).

THE HYPOTENSIVE RESPONSE TO DES-ARG^9-BRADYKININ INCREASES

DURING *E. COLI* SEPTICEMIA IN THE PIG

Matthias Siebeck[1], Eric T. Whalley[3], Hans
Hoffmann[1], Joachim Weipert[2], and Hans Fritz[2]

[1]Chirurgische Klinik Innenstadt und
Chirurgische Poliklinik, [2]Abteilung für
Klinische Chemie und Klinische Biochemie in
der Chirurgischen Klinik, University of Munich
West Germany. [3]Department of Physiological
Sciences, University of Manchester, United
Kingdom

INTRODUCTION

In recent years, two different types of receptors for
kinins have been characterized. It has been shown that the
injection of bacterial lipopolysaccharide from *E. coli* induces
the formation of B_1-receptors for kinins in rabbits within a
few hours. The activation of B_1-receptors by des-Arg^9-brady-
kinin (des-Arg^9-BK) produces hypotension, coronary vasodilation, and stimulation of large arteries and veins isolated and
suspended *in vitro* (Regoli et al., 1981). We have been using a
pig model to study the response of the circulation to the
infusion of live bacteria *in vivo* (Siebeck et al., 1987). In
the present experiment, we have attempted to demonstrate that
the infusion of live *E. coli* in weaned piglets induces an
increased sensitivity of the systemic circulation to bolus
injections of des-Arg^9-BK.

METHODS

Nine weaned piglets (body weight approximately 20 kg) were
studied under anesthesia with pentobarbital and pethidin,
relaxation with pancuronium, and mechanical ventilation. Six
animals received a suspension of freshly cultured *E. coli* (014
B26), $3 \cdot 10^{10}$ cells, as assessed by turbidimetry, in 24 ml
saline over 2 h intravenously. Three animals served as controls
and received 0.9% saline, 24 ml in 2 h. Blood pressure was
measured with a catheter in the carotid artery and a strain
gauge. Solutions of bradykinin (BK) and des-Arg^9-BK (Sigma
Chemical Co., St. Louis, MO) were prepared with isotonic saline
in different dilutions such as to achieve a constant injection
volume of 1 ml. The solutions were made up freshly for each
measurement and were kept on ice. Blood pressure changes were
determined in response to intraarterial bolus injections of BK

(25 ng, 100 ng) and des-Arg^9-BK (1 µg, 10 µg). Measurements
were performed before (0 h) and after (4 h) the induction of
septicemia, or before (0 h) and after (4 h) the start of the
saline infusion in the control animals. The blood pressure
response was determined during the hypotensive phase as the per
cent change in diastolic pressure from baseline level. Means ±
standard deviation were presented. Wilcoxon's test was used to
test differences between 0 h and 4 h measurements, p < 0.05 was
considered significant.

Tab. 1. Blood pressure response in control animals to des-
Arg^9-BK (1 µg, 10 µg) and BK (25 ng, 100 ng) (in per cent
reduction of diastolic pressure, means ± S.D.)

Compound	Dose	0 h	4 h
des-Arg^9-BK	1 µg	1.2 ± 1.0	1.5 ± 1.5
des-Arg^9-BK	10 µg	13.3 ± 6.4	12.0 ± 3.0
Bradykinin	25 ng	12.5 ± 2.3	13.8 ± 1.9
Bradykinin	100 ng	29.2 ± 16.6	26.9 ± 9.9

Tab. 2. Blood pressure response in septic animals to des-
Arg^9-BK (1 µg, 10 µg) and BK (25 ng, 100 ng) (in per cent
reduction of diastolic pressure, means ± S.D.). Asterisk
denotes a significant increase in response.

Compound	Dose	0 h		4 h
des-Arg^9-BK	1 µg	0.0 ± 0.0	*	8.7 ± 2.9
des-Arg^9-BK	10 µg	9.3 ± 3.5	*	17.2 ± 4.1
Bradykinin	25 ng	8.0 ± 5.6		10.1 ± 5.3
Bradykinin	100 ng	30.0 ± 4.6		26.7 ± 6.0

RESULTS

In healthy animals, des-Arg^9-BK 1 µg was ineffective and
the response to des-Arg^9-BK 10 µg approximated 10% (Tab. 1 and
Fig. 2), the response to BK, 25 ng and 100 ng, as shown in
Tab. 1 and Fig. 1), was distinctly above threshold. The blood
pressure response to both peptides remained stable during the
4 h-period in the control animals (Tab. 1, Fig. 1 and 2). Four
h after the onset of septicemia a response to des-Arg^9-BK 1 µg
(Tab. 2 and Fig. 2) was seen. The response to des-Arg^9-BK 10 µg
was nearly doubled, and the response to BK (Tab. 2 and Fig. 1)
was unchanged.

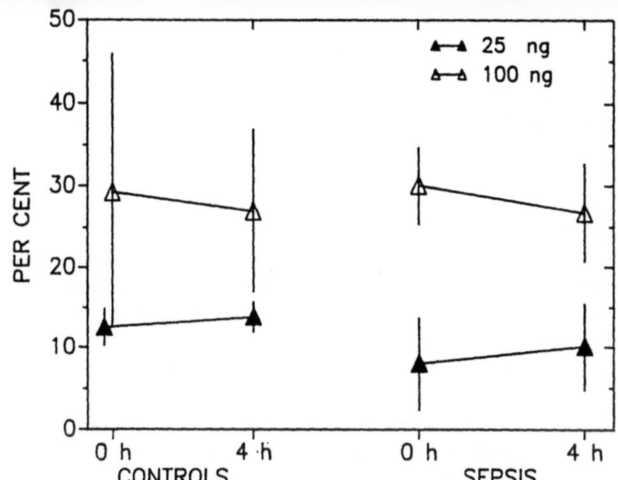

Figure 1. Blood pressure response to **bradykinin**. Abscissa: 0 h: before induction of septicemia. 4 h: 4 h after onset of an infusion of NaCl, 0.9% (control animals, left), or of live *E. coli*, $3 \cdot 10^{10}$ cells in 2 h (septic animals, right). Ordinate: Reduction in blood pressure (per cent change from baseline level, means ± standard deviation) after bradykinin, 25 ng (closed triangle), or bradykinin, 100 ng (open triangle).

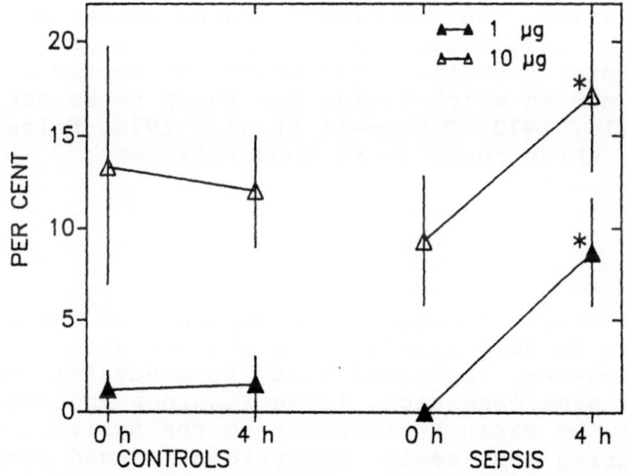

Figure 2. Blood pressure response to **des-Arg^9-bradykinin**. Abscissa: 0 h: before induction of septicemia. 4 h: 4 h after onset of an infusion of NaCl, 0.9% (control animals, left), or of live *E. coli*, $3 \cdot 10^{10}$ cells in 2 h (septic animals, right). Ordinate: Reduction in blood pressure (per cent change from baseline level, means ± standard deviation) after des-Arg^9-BK, 1 μg (closed triangle), or des-Arg^9-BK 10 μg, (open triangle). Asterisk marks a signifikant ($p < 0.05$) difference to the control measurement by Wilcoxon's test.

DISCUSSION

Results from the present study clearly demonstrate that
the sensitivity of the pig cardiovascular system to the selective B_1-receptor agonist des-Arg^9-BK (Regoli & Barabé, 1980)
was significantly increased four hours after receiving an
intravenous infusion of live *E. coli*. An effect was absent in
concurrent control animals. These observations are consistent
with previous studies that have demonstrated the capacity of
several noxious stimuli including lipopolysaccharide from
E. coli and *Salmonella* to induce B_1-receptors in the cardiovascular system of the rabbit when tested *in vivo* and *in vitro*
(Regoli et al., 1981, Marceau et al., 1984). The mechanism
whereby this is brought about is unclear but it is known that
in animal models of bacterial (Bouthillier et al., 1987, McConn
et al., 1983) or endotoxin induced sepsis (Kühne et al., 1985)
activation of the kallikrein-kinin system occurs.

In patients with severe septicemia kinins appear also to
be activated (Aasen et al., 1983, McConn et al., 1983). If
kinins are involved in the expression of B_1-receptors directly
in the vasculature then it can be assumed that it is a B_2-
receptor which is activated since in control animals des-Arg^9-
BK was relatively inactive compared to BK. On the other hand,
it is possible that a variety of other factors activated during
septicemia are also involved. Studies in rabbits by Bouthillier
et al. (1987) have suggested that the macrophage but not
neutrophil activation may be important. It is worthy of note
that induction of B_1-receptors can also be demonstrated *in
vitro* in the pig pulmonary artery (unpublished observation).

In conclusion, the pig offers a good animal model to
investigate the involvement of kinins and the generation of the
kinin B_1-receptor mediating hypotension in septic shock, a
condition in man in which kinins are known to be activated
(Kimball et al., 1972, O'Donnell et al., 1976, Kalter et al.,
1985) and for which there is no good treatment.

SUMMARY

The sensitivity to des-Arg^9-bradykinin of the cardiovascular system was largely increased in piglets with *E. coli*
bacteremia. However, the sensitivity to bradykinin was unchanged under the same condition. These findings indicate the
appearance of the kinin B_1-receptor in the systemic circulation
of the pig during septicemia. Bradykinin induced responses
suggest a stable effect mediated by the classical B_2-receptor.

ACKNOWLEDGEMENT

The authors wish to thank Prof. Dr. Leonhard Schweiberer for
generous support of this work.

REFERENCES

Aasen, A. O., Smith-Erichsen, N., and Amundsen, E., 1983,
    Plasma Kallikrein-Kinin System in Septicemia. Arch. Surg.,
    118:343-345.
Bouthillier, J., Deblois, D., and Marceau, F., 1987, Studies on
    the induction of pharmacological responses to des-Arg^9-
    bradykinin *in vitro* and *in vivo*, Br. J. Pharmac., 92:257-
    264.
Kalter, E. S., Daha, M. R., ten Cate, J. W., Verhoef, J., and
    Bouma, B. N., 1985, Activation and Inhibition of Hageman
    Factor-Dependent Pathways and the Complement System in
    Uncomplicated Bacteremia or Bacterial Shock, J. Infect.
    Dis., 151:1019-1027.
Kimball, H. R., Melmon, K. L., and Wolff, S. M., 1972,
    Endotoxin-induced kinin production in man, Proc. Soc. Exp.
    Biol. Med., 129:1078.
Kühne, H., Schaper, U., Lehmann, B., Dassler, S., and Scheuch,
    D. W., 1985, Zur Aktivierung des Kallikrein-Kinin Systems
    durch Endotoxin im experimentellen Schockmodell der Ratte,
    Z. med. Labor. Diagn., 26:67-70.
Marceau, F., Lussier, A., and St-Pierre, S., 1984, Selective
    induction of cardiovascular responses to des-Arg^9-brady-
    kinin by bacterial endotoxin, Pharmacology, 29:70-74.
McConn, R., Wassermann, F., and Haberland, G., 1983, The kalli-
    krein-kinin system in the acutely-ill: (A) changes in
    plasma kininogen in acutely-ill patients. (B) the efficacy
    of pulmonary clearence of bradykinin, Adv. Med. Biol.,
    156b:1019-1035.
O'Donnell, T. F., Clowes, G. H. A., Talamo, R. C., and Colman,
    R. W., 1976, Kinin activation in the blood of patients
    with sepsis, Surg. Gynecol. Obstet., 143:539-545.
Regoli, D., and Barabé, J., 1980, Pharmacology of bradykinin
    and related kinins, Pharmac. Rev., 32:1-46.
Regoli, D. C., Marceau, F., and Lavigne, J., 1981, Induction of
    B$_1$-receptors for kinins in the rabbit by a bacterial
    lipopolysaccharide, Eur. J. Pharmacol., 71:105-115.
Siebeck, M., Hoffmann, H., Jochum, M., Welter, H. F., and
    Fritz, H., 1987, Therapeutische Effekte der Inhibition
    lysosomaler Proteasen im Schock, Langenbecks Arch. Chir.,
    Suppl.1987:325-328.

Dr. med. Matthias Siebeck, Chirurgische Klinik Innenstadt der
Universität München, Nussbaumstrasse 20, D-8000 München 2,
West Germany.

DEVELOPMENT OF BRADYKININ ANTAGONISTS: STRUCTURE-ACTIVITY RELATIONSHIPS
FOR NEW CATEGORIES OF ANTAGONIST SEQUENCES

Raymond J. Vavrek and John M. Stewart

Biochemistry Department-B126
University of Colorado Medical School
4200 East 9th Avenue, Denver, CO 80262, USA

INTRODUCTION

Three years ago, the first specific, competitive, sequence-related
antagonists of the pharmacological activities of bradykinin (BK, Arg-Pro-Pro-
Gly-Phe-Ser-Pro-Phe-Arg) were described (Vavrek and Stewart, 1985; Stewart
and Vavrek 1986). The replacement of Pro by DPhe at position 7 was the key
to antagonist activity. Modifications at various other positions in the
antagonist sequence increased potency, tissue selectivity, and metabolic
stability, or various combinations of these effects (Stewart and Vavrek,
1987a; Stewart and Vavrek, 1987b; Vavrek and Stewart, 1987a; Vavrek and
Stewart, 1987b). We describe here new classes of BK analogs which have been
designed and synthesized over the past three years. Representative peptides
from most of the new classes we describe have BK antagonist activity.

RESULTS AND DISCUSSION

Table 1 lists 103 representative peptides which were synthesized by
solid-phase methods and assayed in the clasical BK pharmacological assays;
isolated rat uterus (RUT), isolated guinea pig ileum (GPI), and rat blood
pressure (RBP) (Vavrek and Stewart, 1980).

BK may be modified extensively at the N-terminal with amino acids
without significant loss of BK-like agonist activity (Stewart, 1979). Thus
it is not surprising that T-Kinin (Ile-Ser-BK, #2) (Okamoto and Greenbaum,
1983) has full BK activity at somewhat reduced potency. Replacement of the
Ile and Ser residues with DIle and DSer (#3,4) produced selective (for rat
uterus) and potent BK agonist analogs. Similar modifications of the BK
antagonist sequence (7-DPhe-BK, #32) with Ile-Ser at the N-terminus gives
antagonist peptides (#5-12) with broad antagonist spectra. In contrast to
changes at the N-terminus, modifications at the C-terminus of BK, either by
amino acid extension, or by amide or ester formation on the C-terminal Arg
residue, generally destroy BK-like activity. Phyllokinin (#13) is an
exception; the Ile-Tyr(sulfate) addition allows for full activity with about
20% potency. The des-sulfated analogs of phyllokinin (#14-17) exhibit
similar agonist activity and potency. Extension of BK antagonist sequences
at the C-terminus with Ile-Tyr (#18-23) gives a potent GPI antagonist devoid
of any RBP action (#19) and a moderately potent GPI/RBP antagonist (#21).

TABLE 1 - BRADYKININ ANALOGS[a]

	ANALOG		RUT	GPI	RBP-IA	RBP-IV	%DEST
1.	BRADYKININ	BK	100	100	100	100	99
2.	"T-KININ"	Ile-Ser-BK	66	52	90	158	95
3.		DIle-Ser-BK	271	11	10	48	82
4.		Ile-DSer-BK	112	11	2	11	90
5.		Ile-Ser-[DPhe^7]-BK	AG	ANT(7)	0	0	–
6.		DIle-Ser-[DPhe^7]-BK	ANT(6)	ANT(3)	I(B)	I(B)	–
7.		Ile-DSer-[DPhe^7]-BK	0	ANT(6)	I(B)	I(B)	–
8.		DIle-DSer-[DPhe^7]-BK	ANT(2)	ANT(6)	I(B)	I(B)	–
9.		Ile-Ser-[Hyp^3-DPhe^7]-BK	AG	ANT(5)	I(B)	I(B)	–
10.		DIle-Ser-[Hyp^3-DPhe^7]-BK	ANT(6)	MXD	I(B)	I(B)	–
11.		Ile-DSer-[Hyp^3-DPhe^7]-BK	ANT(4)	0	I(B)	I(B)	–
12.		DIle-DSer-[Hyp^3-DPhe^7]-BK	0	0	I(B)	I(B)	–
13.	PHYLLOKININ	BK-Ile-Tyr(SO$_4$)	25	20	14		85
14.		BK-Ile-Tyr	26	21	6	103	61
15.		DArg-BK-Ile-Tyr	25	34	12	189	47
16.		Lys-Lys-BK-Ile-Tyr	18	21	9	497	0
17.		DLys-Lys-BK-Ile-Tyr	5	1	5	165	0
18.		[DPhe^7]-BK-Ile-Tyr	0.6	MXD	0.2	2	70
19.		DArg-[DPhe^7]-BK-Ile-Tyr	0.7	6.2(3)	0	0	–
20.		[Thi^{5,8}-DPhe^7]-BK-Ile-Tyr	0.5	MXD	0.1	8	0
21.		DArg-[Thi^{5,8}-DPhe^7]-BK-Ile-Tyr	0.3	5.8(8)	I(B)	I(B)	–
22.		[Hyp^3-Thi^{5,8}-DPhe^7]-BK-Ile-Tyr	0.1	MXD	0	0	–
23.		DArg-[Hyp^3-Thi^{5,8}-DPhe^7]-BK-Ile-Tyr	0.02	6.7(5)			
24.		[DPhe^7]-BK-DIle-Tyr	0	0	0.3	2	75
25.		DArg-[DPhe^7]-BK-DIle-Tyr	0	0	0	0	–
26.		[Thi^{5,8}-DPhe^7]-BK-DIle-Tyr	0	0	0.2	2	55
27.		DArg-[Thi^{5,8}-DPhe^7]-BK-DIle-Tyr	0	0	0	0	–
28.		[Thi^{5,8}-DPhe^7]-BK-NH$_2$	0.02	0	0.05	2	52
29.		Ac-[Thi^{5,8}-DPhe^7]-BK-NH$_2$	0	0	I(B)	I(B)	–
30.		DArg-[Thi^{5,8}-DPhe^7]-BK-NH$_2$	0	0	I(P)	I(P)	–
31.		Lys-Lys-[Thi^{5,8}-DPhe^7]-BK-NH$_2$	0.02	0	DPRS	DPRS	–
32.		[DPhe^7]-BK	4	5.9(5)	2	4	36
33.		[DPhe^7-Pro^8]-BK	ANT(2)	6.2(5)	0	0	–
34.		DArg-[DPhe^7-Pro^8]-BK	5.9(6)	6.6(6)	I(B)	I(B)	–
35.		[Hyp^3-DPhe^7-Pro^8]-BK	5.7(6)	5.6(7)	I(B)	I(B)	–
36.		DArg-[Hyp^3-DPhe^7-Pro^8]-BK	6.3(7)	6.0(6)	I(B)	I(B)	–
37.		[DPhe^7-Hyp^8]-BK	0	5.2(6)	0	0	–

	ANALOG	RUT	GPI	RBP-IA	RBP-IV	%DEST
38.	DArg-[DPhe^7-Hyp^8]-BK	0	I(7)	I(B)	I(B)	–
39.	[Hyp^3-DPhe^7-Hyp^8]-BK	I(5)	0	0	0	–
40.	DArg-[Hyp^3-DPhe^7-Hyp^8]-BK					
41.	[DPhe^1-DPhe^7-Pro^8]-BK	0	0	0	0	–
42.	[DThi^1-DPhe^7-Pro^8]-BK	0	0	0	0	–
43.	[DNal^1-DPhe^7-Pro^8]-BK	0	0	0	0	–
44.	[des-Pro^2-Hyp^3-DPhe^7]-BK	0	0	0	0	–
45.	DArg-[des-Pro^2-Hyp^3-DPhe^7]-BK	5.9(9)	0	I(B)	I(B)	–
46.	[des-Pro^{2,3}-DPhe^7]-BK	0	0	0	0	–
47.	DArg-[des-Pro^{2,3}-DPhe^7]-BK		I(4)	I(B)	I(B)	–
48.	[des-Pro^2,Gly^4-Hyp^3-DPhe^7]-BK	0	0	0	0	–
49.	DArg-[des-Pro^2,Gly^4-Hyp^3-DPhe^7]-BK	0	0	0	0	–
50.	[Hyp^3-des-Gly^4-DPhe^7]-BK	0	0	0	0	–
51.	DArg-[Hyp^3-des-Gly^4-DPhe^7]-BK	0/I	0			
52.	[Phe^2-des-Pro^3-DPhe^7]-BK	0	0	0	0	–
53.	DArg-[Phe^2-des-Pro^3-DPhe^7]-BK	5.6(3)	0	PRS	PRS	–
54.	[DPhe^1-des-Pro^2-Hyp^3-DPhe^7]-BK	0	0	0	0	–
55.	[DNal^1-des-Pro^2-Hyp^3-DPhe^7]-BK	0	0	0	0	–
56.	[DArg^1-des-Pro^2-Hyp^3-DPhe^7]-BK	0	0	I(B)	I(B)	–
57.	[Bz^1-Hyp^3-DPhe^7]-BK	0	5.4(4)	0	0	–
58.	[PBA^1-Hyp^3-DPhe^7]-BK	0	0	0	0	–
59.	[PBA^1-des-Pro^2-DPhe^7]-BK	0	5.2(7)	ins	ins	–
60.	[Hyp^3]-BK	100	35	85	300	94
61.	[DPhe^1-Hyp^3]-BK	0	0	0	0	–
62.	[DTyr^1-Hyp^3]-BK	0.1	0	0	0	–
63.	[CDF^1-Hyp^3]-BK	0	0	AG	AG	75
64.	[DNal^1-Hyp^3]-BK	0.1	0	0	0	–
65.	[Bz^1-Hyp^3]-BK	0	0	0	0	–
66.	[PBA^1-Hyp^3]-BK	0	0	0	0	–
67.	DArg-[DPhe^1-Hyp^3]-BK	0.1	0	AG	AG	50
68.	DArg-[DTyr^1-Hyp^3]-BK	0.1	0	AG	AG	63
69.	DArg-[CDF^1-Hyp^3]-BK	0.1	0			
70.	[DPhe^1-Thi^{5,8}-DPhe^7]-BK	0	0	I(B)	I(B)	–
71.	[DThi^1-Thi^{5,8}-DPhe^7]-BK	0	0	0	0	–
72.	[DPal^1-Thi^{5,8}-DPhe^7]-BK	0	0	0	0	–
73.	[DNal^1-Thi^{5,8}-DPhe^7]-BK	5.6(8)	0	I(B)	I(B)	–
74.	[DNal^1-DPhe^7]-BK	5.4(6)	0	I(B)	I(B)	–
75.	DArg-[DNal^1-DPhe^7]-BK	5.6(5)	0	I(B)	I(B)	–
76.	[CDF^1-DPhe^7]-BK	5.0(6)	0	I(B)	I(B)	–
77.	DArg-[CDF^1-DPhe^7]-BK	5.4(8)	0	I(B)	I(B)	–

(Continued)

	ANALOG	RUT	GPI	RBP-IA	RBP-IV	%DEST
78.	$[\text{DNal}^1\text{-Hyp}^3\text{-DPhe}^7]$-BK	0	0.1	0	0	–
79.	$[\text{CDF}^1\text{-Hyp}^3\text{-DPhe}^7]$-BK	MXD	0	I(B)	I(B)	–
80.	$[\text{DTyr}^1\text{-Hyp}^3\text{-DPhe}^7]$-BK	5.1(6)	0	I(B)	I(B)	–
81.	$[\text{FDF}^1\text{-Hyp}^3\text{-DPhe}^7]$-BK	ANT(3)	0	I(B)	I(B)	–
82.	$[\text{DVal}^1\text{-Hyp}^3\text{-DPhe}^7]$-BK	0	0	0	0	–
83.	$[\text{DIle}^1\text{-Hyp}^3\text{-DPhe}^7]$-BK	5.0(2)	0	0	0	–
84.	$[\text{Bz}^1\text{-Hyp}^3\text{-DPhe}^7]$-BK	0	5.4(4)	0	0	–
85.	$[\text{PBA}^1\text{-Hyp}^3\text{-DPhe}^7]$-BK	MXD	0	0	0	–
86.	DArg-$[\text{DNal}^1\text{-Hyp}^3\text{-DPhe}^7]$-BK	5.9(6)	0	I(B)	I(B)	–
87.	DArg-$[\text{CDF}^1\text{-Hyp}^3\text{-DPhe}^7]$-BK	5.8(8)	0	I(B)	I(B)	–
88.	DArg-$[\text{DTyr}^1\text{-Hyp}^3\text{-DPhe}^7]$-BK		ANT(2)	I(B)	I(B)	–
89.	DArg-$[\text{FDF}^1\text{-Hyp}^3\text{-DPhe}^7]$-BK	5.7(4)	0	I(B)	I(B)	–
90.	DArg-$[\text{DVal}^1\text{-Hyp}^3\text{-DPhe}^7]$-BK	5.4(4)	0	0	0	–
91.	DArg-$[\text{DIle}^1\text{-Hyp}^3\text{-DPhe}^7]$-BK	5.4(2)	0	0	0	–
92.	$[\text{Thi}^{5,8}\text{-DPhe}^7\text{-DArg}^9]$-BK	0.01	0	0.1	0.6	77
93.	Ac-$[\text{Thi}^{5,8}\text{-DPhe}^7\text{-DArg}^9]$-BK	0	0	0	0	–
94.	DArg-$[\text{Thi}^{5,8}\text{-DPhe}^7\text{-DArg}^9]$-BK	0	0	I(B)	I(B)	–
95.	Lys-Lys-$[\text{Thi}^{5,8}\text{-DPhe}^7\text{-DArg}^9]$-BK	0	0	0.2	14	0
96.	$[\text{Thi}^{5,8}\text{-DPhe}^7\text{-DArg}^9]$-BK-$NH_2$	0.01	0	0.1	0.9	61
97.	Ac-$[\text{Thi}^{5,8}\text{-DPhe}^7\text{-DArg}^9]$-BK-$NH_2$	0	0	I(B)	I(B)	–
98.	DArg-$[\text{Thi}^{5,8}\text{-DPhe}^7\text{-DArg}^9]$-BK-$NH_2$	0.003	0	I(B)	I(B)	–
99.	Lys-Lys-$[\text{Thi}^{5,8}\text{-DPhe}^7\text{-DArg}^9]$-BK-$NH_2$	0	0	0.2	14	0
100.	$[\text{Hyp}^3\text{-DPhe}^7\text{-Phe}^9]$-BK	0	MXD	0	0	–
101.	DArg-$[\text{Hyp}^3\text{-DPhe}^7\text{-Phe}^9]$-BK	6.1(5)	5.2(6)	I(B)	I(B)	–
102.	$[\text{DArg}^1\text{-Hyp}^3\text{-DPhe}^7\text{-Phe}^9]$-BK	0	0	0	0	–
103.	DArg-$[\text{DArg}^1\text{-Hyp}^3\text{-DPhe}^7\text{-Phe}^9]$-BK	6.3(6)	5.0(6)	I(B)	I(B)	–

[a]. Biological activities of BK analogs on rat uterus (RUT) and guinea pig ileum (GPI), and on rat blood pressure (RBP) by intraarterial (IA) or intravenous (IV) administration. Apparent pulmonary destruction (%DEST) for RBP agonist analogs is calculated from the IA and IV potencies. Agonist potency is relative to BK = 100%. AG indicates uncalculated agonist activity. Antagonist activity on smooth muscle is indicated by pA_2 values, or by ANT where antagonist is not calculated, followed by the number of tissues in parentheses. Antagonist activity in RBP is indicated by I(B), where a 50% reduction of the response of an ED(25mm) dose of BK is produced following bolus administration of BK plus antagonist, or I(P) where less than 50% reduction is produced. DPRS indicates depressor effect. MXD indicated mixed AG/ANT activity. Abbreviations: ins = insoluble, Bz = benzoyl, CDF = parachloro-DPhe, DNal = beta-2-naphthyl-DAla, DPal = beta-3-pyridyl-DAla, DThi = beta-2-thienyl-DAla, FDF = parafluoro-DPhe, Hyp = trans-4-hydroxy-Pro, Nal = beta-2-naphthyl-Ala, PBA = phenylbutyryl, and Thi = beta-2-thienyl-Ala.

A DIle residue in the C-terminal dipeptide extension (#24-27) destroys most biological activity. The simple amide (#28) of one of the most potent BK antagonists is devoid of biological activity, thus apparently following conventional wisdom on C-terminal modification of BK analogs. However, additional modifications at the N-terminal (#29,30) permit antagonist activity in the RBP assay.

Most approachs to classical BK structure-activity relationships (SAR) included tandem replacement of the Phe residues at positions 5 and 8. This was done with the first BK antagonist (#32) when both Phe residues were replaced with thienylalanine (Thi) to produce the first potent and generally useful BK antagonist (Vavrek and Stewart, 1985). Other tandem replacements at the Phe positions have been unexciting. Replacement of both Phe residues with Pro residues (analogs not listed), a strategy loosely based on the reverse of replacing both Pro residues at positions 2 and 3 with Phe (Stewart and Vavrek, 1987b) to give highly selective BK antagonists, and the seminal modification of replacing Pro at position 7 with DPhe to give the first BK antagonist, gives totally inactive peptides. However, single replacement of Phe at position 8 with Pro in antagonist sequences gives quite potent antagonists in all of our assays (#33-36), with peptide #34 possessing the highest potency described for antagonizing BK activity on the GPI. The hydroxyproline (Hyp) analogs of #33-36 (#37-40) show similar antagonist activity with some reduced potency.

An examination of the requirements for the residue at position one of BK and BK-like agonist analogs (Arg in the native sequence) led to a series of D-aromatic amino acid-containing BK sequences at position one (#61-64), and two des-amino BK analogs (#65-66) based on aromatic residues at position 1. None of these had BK-like agonist or antagonist activity, confirming the traditional wisom of the requirement for a basic residue at position one for BK agonist activity. However, D-aromatic amino acid substitution for Arg at position one in an antagonist peptide sequence containing Thi (#70-73) showed that Arg is not necessary in BK antagonist peptides. When similar antagonist sequences with D-aromatic amino acid residues at position one, but lacking Thi, were made (#74-81) an new general family of antagonist peptides was produced. These antagonists are completely ineffective against BK in the GPI assay, but are antagonists in th RUT and RBP assays. D-aliphatic amino acid substitution at position one in a closely related peptides gave analogs (#82,83) devoid of both GPI and RBP activity, although the DIle analog (#83) is a weak BK antagonist in the uterus assay. In a quite remarkable finding, the des-amino analog #84 is a specific BK antagonist in the GPI assay. The addition of a DArg residue to the D-aliphatic amino acid-containing analogs (#86-91) increases antagonist potency.

If the Arg residue at position one is not necessary for BK antagonist activity, and can be replaced by an aromatic amino acid, the same might hold at position nine. Peptides #100-103 demonstrate that BK antagonists of good potency do not require an Arg residue at the C-terminus.

Peptides #92-95 demonstrate that changing the configuration of the Arg residue at position nine in antagonist sequences generally eliminates antagonist properties (but #94 is an antagonist in the RBP assay). A combination of C-terminal amide and a DArg residue at position nine (#96-99) is only moderately more interesting for the production of antagonist peptides.

Finally, a series of deletion analogs of BK antagonist peptide sequences was synthesized and assayed (#44-56). Four of the internally shortened peptides (#45,47,53,56) antagonize BK activity in one or more assay. Peptides 47 and 56 contain only eight amino acid residues in their sequence, and represent the first true antagonists of BK which contain less than nine amino acids.

ACKNOWLEDGEMENTS

The authors thank Virginia Callaway for the amino acid analyses, and Frances Shepperdson, Garima Vashistha and Irma Albinana for the bioassays. This research was supported by grants from the NHLBI-NIH (#HL-26284) and from Nova Pharmaceutical Corporation.

REFERENCES

Okamoto, H., and Greenbaum, L. M., 1983, Isolation and structure of T-kinin, Biochem. Biophys. Res. Commun., 112:701.

Stewart, J. M., 1979, Chemistry and biologic activity of peptides related to bradykinin, in: "Handbook of Experimental Pharmacology", Volume XXV Supplement, E. G. Erdos, ed., Springer Verlag, Heidelberg.

Stewart, J. M. and Vavrek, R. J., 1986, Bradykinin competitive inhibitors for classic kinin systems, in: "Kinins IV", L. M. Greenbaum and H. Margolius, eds., Plenum Press, New York.

Stewart, J. M. and Vavrek, R. J., 1987a, Bradykinin competitive antagonists: design and activities, in: "Enzymes and Enzyme Inhibitors", R. L. Schowen and A. Barth, eds., Pergamon Press, Berlin.

Stewart, J. M. and Vavrek, R. J., 1987b, Design of bradykinin antagonists, in: "Proceedings of the 10th American Peptide Symposium", G. R. Marshall, ed., ESCOM Science Publishers, The Netherlands (in press).

Vavrek, R. J. and Stewart, J. M., 1980, Bradykinin analogs containing α-aminoisobutyric acid (Aib), Peptides 1:231.

Vavrek, R. J. and Stewart, J. M., 1985, Competitive antagonists of bradykinin, Peptides 6:161.

Vavrek, R. J. and Stewart, J. M., 1987a, Bradykinin antagonists containing hydroxyproline, in: "Peptides 1986", D. Theodoropoulos, ed., W. de Gruyter, Berlin.

Vavrek, R. J. and Stewart, J. M., 1987b, Bradykinin antagonists modified at the proline positions: heterocyclic residues at positions two and three, in: "50th Anniversary of the Nobel Prize of A. Szent-Gyorgi", B. Penke and A. Torok, eds., W. de Gruyter, Berlin (in press).

TISSUE SELECTIVITY OF NOVEL SPECIFIC AND COMPETITIVE ANTAGONISTS OF
NEUROKININ B ON ISOLATED SMOOTH MUSCLES

Shigeru Naminohira, Yoshiki Uchida, Keiko Okimura, Katsuro
Kurosawa, Takeshi Sakai, Naoki Sakura and Tadashi Hashimoto

School of Pharmacy, Hokuriku University, Ho-3
Kanagawa-machi, Kanazawa 920-11, Japan

In study[1,2] on neurokinin B (NKB) related peptides, we have
developed specific substance P, neurokinin A and eledoisin antagonists as
well as specific NKB antagonists. Therefore, our study suggests that, in
mammalian smooth muscles, there coexist not only each receptor specific for
substance P, neurokinin A and NKB, but also one specific for eledoisin (or
eledoisin-like peptide) of non-mammalian origin.

In the present paper we describe: a) specific and tissue-selective
NKB and kassinin antagonists, and b) a novel method for the classification
of NKB receptor subtypes by the molecular recognition using specific and
competitive NKB antagonist.

SPECIFIC AND TISSUE-SELECTIVE NKB AND KASSININ ANTAGONISTS

Three NKB analogs (Fig. 1), $[Arg^3, Gly^6, D\text{-}Trp^8, Nle^{10}]$-NKB (3-10),
$[D\text{-}Arg^3, D\text{-}Ala^6, Leu^{10}]$-NKB (3-10) and $[Arg^3, Gly^6, D\text{-}Ala^8, Leu^{10}]$-NKB (3-
10) were tested for agonistic activity and for their ability to antagonize
the myotropic actions of NKB, neurokinin A, substance P, eledoisin,
physalaemin and kassinin in isolated guinea-pig ileum, guinea-pig urinary
bladder, rat vas deferens, rat duodenum and rat portal vein preparations.

$$
\begin{array}{lll}
 & & 136810 \\
\text{NKB} & & \text{H-Asp-Met-His-Asp-Phe——Phe-Val——Gly-Leu-Met-NH}_2 \\
\text{I} & [Arg^3,Gly^6,D\text{-}Trp^8,Nle^{10}]\text{-NKB (3-10)} & \text{H-\underline{Arg}-Asp-Phe——\underline{Gly}-Val-\underline{D\text{-}Trp}-Leu-\underline{Nle}-NH}_2 \\
\text{II} & [D\text{-}Arg^3,D\text{-}Ala^6,Leu^{10}]\text{-NKB (3-10)} & \text{H-\underline{D\text{-}Arg}-Asp-Phe-\underline{D\text{-}Ala}-Val——Gly-Leu-\underline{Leu}-NH}_2 \\
\text{III} & [Arg^3,Gly^6,D\text{-}Ala^8,Leu^{10}]\text{-NKB (3-10)} & \text{H-\underline{Arg}-Asp-Phe——\underline{Gly}-Val-\underline{D\text{-}Ala}-Leu-\underline{Leu}-NH}_2
\end{array}
$$

Fig. 1. Amino acid sequences of NKB and its related peptides

The methods used for experiments were essentially the same as those previously described.[1] NKB, neurokinin A, substance P, eledoisin, physalaemin, kassinin and the NKB analogs were cumulatively (50–100 µl volumes per each application) applied up to the concentration of 10^{-6} M to test their agonistic activities. But the contractile effects of substance P and physalaemin in rat vas deferens preparation were not measured, since the peptides are practically inactive in this preparation. The antagonistic effects of the NKB analogs were tested at concentration of 2×10^{-6} M against each neurokinin or tachykinin, which was added cumulatively at concentration of 10^{-10} – 10^{-6} M. The antagonistic effects of the NKB analogs were assessed from the analysis of the cumulative dose-response curves with three concentrations (10^{-6} M, 3×10^{-6} M and 10^{-5} M) of the NKB analogs against neurokinin or tachykinin. The pharmacological parameters of α (an intrinsic activity), pA_2 (a negative logarithm of the dissociation constant of an antagonist) or x (empirical x-intercept of the line of Schild plot in the case of complex antagonism) and Schild plot were used to characterize the NKB analogs. The results are summarized in Table 1.

$[Arg^3, Gly^6, D\text{-}Trp^8, Nle^{10}]$-NKB (3-10) parallelly shifted the concentration-response curve (Fig. 2A) of kassinin only in rat portal vein preparation towards higher concentrations, suggesting competitive antagonism. Slope value (−0.88 ± 0.13) of the Schild plot (Fig. 2B)

Table 1. Biological properties of the NKB related peptides
in isolated smooth muscles*,**

Analog	Guinea-pig ileum α	x NKB	x PH	Guinea-pig urinary bladder α	x NKB	x PH	x KA	Rat vas deferens α	x NKB	x NKA	x KA
I	—	5.69	5.05	—	—	5.18	5.30	—	—	6.06	4.65
II	<0.1	5.01	—	—	—	—	—	—	4.28	—	—
III	—	4.74	—	—	5.14	—	—	—	—	—	4.68

Analog	Rat duodenum α	x NKB	x NKA	x SP	x PH	Rat portal vein α	x NKA	x SP	x KA
I	—	4.79	5.38	4.62	4.53	—	—	—	5.52
II	—	—	—	—	—	—	—	—	—
III	—	—	—	5.33	3.71	—	5.14	4.40	—

α: Maximum contraction by each NKB analog (1 µmol/l)/maximum contraction by NKB (1 µmol/l), in the same preparation.
*: NKB, neurokinin B; NKA, neurokinin A; SP, substance P; PH, physalaemin; ED, eledoisin; KA, kassinin.
**: All NKB analogs failed to antagonize the response(s) to NKA, SP, ED and KA in guinea-pig ileum, NKA, SP and ED in guinea-pig urinary bladder, ED in rat vas deferens, ED and KA in rat duodenum, and NKB, PH and ED in rat portal vein tissues.
x: pA_2 in the case of KA at analog I in rat portal vein and KA at analog III in rat vas deferens preparations.

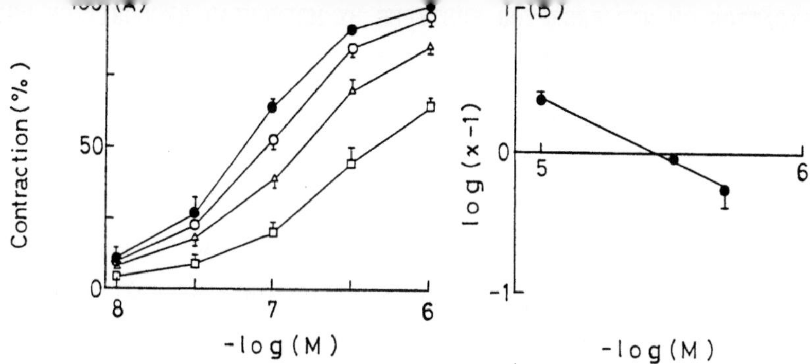

Fig. 2. Effects of [Arg^3, Gly^6, D-Trp^8, Nle^{10}]-NKB (3-10) on the contractile responses to kassinin (A) in isolated rat portal vein. ●, kassinin alone, ○, △, □, in the presence of 2, 3 and 10 μmol/l [Arg^3, Gly^6, D-Trp^8, Nle^{10}]-NKB (3-10), respectively. Contractile response is expressed in % of the maximum response to kassinin in the same preparation. Symbols and bars indicate means ± SE of 4 determinations. Schild plot (B) for the antagonism between [Arg^3, Gly^6, D-Trp^8, Nle^{10}] -NKB (3-10) and kassinin. Abscissa: negative logarithm of molar concentration of [Arg^3, Gly^6, D-Trp^8, Nle^{10}]-NKB (3-10). Ordinate: logarithm of (concentration ratio -1). The line was fitted to the data by linear regression analysis.

calculated from the results of experiments with three concentrations of each of the NKB analog was not significantly different from unity, also suggesting a compeptitive antagonism. The antagonisms of the NKB analog in guinea-pig ileum, guinea-pig urinary bladder, rat duodenum and rat vas deferens preparations were non-specific.

[D-Arg^3, D-Ala^6, Leu^{10}]-NKB (3-10) acted as a specific antagonist against NKB in guinea-pig ileum and rat vas deferens preparations. No antagonistic effect of [D-Arg^3, D-Ala^6, Leu^{10}]-NKB (3-10) against six neurokinin and tachykinin peptides was observed in guinea-pig urinary bladder, rat duodenum, or rat portal vein preparation.

[Arg^3, Gly^6, D-Ala^8, Leu^{10}]-NKB (3-10) exerted an antagonistic effect against NKB in guinea-pig ileum and urinary bladder preparations, but not against other neurokinin and tachykinin peptides. A specific and competitive antagonism of this NKB analog to kassinin was observed in rat vas deferens preparation.

The specific antagonism against kassinin gives support to the conception that there coexist tachykinin (or tachykinin-like peptides) receptors in addition to NKB, neurokinin A and substance P receptors in smooth muscles of mammal.

CLASSIFICATION OF NKB RECEPTOR SUBTYPES BY MOLECULAR RECOGNITION USING
SPECIFIC AND COMPETITIVE NKB ANTAGONIST

NKB molecule can be distinguished from other neurokinin and tachykinin
molecules by NKB receptor on interactions of a specific NKB antagonist and
these peptides with the receptor. On our recent study[3] using a specific
and competitive antagonist, [Gly^6]-NKB (3-10), it was revealed that Asp^4
and Phe^5 in NKB may be essential for the molecular recognition of a peptide
as a NKB molecule for NKB-1 receptor subtype in isolated guinea-pig ileum,
while Asp^1, Met^2 and His^3 of NKB may be less important.

This part deals with the molecular recognition of another NKB receptor
subtype (NKB-2 receptor), which has been verified using an antagonist, and
discrepancy between the recognition sites of NKB molecule for the NKB
receptor subtypes. We studied the mode of action of the specific and
competitive NKB antagonist, [Arg^3, Gly^6, $D-Trp^8$]-NKB (3-10),[2] against four
NKB related peptides (Fig. 3) in isolated guinea-pig ileum, and compared it
with that against NKB.

[Arg^3,Gly^6,$D-Trp^8$]-NKB (3-10)	H-Arg-Asp-Phe-Gly-Val-D-Trp-Leu-Met-NH$_2$
NKB (3-10)	H-His-Asp-Phe-Phe-Val——Gly-Leu-Met-NH$_2$
NKB (4-10)	H-Asp-Phe-Phe-Val——Gly-Leu-Met-NH$_2$
[Gly^4]-NKB (3-10)	H-His-Gly-Phe-Phe-Val——Gly-Leu-Met-NH$_2$
[Gly^5]-NKB (3-10)	H-His-Asp-Gly-Phe-Val——Gly-Leu-Met-NH$_2$

Fig. 3.   Amino acid sequences of NKB antagonist and NKB related peptides

The method and the pharmacological parameters used were the same as
those described above. The NKB related peptides possess the following
relative potencies expressed as a fraction of the potency of NKB (NKB = 1):
NKB (3-10) 0.68,[4] NKB (4-10) 0.07,[4] [Gly^4]-NKB (3-10) 0.42[5] and [Gly^5]-
NKB (3-10) 1.92.[5] The results are presented in Table 2.

Table 2. Antagonistic potency of [Arg^3,Gly^6,$D-Trp^8$]-NKB (3-10)
in inhibiting contractile response to NKB related peptides

NKB related peptide	x-intercept*	Slope
NKB (3-10)	5.25 ± 0.24	−1.13 ± 0.24
NKB (4-10)	——	——
[Gly^4]-NKB (3-10)	——	——
[Gly^5]-NKB (3-10)	5.70 ± 0.47	−0.64 ± 0.20

* pA_2 value in the case of NKB (3-10)

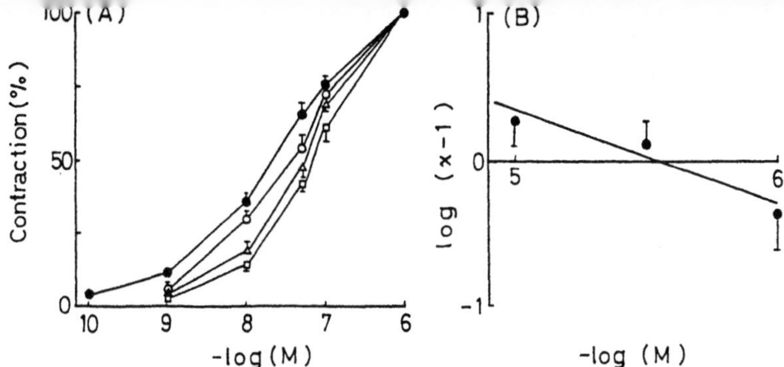

Fig. 4. Effects of [Arg^3, Gly^6, D-Trp^8]-NKB (3-10) on the contractile responses to NKB (3-10) (A) in isolated guinea-pig ileum. ●, NKB (3-10) alone, ○, △, □, in the presence of 1, 3 and 10 μmol/l [Arg^3, Gly^6, D-Trp^8]-NKB (3-10), respectively. Contractile response is expressed in % of the maximum response to NKB (3-10) in the same preparation. Symbols and bars indicate means ± SE of 4 determinations. Schild plot (B) for the antagonism between [Arg^3, Gly^6, D-Trp^8]-NKB (3-10) and NKB (3-10). Abscissa: negative logarithm of molar concentration of [Arg^3, Gly^6, D-Trp^8]-NKB (3-10). Ordinate: logarithm of (concentration ratio -1). The line was fitted to the data by linear regression analysis.

The NKB antagonist caused a parallel shift of the concentration-response curve for NKB (3-10) to the right, in a concentration-dependent manner (Fig. 4A). A Schild plot gave a straight line the slope of which was not significantly different from unity (Fig. 4B), indicating competitive antagonism. The NKB antagonist also shifted the concentration-response curve for [Gly^5]-NKB (3-10), but did not cause a parallel shift of the concentration-response curve toward a higher concentration in a dose-dependent manner. The slope was significantly lower than unity, indicating complex antagonism. On the other hand, the NKB antagonist did not antagonize the response to NKB (4-10) or [Gly^4]-NKB (3-10).

On the interactions of the NKB antagonist, [Arg^3, Gly^6, D-Trp^8]-NKB (3-10), and NKB (3-10) or [Gly^5]-NKB (3-10) with NKB-2 receptor, the antagonistic activity remained complete. In other words, the deletion of Asp^1 and Met^2 in NKB does not effect markedly the interaction with the NKB-2 receptor, which was confirmed by the antagonistic activity of the NKB antagonist. Besides, the replacement of Phe^5 with Gly moiety does not confer the loss of the interaction. From these findings, it is suggested that the NKB-2 receptor may recognize NKB (3-10) and [Gly^5]-NKB (3-10) as a NKB molecule.

In contrast to experiments with the above NKB related peptides, the

NKB antagonist did not antagonize the response to $[Gly^4]$-NKB (3-10) or NKB (4-10). These results indicate that the NKB-2 receptor may not be able to recognize $[Gly^4]$-NKB (3-10) or NKB (4-10) as a NKB molecule by the replacement of the acidic side chain at Asp^4 with hydrogen or the deletion of His^3. The experiments demonstrate that $[Gly^4]$-NKB (3-10) interacts with a neurokinin receptor or with a NKB receptor subtype that is not blocked by the NKB antagonist.

In summary, Asp^1, Met^2 and Phe^5 moieties in NKB seem to be less important for the molecular recognition of the NKB-2 receptor in guinea-pig ileum. Besides, this study demonstrated that the side chains of the amino acid residues at positions 3 and 4 in NKB may be essential for a peptide which can be recognized as a NKB molecule by the NKB-2 receptor. Furthermore, the characteristics in the molecular recognition sites of the NKB receptor subtypes was clearly distinguishable.

REFERENCES

1 Hashimoto,T., Uchida,Y., Naminohira,S. and Sakai,T.:Tachykinin antagonist
  I:Specific, competitive and tissue-selective neurokinin B antagonists on
  contractile activity in smooth muscles, Japan. J. Pharmacol., in press.
2 Sakura,N., Naminohira,S., Uchida,Y., Okimura,K., Kurosawa,K., Sakai.,T.
  and Hashimoto,T.:Specific antagonists of neurokinin B analogs against
  tachykinin receptors, Japan Symposium on Peptide Chemistry, Kobe, 1987.
3 Hashimoto,T. and Uchida,Y.: Neurokinin receptor I:Molecular recognition
  of neurokinin B receptor in isolated guinea-pig ileum using a specific
  and competitive neurokinin B antagonist, Japan. J. Pharmacol. submitted.
4 Osakada,F., Kubo,K., Goto,K., Kanazawa,I. and Munekata,E.:The contractile
  activities of neurokinin A, B and related peptides on smooth muscles,
  Eur. J. Pharmacol., 120, 201-208 (1986).
5 Hashimoto,T., Moro,T. and Uchida,Y.:Neurokinin B analogs substituted with
  glycine, Bull. Chem. Soc. Jpn., 59, 4006-4008 (1986).

COMPETITIVE ANTAGONISTS OF BRADYKININ:

IN VITRO (JUGULAR VEIN) AND IN VIVO (BLOOD PRESSURE RESPONSE) STUDIES

Hans Hoffmann[1], Eric T. Whalley[3], Matthias Siebeck[2],
Joachim Weipert[1], and Hans Fritz[1]

[1]Abteilung für Klinische Chemie und Klinische Biochemie in der
Chirurgischen Klinik Innenstadt
[2]Chirurgische Klinik Innenstadt und Chirurgische Poliklinik
University of Munich, Munich, FRG
[3]Department of Physiological Science, University of
Manchester, Manchester, UK

INTRODUCTION

Antagonists of the action of bradykinin (BK) may be useful in disease
states associated with arterial hypotension and increased vascular permeability. Potent sequence-related BK antagonists were first described by J.
M. STEWART, and R.J. VAVREK in 1985. These compounds have been tested
against BK effects on the rat uterus and guinea pig ileum (Vavrek and
Stewart, 1985) and on the dog carotid artery and dog urinary bladder (Regoli
et al., 1986). In the present study, we have tested three different compounds (B4144, B4146, and B4148) for their antagonist potency against BK in
the rabbit jugular vein and pig blood pressure response.

METHODS

Compounds: B4144 (Arg-Pro-Pro-Gly-Thi-Ser-DPhe-Thi-Arg.TFA), B4146
(Arg-Pro-Hyp-Gly-Thi-Ser-DPhe-Thi-Arg.TFA), and B4148 (Lys-Lys-Arg-Hyp-Pro-
Gly-Thi-Ser-DPhe-Thi-Arg.TFA) were synthesized by R.J. Vavrek and J.M.
Stewart, Denver, Colorado, USA. Bradykinin and Angiotensin II were purchased
from Sigma. Acetylcholine (ACH) was obtained from E.Merck, Darmstadt, FRG.
Concentrated solutions (5 mg/ml) of the peptides were made in 0.9% saline
and stored at -80° C until use.

In vitro studies: Rabbit jugular vein spiral strips (n = 3) were
suspended in 4 ml tissue baths, containing Krebs-Henseleit solution,
maintained at 37° C and gassed with 95 % O_2 and 5 % CO_2. The contraction
force was measured using an isometric transducer. Cumulative concentration-
effect curves were constructed to BK in the absence and presence of various
concentrations of B4144, B4146, and B4148. pA_2 values for each of the three
antagonists were determined against BK according to SCHILD, 1947. The pA_2
value is defined as the negative logarithm of the molar concentration of the
antagonist which reduces the response of an double ED_{50} dose of BK to that
of an ED_{50} dose (the ED_{50} dose produces a half maximal contraction of the
tissue). Data is presented as the mean $\pm$ SD.

<u>In vivo studies</u>: Weaned piglets weighing 17-23 kg were studied under pentobarbital/pethidin anesthesia, relaxation with pancuronium, and were mechanically ventilated. Catheters were inserted into the right carotid artery and the external jugular vein. Systolic and diastolic arterial blood pressure was measured continuously with a Bently Trantec Model 800 transducer, equipped with an amplifier (Sirecust 404, Siemens, Munich, FRG), and a two channel recorder (BD 41, Kipp & Zonen, The Netherlands). Dose-response curves for the hypotensive effect of intraarterial bolus injections of BK (10, 25, 50, 100, and 200 ng) and ACH (500 ng) on arterial pressure were constructed. The blood pressure response was determined as the maximum change in diastolic arterial pressure. The inhibitory potency of the antagonist against BK was evaluated either by

(i) simultaneous intraarterial bolus injections of BK (100 ng) and increasing doses of the antagonists in 6 pigs, or by

(ii) intraarterial bolus injections of BK (25, 50, 100, and 200 ng, 1000 ng) and ACH (500 ng) during continuous infusion of B4146 in three different dosages (8, 16, 32, ug x kg^{-1} x min^{-1}) in 3 pigs.

RESULTS AND DISCUSSION

All three bradykinin analogs tested were found to be potent competitive antagonists of bradykinin on both the rabbit jugular vein strip and the blood pressure response in anesthetized pigs.

Determination of the antagonist potency of B4144, B4146, and B4148 by means of pA_2 calculations indicated similar potency of the three compounds (pA_2 values were between 6.7 and 7.2) (Table 1). The pA_2 values obtained in the rabbit jugular vein are in the same order of magnitude as reported for these antagonists on other smooth muscle preparations (Vavrek and Stewart, 1985; Regoli et al., 1986). The specificity of BK inhibition for all three compounds was demonstrated by the lack of effect on the response towards Angiotensin II (data not shown).

Table 1. BK antagonism on the rabbit jugular vein.
Results are given as pA_2 values (mean $\pm$ SD, n = 3).

Compound		pA_2 value
B4144	$[\text{Thi}^{5,8}, \text{DPhe}^7]$-BK	6.7 $\pm$ 0.07
B4146	$[\text{Hyp}^3, \text{Thi}^{5,8}, \text{DPhe}^7]$-BK	7.1 $\pm$ 0.1
B4148	Lys-Lys-$[\text{Hyp}^2, \text{Thi}^{5,8}, \text{DPhe}^7]$-BK	7.2 $\pm$ 0.1

Table 2. Inhibition of the pig blood pressure response [percent]. Intraarterial bolus injections of bradykinin (100 ng) were given simultaneously with increasing dosages of the antagonists (mean $\pm$ SD, n = 6).

	Dose ratio of BK antagonist to BK			
Compound	50:1	100:1	500:1	1000:1
B4144	11.2 $\pm$ 3.9	23.6 $\pm$ 5.0	56.5 $\pm$ 8.3	72.6 $\pm$ 1.4
B4146	36.3 $\pm$ 7.9	50.3 $\pm$ 13.1	70.3 $\pm$ 12.2	88.1 $\pm$ 4.2
B4148	19.3 $\pm$ 10.8	47.4 $\pm$ 7.0	70.4 $\pm$ 3.8	79.7 $\pm$ 1.1

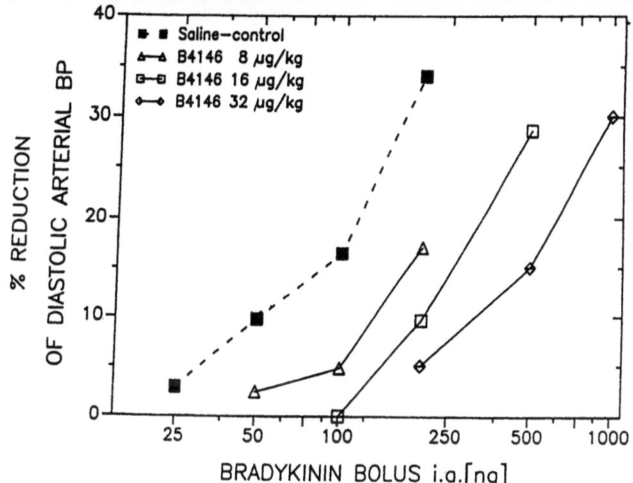

Fig. 1. Depressor effect of intraarterial bolus injections of BK on
diastolic arterial pressure. Dose response curves were constructed without and during continuous infusion of B4146 in 3
different dosages (8, 16, 32, ug x kg^{-1} x min^{-1}) (mean, n = 3).

In the pig blood pressure studies a 50 % inhibition of the depressor
effect of intraarterial bolus injections of BK was achieved when the dose
ratio of BK antagonist to BK was about 100 (B4146, B4148) and 500 (B4144),
respectively (Table 2). This is in a similar range as reported for the rat
blood pressure response (Benetos et al., 1986). Since B4146 had the
strongest inhibitory effect it was selected for additional studies. During
continuous infusion of B4146 a dose dependent right shift of the BK dose
response curve was noted (Fig. 1). At the highest dose given (32 ug x kg^{-1} x
min^{-1}) the inhibition of the depressor effect of intraarterial bolus
injections of BK was about 85 %. Responses to ACH were not significantly
different before and during the antagonist infusion, indicating that the
antagonist is selective. The normal hypotensive response towards BK returned
within 10 min after the end of the antagonist infusion, indicating a short
plasma half live of the antagonist.

The development of BK antagonists offers new approaches to experimental
and therapeutical investigations in kinin related diseases.

REFERENCES

Benetos, A., Gavras, H., Stewart, J.M., Vavrek, R.J., Hatinoglou, S.,
    Gavras, I., 1986, Vasodepressor role of endogenous bradykinin assessed
    by a bradykinin antagonist, Hypertension, 8:971.
Regoli, D., Drapeau, G., Rovero, P., Dion, S., D'Orleans-Juste, P., Barabe,
    J., 1986, The actions of kinin antagonists on B1 and B2 receptor
    systems, Eur J Pharmacol, 123:61.
Schild, H.O., 1947, pA, a new scale for the measurement of drug antagonism,
    Brit J Pharmacol, 2:189.
Vavrek, R.J., Stewart, J.M., 1985, Competitive antagonists of bradykinin,
    Peptides, 6:161.

ACKNOWLEDGMENT

E.T.W. thanks the Alexander von Humboldt Stiftung for financial support.

KININ RECEPTORS IN SMOOTH MUSCLE AND VASCULAR EFFECTS IN SODIUM DEPLETED
RATS

Minoru Yasujima, Keishi Abe*, Kaoru Yoshinaga,
P. Geoffrey Matthews** and Colin I. Johnston***

The Second Department of Internal Medicine, and *Dept of
Clinical Biology and Hormonal Regulation, Tohoku
University School of Medicine, Sendai, Japan
and **Monash University Department of Medicine
Prince Henry's Hospital, Melbourne and
***Melbourne University Department of Medicine
Austin Hospital, Heidelberg, Australia

INTRODUCTION

Bradykinin infused intravenously induces a prominent fall in blood
pressure in all species (Elliot et al. 1960; De Freitas et al. 1964).
This hypotensive peptide, when injected intravenously or into the renal
artery, also causes natriuresis and diuresis probably secondary to
hemodynamic change (Barraclough and Mills 1965; Gill et al. 1965). This
evidence demonstrates that vascular smooth muscle is the most important
target tissue for kinin actions in the regulation of blood pressure and
fluid homeostasis.

Variations in sodium balance induce changes in the myotropic action
of angiotensin II, a potent vasoconstrictor peptide (Reid and Laragh
1965). The administration of a low sodium diet stimulated the renal
kallikrein-kinin system, followed by an increase in urinary excretion of
kallikrein (Geller et al. 1972; Johnston et al. 1976). This evidence
prompted us to investigate the influence of sodium depletion on the
vascular effect of bradykinin.

Furthermore, it has become apparent that a variety of hormones
modulate their own biologic expression through modification of the
activity of their cellular receptors (Kahn 1976). The bradykinin-receptor
interaction has been characterized by inference from indirect studies
using isolated tissues (Barabé et al. 1977). However, these
pharmacological experiments do not localize the specific subcellular
receptors for this hormone, nor are they capable of identifying specific
receptor modifications. There had been few reports on specific bradykinin
direct binding studies using a radiolabeled ligand (Reissmann et al. 1977;
Odya et al. 1980; Yasujima et al. 1984 a).

Therefore, the present investigation was designed to characterize the
influence of sodium depletion on the vasculr effects of bradykinin,
assessed by its blood pressure effect, and to explore the role of changes
in bradykinin receptors on these effects.

MATERIALS AND METHODS

Materials

Bradykinin and analogues were obtained from the Protein Research Foundation (Osaka, Japan). Female Sprague-Dawley rats weighing from 150 to 200g were used. They were injected subcutaneously with 500 µg/kg of stilbesterol dipropionate (May & Baker, Aust. Pty. Ltd., Victoria, 0.01 mmol (p<0.05; compared to controls), respectively. Low sodium diets both for 7 days and for 28 days resulted in a marked increase in urinary excretion of kallikrein (3.38 ± 0.57 mg BK/hr/day compared to 2.23 ± 0.11 mg BK/hr/day on the 7th day; p<0.05 and 3.77 ± 0.64 mg BK/hr/day compared to 2.33 ± 0.22 mg BK/hr/day; p<0.05). Circulating levels of bradykinin in rats with normal sodium diets were 0.74 ± 0.36 ng/ml on the 7th day and 0.60 ± 0.30 ng/ml on the 28th day. Neither 7 days nor 28 days of low sodium diet resulted in any significant changes in circulating levels of bradykinin compared to controls (0.96 ± 0.50 ng/ml on the 7th day and 1.00 ± 0.30 ng/ml on the 28th day).

Blood pressure effect of bradykinin

Fig. 1 depicts the dose response curves to exogenous bradykinin, administered intra-arterially, for the rats on a normal sodium diet compared to rats on low sodium diets for 7 days and 28 days. The hypotensive efect of exogenous bradykinin was greater in the rats on a low sodium diet for 7 days at all doses, than that in the rats on a normal sodium diet. However, there was no significant difference in the hypotensive effect of bradykinin between the rats with low sodium diet for 28 days and the rats on a normal sodium diet.

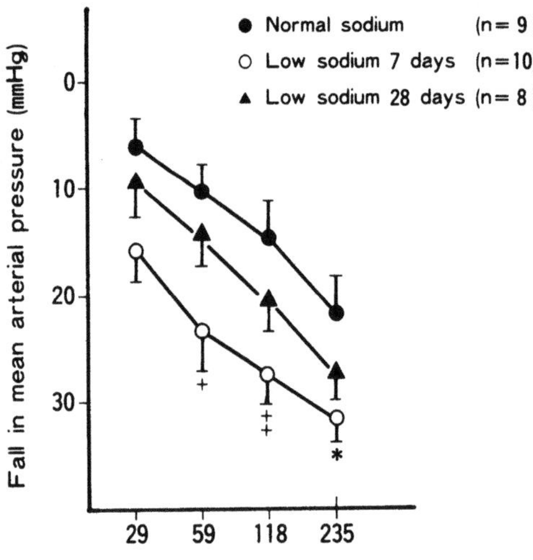

Fig. 1. Change in blood pressure response to exogenous bradykinin in the rats fed on normal sodium diet (● – ●) and low sodium diets for 7 days (o – o) and 28 days (▲ – ▲). Each value indicates the mean ± S.E. of 8-10 animals per group. : Statistical significance at p < 0.02, [+]statistical significance at p < 0.01, and [++]statistical significance at p < 0.001, compared to the value in the rats with normal sodium diet.

The mean overall hypotensive response induced by bradykinin in the rats given a low sodium diet, was 23.1 ± 1.8 mmHg, significantly larger than the value of 12.9 ± 2.2 mmHg found in the rats on a normal sodium diet. For the rats given a low sodium diet for 28 days, the mean overall hypotensive response was 17.0 ± 2.7 mmHg, which was not significantly different from the rats on a normal sodium diet.

Bradykinin receptors

^{125}I-Tyr^8-bradykinin capacity to uterine membranes was enhanced by low sodium diets for 7 days and for 28 days, compared to controls. The ratio of concentration of bradykinin binding sites to 5'-nucleotidase, a marker enzyme of plasma membrane, after low sodium diets of 7 days and 28 days was significantly higher compared to control rats (Table 1). The variation in the number of bradykinin binding sites after low sodium diets of 7 days and 28 days was not associated with alterations in the affinity of binding sites, estimated from the slopes of Scatchard plots (Table 1). In wet weight of uterus, protein content and 5'-nucleotidase activity of Australia) daily for 2 days prior to study.

Sodium depletion

The rats were placed on varying sodium diets for 7 or 28 days before the studies. They were divided in two groups (i) rats receiving a low sodium diet (0.05 mmol/day) with distilled water; (ii) rats receiving a standard diet (0.3 mmol/day) with tap water. The rats were maintained in individual metabolic cages for the last 7 days of the dietary studies. Twenty-four hour urine collections for measurement of volume, sodium and kallikrein content, as an indicator of renal kallikrein-kinin system was made on the day before the experiments. Blood for measurement of circulating levels of bradykinin was obtained by puncture of the abdominal aorta under light ether anesthesia immediately before the bradykinin binding study.

Urinary kallikrein in the rat was measured by an enzyme kinetic method (Johnston et al. 1976). Blood bradykinin was measured by radioimmunoassay as described by Mashford and Roberts (1972). Urinary sodium was measured by flame photometry.

Blood pressure effect of bradykinin

The blood pressure effect of bradykinin was measured as depressor dose response curves to synthetic bradykinin in graded doses from 29 pmol/kg to 235 pmol/kg in rats anesthetized with Inactin® (150 mg/kg ip). A tracheotomy was performed before the carotid artery was cannulated for bradykinin administration and femoral artery was also cannulated for blood pressure measurement. Changes in blood pressure were recorded directly through the catheter in the femoral artery with Statham p23 Db pressure transducers on a Grass model 7C polygraph recorder. The initial hypotensive component of change in blood pressure induced by each dose of bradykinin, was taken as the indicator of direct vascular response to bradykinin. The absolute levels of changes in blood pressure in mmHg was used as the dependent variable. The mean overall responses were calculated as the average of all doese.

Bradykinin receptor binding study

Bradykinin receptor binding studies were performed with ^{125}I-Tyr^8-bradykinin having specific activity of 300 Ci/mmol. The preparation of a uterine smooth muscle subcellular fraction enriched in plasma membrane for the determination of ^{125}I-Tyr^8-bradykinin specific binding, performed as detailed previously (Yasujima et al. 1984a). Specific ^{125}I-Tyr^8-bradykinin binding was determined by the difference between the radioactivity bound in the absence and in the presence of 1000 fold excess of unlabeled bradykinin. The apparent affinity and the number of binding sites were determined by Scatchard plot analysis (Scatchard 1949) of concentration dependent binding dose at the concentrations from 2×10^{-10}M to 1.2×10^{-9}M of ^{125}I-Tyr^8-bradykinin.

5'-Nucleotidase, as a marker enzyme of plasma membrane was measured as described by Song and Bodansky (1967). The unit was expressed as the amount of phosphate liberated from AMP after incubation of 30 minutes. Protein content of subcellular fractions was determined by the method of Lowry et al. (1951).

All data were expressed as mean ± S.E. Differences between groups were evaluated by Student's t-test.

Biochemical parameters

Urinary excretion of sodium in the rats on a normal sodium diet was 0.25 ± 0.05 mmol/day on the 7th day and 0.30 ± 0.05 mmol. on the 28th day. Wherease a low sodium diet for 7 days and for 28 days produced sodium excretions of 0.06 ± 0.03 mmol (p<0.05; compared to ontrols) and 0.02 ± membranes prepared from uterine smooth muscle of the rats fed on low and normal sodium diets, no significant changes were found between the groups.

TABLE 1. Binding parameters of uterine smooth muscle bradykinin receptors after sodium depletion.

		K_D 29°C $(x10^{-10}M)$	Number of binding sites (fmol/mg protein)	(fmol/5'nucleotidase)
7 days	Low sodium	7.3±0.7	58.9±2.0*	781.3±31.0*
(n=6)	Normal sodium	7.1±0.8	44.0±3.7	594.3±40.9
28 days	Low sodium	6.9±0.5	74.5±2.4[+]	1064.5±56.5[+]
(n=5)	Normal sodium	6.6±0.3	44.4±4.5	634.5±64.3

Each value indicates the mean ± S.E. of 6 paired determinations from independent experiments (7 days) and of 5 paired determinations from independent experiments (28 days). *statistical significance at $p < 0.01$, [+]statistical significance at $p < 0.001$.

DISCUSSION

Several possible explanations may account for the changes in the hypotensive effect of bradykinin after sodium depletion. Sodium may have a direct effect on blood pressure response to bradykinin. However, the present study suggests the hormonal changes in kallikrein-kinin system at the effector sites and demonstrates the variation in the number of bradykinin binding sites after sodium depletion. So it is unlikely to regard the change as the direct action of sodium on vascular effects of bradykinin. Strong evidence against the sodium hypothesis in the present study are the observations that the blood pressure response to bradykinin was enhanced in the rats with 7 days of sodium depletion and returned to control levesl in the rats with 28 days depletion.

Recent studies with receptor antagonists of angiotensin II have provided evidence that the increase in angiotensin II during sodium depletion contributes significantly to the maintenance of arterial blood pressure (Johnson and Davis 1973; Coleman et al. 1975). From this evidence, it could be supposed that the vascular effects of bradykinin is modulated by the concomitant vasoconstrictor action of angiotensin II with opposing effects of bradykinin. However, the observation of transient enhancement in the blood pressure response to bradykinin during sodium depletion does not support the hypothesis that angiotensin II might modulate the vascular effects of bradykinin after sodium depletion. Alterations in sympathetic nerve tone after sodium depletion have been reported, followed by increase in the renal vascular response to norepinephrine, with opposite actions of bradykinin on vascular smooth muscle in dogs (Kilcoyne and Cannon 1971). However, this evidence does not explain the change in the vascular effects of bradykinin.

Intra-arterial injection of bradykinin does not provide a result totally free of the effects of kininase action since it is exposed to the plasma kininases for a few seconds before it reaches its site of action, so it could be possible to raise that changes in plasma kininase activity during sodium depletion might modulate the vascular effect of bradykinin. Merrill et al. (1973) reported that a low sodium diet reduced the activity of angiotensin converting enzyme in the kidney which is identical with kininase II responsible for the destruction of bradykinin (Erdös 1975). However, effects of sodium depletion, on plasma kininase activity have not been elucidated in detail. Even if sodium depletion could induce the changes in plasma kininase activity, the present observations that the blood pressure response to bradykinin enhanced in the rats with 7 days of sodium depletion and returned to control levels in the rats with 28 days depletion, would not be fully explained.

The positive linkage between alteration in the blood pressure effect of bradykinin and in the number of bradykinin binding sites in uterine smooth muscle at acute phase of sodium depletion, can raise the possibility that the concentration in bradykinin receptors is a determinant of hormonal action. It could be mentioned that sodium and endogenous bradykinin may affect on vascular effects of bradykinin via influence on the number of bradykinn binding sites at subcellular levels. However, the dissociation between normalized vascular effects of bradykinin and the prolnged increase in the number of bradykinin binding sites at chronic phase of sodium depletion, show that vascular effects of bradykinin is determined not only by the number of binding sites but also other possible mechanisms.

The augmentation of vascular effects of bradykinin after sodium depletion, to be expected to increase in tissues levels of bradykinin, could not be explained by the hypothesis that its vascular effect depends upon the competition between endogenous and exogenous hormone for the same receptor without the change in the number of binding sites. Hence, the present results show the prolonged increase in the number of binding sites during sodium depletion. Therefore, we can put forward the hypothesis that the vascular effects of bradykinin is determined by prior occupancy of endogenous bradykinin at receptor sites. Our results did not exclude all possibilities that post receptor events is involved in the vascular effects of bradykinin.

Concerning the difference in the vascular effects of bradykinin between the rats after 7 days and after 28 days of low sodium diets, it is likely to suppose that the augmentation of the vascular effects of bradykinin after 7 days of low sodium diet indicates the temporal imbalance in receptor occupancy between endogenous bradykinin and the number of bradykinin binding sites. This leads to the hypotehsis that the increase in the number of bradykinin receptors may play an important role in the homeostasis of vascular smooth muscle tone after sodium depletion.

In earlier studies, we showed that the number of uterine smooth muscle bradykinin receptors was decreased by 20 % with prolonged infusion of bradykinin for 2 days (Yasujima et al. 1984b). According to the self regulation thoery (Raff 1976), decreased number of binding sites was expected after sodium depletion which could be considered to enhance the local kallikrein-kinin system. But the contrary was observed. This demonstrates that sodium status per se affect on uterine smooth muscle bradykinin receptors.

In summary, the present study leads to the following conclusions: a) The vascular effects of bradykinin after sodium depletion is mainly determined by prior occupancy of endogenous bradykinin at its receptor sites and is also invovlved in homeostatic mechanisms via the change in the number of binding sites. b) Sodium status per se influences the state of bradykinin receptors in uterine smooth muscle in the rat.

ACKNOWLEDGMENTS

This study was supported by the Grant-in-Aid for Cardiovascular

Disease (60-C-3) from the Ministry of Health and Welfare and for Scientific Research (61132005 and 62570376) from the Ministry of Education, Science and Culture, Japan. We also wish acknowledge the secretarial assistance of Miss J. Okazaki.

REFERENCES

1) Barabé, J., Drouin, J.N., Regoli, D., and Park, W.K., 1977, Receptors for bradykinin in intestinal and uterine smooth muscle. Canad. J. Physiol. Pharmacol., 55:1270.

2) Barraclough, M.A. and Mills, I.H., 1965, Effect of bradykinin on renal function. Clin. Sci., 28:69.

3) Coleman, T.G., Cowley, A.W., and Guyton, A.C., 1975, Angiotensin and the hemodynamics of chronic salt deprivation. Am. J. Physiol., 229:169.

4) De Freitas, F.M., Faraco, E.Z., and De Azavedo, D.F., 1964, General circulating alterations induced by intravenous infusion of synthetic bradykinin in man. Circulation, 29:66.

5) Elliot, D.F., Horton, E.W., and Lewis, G.P., 1960, Actions of pure bradykinin. J. Physiol. (Lond.), 153:473.

6) Erdös, E.G., 1975, Angiotensin converting enzyme. Circ. Res., 36:247.

7) Geller, R.G., Margolius, H.S., Pisano, J. J., and Keiser, H.R., 1972, Effects of mineralocorticoids, altered sodium intake and adrenalectomy on urinary kallikrein in rats. Circ. Res., 31:857.

8) Gill, J.R., Melmon, K.L., Gillespie, L., and Bartter, F.C., 1965, Bradykinin and renal function in normal man: effects of adrenergic blockade. Am. J. Physiol., 209:844.

9) Johnson, J.A., and Davis, J.O., 1973, Effects of a specific competitive antagonist of angiotensin II on arterial pressure and adrenal steroid secretion in dogs. Circ. Res, 32,33:159.

10) Johnston, C.I., Matthews, P.G., and Dax, E.M., 1976, Renin angiotensin and kallikrein kinin systems in sodium homeostasis and hypertension in rats. Clin. Sci. Mol. Med., 51:283s.

11) Kahn, C.R., 1976, Membrane receptors for hormones and neurotransmitters. J.Cell. Biol., 70:261.

12) Kilcoyne, M.M., and Cannon, P.J., 1971, Neural and humoral influences on intrarenal blood flow distribution during thoracic caval occlusion. Am. J. Physiol., 220:1231.

13) Lowry, O.H., Resenbrough, N.J., Farr, A.L., and Randall, R.J., 1951, Protein measurement with the Folin phenol reagent. J.Biol. Chem., 193:265.

14) Mashford, M.L., and Roberts, M.L., 1972, Determination of blood kinin levels by radioimmunoassay. Biochem. Pharmacol., 21:2727.

15) Merrill, J.E., Peach, M.J., and Gilmore, J.P., 1973, Angiotensin I conversion in the kidney and its modulation by sodium balance. Am. J. Physiol., 224:1104.

16) Odya, C.E., Goodfriend, T.L., and Pena, C., 1980, Bradykinin receptor-like binding studied with iodinated analogues. Biochem. Parmacol., 29:175.

17) Raff, M., 1976, Self-regulation of membrane receptors. Nature, 259:265.

18) Reid, W.D., and Laragh, J.H., 1965, Sodium and potassium intake, blood pressure and pressor response to angiotensin. Proc. Soc. Exp. Biol. Med., 120:26.

19) Reissmann, S., Pregelow, I., Liebmann, C., Steinmetzger, H., Jonkova, T., and Arold, H., 1977, Investigations on the mechanism of bradykinin action on smooth muscles. In: Physiology and Pharmacology of Smooth Muscle, edited by M. Papasova & E. Atanassova, Bulgarian Academy of Sciences, Sofia, pp. 208–217.

20) Scatchard, G., 1949, The attractions of proteins for small molecules and ions. <u>Ann.NY Acad. Sci.</u>, 51:660.

21) Song, C.S., and Bodansky, D., 1967, Subcellular localization and properties of 5'-nucleotidase in the rat liver. <u>J. Biol. Chem.</u>, 242:694.

22) Yasujima, M., Matthews, P.G., and Johnston, C.I., 1984a, Bradykinin receptors in rat uterine smooth muscle: studies using radiolabeled ligand binding. <u>Tohoku J. exp. Med.</u>, 144:107.

23) Yasujima, M., Matthews, P.G., and Johnston, C.I., 1984b, Hypotensive effect of captopril and decreased rat uterine bradykinin receptors. <u>Tohoku J. exp. Med.</u>, 144:119.

EFFECT OF THE SUBSTANCE(S) RELEASED *IN VITRO* BY THE INTERACTION OF *BOTHROPS JARARACA* (BJ) VENOM OR TRYPSIN AND BJ PLASMA ON BJ BLOOD PRESSURE AND UTERUS

B.C. Prezoto, E. Hiraichi, F.M.F. Abdalla, A.A.C. Lavras and
Z.P. Picarelli

Serviço de Farmacologia, Instituto Butantan, Caixa Postal 65
05504, São Paulo, SP, Brazil

INTRODUCTION

BJ venom or trypsin decrease blood pressure of various mammalian species, as a consequence of the release of histamine and bradykinin from their
plasmas[1,2]. However, experiments carried on pharmacological preparations
suitable to the assay of mammalian kinins have shown that BJ venom, trypsin
and some other kininogenases, active on mammalian plasmas, were unable to
release kinins from BJ plasma[3]. No evidence could be found that this plasma contained either factor XII, prekallikrein or kininogen; only kallikrein
inhibitors and kininases were there detected.

Birds, too, do not possess factor XII[4], but they do present all the
other components of the kallikrein-kinin system, a kinin beeing released
when glass beads having adsorbed mammalian or aligator factor XII were transferred to their plasma[5,6]. In addition, birds possess their own ornithokal-
likrein-kinin system that is inactive in mammals[5,6,7,8].

Therefore, it was thought worthwhile to investigate the occurrence of
a kallikrein-kinin system specific for snakes, not revealed on pharmacological preparations responsive to mammalian kinins.

A first approach has been made by studying the effects of BJ venom on
the own snake blood pressure. As it occurs in mammals, BJ venom or a kinin-
-releasing enzyme purified from this venom caused hypotension in the own
snake[9]. The effect was tachyphylactic, it was not affected by atropine, but
it turned shorter after treatment of the snake with promethazine associated
with cimetidine and longer after treatment with captopril. These facts indicate that BJ venom hypotensive effect in BJ could be due to the release
of, at least, two substances: a histamine-like and a kinin-like.

The aim of the present work was to study the action of the product(s)
eventually released, either by activating BJ plasma intrinsic kallikrein-
-kinin system or by incubating BJ plasma with trypsin or a fraction from BJ
plasma with a kinin-releasing enzyme purified from BJ venom, on the carotidean blood pressure and the isolated uterus of the own snake.

BJ snakes came from nature and, after a quarantine of at least 15 days, were kept under controlled environmental conditions: 12 hours light/12 hours darkness, 26°C and 65% air humidity.

BJ venom was a pool of crystallized venoms from the Instituto Butantan, presenting an LD50 = 2.4-2.8 μg g^{-1}, *ip*, in mice. From this pool, a fraction VF was obtained by 0.60-0.90 ammonium sulfate saturation and contained an almost three-fold purified kinin-releasing enzyme.

BJ plasma was collected from decapitated snakes in polyethylene tubes containing heparin (2-10 UI ml^{-1} blood) and immediately centrifuged at 8,000 r.p.m., 5-10°C, during 30 minutes. Plasma was used fresh or after storage at -20°C. A fraction GF from BJ plasma, containing globulins, was obtained by 0-0.50 ammonium sulfate saturation.

A purified kininase II (or angiotensin I - converting enzyme ACE) with activity corresponding to 83.3 U ml^{-1}, was obtained from BJ plasma by 0.60-0.80 ammonium sulfate saturation[10].

The following drugs were used throughout: sodium heparine (*Liquemine*, Roche Labs., Brazil); Captopril (*Capoten*, kindly supplied by Squibb Labs. Brazil); angiotensin I and bradykinin (synthetized at the Dept. of Biophysics, Escola Paulista de Medicina, Brazil); acethylcholine hydrochloride, bovine pancreas trypsin (2 x crystallized, type III) and chymotrypsin (3 x crystallized, type II), and glass beads (type I, 75-105 μ)(Sigma Chem. Co., USA); atropine and ammonium sulfate (E. Merck, Germany); ellagic acid (Fluka AG, Switzerland) and sodium pentobarbital (kindly supplied by Abbott Labs., Brazil).

The carotidean blood pressure of adult male rats (280-300 g) and of adult male or female BJ (150-600 g) anesthetized with sodium pentobarbital (90 mg kg^{-1} and 30 mg kg^{-1}, respectively), *ip*, was recorded on a smoked drum with the aid of a mercury manometer. Administration of drugs was made through a polyethylene catheter introduced in the iliac vein of the rats or in the renal vein of the snakes.

Isolated rat uterus was prepared according to Gaddum and Hameed[11]; isolated guinea-pig ileum, as described by Henriques et al.[12]. Pieces of BJ uterus were suspended in Ringer solution for snakes[13] and pigeon oviduct, in Ringer-Locke solution[14].

The release of active substance(s) was investigated either by activating the kallikrein-kinin system of BJ plasma with acid[15], ellagic acid[16] or glass beads[17] or by incubating either BJ plasma with trypsin[17] or 0.4 ml GF with 0.01 ml VF (75 μg protein) and 1.09 ml 0.2M tris-HCl buffer, pH 7.6, containing captopril (5 mg ml^{-1} GF)[18]. The released substance(s) was(ere) assayed on rat or BJ blood pressure, rat or BJ uterus, pigeon oviduct and guinea-pig ileum.

The released substance(s) was(ere) submitted to: a) dialysis against 0.9% NaCl, at 4°C, during 24 hours; b) heating in a boiling water bath, either at pH 10-11 for 5 and 10 minutes, or at pH 1.5-2.0, for 30 and 60 minutes[19]; c) incubation with trypsin or chymotrypsin[19]; d) incubation, at 37°C during 15 minutes, of 0.5 ml of the incubate of BJ plasma and trypsin with 0.3 ml of 25 fold diluted BJ plasma and 0.2 ml 0.05M tris-maleate buffer, pH 7.4, the reaction being interrupted with 1.5 ml boiling Ringer for snakes; e) incubation, at 37°C during 10 minutes, of 0.5 ml of the incubate of BJ plasma and trypsin with 0.15 ml ACE and 0.05 ml of the same buffer, the reaction being stopped with 0.8 ml boiling Ringer for snakes. Similar

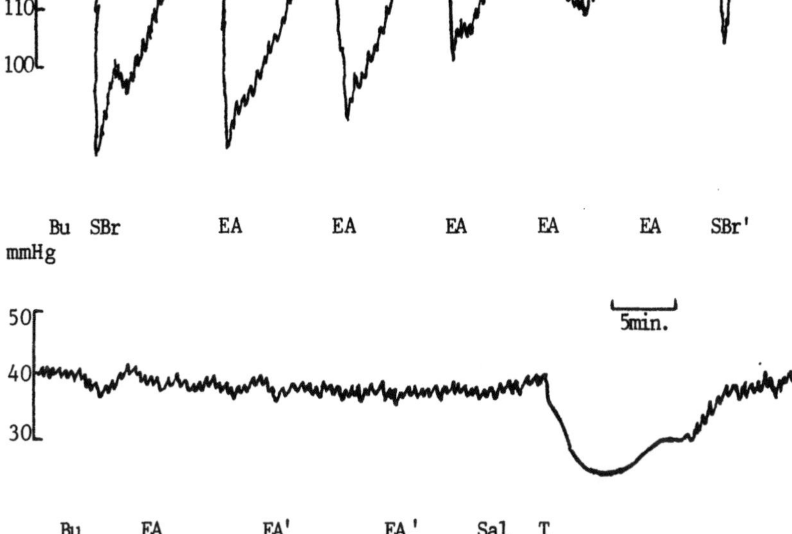

Fig. 1. Effect of ellagic acid (EA) upon rat (above) and *Bo-throps jararaca* (below) carotidean blood pressure. Bu_0.15M tris-HCl buffer, pH 7.35; SBr and SBr'_1.0 and 0.5 µg synthetic bradykinin; EA and EA'_0.22 and 2.2 mg kg^{-1} of ellagic acid in the same buffer; T_ 8 mg kg^{-1} of trypsin in 0.9% NaCl (Sal). The snake was previously treated with 0.5 mg kg^{-1} captopril.

experiments were carried on with 25 fold diluted BJ plasma and ACE, in the presence of captopril (170 µg ml^{-1} plasma or 13.5 µg ml^{-1} ACE).

RESULTS

As described in the literature for mammalian plasma[16], a tachyphylactic hypotensive effect was produced in rats by ellagic acid (0.22 mg kg^{-1}). However, doses of this drug as high as 2.2 mg kg^{-1} did not alter BJ blood pressure (Fig. 1).

Contrary to the decrease in kininogen content observed in mammalian plasma after contact with glass[17], and here confirmed with rat plasma, the kininogen content of BJ plasma rotated in a glass vessel containing glass beads (10 mg ml^{-1} plasma) was shown to be similar to that of BJ plasma kept in a polyethylene vessel.

However, a dialysable substance(s), contracting BJ uterus, was released by incubating BJ plasma at pH 4, 37°C[15], during 4 to 24 hours.

Fraction GF from BJ plasma incubated with VF, in the conditions used by Hamberg[18] for releasing kinins, released a substance(s) which caused hypotension in the own snake (Fig. 2). Similar result was obtained by incubating BJ plasma with trypsin, according to the method of Diniz and Carvalho[17] for the determination of kininogen. The effect of the substance(s) released by this last method, in BJ blood pressure, was potentiated by captopril (0.5 mg kg^{-1}). The substance(s) was(ere) inactive in rat blood pressure (Fig. 2).

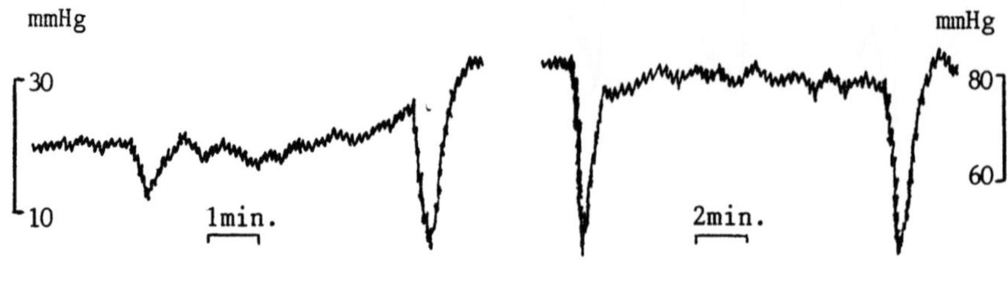

GF	VF	GF + VF	AI	BJpl	T	BJpl + T	SBr	BJpl + T	BJpl	T	SBr
.4 ml	.4 ml	.4 ml	140 ng	.3 ml	.3 ml	.3 ml	1 µg	.3 ml	.3 ml	.3 ml	1 µg

Fig. 2. Effect of the substance(s) released by incubating *Bothrops jararaca* (BJ) plasma (pl) with trypsin (T) or BJpl globulins (GF) with a kinin-releasing enzyme (VF) from BJ venom upon BJ or rat carotidean blood pressure. BJ_150 g; rat_300 g; AI_angiotensin I; SBr-synthetic bradykinin.
The snake was previously treated with 0.5 mg kg^{-1} captopril.

ACh	BJpl + T	BJpl	T	ACh	SBr	BJpl + T	SBr	BJpl	T	SBr	ACh	Ppl + T	Ppl	T	SBr	BJpl + T	ACh
500 ng	.02 ml	.02 ml	.02 ml	500 ng	15 ng	.28 ml	15 ng	.28 ml	.28 ml	15 ng	5 µg	.1 ml	.1 ml	.1 ml	2.5 µg	.2 ml	5 µg

Fig. 3. Effect of the substance(s) released by incubating *Bothrops jararaca* (BJ) plasma (pl) or pigeon plasma (Ppl) with trypsin (T) on BJ or rat uterus and pigeon oviduct. Bath volume 10 ml.
ACh_acetylcholine; SBr_synthetic bradykinin.

This(ese) released substance(s) contracted BJ uterus, a preparation
standardized with acetylcholine (20-400 ng ml^{-1}) in view of its low sensitivity to bradykinin. It (they) was(ere) inactive on rat uterus, showed low
activity on pigeon oviduct (Fig. 3) and, in high doses, caused a weak contraction of the guinea-pig ileum.

The released substance(s) was(ere) dialysable, thermostable in acid but
thermolabile in alkaline pH; it(they) was(ere) inactivated by chymotrypsin,
25 fold diluted BJ plasma or BJ plasma purified kininase II, but not by trypsin. The inactivation of the released substance(s) by diluted BJ plasma or
the purified kininase II was inhibited by a previous incubation of these two
materials with captopril.

DISCUSSION

As it occurs in mammals, BJ venom caused hypotension in the own snake,
an effect that could be due to the release of a histamine-like and a kinin-
-like substance from the snake plasma[9]. This hypothesis was reinforced by the
data showing that trypsin, an enzyme known to release kinins from plasma,
caused effects in BJ blood pressure similar to those produced by BJ venom[20].

The present data, showing no hypotensive effect after administration
of ellagic acid to BJ, confirm previous reports[3,21,22] of absence of factor
XII in snake plasma. They are further reinforced by the results of the experiments in which the intrinsic kallikrein-kinin system was tryed to be activated by contact of BJ plasma with glass. No alteration of the BJ plasma kininogen content was detected on such experiments.

However, treatment of BJ plasma, at pH 4 and 37°C, during 4 to 24 hours,
produced a dialysable substance which contracted BJ uterus.

From similar results obtained with avian plasma[5], it was concluded that,
in spite of having no factor XII, birds possess prekallikrein. Therefore,
the above results indicate that BJ plasma possess prekallikrein, in spite of
lacking factor XII. After BJ plasma activation by acid, the resulting active
enzyme, kallikrein, would cause the release of a kinin-like substance(s),
active only upon pharmacological preparations from the own snake. These results also indicate the presence of substrate(s) for the active enzyme in
BJ plasma.

These data are reinforced by the experiments showing that the release
of a substance(s) hypotensive in BJ and contracting BJ uterus may be elicited
by incubating BJ plasma or its globulins (GF) with trypsin or VF, respectively. As mammalian kinins, this(ese) substance(s) was(ere) dialysable, thermo-
stabile in acid but not in alkaline pH, inactivated by chymotrypsin and BJ
kininases but not by trypsin.

The released substance(s) was(ere) shown to be inactive on rat blood
pressure or uterus and weakly active on pigeon oviduct, this strongly suggesting that it (they) may be different from ornithokinin and from kinins
already described in various animal species.

Purification and characterization of the released substance(s) and extension of these studies to other snake species must be carried on, in
order to stablish if snakes had developed a specific kallikrein-kinin system.

REFERENCES

1 - M. Rocha e Silva, W.T. Beraldo and G. Rosenfeld. Bradykinin, a hypoten-

sive and smooth muscle stimulating factor released from plasma globulin by snake venom and trypsin. <u>Amer. J. Physiol</u>. 156: 261-273 (1949).

2 - T. Suzuki and S. Iwanaga. Snake venoms. <u>Handb. Exper. Pharmacol</u>. XXV: 193-212 (1970).

3 - A.A.C. Lavras, M. Fichman, E. Hiraichi, M.A. Boucault, T. Tobo, P. Schmuziger, L. Nahas and Z.P. Picarelli. Deficiency of kallikrein-kinin system and presence of potent kininase acitivity in plasma of *Bothrops jararaca* (Serpentes, Crotalinae). <u>Ciência e Cultura</u> 31: 168-174 (1979).

4 - O.D. Ratnoff. The biology and pathology of the initial stages of blood coagulation. <u>Progr. Hematol</u>. 15: 204-245 (1966).

5 - E.G. Erdös , J. Miwa and W.J. Graham. Studies on the evolution of plasma kinin: reptilian and avian blood. <u>Life Sci.</u> 6: 2433-2439 (1967).

6 - T. Seki, I. Miwa, T. Nakajima and E.G. Erdös. Plasma kallikrein-kinin system in non mammalian blood: evolutionary aspects. <u>Amer. J. Physiol</u>. 224: 1425-1430 (1973).

7 - E. Werle and J. Hürter. Über Ornitho-kallikrein. I-Mitteilung über kreislaufaktive Substanzen der Vögel. <u>Biochem. Z</u>. 285: 175-191 (1936).

8 - E. Werle and G. Leysath. Über das Moleculargewicht des Plasmakinins von Vögeln. <u>Z. Physiol. Chem</u>. 348: 352-353 (1967).

9 - B.C. Prezoto, Z.P. Picarelli and A.A.C. Lavras. Effect of *Bothrops jararaca* venom on *Bothrops jararaca* blood pressure. <u>Braz.J. Med. Biol</u>. <u>Res</u>. 19: 521A (1986).

10 - A.A.C. Lavras, M. Fichman, E. Hiraichi, T. Tobo and M.A. Boucault. The kininases of *Bothrops jararaca* plasma. <u>Acta physiol. latinoamer</u>. 30: 269-274 (1980).

11 - J.H. Gaddum and K.A. Hameed. Drugs which antagonize 5-hydroxytryptamine. <u>Brit. J. Pharmacol</u>. 9: 240-248 (1954)

12 - O.B. Henriques, Z.P. Picarelli and M.C.F. Oliveira. Partial purification of the plasma substrate for the bradykinin-releasing enzyme from the venom of *Bothrops jararaca*. <u>Biochem. Pharmacol</u>. 11: 707-714 (1962).

13 - K.W. Beyenback. Water-permeable and -impermeable barriers of snakes distal tubules. <u>Amer. J. Physiol.</u> 246: F-290-299 (1984).

14 - J. Crossley, G. Ferrando and H. Eiler. Distribution of adrenergic receptors in the domestic fowl oviduct. <u>Poult. Sci</u>. 59: 2331-2335 (1980).

15 - V. Eisen. Observations on intrinsic kinin-forming factors in human plasma: the effect of acid, acetone, chloroform, heat and euglobulin separation on kinin formation. <u>J. Physiol.</u> 166: 496-513 (1963).

16 - K.M. Gautvik and H. Rugstad. Kinin formation and kininogen depletion in rats after intravenous injection of ellagic acid. <u>Brit. J. Pharmacol</u>. 31: 390-400 (1967).

17 - C.R. Diniz and I.V. Carvalho. A micromethod for determination of bradykinin under several conditions. <u>Ann. N.Y. Acad. Sci.</u> 104: 77-89 (1963).

18 - U. Hamberg and M. Rocha e Silva. On the release of bradykinin by trypsin and snake venoms. <u>Arch. int. Pharmacodyn</u>. 110: 222-238 (1957).

19 - J.L. Prado, R. Monier, E.S. Prado and C. Fromageot. Pharmacologically active polypeptide formed from blood globulin by a cysteine-activated protease from *Clostridium histolyticum*. <u>Biochim. biophys. Acta</u> (Amst.) 22: 87-95 (1956).

20 - B.C. Prezoto and Z.P. Picarelli. Unpublished results.

21 - P. Fantl. A comparative study of blood coagulation in vertebrates. <u>Austral J. Exp. Biol</u>. 39: 403-412 (1961).

22 - L. Nahas, A.S. Kamiguti, F. Betti, I.S.S. Martins and M.I. Rodrigues. Blood coagulation mechanism in the snakes *Waglerophis merreemii* and *Bothrops jararaca*. <u>Comp. Biochem. Physiol</u>. 69A: 739-743 (1983).

Supported by FAPESP and CNPq.

LONG-TERM EFFECTS OF ALDOSTERONE ON KALLIKREIN AND SODIUM IN RATS

Minoru Yasujima, Keishi Abe*, Masaya Tanno, Masahiro
Kohzuki, Masayuki Kanazawa, Kazunori Yoshida, Ken Omata,
Yutaka Kasai, Makito Sato, Kazuhisa Takeuchi, Masao
Hiwatari and Kaoru Yoshinaga

The Second Department of Internal Medicine, and *Dept of
Clinical Biology and Hormonal Regulation, Tohoku University
School of Medicine, Sendai, Japan

INTRODUCTION

It is generally agreed that the renal kallikrein-kinin system is
involved in the regulation of electrolytes and water excretion (Levinsky
1979; Carretero and Scicli 1980). It is well established that kallikrein
in the urine arises within the kidney and its rate of excretion is a
function of renal kallikrein synthesis (Nustad et al. 1975; Levinsky
1979; Carretero and Scicli 1980) although it cannot be excluded that
glandular kallikrein from various origin is excreted in the urine.
Several previous studies have demonstrated that mineralocorticoids could
have a major regulatory influence on renal kallikrein and increase urinary
kallikrein excretion (Levinsky 1979; Carretero and Scicli 1980). That
mineralocorticoids enhance the activity of the renal kallikrein-kinin
system has been inferred from the finding of increased urinary kallikrein
excretion in patients with primary aldosteronism and in patients and
animals receiving sodium-retaining mineralocorticoids. Many efforts have
been addressed to solve complex interactions between sodium intake, sodium
excretion and kallikrein excretion, and aldosterone (Nasjletti and Colina-
Chourio 1975; Nasjletti and Malik 1981). However, the physiological
relevance of mineralocorticoids to the regulation of renal kallikrein-
kinin system has remained to be determined in detail. In addition, the
effect of mineralocorticoids on the excretion of inactive kallikrein has
not been studied whereas it has been recently reported that part of
kallikrein is present in an inactive form which can be activated by
trypsin in the kidney in rats (Yamada and Erdös 1982; Nishimura et al.
1983; Van Leeuwen et al. 1984) as well as in rabbits (Omata et al. 1982)
and human (Corthorn et al. 1979). It would therefore be needed to examine
the long-term effects of moderate dose of aldosterone that can produce
plasma levels similar to those observed in many clinical situations, on
renal kallikrein-kinin system.
In the present study, we assessed the effects of chronic aldosterone
administration on urinary excretion of total, active and inactive
kallikrein in conscious rats.

MATERIALS AND METHODS

Experiments were performed on 28 male Sprague-Dawley rats weighing
from 150 to 250 g. All rats were maintained in a humidity- and

temperature-controlled room, each rat being housed in a metabolic cage
during the study. The metabolic cage was deviced to prevent feces-urine
contact (Model Metabolism Cage ST type, Sugiyamagen Corporation, Tokyo).
The rats were fed on a regular diet (Oriental CMF, 0.24 % of sodium, 0.69
% of potassium, Oriental Yeast, Tokyo) and had free access to tap water.
Studies were performed after a 7 day period of acclimatization to the
housing, feeding and drinking conditions.

Fourteen rats were sodium-loaded and 14 were not. After subsequent 7
day period, each animal was anesthetized with ether, and an Alzet
osmotic minipump (Model 2002, Alza Corporation, Palo Alto, CA, USA),
filled with aldosterone solution or vehicle, was placed in the abdominal
cavity through a middle incision, which was then closed with autoclips.
D-Aldosterone (Wako Pure Chemical Industries Ltd., Osaka) was dissolved in
polyethylene glycol. Seven sodium-loaded and 7 unloaded rats were infused
with aldosterone at a rate of 50 µg/kg/day for up to 10 days. Another
group of rats, 7 sodium-loaded and 7 unloaded, received only polyethylene
glycol. Assuming that aldosterone did not degrade during the study, the
pumps dispensed fluid at the specified rate of approximately 0.5 µl/hr.
The infusion dose was set to induce and maintain a distinct elevation of
circulating levels of aldosterone, and not to affect the blood pressure,
essentially according to the schedule deviced by Garwitz and Jones (1982).
Daily systolic blood pressure was recorded in conscious rats by an
indirect tail cuff method (Pfeffer et al. 1971). The daily fluid intake,
urine volume, urinary sodium excretion and urinary total, active and
inactive kallikrein excretion were determined. Urine was collected into
vessels chilled at 4 °C and kept at -20 °C until the assay. Blood for the
measurements of plasma renin activity and plasma aldosterone
concentration was obtained by decapitation at the termination of each
experiment.

Active kallikrein in urine samples was measured by its kininogenase
activity (kinin releasing capability) using the method of Abe et al.
(1979). Kallikrein activity is expressed as an amount of kinin per ml of
urine generated by the incubation of urine samples with bovine serum low
molecular weight kininogen for 20 min. Total kallikrein was determined by
measuring the kininogenase activity in urine samples after inactive
kallikrein had been activated with trypsin, and inactive kallikrein was
calculated as the difference between total kallikrein (both active and
inactive kallikrein) and active kallikrein (Yasujima et al. 1986).
Urinary concentration of sodium and potassium were measured with a flame
photometer. Plasma renin activity was radioimmunologically determined by
a modification of Haber's method (Abe et al. 1971). Plasma aldosterone
concentration was radioimmunologically measured with a commercial kit
(Dainabot Pharmaceutical Company, Tokyo).

All results were expressed as mean ± S.E.M. Statistical analysis of
the data between groups was performed by two-way analysis of variance for
repeated measurements. Statistically significant differences on each day
were isolated by the unpaired t-test between groups. The significance of
the changes in some parameters between groups was also evaluated using the
unpaired t-test.

RESULTS

In sodium-unloaded rats, intraperitoneal infusion of aldosterone up
to 10 days did not induce any changes in body weight, systolic blood
pressure, urine volume and urinary sodium and potassium excretion when
compared with values in vehicle-infused rats, whereas the plasma
aldosterone concentration was increased from 19.2 ± 1.0 to 30.1 ± 5.2
ng/100 ml (p < 0.05) and the plasma renin activity was reduced from 5.5 ±
0.3 to 1.8 ± 0.4 ng/ml/hr (p < 0.01). Body weight gain in rats receiving
aldosterone for 10 days (51.9 ± 3.3 g) was greater than in vehicle-infused

controls (38.7 ± 4.6 g) ($p < 0.05$). In sodium-loaded rats, the systolic
blood pressure of the aldosterone group began to rise significantly on the
4th day and remained high up to the end of experiment, whereas that of the
vehicle group did not change (Table 1). Concomitantly, intraperitoneal
infusion of aldosterone induced a significant increase in urinary sodium
excretion on the 4th day in sodium-loaded rats, which sustained for up to
the end of experiment. Urinary potassium excretion is transiently
increased during chronic infusion of aldosterone in sodium-loaded rats,
whereas body weight and urine volume did not change.

Table 1. Chronic effects of aldosterone (ALDO) infusion in rats on sodium
loading with 1 % NaCl

Day	0	2	4	6	8	10
SBP (mmHg)						
Vehicle	120.3±2.8	115.7±4.2	118.6±2.3	117.0±4.5	126.7±1.5	121.0±2.0
ALDO	114.7±1.6	117.9±5.1	128.6±3.4*	138.9±3.5**	136.6±3.6*	135.4±2.2**
$U_{Na}V$ (mEq/day)						
Vehicle	4.71±0.29	4.48±0.17	4.32±0.11	4.56±0.36	4.48±0.40	4.30±0.14
ALDO	4.26±0.19	4.04±0.25	5.69±0.57*	6.40±0.34*	6.39±0.42*	5.62±0.49*
U_KV (mEq/day)						
Vehicle	2.59±0.14	2.34±0.11	2.25±0.04	2.48±0.17	2.31±0.17	2.40±0.11
ALDO	2.26±0.13	2.99±0.10*	2.98±0.20**	2.99±0.19	2.80±0.19	2.54±0.15

Results are means ± S.E.. ALDO, aldosterone; SBP, systolic blood
pressure; $U_{Na}V$, urinary sodium excretion, U_KV, urinary potassium
excretion. Analysis of variance for repeated measurements revealed a
significant change in SBP in ALDO-infused rats (n=7) ($p < 0.01$) compared
with control values in vehicle-infused rats (n=7). *$p < 0.05$ and **$p <$
0.01 compared with corresponding values in vehicle-infused rats.

With infusion of aldosterone, the plasma aldosterone concentration was
increased from 12.4 ± 1.0 to 20.7 ± 2.0 ng/100 ml ($p < 0.01$) in sodium-
loaded rats whereas the plasma renin activity was reduced from 3.1 ± 0.3
to 0.7 ± 0.2 ng/ml/hr ($p < 0.01$). Body weight gain in rats receiving
aldosterone for 10 days was not different from that in vehicle-infused
rats on sodium loading with 1 % NaCl.
 Fig. 1 shows the urinary excretion of total, active and inactive
kallikrein in aldosterone- or vehicle-infused rats on regular diets.
Compared with values in vehicle-infused rats, urinary total, active, and
inactive kallikrein excretion increased significantly in rats infused with
aldosterone, although the ratio of active to total kallikrein was not
changed. A significant increase in urinary kallikrein was seen on the 4th
day of implantation of minipumps and the maximal effect was observed on
the 8th and 10th day, although the effect of aldosterone on electrolytes
was evident on the 2nd day of aldosterone infusion.

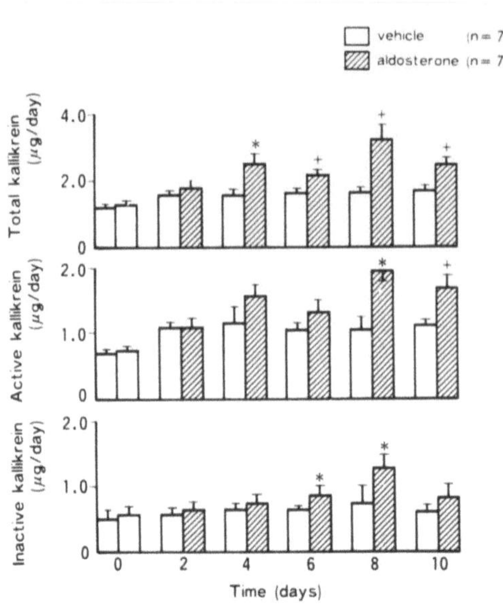

Fig. 1. Urinary kallikrein excretion in rats infused at a rate of 50 µg/kg/day of aldosterone (hatched column) and with vehicle alone (open column) on regular diets. Kallikrein activity is expressed as an amount of kinin per ml of urine generated by the incubation of urine samples with bovine serum low molecular weight kininogen for 20 min. Results are mean ± S.E.M. Analysis of variance for repeated measurements revealed a significant change in urinary total ($p < 0.01$), active ($p < 0.01$) and inactive ($p < 0.01$) kallikrein excretion in aldosterone-infused rats compared with control values in vehicle-infused rats. *$p < 0.05$ and **$p < 0.01$ compared with corresponding values in vehicle-infused rats.

However, in rats on sodium loading with 1% NaCl intraperitoneal infusion of aldosterone at a rate of 50 µg/kg/day did not induce any changes in the urinary excretion of total, active and inactive kallikrein compared with values in vehicle-infused rats.

DISCUSSION

In the present study, we demonstrated that chronic infusion of a subpressor dose of aldosterone induced significant increases in urinary excretion of total, active and inactive kallikrein without any changes in urine volume, and urinary sodium and potassium excretion. However, chronic infusion of the same dose of aldosterone failed to increase urinary excretion of total, active and inactive kallikrein in soidum-loaded rats, although it induced a slight elevation of systolic blood pressure and plasma concentration of aldosterone was significantly higher when compared with that in vehicle-infused rats.

To our knowledge, the effects of chronic aldosterone infusion on urinary total and inactive kallikrein excretion have not been reported in rats, but there have been a few reports that in experimental animals aldosterone induced a sustained increase in urinary active kallikrein excretion on different sodium diets (Fejes-Toth and Nary-Fejes-Toth 1984). In rats on ordinary intakes of sodium, exogenous aldosterone induced significant increases in urinary excretion of total, active and inactive kallikrein, but did not affect the ratio of active to total kallikrein. The concomitant changes in active and inactive enzyme values suggest that increased synthesis might have been responsible for the increase in active kallikrein excretion.

In our previous study (Yasujima et al. 1986), we reported that chronic sodium loading with 1 % NaCl for 6 days increased continuously urinary total, active and inactive kallikrein excretion and chronic infusion of angiotensin II also increased the urinary kallikrein. But the angiotensin II infusion did not induce any changes in urinary kallikrein excretion in sodium-loaded rats, suggesting that angiotensin II might stimulate the synthesis of kallikrein, at least, via the same mechanism as sodium loading does. In the present study, the failure of the increase in urinary excretion of total, active and inactive kallikrein after the chronic infusion of aldosterone was observed in sodium-loaded rats, which suggest again that aldosterone might stimulate the synthesis of kallikrein , at least, via the same mechanism as sodium loading does. Another possible explanation for the failure of aldosterone to increase urinary excretion of total, active and inactive kallikrein in sodium-loaded rats might be that kallikrein excretion had reached its upper limit after sodium loading for 7 days, since the baseline values for urinary kallikrein excretion in the rats on sodium loading are significantly greater than those obtained after aldosterone infusion in the rats on regular diets. However, it was not possible to determine the upper limit of the urinary kallikrein excretion response to aldosterone or sodium loading in the present study, since no assessment was made of the response of urinary kallikrein to graded doses of aldosterone or dietary sodium. In addition, the elevated blood pressure induced by sodium loading might affect the urinary kallikrein excretion response to aldosterone. However the exact mechanism also remains to be elucidated.

It is also interesting to note that until the 4th day of the infusion aldosterone did not induce any increase in urinary kallikrein excretion whereas aldosterone had already induced a change in the ratio of urinary sodium to potassium on the 2nd day of treatment. The animals on the ordinary intakes of sodium escaped from the effect of aldosterone by the 6th day of treatment, associated with the progressive increase in urinary kallikrein excretion, suggesting a involvement of renal kallikrein in the escape phenomenon as suggested previously (Marin-Grez et al. 1973; Zipser et al. 1978). In contrast, no significant changes were observed in urinary kallikrein excretion during the administration of aldosterone in sodium-loaded rats, whereas the escape phenomenon from the effect of aldosterone occurred more promptly in sodium-loaded rats than in rats on ordinary intakes of sodium, associated with the increase in systolic blood pressure. These results may represent that renal kallikrein-kinin system can counteract the sodium-retaining effect of aldosterone to some extents. In addition, the elevation of blood pressure could occur when the effect of aldosterone overcome the activity of renal kallikrein-kinin system, which may in turn contribute to the natriuresis. However, the exact mechanism underlying the escape phenomenon from the effect of aldosterone remains to be determined.

In summary, the present results suggest that aldosterone might stimulate the synthesis or release of kallikrein, at least partly, via the same pathway as sodium loading does. However no direct evidence was obtained from the present experiments on the possible physiological role of aldosterone in the regulation of urinary kallikrein excretion.

ACKNOWLEDGEMENTS

This study was supported by the Grant-in-Aid for Cardiovascular Disease (60-C-3) from the Ministry of Health and Welfare and for Scientific Research (61132005 and 62570376) from the Ministry of Education, Science and Culture, Japan. We also wish acknowledge the secretarial assistance of Miss J. Okazaki.

References

1. Abe, K., Otsuka, Y., Saito, T., Chin, B.S., Aoyagi, H., Miyazaki, S., Irokawa, N., Seino, M., and Yoshinaga, K., 1971, Measurement of plasma renin activity by angiotensin I radioimmunoassay: A modification of Haber's method. Jap. Circ. J., 29:1349.
2. Abe, K., Kato, H., Sakurai, Y., Ito, T., Saito, K., Haruyama, T., Otsuka, Y., and Yoshinaga, K., 1979, Estimation of urinary

kininogenase activity using bovine serum low molecular weight kininogen. In: <u>Kinin II</u>, edited by S. Fujii, H. Moria and T. Suzuki, Plenum Publishing Corporation, New York, pp.105-114.

3. Carretero, O.A., and Scicli A.G., 1980, The renal kallikrein-kinin system. <u>Am. J. Physiol.</u>, 238: F247.

4. Corthorn, J., Imanari, T., Yoshida, H., Kaizu, T., Pierce, J.V., and Pisano, J.J., 1979, Isolation of prokallikrein from human urine. <u>Adv. Exp. Med. Biol.</u>, 120B:575.

5. Fejes-Toth, G., and Naray-Fejes-Toth, A., 1984, Effect of aldosterone on urinary kallikrein and prostaglandin excretion in the rat. <u>J. Physiol.</u>, 354:79.

6. Garwitz, E.T., and Jones, A.W., 1982, Aldosterone infusion into the rat and dose-dependent changes in blood pressure and atrial ionic transport. <u>Hypertension</u>, 4:374.

7. Levinsky, N.G., 1979, The renal kallikrein-kinin system. <u>Circ. Res.</u>, 44:441.

8. Marin-Grez, M., Oza, N.B., and Carretero, O.A., 1973, The involvement of urinary kallikrein in the renal escape from the sodium retaining effect of mineralocorticoids. <u>Henry Ford Hosp. Med. J.</u>, 21:85.

9. Nasjletti, A., and Colina-Chourio, J., 1975, Interaction of mineralocorticoids, renal prostaglandins and the renal kallikrein-kinin system. <u>Fed. Proc.</u>, 35:189.

10. Nasjletti, A., and Malik, K.U., 1981, The renal kallikrein-kinin and prostaglandin systems interaction. <u>Ann. Rev. Physiol.</u>, 43:597.

11. Nishimura, K., Shimizu, H., and Kokubu, T., 1983, Existence of prokallikrein in the rat: Its biochemical properties compared to three active glandular kallikreins from the kidney, serum and urine of the rat. <u>Hypertension</u>, 5:205.

12. Nustad, K., Vaaje, K., and Pierce, J.V., 1975, Synthesis of kallikreins by rat kidney slices. <u>Br. J. Pharmacol.</u>, 53:229.

13. Omata, K., Carretero, O.A., Scicli, A.G., and Jackson, B.A., 1982, Localization of active and inactive kallikrein (kininogenase activity) in isolated tubular segments of the rabbit nephron. <u>Kidney Int.</u>, 22:602.

14. Pfeffer, J.M., Pfeffer, M.A., and Frohlich, E.D., 1971, Validity of an indirect tail-cuff method for determining systolic arterial pressure in unanesthetized normotensive and spontaneously hypertensive rats. <u>J. Lab. clin. Med.</u>, 78:957.

15. Van Leeuwen, B.H., Grinblat, S.M., and Johnston C.I., 1984, Release of active and inactive kallikrein from the isolated perfused rat kidney. <u>Clin. Sci.</u>, 66:201.

16. Yamada, K., and Erdös, E.G., 1982, Kallikrein and prekallikrein in the isolated basolateral membrane of rat kidney. <u>Kidney Int.</u>, 22:231.

17. Yasujima, M., Abe, K., Tanno, M., Kohzuki, M., Omata, K., Kasai, Y., Kudo, K., Tsunoda, K., Sato, M., Chiba, S., and Yoshinaga, K., 1986, Effects of sodium and angiotensin II on urinary active and inactive kallikrein in rats. <u>J. Hypertension</u>, 4:13.

18. Zipser, R.D., Zia, P., Stone, R.A., and Horton, R., 1978, The prostaglandin and kallikrein-kinin systems in mineralocorticoid escape. <u>J. Clin. Endocrinol. Metab.</u>, 47:996.

ACTIVATION OF INACTIVE KALLIKREIN IN THE RAT KIDNEY

DURING LOW SODIUM INTAKE

Masanori Takaoka, Motokazu Ohyama, Masatsugu Nakamura,
Mikio Nishii and Shiro Morimoto

Department of Pharmacology, Osaka University of
Pharmaceutical Sciences, 2-10-65 Kawai, Matsubara
Osaka 580, Japan

SUMMARY

A method was developed to measure the protease responsible for
activation of inactive kallikrein in the rat kidney. The renal protease
was evaluated by incubating the purified rat urinary inactive kallikrein
with the renal cortical extract in the presence of cysteine at pH 5.0.
The renal cortical extract produced a dose- and time-dependent activation
of the inactive kallikrein. Levels of the renal protease responsible for
activation of inactive kallikrein remained unchanged with dietary sodium
restriction. On the other hand, urinary excretion of total, active, and
inactive kallikrein increased significantly during low sodium intake,
with no change in the ratio of active to total kallikrein. These results
suggest that low sodium intake stimulates the biosynthesis of inactive
kallikrein but not the activation of this kallikrein precursor in the
kidney.

INTRODUCTION

Urinary kallikrein is a tissue kallikrein (EC 3.4.21.35) which seems
to be synthesized in the kidney. [1,2] The level of urinary kallikrein is
measured as an index of changes in renal kallikrein production, mainly
regulated by the synthesis and activation of the kallikrein precursor.
Although low sodium intake increases the urinary excretion of kallikrein [3-5] and the rate of renal kallikrein synthesis, [6] there are no
available data showing whether low sodium intake alters the activation
process of kallikrein precursor in the kidney.

The presence of an inactive form of kallikrein has been demonstrated
in human and rat urine. [7-9] The inactive kallikrein is probably a
precursor and of renal origin. [10] We also found that the rat kidney
cortex contains protease(s) responsible for activation of inactive
kallikrein and that the protease has properties compatible with those of
a thiol protease. [11] We developed a method to measure the protease
responsible for activation of inactive kallikrein in the kidney and
examined the level of the protease in rats fed a normal or low sodium
diet. The extent of urinary excretion of total, active, and inactive
kallikrein during low sodium intake is described herein.

MATERIALS AND METHODS

Animal experiments and sample preparation

Male Wistar rats weighing about 170 g were used. The experimental animals were maintained on a sodium-deficient diet (no sodium and 124 meq potassium/Kg diet) and distilled water, while the control animals were given a normal sodium diet (104 meq sodium and 124 meq potassium/Kg) and tap water. These diets were obtained from Clea Japan Inc. All rats were placed in individual stainless-steel metabolic cages and maintained on a normal or low sodium intake. After 2 weeks, 24 h urine sample was collected from each rat. The rats were fasted during the collection period but were allowed free access to drinking water. After urine collection, the rats were anesthetized with pentobarbital sodium (40 mg/Kg, i.p.) and a bilateral nephrectomy was done. The kidney cortex was removed from the medulla, minced and homogenized with 50 mM sodium acetate buffer (pH 5.0) containing 1 mM EDTA and 0.2% Triton X-100 (1:3 w/v) at 4° C for 90 sec. The homogenate was centrifuged at 105,000 x g at 4° C for 60 min. The resulting supernatant was dialyzed against 50 mM sodium acetate buffer (pH 5.0) containing 1 mM EDTA at 4° C for 18 h and was used as the renal cortical extract. An arterial blood sample was withdrawn through the aorta with a syringe and needle made wet with heparin and then immediately centrifuged at 3,000 rpm at 4° C for 15 min.

Analytical methods

Sodium and potassium concentrations in the plasma and urine were measured by flame photometry. The plasma aldosterone concentration was measured by radioimmunoassay using a commercial kit (Green Cross Co.). Protein concentration was determined according to Lowry et al. [12] using bovine serum albumin as the standard.

Total, active, and inactive kallikrein was measured in urine after removal of the non-kallikrein arginine esterases [13,14] by a modification of the method of McPartland et al. [13] The urine sample obtained from individual rats was first dialyzed against distilled water and then against two changes of 10 mM sodium phosphate buffer (pH 7.0) for 48 h at 4° C. 2-4 ml of the dialyzed urine was applied to a DEAE cellulose minicolumn (0.75 x 4.5 cm) equilibrated with the above buffer. Non-kallikrein arginine esterases were eluted from the column with 10 ml of the same buffer, followed by 6 ml of the same buffer containing 0.1 M NaCl. Active and inactive kallikreins were eluted with 6 ml of 0.5 M NaCl in the column-equilibrating buffer. The recoveries of partially purified urinary active and inactive kallikreins were 98.5 ± 2.1% and 97.9 ± 1.2%, respectively. The enzyme activity of active kallikrein was determined by the method of Morita et al. [15] using Pro-Phe-Arg-4-methylcoumaryl-7-amide as the substrate. Total kallikrein was detected by measuring the kallikrein activity after trypsin treatment. [7] Inactive kallikrein was calculated as the difference between total and active kallikrein. The kallikrein activity was expressed in terms of amidolytic units (AU) equivalent to μmoles of the substrate hydrolyzed per min during incubation at 37° C.

The protease responsible for activation of inactive kallikrein in the rat kidney was measured using a procedure modified from that described. [11] A mixture of 50 μl each of the renal cortical extract and 0.2 M sodium acetate buffer (pH 5.0) containing 40 mM cysteine was incubated at 37° C with 20 μl of purified urinary inactive kallikrein (120 mAU/ml). [7] The reaction was terminated by the addition of 80 μl of iodoacetate (2.5 mM) in 0.1 M Tris-HCl buffer (pH 8.0) containing 0.15 M NaCl. As the renal cortical extract contains a small amount of amidolytic activity, the active kallikrein generated from the purified inactive kallikrein by the renal cortical extract was assessed by subtracting the endogenous amidolytic activity in the renal cortical extract from the total amidolytic activity in the reaction mixture. The activation of purified inactive kallikrein by the renal cortical extract was expressed in terms of kallikrein amidolytic activity generated per min during incubation at 37° C. Using this method, we found that the activation of inactive kallikrein by the renal cortical extract (0.5 - 1.25 mg of protein/ml) increased linearly with the incubation time up to 30 min (Figure 1). Therefore, the incubation for activation of the inactive kallikrein was performed with the renal cortical extract at 1.0 mg protein/ml for 20 min.

All results are expressed as mean ± S.E. Statistical analysis was performed using Student's $\underline{t}$ test. Differences were considered significant at $\underline{p} < 0.05$.

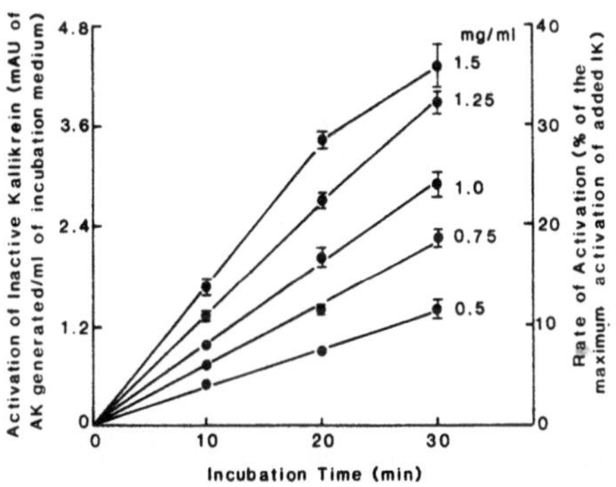

Figure 1

Activation of inactive kallikrein by the renal cortical extract. Purified inactive kallikrein was incubated with the renal cortical extract (0.5–1.5 mg protein/ml) prepared from rats on normal sodium intake, as described in METHODS. The incubation medium was then assayed for kallikrein activity. Points and bars represent the mean ± S.E. of five rats.

RESULTS

After a 2 week experimental period, no significant difference could be detected in average body weight or kidney weight between the control and experimental rats. Although low sodium intake significantly increased plasma aldosterone concentrations and decreased urinary sodium excretions, it had no effect on plasma sodium or potassium levels, urine volume and urinary potassium excretion (Table I).

Table I   Effect of low sodium intake on PAC, P_{Na}, P_K, UV, $U_{Na}V$, and U_KV

	PAC	P_{Na}	P_K	UV	$U_{Na}V$	U_KV
	(ng/ml)	(meq/1)		(ml/day/100 g BW)	(meq/day/100 g BW)	
Control	0.70 ±0.03	144 ±1.1	4.02 ±0.1	9.52 ±1.5	0.29 ±0.03	0.46 ±0.02
Low Na	3.25*** ±0.28	140 ±2.0	3.77 ±0.1	9.82 ±1.4	0.02*** ±0.002	0.50 ±0.03

Each value represents the mean ± S.E. of six rats. Abbreviations: PAC, plasma aldosterone concentration; P_{Na}, plasma sodium concentration; P_K, plasma potassium concentration; UV, urinary volume; $U_{Na}V$, urinary sodium excretion; U_KV, urinary potassium excretion. *** $\underline{p} < 0.001$ compared with the values in the control.

Urinary excretion of total, active, and inactive kallikrein was respectively about 2.5-fold higher in rats maintained on low sodium intake than normal sodium intake (Figure 2). However, there was no significant change in the ratio of active to total kallikrein between the two groups (normal sodium intake, 70.0 ± 1.8%; low sodium intake, 71.9 ± 2.0%). We next examined the level of the protease responsible for activation of inactive kallikrein in kidney of rats fed normal or low sodium diet (Table II). No significant change in the activation rate of inactive kallikrein by the renal cortical extract was observed between the control and low sodium groups.

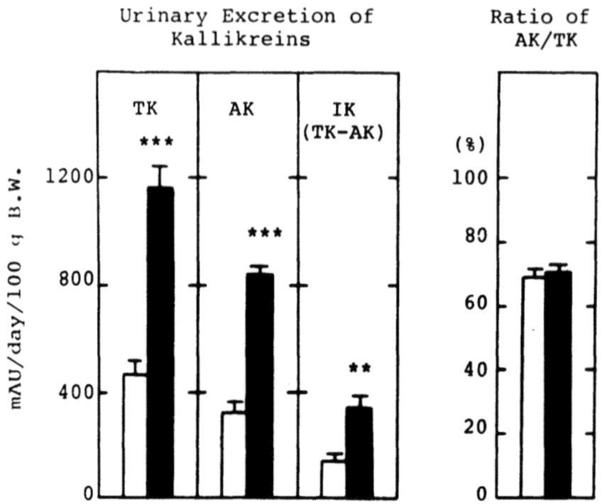

Figure 2   Total, active, and inactive kallikrein in the urine of rats on low sodium intake. Abbreviations: TK, total kallikrein; AK, active kallikrein; IK, inactive kallikrein. ☐ , control; ▓ ,low sodium. Columns and bars represent the mean ± S.E. of six rats. ** p<0.01; *** p<0.001 compared with the values in the control.

Table II   Activation of inactive kallikrein by the renal cortical extract from rats on low sodium intake

	Protein	Activation of inactive kallikrein
	(mg/ml of extract)	(mAU of AK generated/min/ mg protein of extract)
Control	6.38 ± 0.14	0.45 ± 0.02
Low Na	6.51 ± 0.16	0.42 ± 0.04

Each value represents the mean ± S.E. of six rats. The renal extract (1.0 mg protein/ml) was incubated with purified urinary inactive kallikrein (120 mAU/ml), as described in METHODS.

DISCUSSION

It is generally accepted that low sodium intake stimulates the renin-angiotensin-aldosterone system, [16] and the increased aldosterone secretion is associated with an increase in urinary kallikrein excretion.[4,5] An increase in the relative rate of kallikrein synthesis in the rat kidney by dietary sodium restriction was also observed by Miller et al., [6] in in vivo studies using [^{35}S] methionine labelling. Our present study showed that low sodium intake resulted in an increased urinary excretion of total, active, and inactive kallikrein, and these changes were accompanied by a significant increase in plasma aldosterone concentrations. All these findings taken together suggest that the increased endogenous aldosterone by low sodium intake stimulates the production of both active and inactive kallikrein in the kidney, with resulting increases in the urinary excretion of the two kallikreins.

We calculated the ratio of active to total kallikrein for each urine sample and found that about 70% of the total urinary kallikrein in rats on a normal sodium intake is present in the active form. The value is similar to findings obtained in rat urine by other investigators [17,18] and is relatively high, compared with data on human and rabbit urine (about 40%). [19-21]. A species difference may exist in the activation of inactive kallikrein in the kidney, but the question requires further investigation. The present study also showed no significant change in the ratio of active to total kallikrein in the urine of rats on a low sodium intake, as was noted in the rabbit urine. [21] Therefore, the activation rate of inactive kallikrein in the kidney is not altered by dietary sodium restriction. For confirmation, we examined the level of the protease responsible for activation of inactive kallikrein in the kidney of rats on low sodium intake, in comparison with those on a normal intake.

Our previous study [11] showed that an extract from the rat kidney cortex activated purified inactive kallikrein at the optimum pH of 5.0, and the activation was suppressed by the renal cortical extract pre-treated with thiol protease inhibitors. SH-containing compounds such as cysteine or dithiothreitol stimulated activation by the renal cortical extract (not shown). On the basis of these observations, an assay procedure was developed to measure quantitatively the protease responsible for activation of inactive kallikrein in the rat kidney. Using this assay, we found that the renal protease is not altered by dietary sodium restriction. Therefore, low sodium intake has no apparent effect on the activation process of inactive kallikrein in the rat kidney.

In conclusion, the present study suggests that an increase in endogenous aldosterone seen with a low sodium intake stimulates the production of renal kallikrein, presumably at the process of biosynthesis but not by activation of the kallikrein precursor.

ACKNOWLEDGEMENT

This study was supported in part by a grant-in-Aid for Scientific Research from the Ministry of Education, Science and Culture of Japan.

REFERENCES

1. K. Nustad, The relationship between kidney and urinary kininogenase, Brit. J. Pharmacol. 39:73 (1970)
2. K. Nustad, K. Vaaje, and J. V. Pierce, Synthesis of kallikrein by rat kidney slices, Brit. J. Pharmacol. 53:229 (1975)
3. R. G. Geller, H. S. Margolius, J. J. Pisano, and H. R. Keiser, Effect of mineralocorticoids, altered sodium intake and adrenal-ectomy on urinary kallikrein in rats, Circ. Rec. 31:857 (1972)
4. H. S. Margolius, D. Horwitz, R. G. Geller, R. W. Alexander, J. R. Gill Jr, J. J. Pisano, H. R. Keiser, Urinary kallikrein excretion

in normal man: relationship to sodium intake and sodium retaining steroids, Circ. Res. 35:812 (1974)

5. A. Mimran, G. Baudin, D. Casellas, and D. Soulas, Urinary kallikrein and changes in endogenous aldosterone in the rat, Eur. J. Clin. Invest. 7:497 (1977)

6. H. Miller, J. Chao and H. S. Margolius, Tissue kallikrein synthesis and its modification by testosterone or low dietary sodium, Biochem. J. 218:37 (1984)

7. M. Takaoka, H. Okamura, T. Iwamoto, C. Ikemoto, Y. Mimura, and S. Morimoto, Purification to apparent homogeneity of inactive kallikrein from rat urine, Biochem. Biophys. Res. Commun. 122:1282 (1984)

8. Y. Takada, R.A. Skidgel, and E. G. Erdos, Purification of human urinary prokallikrein: Identification of the site of activation by the metalloproteinase thermolysin, Biochem. J. 232:851 (1985)

9. A. Irie, S. Takahashi, Y. Katayama, K. Ito, and Y. Miyake, Human urinary prokallikrein: Rapid purification and model activation by trypsin, Biochemistry Int. 13:375 (1986)

10. H. Okamura, M. Takaoka, T. Iwamoto, and S. Morimoto, Renal inactive kallikrein as the possible origin of urinary inactive kallikrein in the rat, J. Pharm. Dyn. 8:175 (1985)

11. M. Takaoka, H. Okamura, Y. Kuribayashi, H. Matsuoka, and S. Morimoto, Activation of urinary inactive kallikrein by an extract from the rat kidney cortex, Life Sci. 37:1015 (1985)

12. O. H. Lowry, N. J. Rosebrough, A. L. Farr, and R. J. Randall, Protein measurement with the Folin phenol reagent, J. Biol. Chem. 193:265 (1951)

13. R. P. McPartland, D. L. Sustarsic, and J. P. Rapp, Evidence for an androgen-dependent urinary arginine esterase in the rat: Separation from other urinary arginine esterases including kallikrein, Endocrinology 108:1634 (1981)

14. J. Chao, Purification and characterization of rat urinary esterase A; a plasminogen activator, J. Biol. Chem. 254:7287 (1983)

15. T. Morita, H. Kato, S. Iwanaga, K. Takada, T. Kimura, and S. Sakakibara, New fluorogenic substrates for α-thrombin, factor Xa, kallikrein, and urokinase, J. Biochem. 82:1495 (1977)

16. N. R. Levens, M. J. Peach, and R. M. Carey, Role of the intrarenal renin-angiotensin system in the control of renal function, Circ. Res. 48:157 (1981)

17. M. S. Weinberg, N. B. Oza, and N. G. Levinsky, Components of the kallikrein-kinin system in rat urine, Biochem. Pharmacol. 33:1779 (1984)

18. R. Garcia, G. Thibault, and J. Genest, Lymphatic, renal, and urinary kallikreins in the rat, Am. J. Physiol. 247:R29 (1984)

19. J. J. Pisano, J. Corthorn, K. Yates, and J. V. Pierce, The kallikrein-kinin system in the kidney, Contr. Nephrol. 12:116 (1978)

20. N. B. Oza, W. Lieberthal, D. B. Bernard, and N. G. Levinsky, Antibody that recognizes total human urinary kallikrein: Radioimmunological determination of inactive kallikrein, J. Immunol. 126:2361 (1981)

21. K. Omata, O. A. Carretero, S. Itoh, and A. G. Scicli, Active and inactive kallikrein in rabbit connecting tubules and urine during low and normal sodium intake, Kidney Int. 24:714 (1983)

URINARY KALLIKREIN EXCRETION IN NEUROGENIC HYPERTENSION IN THE DOGS :

POSSIBLE RELATIONSHIP BETWEEN KALLIKREIN EXCRETION AND CATECHOLAMINES

Philippe Valet, Jean-Loup Bascands*, Christiane Pécher*,
Jean-Pierre Moatti**, Jean-Louis Montastruc and Jean-Pierre
Girolami*

Laboratoire de Pharmacologie Medicale et Clinique, *INSERM U
133, **Laboratoire de Biochimie, Faculté de Médecine
31062 Toulouse, France

INTRODUCTION

The contribution of the vasodepressive systems in the pathogenesis of
hypertension remains unclear. One of the earliest model for experimental
hypertension was provided by denervation of arterial baroreceptors (1).
Using this surgical procedure several investigators induced significant
hypertension in dogs (2-3), rabbits (4). A transient hyperadrenergic activity has been suggested as a possible mechanism of this hypertensive model.
Whether the development of this model of hypertension induced renal disturbances or not is poorly documented. Renal excretory functions are markedly
modified during hypertensive diseases. With respect to the renal kallikrein kinin system, it is now well admitted that the urinary kallikrein
excretion is generaly decreased in hypertensive states either in men or in
animals. One exception is mineralocorticoid-dependent hypertension where
urinary kallikrein is frequently increased or in some cases normal (5-6).
Thus, in this study, we investigated urinary kallikrein excretion in relation with the development of neurogenic hypertension in the dog. The main
objectives of this protocol were :

1- to study the long term pattern of urinary kallikrein excretion over 8
months in a neurogenic hypertensive model.
2- to assess some possible renal targets during the development of this
experimental model.
3- to investigate the possible relationships between the urinary excretion
of kallikrein, the level of catecholamines and urinary sodium excretion.

MATERIALS and METHODS

*SINOARTIC DENERVATION (SAD)

Six dogs of either sex weighing 12-25 kg were studied. SAD involved
two successive surgical procedures. This time interval was always respec-
ted since previous experiments showed that one time bilateral surgery was
associated with a very high rate of mortality.

*BLOOD PRESSURE AND HEART RATE MEASUREMENT IN CONSCIOUS DOGS

Several days before any experiment, dogs were trained to stand still for 3 to 4 hours and direct blood pressure was recorded. Blood samples were obtained at the same hour in dogs deprived of food for 12 hours. The animals were acclimatized for 3 days in individual cages and the urine volume of the 2 following days was measured. The present experiments were repeated 2,4,16 and 32 weeks after SAD.

* CATECHOLAMINE ASSAYS

Norepinephrine and epinephrine were assayed by high pressure liquid chromatography using electrochemical detection. In these conditions our detection limit was 0.3 nM.

* KALLIKREIN MEASUREMENT

Urinary kallikrein activities were estimated either by the amidolytic activity (nMoles S2266) or by the kininogenase activity (ng bradykinin).

* BIOCHEMICAL ASSAYS

Plasma renin activity and plasma aldosterone concentration were measured with commercial radio-immunoassays kits. Urinary creatinine was assayed with a colorimetric method and urinary sodium concentration with a flame photometer.

* STATISTICAL ANALYSIS

All data are mean ± s.e.m. Statistical analysis were performed using analysis of variance and Student's t test for paired comparison. Each animal served as its own control. Correlation tests were made using Fisher and Yates table.

RESULTS

The cardiovascular parameters were always measured after a resting period of 60 min in conscious dogs. During the control period (before SAD) mean values of systolic and diastolic blood pressure were respectively 157 ± 6.5 and 68.3 ± 3.2 mmHg. Two weeks after SAD, systolic and diastolic values were respectively over 205 mmHg and 112 mmHg and then remained stable until the 32th week (Figure 1).

We show on Figure 2 an increase in plasma catecholamines level during the first month reaching the maximal values : 3.53 ± 0.7 nM for Epinephrine and 6.04 ± 1.1 nM for Norepinephrine. Then we noticed a progressive decrease not significantly different from controls values.

After a significant decrease (58%) in PRA during the first two weeks; the PRA values slowly returned to control values at the 16th week. Plasma aldosterone concentration exhibited at the 2nd week a significant decrease (43%) observed until the end of the study (Figure 3).

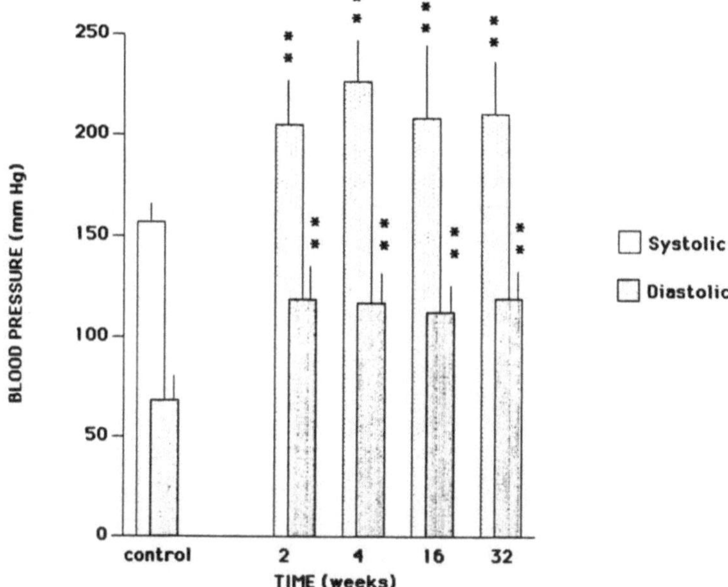

FIGURE 1 . Time course of systolic and diastolic blood pressure (mmHg) before and after sinoaortic denervation in conscious dogs measured at 2, 4,16 and 32 weeks. n = 7 dogs. ** p < 0.01.

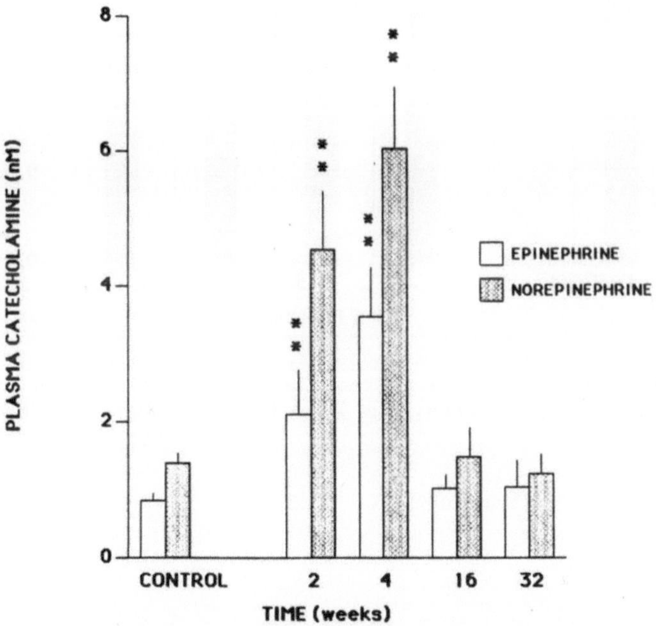

FIGURE 2 . Time course of plasma catecholamines (epinephrine and norepine-phrine) (nM) before and after sinoaortic denervation in conscious dogs measured at 2,4,16 and 32 weeks. n = 7 dogs. * p < 0.05, ** p < 0.01.

On Figure 4, amidolytic and kininogenase activity show the same biphasic evolution. First, two weeks after SAD urinary kallikrein exhibited a significant increase (amidolytic activity : 330.1 $\pm$ 86.3 vs control 158 $\pm$ 31.3 nmoles/min/mg creat, $p < 0.01$ and kininogenase activity : 5.16 $\pm$ 2.62 vs control 0.75 $\pm$ 0.19 ug BK/min/mg creat $p < 0.01$). This increase in kallikrein excretion at week 2 was highly correlated with the norepinephrine level ($r = 0.877$, $p < 0.01$). Then kallikrein excretion decreased progressively reaching the minimal value at the 32th week (amidolytic activity : 22.4 $\pm$ 10 nmoles/min/mg creat, $p < 0.01$ and kininogenase activity: 0.11 $\pm$ 0.03 ug BK/min/mg creat $p < 0.01$).

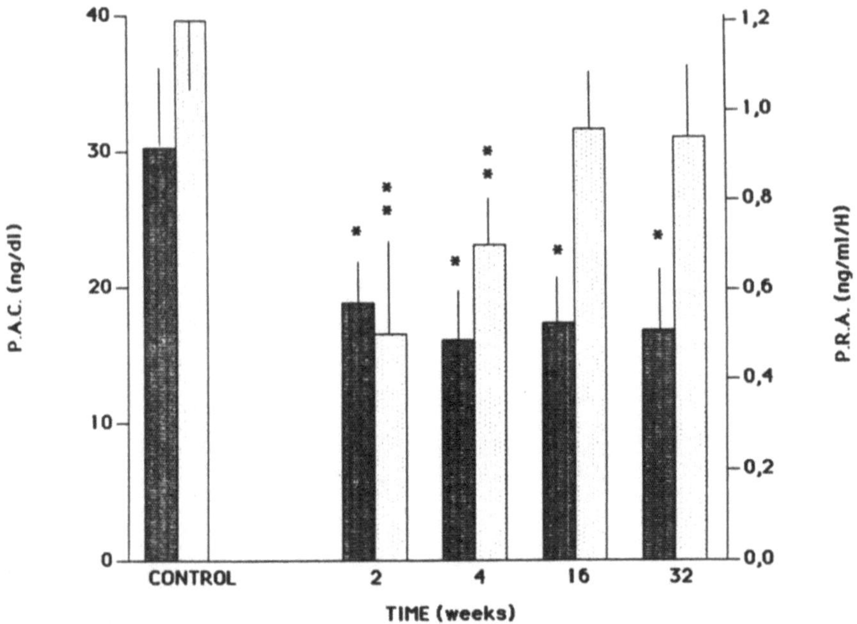

FIGURE 3 . Time course of plasma aldosterone (ng/dl) and plasma renin activity (ng/ml/h) before and after sinoaortic denervation in conscious dogs measured at 2,4,16 and 32 weeks. n = 7 dogs. * p < 0.05, ** p < 0.01.

- In our study urinary sodium excretion exhibited a permanent increase from the 4th week up to the 32th week compared to control values (22.7 $\pm$ 5.5 vs control 3.2 $\pm$ 0.5 mEq/24/kg $p < 0.001$). From week 4 to week 32, the increase in urinary sodium excretion was inversely correlated with the decrease in UKE ($r = 0.615$, $n = 21$ $p < 0.01$).

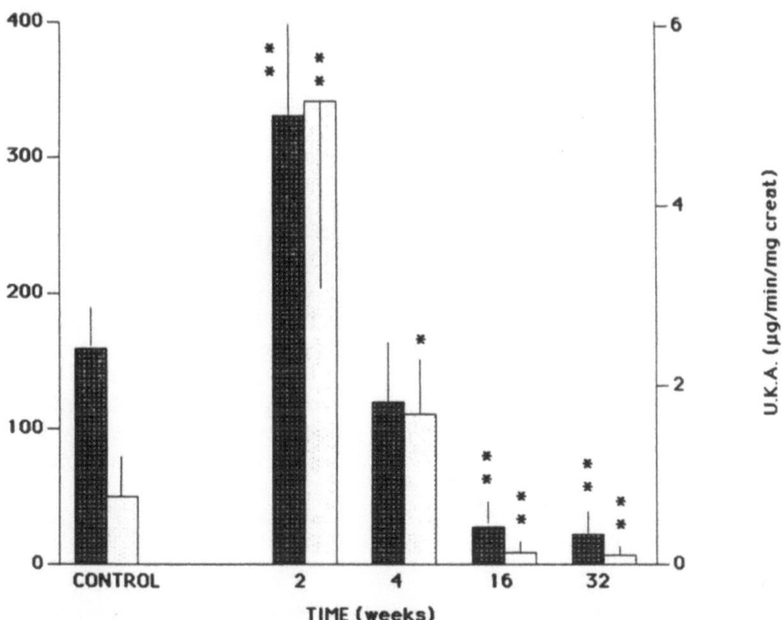

FIGURE 4 . Time course of urinary kallikrein (amidolytic nmole/min/mg creat)
and kininogenasic activities (ug/min/mg creat) before and after sinoaortic
denervation in conscious dogs measured at 2,4,16 and 32 weeks. n = 7 dogs.
* p < 0.05, ** p < 0.01.

DISCUSSION

Our study investigates for the first time the long term urinary excretion of kallikrein in sinoaortic denervated hypertensive dogs.

Under our experimental conditions, SAD dogs exhibited a significant
and permanent rise in blood pressure recorded at regular time interval.
Urinary kallikrein excretion exhibited a biphasic pattern : the initial
increase observed two and four weeks after bilateral denervation was followed by a significant decrease below base line values after the fourth week
which remained at this lower level throughout the period of study.

The four weeks following bilateral denervation are mainly characterized by an increase in sympathetic tone as attested by high plasma catecholamine levels. Therefore the transient increase in urinary kallikrein
excretion may be linked to this sympathetic hyperactivity. This hypothesis
is supported by a positive significant correlation between the increase in
urinary kallikrein excretion and the elevation in plasma catecholamines.
This correlation was not observed during the control period and disappeared in the last periods of study i.e. after the 4th week. Although the relationships between the sympathetic system and kallikrein are poorly explored, our hypothesis is consistent with previous data : relationships between urinary kallikrein and plasma catecholamines have been already described in patients suffering from pheochromocytoma which exhibited high levels
of urinary kallikrein (7). Sympathetic nerve stimulation of the salivary
submandibular gland resulted in a significant decrease in kallikrein tissue
content in rat (8).

It is well known that urinary kallikrein is synthetized by the kidney
(9) and in this respect, variations in urinary kallikrein may reflect dys-
functions in the tissue. This observation is of interest because, to our
knowledge, no renal effects have been so far reported in this model of hypertension. In addition, the observed natriuresis supports also the possibility of renal dysfunction in this hypertensive model.

Finally, the original data of this study was to describe in the same
animal a transient increase followed by a decrease in urinary kallikrein
excretion during the time course of hypertension. The transient increase
in kallikrein excretion could be related to an hyperadrenergic activity.
The subsequent decrease observed in urinary kallikrein excretion also suggests possible renal dysfunction in this model and is consistent with the
alterations of renal kallikrein system observed in other models of hypertension. Such a biphasic pattern during the establishment of hypertension
in neurogenic hypertensive dogs suggests that changes in urinary kallikrein
excretion are rather a secondary effect of hypertension than a physiopatho-
genic factor.

REFERENCES

1- E. Koch, H. Mies, Chronischer arterieller Hockdruck durch experimentel-
   le Dauerausschaltung der Bluutdruckzzuglerr. _Krankleitsforsch._
   7 : 241 (1929).
2- C.M. Ferrario, J.W. Mc Cubbin, I.H. Page, Hemodynamic characteristics
   of chronic experimental neurogenic hypertension in unanesthetized
   dogs. _Circ. Res._ 24 : 911 (1969).
3- C.S. Ito, A.M., Hypertension following arterial baroreceptor denervation in unanesthetized dog. _Circ. Res._ 48 : 576 (1981).
4- N. Alexander, V. De Quattro, Regional and systemic hemodynamic patterns
   in rabbits with neurogenic hypertension. _Circ. Res._ 35 : 636 (1974).
5- A.G. Scicli, O.A. Carretero, Renal kallikrein-kinin system. _Kidney Int._
   29 : 120 (1986).
6- H.S. Margolius, The kallikrein-kinin system and the kidney. _Ann. Rev._
   Physiol. 46 : 309 (1984).
7- H.S. Margolius, R.G. Geller, W. de Jong, J.J. Pisano, A. Sjoerdsma,Uri-
   nary kallikrein excretion in hypertension. _Circ. Res. Suppl.II_ : 125
   (1972).
8- T.B. Orstavik, K.M. Gautvik, Regulation of salivary kallikrein secretion in the rat submandibular gland. _Acta Physiol. Scand._ 100 : 33
   (1977).
9- K. Nustad, V. Kirstein, J.V. Pierce, Synthesis of kallikreins by rat
   kidney slices. _Br. J. Pharmacol._ 53 : 229 (1975).

GLANDULAR KALLIKREIN, RENIN AND ANGIOTENSIN CONVERTING ENZYME OF DIABETIC

AND HYPERTENSIVE RATS

Hiroshi Handa, Shoki Sakurama, Shoichi Nakagawa,
Taro Yasukouchi,* Wataru Sakamoto** and Hiroshi Izumi***

The Second Department of Internal Medicine, School of
Medicine, **Department of Biochemistry, School of Dentistry
Hokkaido University, Sapporo
*Department of Internal Medicine, School of Dentistry
Higashi Nippon Gakuen University, Tobetsu
***Department of Physiology, School of Dentistry, Tohoku
University, Sendai, Japan

ABSTRACT

To clarify the relationship between kallikrein-kinin and renin-
angiotensin systems, glandular kallikrein, renin and angiotensin converting
enzyme in the submandibular gland, the kidney and plasma were investigated
in streptozotocin diabetic and spontaneously hypertensive rats.

Kallikrein content in the submandibular gland, the kidney and plasma of
diabetic rats was found to be decreased compared with nondiabetic controls.
Renin activity in diabetic rats was also reduced in the submandibular gland,
but the activity showed no significant changes in the kidney and plasma.
The activity of angiotensin converting enzyme (ACE) in plasma significantly
increased in diabetic rats.

On the other hand, kallikrein content in hypertensive rats was
depressed in the kidney, while the content was unchanged in the
submandibular gland and plasma. Renin activity in hypertensive rats was
found to be higher than that of normotensive rats in the submandibular
gland, but the activity showed no remarkable changes in the kidney and
plasma. ACE activity in plasma markedly decreased in hypertensive rats in
contrast to diabetic rats.

In hypertensive-diabetic rats, changes in the levels of these
enzymes in tested materials were similar to those of diabetic rats.

From these results it is reasonable to assume that (1) reduced
kallikrein generation and elevated ACE activity may induce impaired kinin
formation and contribute to the development of diabetes mellitus apart from
the presence of hypertension and (2) low kallikrein content in the kidney
could cause hypertension.

INTRODUCTION

Glandular kallikrein is thought to be involved in the regulation of
blood pressure and electrolyte balance, and the pathogenesis of
hypertension.[1] Decrease in the urinary excretion of kallikrein has been
reported in experimental and clinical hypertension.[2,3] In addition,

glandular kallikrein is reported to be utilized during glucose uptake in peripheral tissues.[4] On the other hand, renin is also one of the major blood pressure-regulating factors as well as kallikrein and is involved in the etiology of hypertension.[5]

Angiotensin converting enzyme (ACE) is known to convert angiotensin I, which is liberated from angiotensinogen by renin, to vasoactive peptide angiotensin II and to inactivate kinin released from kininogen by kallikrein.[6] Therefore, it is apparent that there is a close interaction between the kallikrein-kinin system and the renin-angiotensin system. However, not much has been known about the changes in kallikrein content, renin activity and ACE activity in tissues and plasma in diabetes mellitus and hypertension.

In the present study, we measured the contents of kallikrein, renin and angiotensin converting enzyme in the submandibular gland, kidney and plasma in diabetic and hypertensive rats and discussed the possibility of the pathogenic influence of kallikrein, renin and ACE in diabetes mellitus and hypertension.

MATERIAL AND METHODS

Male Wistar strain rats, spontaneously hypertensive rat strain and Wistar-Kyoto strain (7-8 weeks old and weighing 150-200 g) were used in these experiments. Diabetes was induced by injecting streptozotocin intravenously (70 mg/kg). 28 days after the injection, the blood of treated and control rats were obtained by cardiac puncture with 1/9 volume of 3.8% (w/v) trisodium citrate. After blood sampling, the kidney and the submandibular gland were removed from each animal, washed in saline and frozen at -30°C to be stored for later use. Plasma glucose concentration was determined by the glucose oxidase method[7] and systolic blood pressure was measured by the tail-cuff method. Protein was determined by the method of Lowry et al.[8] The homogenates of the submandibular gland and the kidney were prepared in 10 mmol/l sodium phosphate buffer (pH 6.0), using a Polytron homogenizer. Homogenates were centrifuged at 4°C for 20 min at 10,000 rpm. The supernatant was used for the measurement of kallikrein and renin.

The content of glandular kallikrein in the submandibular gland and the kidney were measured by enzyme immunoassay as described previously.[9]

Kallikrein concentration in plasma was determined by radioimmunoassay as follows: the reaction mixture contained 0.1 ml of ^{125}I-kallikrein, 0.1 ml of the sample, 0.1 ml of rabbit anti-kallikrein serum and 0.2 ml of base buffer (15 mM phosphate buffer, pH 7.4, containing 0.15 M NaCl, 0.02% sodium azide and 0.2% bovine serum albumin). After incubation at 4°C for 24 hr, 0.1 ml of goat anti-rabbit gammaglobulin serum was added and incubated again at 4°C overnight. The reaction mixture was centrifuged and the supernatant was discarded. The radioactivity of the precipitate was counted on a gamma scintillation counter.

Renin activity was measured by the rate of generation of angiotensin I in nephrectomized rat plasma as described previously.[10]

The activity of angiotensin-converting enzyme was assayed in a 125 ul incubation mixture containing 150 mM Tris-HCL buffer (pH 7.4), 450 mM NaCl and 1.0 mM hippuryl-histidyl-leucin (HHL). The reactions were initiated by the addition of plasma (25 μl) and the reaction mixture was incubated at 37°C for 30 min. Then, the reactions were terminated by the addition of 75 ul of 1 N HCl. The hippuric acid liberated from HHL was determined by the HPLC analysis system.

Table 1. The levels of blood glucose and systolic blood pressure of control, diabetic and hypertensive rats

	Blood pressure (mmHg)	Blood glucose (mmol/l)
Wistar strain		
Control (n=11)	N.D.	7.7 ± 1.2*
Diabetic (n=10)	N.D.	21.7 ± 2.4
Wistar-Kyoto strain		
Normotensive (n=10)	99 ± 6*	7.5 ± 0.6
Hypertensive (n=10)	185 ± 12	6.4 ± 0.9
Hypertensive+Diabetic (n=6)	192 ± 15	22.0 ± 2.2

* Standard deviation; N.D., not determined.

RESULTS

Blood Glucose and Blood Pressure in Diabetic and Hypertensive Rats

Table 1 shows the levels of blood glucose and systolic blood pressure in control, diabetic and hypertensive rats. Diabetic rats showed a marked rise in blood glucose levels. Systolic blood pressure of hypertensive rats was significantly elevated compared with the controls.

Glandular Kallikrein Content in the Submandibular Gland, the Kidney and Plasma

As shown in table 2, kallikrein content in the submandibular gland in diabetics, which include only diabetic and hypertensive-diabetic rats, was markedly reduced compared with that of the controls. Kallikrein content in the kidney also decreased in diabetics. Plasma concentration of kallikrein in diabetic rats was significantly lower (11.8 ± 2.9 ng/ml) than that of the controls (15.3 ± 2.3). In contrast to diabetics, kallikrein contents in the submandibular gland and plasma of hypertensive rats were scarcely changed, while the content was significantly reduced in the kidney.

Renin Activity in the Submandibular Gland, the Kidney and Plasma

As shown in table 3, renin activity in the submandibular gland was markedly reduced in diabetics compared to that of the controls but the activity in the kidney and plasma showed no differences between diabetics and controls. Renin activity in the submandibular gland increased in hypertensive rats, whereas no significant changes in the activity were found in the kidney and plasma.

Table 2. Glandular kallikrein content in the submandibular gland, the kidney and plasma of control, diabetic and hypertensive rats

	Submandibular gland (ug/mg protein)	Kidney (ng/mg protein)	Plasma (ng/ml)
Wistar strain			
Control (n=11)	73.5 ± 27.2*	8.1 ± 1.1*	15.3 ± 2.3*
Diabetic (n=10)	17.4 ± 9.9	4.6 ± 2.0	11.8 ± 2.9
Wistar-Kyoto strain			
Normotensive (n=10)	66.3 ± 7.0	8.0 ± 1.3	14.7 ± 2.9
Hypertensive (n=10)	78.4 ± 8.0	5.9 ± 1.2	16.9 ± 3.3
Hypertensive+			
Diabetic (n=6)	20.4 ± 6.4	3.7 ± 2.3	13.6 ± 3.9

* Standard deviation

Table 3. Renin activity in the submandibular gland, the kidney and plasma of control, diabetic and hypertensive rats

	Submandibular gland (ng Ang. I/h/mg protein)	Kidney (ng Ang. I/h/mg protein)	Plasma (ng Ang. I/h/ml)
Wistar strain			
Control (n=11)	108.4 ± 22.1*	946 ± 139*	80.3 ± 30.9*
Diabetic (n=10)	20.9 ± 6.5	1175 ± 149	87.5 ± 6.5
Wistar–Kyoto strain			
Normotensive (n=10)	89.7 ± 13.3	N.D.	89.6 ± 8.4
Hypertensive (n=10)	152.7 ± 14.5	893 ± 177	94.3 ± 9.8
Hypertensive + Diabetic (n=6)	33.0 ± 9.6	901 ± 113	84.1 ± 6.1

* Standard deviation ; N.D., not determined.

Activity of ACE in Plasma

The data of ACE activity in plasma are shown in table 4. ACE activity in plasma was as follows: 3.40 ± 0.75 and 3.35 ± 0.40 Hip-Acid μmol/ml/hr in normal rats (Wistar and Wistar-Kyoto strains), 4.71 ± 0.46 in diabetic Wistar strain rats, 1.48 ± 0.16 in hypertensive rats and 2.05 ± 0.54 in hypertensive-diabetic rats respectively. The activity of ACE was significantly elevated in diabetics but conversely reduced in only hypertensive rats.

DISCUSSION

Kallikrein-kinin and renin-angiotensin systems have been known to be involved in the pathogenesis of diabetes mellitus and hypertension.[1,5] We have reported that streptozotocin diabetic rats showed low kallikrein content in the pancreas as well as in the submandibular gland and the kidney and presumed that depressed kallikrein production in the pancreas may contribute to reduced insulin production in diabetes mellitus,[9] since glandular kallikrein is reported to accelerate insulin generation in the pancreas by converting proinsulin to insulin.[15]

In this study, the kallikrein content in the kidney, submandibular gland and plasma were significantly reduced in diabetic rats. Margolius et al.[11] reported that streptozotocin diabetic rats showed low urinary kallikrein excretion, which could be prevented by insulin administration. Furthermore, Hayashi et al.[13] observed that the reduced urinary excretion of kallikrein was followed by increased systolic blood

Table 4. Angiotensin converting enzyme activity in plasma of control, diabetic and hypertensive rats

	Angiotensin-converting enzyme activity (Hip-Acid μmol/ml/h)
Wistar strain	
Control (n=11)	3.40 ± 0.75*
Diabetic (n=10)	4.71 ± 0.46
Wistar-Kyoto strain	
Normotensive (n=10)	3.35 ± 0.40
Hypertensive (n=10)	1.48 ± 0.16
Hypertensive+Diabetic (n= 6)	2.05 ± 0.54

* Standard deviation

pressure. Although blood pressure in diabetic rats was not measured in the present study, it was determined that kallikrein content in diabetic rats is reduced not only in the kidney but also in the submandibular gland and plasma. As glandular kallikrein in plasma is thought to be released mainly from the submandibular gland in rats,[12] it seems possible that low kallikrein concentration in plasma reflects the decreased production of kallikrein in the organ. The activity of ACE was found to be elevated in diabetic rats as observed by Lieberman et al.[16] Therefore, it is expected that depressed kallikrein generation may result in decreased release of the kinin, which is liberated from kininogen by kallikrein, and/or the liberated kinin may be rapidly inactivated by ACE in diabetes mellitus. In correlation with the low kallikrein content, the low renin activity in the submandibular gland was found in diabetic rats. From the fact that kallikrein is a potent activator of prorenin,[14] low renin activity may be due to reduced kallikrein generation in the submandibular gland and it is thought that glandular kallikrein in the submandibular gland may regulate the generation of renin in the organ.

In hypertensive rats, low kallikrein content was found in the kidney. The low content in the kidney may be the cause of the decreased urinary excretion of kallikrein in hypertensive rats as observed by other investigators.[3] Although changes in renin activity in plasma were reported in hypertension cases,[5] the renin activity of the kidney and plasma in hypertensive rats showed slight differences compared with the controls in the present study. Contrary to diabetic rats, ACE activity was reduced in hypertensive rats as reported by Polsky-Cynkin et al.[17] Therefore, it is proposed that the production of vasoactive peptide angiotensin II, generated from angiotensin I by ACE, is expected to be depressed in hypertensive rats. Consequently, it is assumed that reduced kallikrein formation in the kidney plays a role in the etiology of hypertension in spontaneously hypertensive rats.

Hypertensive-diabetic rats showed similar changes in content of kallikrein and activity of renin to those of just diabetic rats. ACE activity in plasma of hypertensive rats was found to increase by inducing diabetes, while the activity was depressed in hypertensive rats. The elevated levels of ACE activity in diabetes may come from diffuse vascular damage as mentioned by Lieberman et al.[16]

In conclusion, changes in levels of kallikrein, renin and ACE of hypertensive rats were revealed to be less remarkable than those of diabetic rats, although these enzymes are generally thought to be involved in the etiology of hypertension. This may imply that other factors contribute to hypertension in spontaneously hypertensive rats. Further investigations should be required to clarify the role of kallikrein-kinin system in diabetes mellitus, including the measurements of kinin and kininogen in plasma and several organs.

ACKNOWLEDGEMENTS

This research was supported in part by a grant-in-aid from the Ministry of Education, Science and Culture.

REFERENCES

1. M. Schachter, Kallikreins (kininogenases)-a group of serine proteases with bioregulatory action, Pharmacol. Rev. 31:1 (1980).
2. H. S. Margolius, D. Horwitz, J. J. Pisano, and H. R. Keiser, Urinary kallikrein excretion in hypertensive man, Circ. Res. 35:820 (1974).

3. R. G. Geller, H. S. Margolus, J. J. Pisano, and H. R. Keiser, Urinary kallikrein excretion in spontaneously hypertensive rats, Circ. Res. 36, Sup.I:103 (1975).

4. M. Wicklmayr, G. Dietze, L. Mayer, I. Böttger and J. Grunst, Evidence for an involvement of kinin liberation in the priming action of insulin on glucose uptake into skeletal muscle, FEBS Lett. 98:61 (1979).

5. F. R. Bühler, Renin, renin inhibition and antihypertensive therapy, Clin. Exper. Hypertension, A5(7/8):1395 (1978).

6. E. G. Erdös, Conversion of angiotensin I to angiotensin II, Am. J. Med. 31:749 (1976).

7. H. U. Bergmeyr, and E. Bernt, Determination of glucose with glucose oxidase and peroxidase, in "Methods in Enzymatic Analysis vol 3," H. U. Bergmeyer, ed., Academic Press, New York (1947).

8. D. H. Lowry, N. J. Rosebrough, A. L. Farr, and R. J. Randall, Protein measurement with Folin phenol reagent, J. Biol. Chem. 193:265 (1951).

9. W. Sakamoto, K. Yoshikawa, O. Nishikaze, H. Handa, A. Hirayama, and S. Uehara, Glandular kallikrein content in tissues of diabetic and hypertensive rats measured by enzyme immunoassay, J. Clin. Chem. Clin. Biochem. 23:521 (1985).

10. W. Sakamoto, K. Yoshikawa, A. Yokoyama, M. Kohri, H. Handa, S. Uehara, A. Hirayama, and H. Izumi, Glandular kallikrein, renin and tonin in tissues of diabetic and hypertensive rats, J. Clin. Chem. Clin. Biochem. 24:437 (1986).

11. R. K. Mayfield, H. S. Margolius, G. S. Bailey, D. H. Miller, D. A. Sens, J. Squires, and D. H. Namm, Urinary and renal tissue kallikrein in the streptozotocin-diabetic rat, Diabetes 34:22 (1985).

12. W. J. Lawton, D. Pround, M. E. Frech, J. V. Pierce, H. R. Keiser, and J. J. Pisano, Characterization and origin of immunoreactive glandular kallikrein in rat plasma, Biochem. Pharmacol. 30:1731 (1981).

13. M. Hayashi, S. Senda, I. Saito, W. Kitajima, and T. Saruta, Changes in blood pressure, urinary kallikrein and urinary prostaglandin E in rats with streptozotocin-induced diabetes, Naunyn Schmiedebergs Arch. Pharmacol. 322:290 (1983).

14. J. E. Sealey, S. A. Atlas, J. H. Lararh, N. B. Oza, and J. W. Ryan, Human urinary kallikrein converts inactive to active renin and is a possible physiological activator of renin, Nature 275:144 (1978).

15. O. ole-Moiyoi, D. C. Seldin, J. Spragg, G. S. Pinkus and K. F. Austin, Sequential cleavage of proinsulin by human pancreatic kallikrein and a human pancreatic kininase, Proc. Natl. Acad. Sci. USA 76:3612 (1979).

16. J. Lieberman, and A. Sastre, Serum angiotensin converting enzyme: evaluations in diabetes mellitus, Ann. Intern. Med. 93:825 (1980).

17. R. Polsky-Cynkin, S. Reichlin, and B. L. Fanburg, Angiotensin-1-converting enzyme activity in the spontaneously hypertensive rat, Proc. Soc. Exper. Biol. Med. 164:242 (1980).

ROLE OF RENAL KALLIKREIN IN THE INCREASED FRACTIONAL SODIUM EXCRETION IN THE RAT REMNANT KIDNEY MODEL OF CHRONIC RENAL FAILURE

Masayuki Kanazawa, Keishi Abe*, Minoru Yasujima,
Kazunori Yoshida, Masahiro Kohzuki, Masaya Tanno, Yutaka Kasai,
Ken Omata, Makito Sato, Kazuhisa Takeuchi, Masao Hiwatari and
Kaoru Yoshinaga

The Second Department of Internal Medicine, and *Dept of
Clinical Biology and Hormonal Regulation, Tohoku University
School of Medicine, Sendai, Japan

ABSTRACT

To assess the potential role of renal kallikrein-kinin system in
enhancing sodium excretion per nephron in chronic renal failure, we
studied urinary excretion of active and inactive kallikrein for 3 weeks in
Wistar-Kyoto rats subjected to 5/6 nephrectomy (5/6), 1/2 nephrectomy
(1/2) or sham operation (Sham). We determined urinary active and inactive
kallikrein by measuring kallikrein activity using a kininogenase assay
before and after treatment with trypsin (200 µg/ml). Fractional sodium
excretion was significantly increased in 5/6-rats as compared with 1/2- or
sham-rats. On the contrary, urinary active kallikrein excretion per
nephron was not different in the three models whereas a significant rise
in urinary inactive kallikrein excretion per nephron was found in 5/6-rats
as compared with 1/2- or sham-rats. Urinary total kallikrein excretion per
nephron was significantly increased in 5/6-rats as compared with sham-
rats. In addition, no correlation was found between fractional sodium
excretion and urinary active kallikrein excretion corrected for creatinine
clearance (Ccr) in 5/6-rats. These results indicate that decreased
excretion of renal active kallikrein may not play a significant role in
the increased sodium excretion per nephron in the rat remnant kidney model
of chronic renal failure. Furthermore, it is suggested that in this model
of rat there might be impaired production of renal active kallikrein
although its exact mechanism remains to be determined.

INTRODUCTION

It is generally accepted that the normal kidney possesses a
remarkable ability to maintain constancy of extracellular fluid volume and
sodium balance. When the glomerular filtration rate is reduced as seen in
chronic renal failure, fractional excretion of sodium must increase to
maintain sodium balance. Previous studies have demonstrated that four
times higher values for fractional sodium excretion were found in patients
with advanced renal disease (Abe et al.1981). However, the physiological
mechanisms responsible for this adaptation in sodium excretion per nephron
in chronic renal failure have not been elucidated. On the other hand,

renal kallikrein is a component of the vasoactive peptide system called
the kallikrein-kinin system and this system has important physiological
functions, including modulation of salt and water transport in the kidney
(Levinsky,1979, Carretero,1980). Stein et al.(1972) reported that intraarterial bradykinin reduces proximal reabsorption of sodium and water in
the dog. Marin-Grez (1974) reported that the fractional excretion of
sodium and water was lower in antibradykinin-treated rats. In addition,
sodium loading produced a sustained increase in urinary active as well as
inactive kallikrein excretion in rats (Yasujima et al.1986), and urinary
active kallikrein increases during saline infusion in dogs (Marin-
Grez,1972) and rats (Godon et al.1974). These reports suggest that
kallikrein may be involved in the regulation of renal sodium excretion. On
the contrary, it was shown that sodium loading induced an acute fall in
urinary kallikrein excretion which was prolonged for the experimental
period of 28 days (Johnston et al.1976). Bönner et al.(1981) also reported
that sodium loading caused a decrease in urinary kallikrein excretion in
rat. Furthermore, Lieberthal et al.(1983) reported that dietary sodium
restriction increased the excretion of total kallkrein determined by a
direct radioimmunoassay in man, whereas inactive kallikrein excretion was
unchanged and acute volume expansion with saline did not alter the
excretion of either active or inactive kallikrein. Thus, previous reports
concerning the roles of renal kallikrein in renal sodium handling have
been conflicting. Therefore, in the present study, to investigate the
potential role of renal kallikrein-kinin system in enhancing fractional
sodium excretion in chronic renal failure , we studied urinary excretion
of active and inactive kallikrein in the rat remnant kidney model of
chronic renal failure.

MATERIALS AND METHODS

    Male Wistar-Kyoto rats (WKY) were subjected to 5/6 nephrectomy (n=12)
by infarction of 2/3 of the right kidney at 7 weeks of age and removal of
the left kidney at 8 weeks or to 1/2 nephrectomy (n=6) by removal of the
left kidney at 8 weeks or to sham operation (n=7) at 8 weeks. Animals were
housed in individual metabolic cages in a humidity- and temperature-
controlled room and fed a regular diet (Oriental CMF, 0.24 % of sodium,
0.69 % of potassium) and given ad libitum access to tap water. Studies
were performed after a 7-day period of acclimatization to the housing,
feeding, and drinking conditions and were continued for up to 3 weeks.
    Daily systolic blood pressure was recorded in conscious rats by an
indirect tail-cuff method (Pfeffer et al.1971).
    The daily urinary kallikrein excretion, urine volume, urinary sodium
excretion were determined.
    At the end of the study rats were killed by rapid decapitation and
trunk blood was collected for determination of serum creatinine (Scr),
blood urea nitrogen (BUN), serum sodium concentration and plasma
aldosterone concentration (PAC), and creatinine clearance (Ccr) was
calculated.
    The active kallikrein in urine samples was measured by its
kininogenase activity (kinin releasing capability) using the mothod of Abe
et al.(1979). Briefly, duplicate aliquots of 20 µl of urine samples were
incubated with 4 µg of purified bovine serum low molecular weight
kininogen as substrate (generously supplied by Dr H. Kato, Fukuoka, Japan)
in the presence of 1-10 phenanthroline (3 mmol/l), disodium ethylene
diaminetetraacetic acid (EDTA, 30 mmol/l) to inhibit kininases and
neomycin (0.1 %) as an antibacterial agent. The incubation volume was
adjusted to 400 µl with 0.1 mol/l phosphate buffer, pH 8.5. The samples
were incubated at 37 °C for 20 min and the reaction was stopped by heating
in a boiling water bath for 5 min. The samples were then diluted with 1 ml
of ice cold 0.1 mol/l Tris-HCl buffer, pH 7.4, and the generated kinins
were radio-immunologically measured by a modification of the method of

Carretero et al.(1976). Rabbit antibradykinin serum was generously supplied by Dr O.A. Carretero (Detroit, USA). Kallikrein activity is expressed as the amount of kinin/ml urine as generated by the incubation of urine samples with bovine serum low molecular weight kininogen for 20 min. Total kallikrein was determined by measuring the kininogenase activity in urine samples after inactive kallikrein had been activated with trypsin, and inactive kallikrein was calculated as the difference between total kallikrein and active kallikrein. To activate the inactive kallikrein, duplicate 10 µl aliquots of urine samples were incubated with 2 µg trypsin for 30 min at 37 °C. The reaction was stopped by adding 100 µg soybean trypsin inhibitor (SBTI). The incubation volume was adjusted to 400 µl with 0.1 mol/l phosphate buffer, pH 8.5, and the mixture was incubated for more than 2h at room temperature. Kininogenase activity was then measured as described above. To determine the optimal amount of trypsin needed to activate urinary inactive kallikrein in the preliminary experiments, the pooled rat urine (10 µl) from 10 normal rats was incubated with trypsin at doses of 0.1, 0.5, 2, 5 and 10 µg for 30 min at 37 °C. The reaction was stopped by adding 100 µg SBTI. The maximum activation of urinary inactive kallikrein by trypsin was observed at a concentration of 0.2 µg/ml, and the dose of SBTI used completely inhibited the kininogenase activity of trypsin used. Furthermore, we confirmed that the doses of trypsin and SBTI used in the present experiment did not affect the radio-immunoassay of kinins.

Urinary and serum sodium cncentrations were measured with a flame photometer.

Scr and BUN were measured with an autoanalyzer.

PAC was measured with a commercial radioimmunoassay kit (Cer Ire Serin). This method was sensitive to 10 pg of aldosterone.

All results were expressed as the mean ± SEM. The significance of difference between mean values was evaluated by Student's t-test, and statistical significance was defined as $P < 0.05$.

RESULTS

Systolic Blood Pressure

Systolic blood pressure was not different in the three models throughout the 3 week experimental period. Two and four weeks after surgery average values of systolic blood pressure were 130 ± 2.7 mmHg and 134 ± 2.2 mmHg in 5/6-rats, 129 ± 5.3 mmHg (n.s.) and 138 ± 3.7 mmHg (n.s.) in 1/2-rats, 130 ± 6.2 mmHg (n.s.) and 132 ± 2.6 mmHg (n.s.)in sham-rats, respectively.

Renal Function

Significantly higher concentrations of Scr and BUN were found in 5/6-rats than those of 1/2- or sham-rats at four weeks after surgery. Average Scr and BUN concentrations were 0.71 ± 0.12 mg/dl and 45.8 ± 8.0 mg/dl in 5/6-rats, 0.27 ± 0.03 mg/dl (P<0.05) and 8.3 ± 1.7 mg/dl (P<0.01) in 1/2-rats, 0.17 ± 0.03 mg/dl (P<0.01) and 7.3 ± 1.2 mg/dl (P<0.01) in sham-rats, respectively. Average values of Ccr were 0.89 ± 0.13 ml/min in 5/6-rats, 1.99 ± 0.14 ml/min (P<0.001) in 1/2-rats, 3.3 ± 0.52 ml/min (P<0.01) in sham-rats. Therefore, markedly impaired renal function was found in 5/6-rats as compared with 1/2- or sham-rats.

Urinary Excretion of Sodium

Urinary excretion of sodium was not different in the three models throughout the 3 week experimental period. Two and four weeks after surgery average values of urinary excretion of sodium were 0.60 ± 0.07 mEq/day and 0.63 ± 0.06 mEq/day in 5/6-rats, 0.60 ± 0.14 mEq/day (n.s.)

and 0.59 ± 0.06 mEq/day (n.s.) in 1/2-rats, 0.56 ± 0.09 mEq/day (n.s.) and 0.62 ± 0.07 mEq/day (n.s.) in sham-rats, respectively.

Fractional Sodium Excretion

Fractional sodium excretion was significantly increased in 5/6-rats as compared with 1/2- or sham-rats. Average values of fractional sodium excretion were 0.34 ± 0.03 % in 5/6-rats, 0.16 ± 0.02 % (P<0.001) in 1/2-rats, 0.1 ± 0.01 % (P<0.001) in sham-rats. Three times higher value in fractional sodium excretion was found in 5/6-rats than that of sham-rats.

Urinary Excretion of Active and Inactive Kallikrein and Corrected Values of Urinary Excretion of Them

Significantly lower values of urinary excretion of active and inactive kallikrein were found, and the ratio of active to total kallikrein were found lower in 5/6-rats than those of sham-rats. Four weeks after surgery average values of urinary active and total kallikrein excretion were 3.6 ± 1.1 µg/day and 10.1 ± 1.6 µg/day in 5/6-rats, 9.0 ± 3.2 µg/day (n.s.) and 20.7 ± 5.3 µg/day (n.s.) in 1/2-rats, 10.2 ± 2.4 µg/day (P<0.05) and 18.3 ± 3.4 µg/day (P<0.05) in sham-rats, respectively. Urinary excretion rate of kallikrein was corrected for Ccr to compare with fractional sodium excretion. Urinary active kallikrein excretion corrected for Ccr was not different in the three models whereas a significant rise in urinary inactive kallikrein excretion corrected for Ccr was found in 5/6-rats as compared with 1/2- or sham-rats. Urinary total kallikrein excretion corrected for Ccr was significantly increased in 5/6-rats as compared with sham-rats. Four weeks after surgery average values of urinary total, active and inactive kallikrein corrected for Ccr were 7.9 ± 1.2 µg/l, 2.8 ± 0.8 µg/l and 5.1 ± 0.6 µg/l in 5/6-rats, 7.2 ± 1.9 µg/l (n.s.), 3.1 ± 1.1 µg/l (n.s.) and 2.3 ± 0.7 µg/l (P<0.05) in 1/2-rats, 3.8 ± 0.7 µg/l (P<0.05), 2.1 ± 0.5 µg/l (n.s.) and 7.1 ± 1.3 µg/l (P<0.001) in sham-rats, respectively.

Relationship between Fractional Sodium Excretion and Urinary Active Kallikrein Excretion Corrected for Ccr

No significant correlation was found between fractional sodium excretion and urinary active kallikrein excretion corrected for Ccr in 5/6-rats (r=0.35211), 1/2-rats (r=-0.38085), sham-rats (r=0.48545), and all of three models (r=0.24300).

PAC

PAC was not different in the three models. Four weeks after surgery average values of PAC were 45.2 ± 4.3 ng/dl in 5/6-rats, 34.0 ± 3.4 ng/dl (n.s.) in 1/2-rats, 33.1 ± 6.9 ng/dl (n.s.) in sham-rats.

DISCUSSION

In the present study, significantly lower values of urinary excretion of active and inactive kallikrein were found, and the ratio of active to total kallikrein were found lower in 5/6-rats than those of sham-rats. It may be postulated that the presence of protein in the urine may explain the lower value of urinary kallikrein excretion in this model, since a large amount of protein induced by reduced renal mass was excreted into the urine. However, we could exclude this possibility by showing no influence of protein on the kininogenase assay in our method in preliminary experiments. In addition, the present results for the ratio of inactive to total kallikrein in urine of sham-rats are similar to those reported previously (Nishimura et al.1983, Van Leeuwen et al.1984). The decrease in urinary excretion of active kallikrein is consistent with the finding of Croxatto et al.(1970), who reported that the group of uninephrectomized Wistar rats with a figure-of-8-ligature in the remnant kidney showed an invariably striking fall in the urinary kallikrein-like activity. On the other hand, Vergara et al.(1983) reported that in hypertensive one-kidney pole-ligated rats the total urinary kallikrein did not differ from that excreted by solely uninephrectomized rats. In our experiment, urinary excretion of total kallikrein was not different in 5/6- and 1/2-rats. However, significantly lower value of urinary excretion of total kallikrein was found in 5/6-rats than that of sham-rats. Accordingly, it is suggested that in 5/6-rats the renal ability to produce kallikrein may be impaired due to reduced renal mass. Furthermore, it is suggested that the ability to activate kallikrein may be attenuated, but the exact mechanisms remain to be determined.

What is responsible for this increment of fractional sodium excretion ? Urinary active kallikrein excretion per nephron was not different in the three models whereas a significant rise in inactive and total kallikrein excretion per nephron was found in 5/6-rats as compared with 1/2- or sham-rats. Furthermore, a significant correlation was not found between fractional sodium excretion and urinary active kallikrein excretion per nephron in 5/6-rats. Therefore, it is unlikely to support the possibility that the decreased excretion of urinary active kallikrein may be involved in the increased fractional sodium excretion in this model of rat. Previously, Abe et al.(1981) reported that in half of the patients with advanced renal disease a positive correlation was found between kallikrein excretion corrected for Ccr and fractional sodium excretion. On the other hand, in the remaining half of the patients an inverse relationship was found between the two, low values of urinary kallikrein excretion occurring in patients with exaggerated sodium excretion. At the moment, we have no explanation for the discrepancy between the present results and data reported previously although it may be due to the differences in the objects studied.

Blood pressure was not different in the three models and did not show any changes throughout the 3 week experimental period. Moreover, there was no significant difference in PAC. These results suggest that blood pressure and aldosterone may not play a significant role in the increased sodium excretion per nephron in this model of rat.

In conclusion, it was indicated that the renal ability to activate kallikrein may be attenuated in the rat remnant kidney model of chronic renal failure due to reduced renal mass, and also indicated that the ability to produce kallikrein may be impaired in this model of rat. Furthermore, the present result suggests that the decreased excretion of urinary active kallikrein may not be involved in the physiologic mechanisms responsible for the adaptation in sodium excretion per nephron in chronic renal failure. On the other hand, it remains to be determined whether other substances such as renal prostaglandin and atrial natriuretic peptide may be involved in the exaggerated natriuresis in chronic renal failure or not.

ACKNOWLEDGEMENTS

This study was supported by a Grant-in-Aid for Cardiovascular Disease (60-C-3) from the Ministry of Health and Welfare and for Scientific Research (61132005 and 62570376) from the Ministry of Education, Science and Culture, Japan, and by the Miyagi Prefectural Kidney Association. We wish to acknowledge the excellent technical assistance of Miss Keiko Shiraishi, Miss Michiko Okamoto, Miss Naeko Nakagawa, and the secretarial assistance of Miss Junko Okazaki.

REFERENCES

Abe, k., Kato, H., Sakurai, Y., Ito, T., Saito, K., Haruyama, T., Otsuka, Y., and Yoshinaga, K.,1979,Estimation of urinary kininogenase activity using bovine serum low molecular weight kininogen, In Kinin II edited by Fijii, S., Moriya, H., Suzuki, T., New York: Plenum Publishing Corporation, pp 105-114.

Abe, K., Imai, Y., Sato, M., Haruyama, T., Sato, K., Hiwatari, M., Kasai, Y., Itoh, S., Yasujima, M., Seino, M., and Yoshinaga, K., 1981, Exaggerated fractional sodium excretion in hypertension with advanced renal disease: the role of renal prostaglandin and kallikrein, Clin Sci,61:327s-330s.

Bönner, G., Autenrieth, R., Marin-Grez, M., Rascher, W., and Gross, F.,1981, Effect of sodium loading, deoxycorticosterone acetate, and corticosterone on urinary kallikrein excretion, Hormone Res, 14:87-94.

Carretero, O.A., Oza, N.B., Piwonska, A., Ocholik, T., and Scicli, A.G., 1976, Measurement of urinary kallikrein activity by kinin radioimmunoassay , Biochem Pharmacol, 25: 2265-2270.

Carretero, O.A., and Scicli, A.G., 1980, The renal kallikrein- kinin system, Am J Physiol, 238:F247-F255.

Croxatto, H.R., and San Martin, M., 1970, Kallikrein-like activity in the urine of renal hypertensive rats, Experientia, 26:1216-1217.

Godon, J.P., and Damas, J., 1974, The kallikrein-kinin system in normal and glomerulonephritic rats, Arch Int Physiol Biochem, 82:273-277.

Johnston, C.I., Matthews, P.G., and Dax, E., 1976, Renin-angiotensin and kallikrein-kinin system in sodium homeostasis and hypertension in rats, Clin Sci Mol Med, 51:283s-286s.

Lieberthal, W., Oza, N.B., Arbeit, L., Bernard, D.B., and Levinsky, N.G., 1983, Effects of alterations in sodium and water metabolism on urinary excretion of active and inactive kallikrein in man, J Clin Endocrinol Metab, 56:513-519.

Marin-Grez, M., 1974, The influence of antibodies against bradykinin on isotonic saline diuresis in the rat, Pfluegers Arch, 350:231-239.

Marin-Grez, M., Cottone, P., and Carretero, O.A., 1972, Evidence for an involvement of kinins in regulation of sodium excretion, Am J Physiol, 223:794-796.

Nishimura, K., Shimizu, H., and Kokubu, T.,1983, Existence of prokallikrein in the rat: its biochemical properties compared to three active glandular kallikreins from the kidney , serum and urine of the rat, Hypertension, 5:205-210.

Pfeffer, J.M., Pfeffer, M.A., and Frohlich, E.D., 1971, Validity of an indirect tail-cuff method for determining systolic arterial pressure in unanesthetized normotensive and spontaneously hypertensive rats, J Lab Clin Med, 78:957-962.

Stein, J.H., Congbalay, R.C., Karsh, D.L., Osgood, R.W., and Ferris, T.F., 1972, The effect of bradykinin on proximal tubular sodium reabsorption in the dog: evidence for functional nephron heterogeneity, J Clin Invest, 51:1709-1721.

Van Leeuwen, B.H., Grinblat, S.M., and Johnston, C.I., 1984, Release of active and inactive kallikrein from the isolated perfused rat kidney, Clin Sci, 66:201-215.

Vergara, M., and Corthorn, J., 1983, Urinary excretion of activatable kallikrein in one-kidney pole-ligated hypertensive rats, J Hypertension, 1:387-391.

Yasujima, M., Abe, K., Tanno, M., Kohzuki, M., Omata, K., Kasai, Y., Kudo, K., Tsunoda, K., Sato, M., Chiba, S., and Yoshinaga, K.,1986, Effects of sodium and angiotensin II on urinary active and inactive kallikrein in rats, J Hypertension, 4:13-18.

ALDOSTERONE, KALLIKREIN, KININASE I AND II IN NORMAL AND HYPERTENSION

COMPLICATED PREGNANCY

S.Ferrazzani*,P.Leardi*,D.L.Magnotti*,S.De Carolis.*,
E.Moneta.**,G.Porcelli#,A.R.Volpe #, E.Menini##, and I.Liberale ##

* Istituto di Clinica Ostetrica e Ginecologica, # Centro
Chimica dei Recettori C.N.R., Istituto di Chimica
##Servizio Analisi Ormonali, Istituto di Chimica Biologica
Facoltà di Medicina e Chirurgia, Università Cattolica, Rome
(Italy)
** 2ª Clinica Ostetrica e Ginecologica Università di
Modena, Moden (Italy)

INTRODUCTION

Increasing interest has recently been concentrated on investigations of the integration between the renin-angiotensin-aldosterone
(RAAS), kallikrein-bradykinin (KBS), and prostaglandin (PS) systems.
It is, in fact, generally agreed that these systems may be a single complex in constant dynamic equilibrium for maintaining homeostasis
of the body fluids.
In physiological pregnancy the RAAS is found to be activated, but,
despite this, diastolic arterial pressure tends to decrease, thus indicating a drop in peripheral resistance. Stimulation of this system
would produce a collateral increase in arterial tone with consequent
hypertension, were it not for the simultaneous activation of the PS
that has a contrary effect.
The PS is activated directly by the action of angiotensin II on
phospholipases A_2 and C and on the diglyceride lipase at the level of
the arterial wall.
Similarly, the KBS is found to be hyperactive in pregnancy, at
least up to the time of maximum pressure decrease which appears to coincide with the 20th week, then return to pre-pregnancy levels[1].
It is likely that the interrelation may be altered during both
normal and hypertension complicated pregnancy and that onset of pre-
eclampsia may produce imbalance between the pressor and depressor systems.
This investigation aims to establish whether there are, in normal
and complicated by hypertension pregnancy, any important changes in
these homeostatic systems that can be explained pathogenetically, and
whether such changes are related to any indices of maternal or foetal
wellbeing, in order to detect in due time any deviations from the normality.

MATERIALS AND METHODS

The study was made on 19 pre- and post-partum patients with proteinuric pre-eclampsia (PP), 10 patients with chronic hypertension (CH), and 10 with not-proteinuric gestational hypertension (GH)[2]. For the purposes of comparison, 22 patients admitted for reasons not involving haemodynamic, metabolic or cardiac conditions were considered as controls (CO).

All the hypertensive patients were under α-methyl-dopa treatment. Only after the end of the study were other antihypertensive drugs used. No diuretics were administered.

During the 24 hours prior to investigation, each patient was predominantly confined to bed, received no liquids by phleboclysis and was on a standard sodium-normal diet. Samples were taken after at least eight hours bedrest, between 8 and 8.30 a.m. while fasting. Completeness of the urine collection over 24 hours was checked by simultaneous assay of creatininuria.

Urinary kallikrein activity was assessed as the capacity of the enzyme to hydrolyze the Pro-Phee-Arg.MCA as described by Morita et al (1977)[3] and expressed in units (Us).

Plasma and urinary kininase I and II, expressed in KUs, were dosed using the method of Porcelli et al (1987)[6].

Plasma aldosterone was measured by radioimmunoassay using antibody-coated tubes and a ^{125}I tracer (Coat-A-Count kit, Diagnostic Products Corporation, Los Angeles, CA).

Urinary aldosterone was determined with the same technique after acid hydrolysis of the 18-glucosiduronate and extraction of the free steroid into ethyl acetate.

All the other biochemical and haematological data were assessed by automatic methods that are of routine in the Central laboratory of this Hospital.

The statistical methods used were: the Mann-Whitney/Wilcoxon rank sum test to compare the means of independent samples, linear correlation by the method of least squares with the appropriate Pearson correlation coefficient, after logarithmical transformation whenever necessary. Values of $P<0.05$ were considered significant.

RESULTS

COMPARISON OF THE GROUPS STUDIED

Table I shows the plasma and urinary levels of the parameters assessed pre-partum in the various groups of patients.

As can be seen, there is a remarkable range of variability between the single parameters in each group.

In group PP there is a significant difference as compared with the controls in plasma aldosterone levels and in the urinary levels of aldosterone and kallikrein respectively.

After 4-6 days post partum there was no longer any significant difference between the various groups, as is shown in Table II.

When comparison is made of the parameters studied pre- and post-partum, it can be seen that plasma and urinary aldosterone rapidly return to the normal limits for non-gestational conditions just a few days (4-6) post partum, and the other parameters present no tendency to change. The only exception is for urinary kallikrein in chronic hypertension, which is significantly reduced during the immediate post-partum period (Table III).

This statistic should, however, be considered in the light of the reduced number of post-partum samples.

TABLE I   PRE-PARTUM

	PROTEINURIC PRE-ECLAMPSIA	GESTATIONAL HYPERTENSION	CHRONIC HYPERTENSION	CONTROLS
Plasma Aldosterone	*n=16 *	n=9	n=8	n=19
pg/ml	240.4 (54-537)	380.8 (136-720)	414.9 (232-951)	400.9 (186-1058)
Urinary Aldosterone	n=16 ***	n=9	n=8	n=19
mg/ml	40.2 (4.8-128.3)	78.4 (6.3-229.1)	102.3 (39.7-182.5)	135.4 (55.9-433.6)
Urinary Kallikrein	n=14 **	n=10	n=10	n=22
Us.	132 (25.3-363.1)	189.4 (0-418)	493.9 (70-1696)	399.1 (0-3150)
Urinary Kininase I	n=14	n=10	n=10	n=22
K.Us.	595.8 (285-1564)	473.1 (144-874)	541.9 (78-1328)	498.1 (129-1098)
Urinary Kininase II	n=14	n=10	n=10	n=22
K.Us.	1651 (501-3568)	1827 (798-3620)	1382 (430-2476)	1350 (446-2923)
Plasma Kininase I	n=13	n=3	n=7	n=12
K.Us.	13.6 (8.3-19.9)	13.3 (11.45-15.3)	14.6 (9.3-19.1)	13.9 (9.96-19.42)
Plasma Kininase II	n=13	n=3	n=7	n=11
K.Us.	7.8 (5.06-10.45)	10.1 (8.3-11.95)	8.02 (5.81-10.7)	8.03 (3.98-10.95)

* number of patients, mean and (range) are given.

* = P significance value versus controls (Wilcoxon rank sum test). * P<0.05; ** P<0.02; *** P<0.001

TABLE II   POST-PARTUM

	PROTEINURIC PRE-ECLAMPSIA	GESTATIONAL HYPERTENSION	CHRONIC HYPERTENSION	CONTROLS
Plasma Aldosterone	*n=14	n=6	n=3	n=8
pg/ml	49.1 (10-237)	43.3 (26-69)	52 (28-86)	52.5 (23-72)
Urinary Aldosterone	n=15	n=6	n=3	n=7
µg/ml	5.2 (2.2-15.4)	14.4 (3.7-38.2)	6.8 (3.9-8.5)	10.1 (3.6-21.6)
Urinary Kallikrein	n=14	n=7	n=3	n=5
Us.	96 (0-266)	111.2 (8-336.5)	62.6 (30-83.8)	402.6 (0-614)
Urinary Kininase I	n=15	n=7	n=3	n=6
K.Us.	629.3 (178-1176)	435.9 (121-953)	719.4 (580.3-986)	440.8 (58-1189)
Urinary Kininase II	n=15	n=7	n=3	n=6
K.Us.	1583 (506-2812)	1782 (324-3473)	1077 (503-1851)	1086 (137-3312)
Plasma Kininase I	n=15	n=3	n=3	n=2
K.Us.	13.65 (5.9-21.9)	12.45 (11.9-13.3)	13 (10.4-16.8)	11.1 (7.6-14.6)
Plasma Kininase II	n=15	n=3	n=3	n=2
K.Us.	7.3 (3.3-10.95)	7.8 (6.4-10)	6.9 (5.1-8.7)	7.84 (7.8-7.88)

* number of patients, mean and (range) are given. * = P significance value versus controls (Wilcoxon rank sum test). * P<0.05; ** P<0.02; *** P<0.001

	PROTEINURIC PRE-ECLAMPSIA	GESTATIONAL HYPERTENSION	CHRONIC HYPERTENSION	CONTROLS
Plasma Aldosterone pg/ml	*n=16 *** 240.4 (54-537) n=1 49.1 (10-237)	n=9 *** 380.8 (136-720) n=3 43.3 (26-69)	n=8 ** 414.9 (232-951) n=8 52 (28-86)	n=19 *** 400.9 (186-1058) n=7 52.5 (23-72)
Urinary Aldosterone µg/ml	n=16 *** 40.2 (4.8-128.3) n=15 5.2 (2.2-15.4)	n=9 78.4 (6.3-229.1) n=6 14.4 (3.7-38.2)	n=8 ** 102.3 (39.7-182.5) n=3 6.8 (3.9-8.5)	n=19 *** 135.4 (55.9-433.6) n=7 10.1 (3.6-21.6)
Urinary Kallikrein Us.	n=14 132 (25.3-363.1) n=14 96 (0-266)	n=10 189.4 (0-418) n=7 111.2 (8-336.5)	n=10 * 493.9 (70-1696) n=3 62.6 (30-83.8)	n=22 399.1 (0-3150) n=5 402.6 (0-614)
Urinary Kininase I K.Us.	n=14 595.8 (285-1564) n=15 629.3 (178-1176)	n=10 473.1 (144-874) n=7 435.9 (121-953)	n=10 541.9 (78-1328) n=3 719.4 (580.3-986)	n=22 498.1 (129-1098) n=6 440.8 (58-1189)
Urinary Kininase II K.Us.	n=14 1651 (501-3568) n=15 1583 (506-2812)	n=10 1827 (798-3620) n=7 1782 (324-3473)	n=10 1382 (430-2476) n=3 1077 (503-1851)	n=22 1350 (446-2923) n=6 1086 (137-3312)
Plasma Kininase I K.Us.	n=13 13.6 (8.3-19.9) n=15 13.65 (5.9-21.9)	n=3 13.3 (11.45-15.3) n=3 12.45 (11.9-13.3)	n=7 14.6 (9.3-19.1) n=3 13 (10.4-16.8)	n=12 13.9 (9.96-19.42) n=2 11.1 (7.6-14.6)
Plasma Kininase II K.Us.	n=13 7.8 (5.06-10.45) n=15 7.3 (3.3-10.95)	n=3 10.1 (8.3-11.95) n=3 7.8 (6.4-10)	n=7 8.02 (5.81-10.7) n=3 6.9 (5.1-8.7)	n=11 8.03 (3.98-10.95) n=2 7.84 (7.8-7.88)

* number of patients, mean and (range) are given. * = P values for the difference
between pre-partum and post-partum mean (Wilcoxon rank sum test). * P<0.05; ** P<0.02; *** P<0.001

RELATIONSHIP BETWEEN THE PARAMETERS STUDIED AND RENAL FUNCTION

The following parameters directly or indirectly relevant to pre- and post-partum renal function were taken into consideration: plasma and urinary potassium, plasma and urinary sodium, creatininaemia, 24-hour creatinine clearance, urea nitrogen, and plasma and urinary uric acid.

A highly-significant positive linear correlation between pre-partum plasma and urinary aldosterone (n=53,r=0.67,P<0.0001) was found confirming that the metabolite measured in urine corresponds to the plasma level.

Plasma aldosterone also showed, in our pre-partum patients, a significant positive correlation with urinary kallikrein (n=51,r=0.47, P=0.01).

The negative correlation between aldosteronaemia and aldosteronuria with the pre-partum uricaemia should also be noted (respectively n=50,r=-0.31,P=0.03; n=50,r=-0.47,P=0.0006).

Pre-partum plasma aldosterone correlates positively with creatinine clearance, both in the controls and in PP group, but not in the other groups considered (respectively: n=7,r=0.84,P=0.02; n=12,r=0.65,P=0.02); while aldosteronuria correlates negatively with urea nitrogen (n=52,r=0.42,P=0.002) in all the patients considered.

Lastly; a correlation between urinary kininase II and pre-partum potassium is also to be noted (n=52,r=0.29,P=0.04).

RELATIONSHIP BETWEEN THE PARAMETERS STUDIED AND ARTERIAL PRESSURE

The systolic and diastolic pressures on the morning on which the blood sample was collected were taken into consideration and also the mean of systolic and diastolic pressures for the previous 24 hrs.

None of the parameters was related to the morning pressures, but both aldosteronaemia and aldosteronuria were negatively correlated with the mean calculated on the pressures over the previous 24 hrs., pre-partum but not post-partum (aldosteronuria/systolic pressure n=49,r=-0.37, P=0.009; aldosteronuria/diastolic pressure n=49,r=-0.42,P=0.002; plasma aldosterone/diastolic pressure n=49,r=-0.30,P=0.04).

The mean systolic pressure over the previous 24 hrs. showed no significant relation to plasma aldosterone.

RELATIONSHIP BETWEEN THE PARAMETERS STUDIED AND FOETAL DEVELOPMENT

Highly significant positive relations were detected between pre-partum plasma and urinary aldosterone on the one hand, and weight at birth on the other (plasma ald./weight at birth n=51,r=0.45,P=0.001; urinary ald./weight at birth n=51,r=0.63,P=0.0001).

Lastly, it was observed that there is no correlation either between plasma kininase I and urinary kininase I or between plasma kininase II and urinary kininase II, but the relation between kininase I and kininase II is highly significant both in plasma and urine (respectively n=35,r=47,P=0.004; n=57,r=0.58,P=0.0001).

DISCUSSION

From comparison between the various groups studied it appears appropriate to emphasize that only patients with proteinuric pre-eclampsia showed more evident deviations from the normality, with significant reduction of urinary kallikrein activity, of plasma and urinary aldosterone as has already been reported in the literature[7,8].

Relatively low levels of plasma and urinary aldosterone may be the result of decreased stimulation of adrenal gland by angiotensin II and III.

The apparently paradoxical cause of such an inhibition might be a decrease in the production of kidney prostaglandin, as observed recently a decreased urinary excretion of PGE_2 in patients with proteinuric pre-eclampsia[8,9].

Other mechanisms may, however, be involved, including a possible interaction with the KBS. It was observed that aldosterone influences the production of kinin at kidney level[10].

Other authors have recently reported a reduction of urinary kallikrein in gestosis[1,3,11] that mirrors that of aldosterone and the various components of the RAAS.

As regards the converting enzyme or kininase II, no significant difference was detected between the various groups. This enzyme has recently been studied regarding the specific role it plays within these systems. Several authors have reported reduction of its plasma activity in pregnancy vs. non-pregnant patients[12,13]. The majority of authors have failed to find any difference between gestosis and normal pregnancies[13,14] perhaps because the converting enzyme influences both the RAAS and the KBS at pulmonary level. Any determination of its level in peripheral blood would thus appear to be inadequate[14]. Other authors have detected a reduction in the activity of this enzyme[15], possibly connected with kidney damage.

From 4 to 6 days post partum there is no longer any detectable difference between the various groups and the return of these parameters to non-pregnant levels is seen to be rapid only for plasma and urinary aldosterone, which are the only parameters that undergo changes. Regarding kallikrein, no changes were detected during the post-partum period, probably because of the fact already reported that kallikrein excretion is reduced during the third trimester of pregnancy and remains so during the first 10 post-partum days.

The presence of a positive correlation between plasma aldosterone and urinary kallikrein activity during pregnancy appears to be highly significant, since the renal and urinary levels of kallikrein increase in cases of primary hyperaldosteronism and ADH hyperincretion outside pregnancy. The physiopathological significance of these observation is however not clear.

The haemodinamics of pregnancy would appear to involve a condition of hyperaldosteronism without hypertension, as can be detected in the rare Bartter's syndrome in which hyperaldosteronism appears to be connected with increased renal production of natriuretic prostaglandin.

The negative relation between plasma and urinary aldosterone and uricaemia is of some interest because of the importance given to this product of purine catabolism during gestosis in connection with the existing link between this parameter and foetal prognosis. The relation between aldosterone and uric acid may perhaps be mediated by changes in kidney function, as is shown by the simultaneous significant relation between plasma aldosterone and creatinine clearance, both in the controls and in patients with proteinuric pre-eclampsia, and between urinary aldosterone and urea nitrogen in all the patients.

The significant relation between urinary kininase II and plasma kalaemia would be easy to explain if a simultaneous relation had been found between that electrolyte and plasma and urinary aldosterone. But, since this has not been detected, its significance might also be the result of statistic fluctuation.

The negative relations between plasma and urinary aldosterone and mean systolic and diastolic arterial pressure over 24 hours, which are not found when pressure is taken once in the morning, is evidence of the relative validity of this way of measuring pressure as is now generally accepted. The fact that pressure levels are higher in those patients with the lowest amounts of this mineralcorticoid hormone suggests that there is probably a secondary inhibition of the hormone during hypertension, although this occurs only in PP cases and not in other hypertensive conditions studied here. This might be explained by the fact that there is a close relation between the KBS, the RAAS, arterial pressure and the hydroelectrolytic balance. Sodium restriction increases the production of kallikrein in the same way as that of renin, and there is an inverse relationship between urinary kallikrein and arterial pressure. The extreme pressure levels and excessive sodium retention typical of proteinuric pre-eclampsia might, on the contrary, inhibit each of the two systems.

These data also emphasize that weight at birth goes hand-inhand with the plasma and urinary levels of aldosterone. The plasma levels of this hormone are higher when weight at birth is normal, in controls and in the GH and CH groups, but lower when there is greater prevalence of foetal growth retardation as in the PP group. The presence of such a relation does not necessarily mean that there is a direct connection, but the relation might be mediated by volaemia.

It is well known that weight at birth is in proportion to volaemia
and that this parameter is controlled by aldosterone secretion.

In conclusion, it is confirmed that there is marked activation of
aldosterone secretion both in normal and hypertension complicated pregnancies, but there is also a very marked decrease in the mineral-
corticoids levels in case of proteinuric pre-eclampsia.

Urinary secretion of kallikrein also appears to decrease, but only
in cases of proteinuric pre-eclampsia. This suggests that there may be
a different pathogenesis for this condition from that of other forms of
hypertension in pregnancy.

REFERENCES

1. B.E. Karlberg, G. Ryden and K. Wichman, "Changes in the renin-angiotensin-aldosterone and kallikrein-kinin systems during normal
   and hypertensive pregnancy," Acta Obstet. Gynecol. Scand. Sup-
   pl.118, 17-24 (1984)
2. D.A. Davey, I. Mac Gillivray, "The classification and definition of
   the hypertensive disorders of pregnancy," Clin. and Exper. Hyper.
   in Pregnancy, B5(1),97-133 (1986)
3. T. Morita, H. Kato, S. Iwanaga, "Kallikrein activity determined by
   fluorimetric method," J. Biochem. Vol.82, 1495 (1977)
4. J. Lieberman, "Elevation of serum angiotensin-converting enzyme
   (ACE) levels in sarcoidosis," Am. J. Med. 59,365 (1975)
5. G. Porcelli, M. Di Iorio, A.R. Volpe, "Kininase I and Kininase II
   assay by liquid chromatography", J. of Chromatography (1986)
6. G. Porcelli, M. Di Iorio, A.R. Volpe, "Determination of kininase I
   and kininase II activities in human urine in high-performance
   liquid chromatography," J. of Chromatography 414,423-428 (1987)
7. R.D. Gordon, E.M. Symmonds, E.G. Wilmhurst, "Plasma renin activity,
   plasma angiotensin and plasma urinary electrolytes in normal and
   toxaemic pregnancy," Clin. Sci. Mol. Med.,45:115 (1973)
8. W.H. Bay & T.F. Ferris, "Factors controlling plasma renin and aldosterone during pregnancy," Hypertension,1:410 (1979)
9. E.B. Pedersen, N.J. Christensen, P. Christensen, "Pre-eclampsia. A
   state of prostaglandin deficiency. Urinary prostaglandin excretion, the renin-aldosterone system and circulating catecholamines
   in pre-eclampsia," Hypertension,5:105 (1983)
10.H.S. Margolius, D. Horwitz, R.G. Geller, "Urinary kallikrein in normal subjects: relationships to sodium intake and to sodium retaining steroids," Circ. Res.,35:812 (1974)
11.M. Hiruta, N. Furuhashi, M. Tanaka, T. Takahashi, H. Kono, K. Takahashi, M. Suzuki, "Urinary kallikrein quantity and activity of
   hypertensive gestosis in third trimester," in:"Perinatal care and
   gestosis", M. Suzuki, N. Furuhashi ed., 491-494 (1985)
12.J.N. Oats, F. Broughton Pipkin and E.M. Symonds, "Angiotensin-converting enzyme and the renin-angiotensin system in normotensive
   primigravid pregnancy," Clin. Exp. Hyper. in Pregnancy,B1(1),73
   (1982)
13.A.B. Rasmussen, E.B. Pedersen, F.K. Romer, P. Johannesen, S. Kris-
   tensen, J.G. Lauritsen and M. Wohlert, "The influence of normotensive pregnancy and pre-eclampsia on angiotensin-converting
   enzyme," Acta Obst. Gynec. Scand., 62:341-344 (1983)
14.T. Hira, Y. Nagata, Bradykinin in toxemic pregnancy, in:"Perinatal
   care and gestosis", M. Suzuki, N. Furuhashi ed., 369-372 (1985)
15.J.N. Oats, P.A. Long, L.A. Beaton, H.M. Andersen, "Ace in pregnancies complicated by hypertension and chronic renal disease,"
   Clin. Exp. Hyper. in Pregnancy,B3(1),31-41 (1984)

KININ-KININASE SYSTEM IN DRUG ADDICT WOMAN

IN PREGNANCY AND PUERPERIUM

A. Virgolino, G. Noia, M. De Santis, A.R. Volpe,
*M. Di Iorio, *G. Porcelli and *U. Bellati

Departments of Obstetrics and Gynaecology and Chemistry
Chemical Receptors Center
Catholic University, Via P. Sacchetti 664, Rome, Italy

The kinin-kininase system contributes, in close connection to the
renina-angiotensin and prostaglandin systems, to the local and systemic
vasal tone regulation (YLITALO, 1983)[1].

This same kinin-kininase system is also involved in psycho-physic
stress reaction (PORCELLI, 1984)[2]. This correlation between the
vasomotory and neuroendocrine systems was confirmed by the presence of a
great deal of kininogenase activity (kallikrein) at the hypothalamic
level (SCICLI, 1984)[3].

In opioid (heroin, methadone) drug addiction the alteration of the
hypothalamo-hypophysis-adrenal axis is well known both under clinical and
experimental conditions (FACCHINETTI, 1984; BUCKINGHAM, 1984)[4,5]; the
preliminary influence of these drugs on the kinin-kininase system has
also been shown (NOIA, 1986)[6].

A transitory arterial hypertension state in newborn babies of drug
addict women was reported in literature (ROSEN, 1982)[7]; as the kinin-
kininase system contributes, together with the prostaglandin system, to
the physiologic adaptation of neonatal circulation (MELMON, 1968)[8], we
proposed checking the parameters of urinary Kallikrein, Kininase I and
Kininase II (A.C.E.) in drug addict women in pregnancy and puerperium.

MATERIALS AND METHODS

In 13 drug addict (D.A.) women in pregnancy in the 32nd - 40th week
and in 9 D.A. women in puerperium on the 3rd - 4th day after vaginal
eutocic birth, we assessed the quantity of Kallikrein, Kininase I and
Kininase II present in their urine taken during the night, the initial
and final collection hours being noted, so as to obtain a unit expressed
as the quantity of enzymic activity present in 1 ml of urine excreted in
1 hour, hydrolizing a specific substrate in 1 minute (U = nM/min/ml/h).

For some D.A. patients in pregnancy several assessments were made,
so that the total number of urine samples examined was 18; in puerperium,
instead, each assessment corresponded to a single case of drug addiction

(total = 9).   In 9 D.A. women the assessments of urinary Kallikrein,
Kininase I and II were made both in the last weeks of pregnancy and the
first days of puerperium.

All the D.A. patients were under treatment with methadone orally or
intramuscularly, according to a detoxication program carried out in
hospital.

The control cases (13 women in the 36th – 40th week of pregnancy, 22
puerperae on the 3rd – 4th day after vaginal eutocic birth) were free
from hypertensive and haemovascular pathologies, like all the D.A.
patients.

Urinary Kallikrein was ascertained by Morita's method (1977)[9].

Urinary Kininase I and II (A.C.E.) were ascertained by Porcelli's
method (1987)[10].

RESULTS AND CONCLUSIONS

As is shown in figures 1, 2 and 3, the average urinary excretion
value of Kallikrein and Kininase I in pregnancy is higher in the D.A.
women than in the controls, whereas the value of Kininase II in D.A.
women almost coincides with that of the controls. However, the wide
distribution of the single values of Kallikrein and Kininase I does not
make this result statistically significant.

In the D.A. puerperae the average value of Kallikrein and Kininase I
and II is lower than in the controls, even if it is not significant
statistically.

The systemic arterial pressure did not show any changes compared
with the controls both in the drug addict women in pregnancy and in
puerperium, in spite of the above-mentioned changes in the average values
of urinary Kallikrein, Kininase I and Kininase II compared with the
controls.

This result shows that the kinin-kininase system keeps its balance
even under conditions of opioid addiction: in pregnancy, the increase of
Kallikrein is accompanied predominantly by the increase of Kininase I; in
puerperium, the decreased urinary excretion of Kallikrein is accompanied
by a contemporary decrease of both (I and II) urinary Kininases.

The change of urinary excretion of Kallikrein, Kininase I and II in
the drug addict women was more evident in the transition from pregnancy
to post-partum. In fact, whereas in the control patients the
distribution of the values of all the above-mentioned activities (the
kininogenase and kininase ones) remained almost unchanged between
pregnancy and puerperium, on the contrary in the D.A. patients a sharp
decrease of the average value was noted in puerperium compared with that
in pregnancy.

In particular, in the D.A. women who were tested both in pregnancy
and the first 3-4 days of puerperium (9 cases: see Table 1), a general
trend towards the decrease of both kininogenase (Kallikrein) and kininase
(Kininase I and II) activities in urine could be noted, with greater
statistic significance in the Kallikrein change (p < 0.0256).

Apparently, this decrease in the activities of the main enzymic
factors of the kinin-kininase system in the urine of the D.A. women in

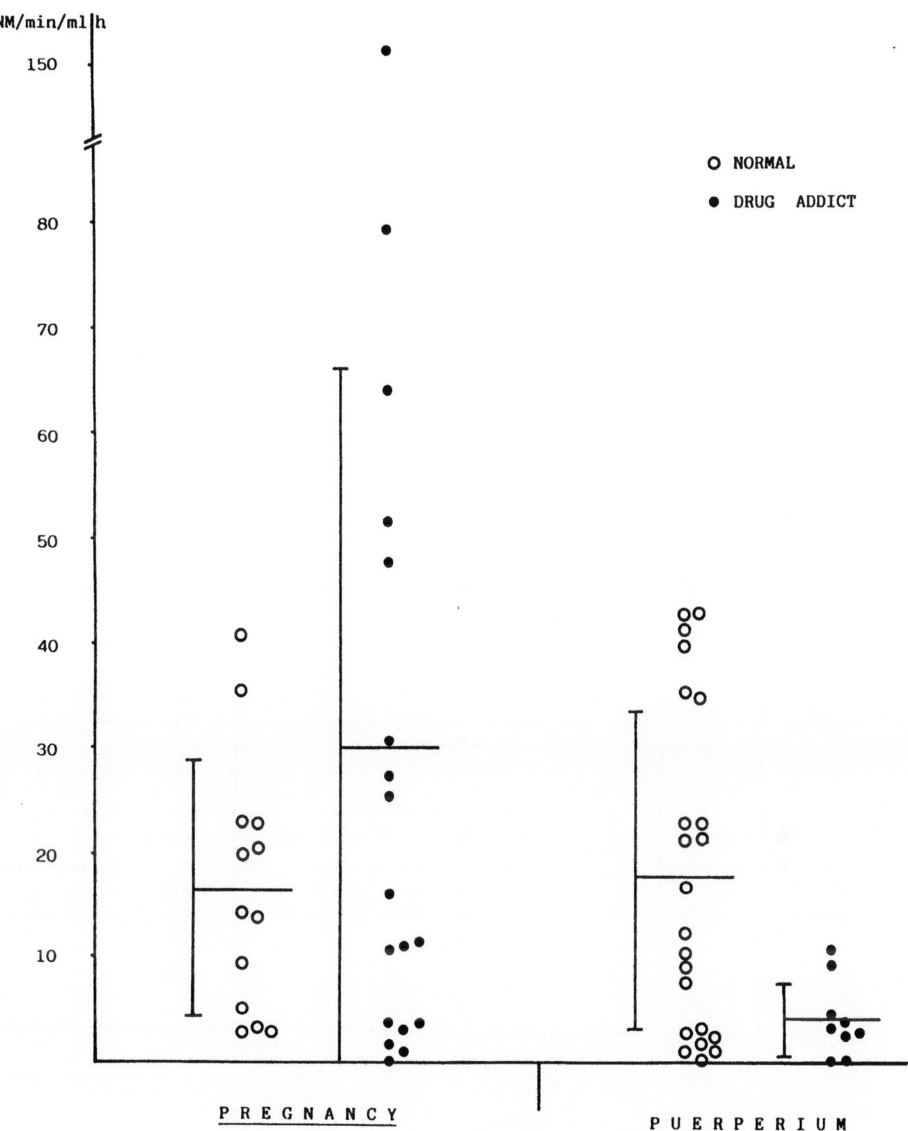

Figure 1. Urinary Kallikrein

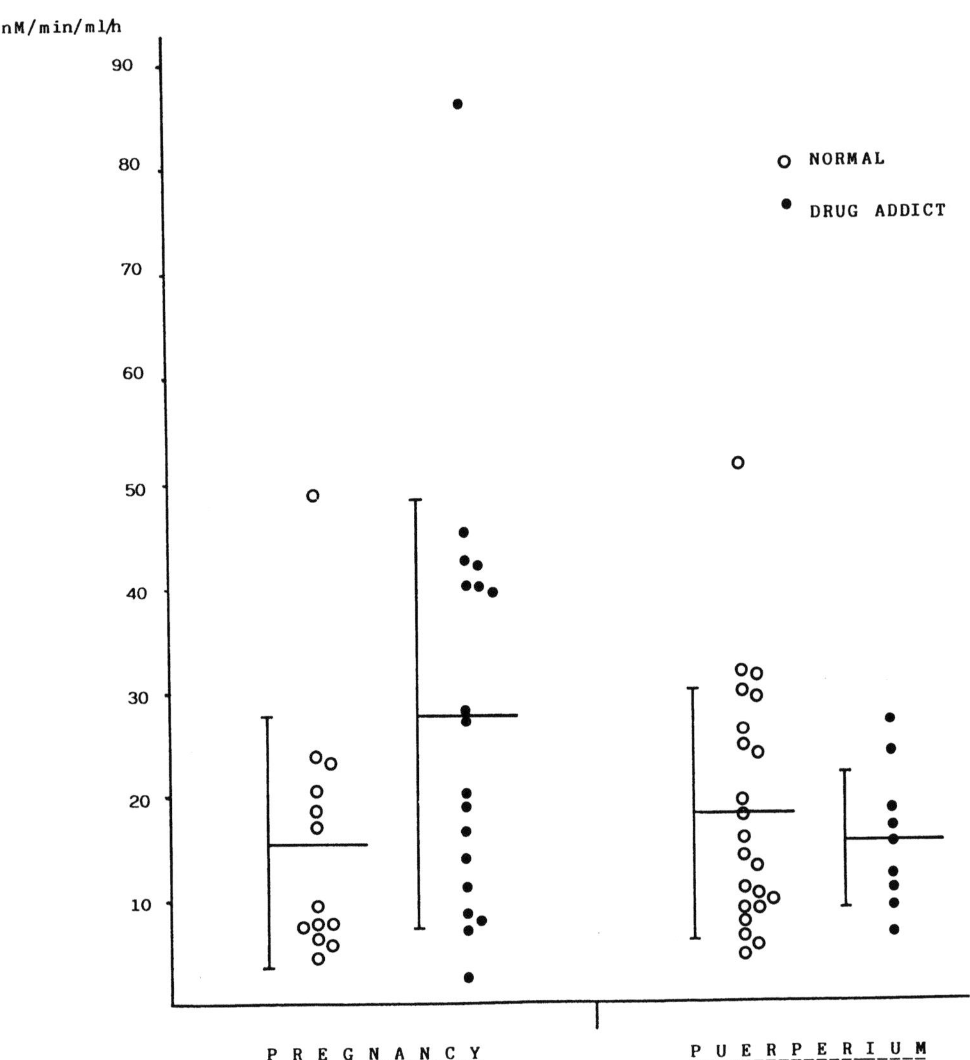

Figure 2. Urinary Kininase I

466

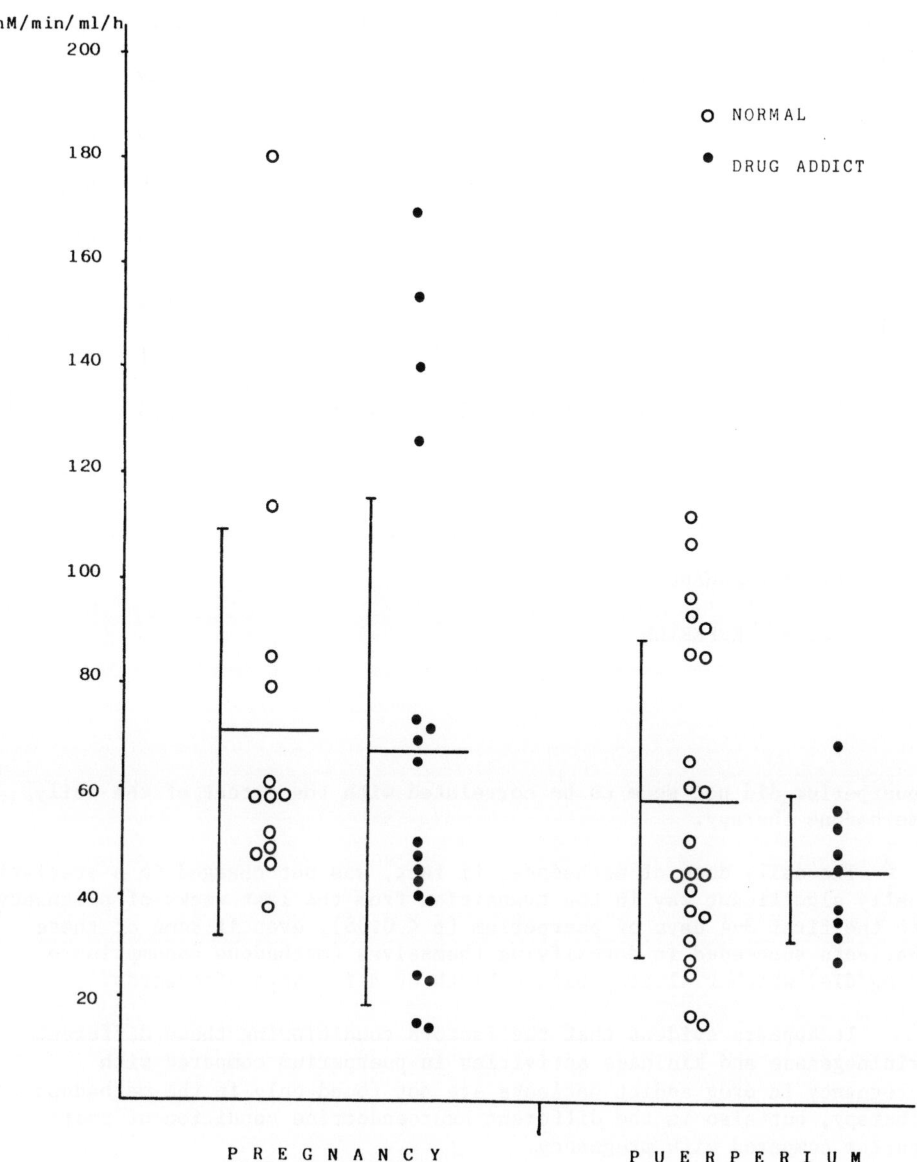

Figure 3. Urinary Kininase II

TAB. 1

CASE N.	Methadone mg/die		KALLIKREIN nM/min/ml/h		KININASE I nM/min/ml/h		KININASE II nM/min/ml/h	
	Pr.	P.	Pr.	P.	Pr.	P.	Pr.	P.
1	40	30	0	4.6	20.1	15.4	65.0	36.0
2	25	15	27.2	0	2.5	16.7	13.9	52.3
3	15	15	63.6	19.5	28.3	208.1	49.6	272.0
4	12	6	79.0	3.2	86.1	18.5	169.8	68.5
5	1	6	51.4	3.2	42.1	18.5	140.0	68.5
6	5	0	10.9	3.5	11.0	9.1	39.3	35.2
7	0	0	15.9	3.5	8.8	9.1	24.1	35.2
8	9	5	10.6	2.8	42.6	23.6	40.6	56.2
9	0	0	3.5	2.6	39.6	6.6	69.1	27.3

Pr. = PREGNANCY

P. = PUERPERIUM

puerperium did not seem to be correlated with the extent of the daily methadone therapy.

The daily dose of methadone, in fact, was not changed in a statistically significant way in the transition from the last weeks of pregnancy to the first 3-4 days of puerperium ($p < 0.08$), even if some of these patients succeeded in detoxifying themselves (methadone assumption = 0 mg/die) whether already before birth or a few days afterwards.

It appears evident that the factors conditioning these different kininogenase and kininase activities in puerperium compared with pregnancy in drug addict patients are not found only in the methadone therapy, but also in the different neuroendocrine condition of postpartum compared with pregnancy.

The study now in progress concerning the kinin-kininase system in the neonatal aspect, and the clinical check of blood pressure values in children of drug addict women may show the possible consequences on them of the changes in the kinin-kininase system which were noted in their drug addict mothers.

REFERENCES

1 - YLITALO P. "Relation of Renin-Angiotensin System to Kallikrein-
    Kinin and Prostaglandin Systems in hypertension".
    Acta Medica Scandinavica (Suppl.), 1983; 677: 36-39.

2 - PORCELLI G., BOTTA B., DI IORIO M., RANIERI M., VOLPE A.R.
    "Kallikrein and Kininase excretion in football players after
    psychophysical stress".
    Kinin '84 Savannah - International Congress, Oct. 21-25, 1984,
    (abstract on page 107).

3 - SCICLI A.G., FORBES G., NOLLY H., DUJOVNY M., CARRETERO O.A.
    "Kallikrein-Kinins in the central nervous system".
    Clin. and Exper. - Theory and Practice, 1984, A6 (10-11): 1731-1738.

4 - FACCHINETTI F., GRASSO A., PETRAGLIA F., PARRINI D., VOLPE A. and
    GENAZZANI A.R. "Impaired circadian rhythmicity of beta-lipotrophin,
    beta-endorphin and ACTH in Heroin addicts".
    Acta Endocrinologica, 1984, 105: 149-155.

5 - BUCKINGHAM J.C., COOPER T.A. "Differences in hypothalamo-pituitary-
    adrenocortical activity in the rat after acute and prolonged treat-
    ment with morphine".
    Neuroendocrinology, 1984, 38: 411-417.

6 - NOIA G., VIRGOLINO A., ROSATI P., VOLPE A.R., PORCELLI G.,
    BELLATI U. "The Kinin-Kininase System in neuro-endocrine balance of
    drug addict women in pregnancy".
    Psychiatry Research, Vol. 16, No. 4, Special Suppl., 1986/82.

7 - ROSEN T.S., and JOHNSON H.L. "Children of methadone-maintained
    mothers: follow-up to 18 months of age".
    J. Pediatrics, 1982, 101 (2): 192-196.

8 - MELMON K.L., CLINE M.J., HUGHES T., and NIES A.S. "Kinins: possible
    mediators of neonatal circulatory changes in man".
    J. Cl. Investigation, 1968, 47: 1295-1302.

9 - MORITA T., KATO H., IWANAGA S., TAKADA K., KIMURA T. and
    SAKAKIBARA S. "New fluorogenic substrates for alfa-thrombin, factor
    Xa, Kallikreins and urokinase".
    J. Biochem., 82, 1977: 1495-1498.

10 - PORCELLI G., DI IORIO M. and VOLPE A.R. "Determination of kininase I
    and kininase II activities in human urine by high-performance liquid
    chromatography".
    Journal of Chromatography, 1987, 414: 423-428.

KALLIKREIN-KININ SYSTEM IN NEWBORNS OF THE DRUG ADDICTED

E.Salvaggio*, C.Fundarò*, A.M.Falasconi*, A.Parigi*, P.De
Sole⁀, P.Ferrara*, A.R.Volpe⁀, and G.Porcelli⁀

* Department of Pediatrics, ⁀Center of Receptor Chemistry
C.N.R., Department of Chemistry, ⁀Department of Chemical
Chemistry - Catholic University, School of Medicine - Rome
Italy

INTRODUCTION

A lot of experimental and clinical studies have investigated, in the
last year, the interrelations between Kallikrein-Kinin system and hydroelectrolytic balance, etiopathogenesis of hypertension, coagulation mechanisms and physiopathology of diabetes mellitus. Kallikrein releases kinins
from kininogens and is present in the human body as Kallikrein and prekallikrein. The Kininases, proteolitic enzymes that inactive vasoactive Kinins,
are the point of arrive. Actually, we have sophisticated methodics to dose
the components of this system, which allowed to study this system clinically, besides experimentally, also in Pediatrics and in Neonatology[2,4,5,6,7].
Numerous studies showed that perinatal stress causes an activation of Kallikrein-Kinin system. Drug addiction during pregnancy in particular determines
a remarkable level of perinatal stress. It results both from birth-related
stress and from typical addiction-related changes of mother and fetus. The
aim of the present study is to evaluate perinatal activation of K-K system
in newborns of drug addicted mother in order to obtain valuable data on the
degree of perinatal stress in this particular condition.

MATERIALS AND METHODS

The study was performed in 17 newborns (12 males and 5 females) of mothers which abused of heroin and/or methadone during pregnancy, admitted in the
Pediatric Clinic of "Università Cattolica del Sacro Cuore" in Rome. Gestational age ranged from 34 to 42 weeks (mean ± sd: 38.6 ± 2.1). Birth weight
ranged from 1830 to 4100 gms (mean ± sd: 2909 ± 575). 12 mothers were on
methadone at the time of delivery, 4 assumed heroin and 1 had discontinued
heroin more than 3 weeks before delivery.

Table 1. Neonatal data

	FD (n=17) n (%)	CONTROLS (n=31) n (%)
males	12 (70.6)	18 (58.1)
females	5 (29.4)	13 (41.9)
prematures	2 (11.7)	3 (9.7)
cesarean section	6 (35.3)	5 (16.1)
meconium stained amniotic fluid	6 (35.3)	6 (19.3)
Apgar score 7	3 (17.6)	1 (3.2)
weight 2500 gms	4 (23.5)	1 (3.2)
neonatal pathology:		
infections	4 (23.5)	0 (0.0)
hypocalcemia	4 (23.5)	0 (0.0)
jaundice	1 (5.9)	31 (100)
drug withdrawal	15 (88.2)	0 (0.0)

A control group was selected of 31 newborns (18 males and 13 females) born of mothers that used no drug during pregnancy, affected by hyperbilirubinemia and treated with phototherapy and without any other neonatal problem (a previous study has assessed that newborns with jaundice have a normal Kallikrein and Kininase activity) . The gestational age ranged from 34 to 42 weeks (mean ± sd: 39.2 ± 2.7) and birth weight varied from 2480 to 4220 gms (mean ± sd: 3345 ± 425). All the newborns were evaluated for kind of delivery, Agpar score, presence of meconium stained amniotic fluid and neonatal pathology. The newborns of the study group were observed for the detection of symptoms of withdrawal and were treated according to the criteria proposed by L.P. Finnegan. We used methadone as pharmacological agent. Neonatal withdrawal was classified as absent (0), mild (+), moderate (++),severe (+++). Blood pressure was measured during the first week of life. Kallikrein and Kininase I and II dosages were performed on urine collected with sterilized plastic bags during the first week of life and were repeated during the second week of life and later up till the 60th day of life. The samples of urine were than poured into vials containing toluene and stored at +4°C. Urinary

Table 2. Urinary data

days of life	patients	Kallikrein (u) m ± sd	K I (u) m ± sd	K II (u) m ± sd
0 - 7	FD	0.54 ± 0. 8	3.82 ± 3.46	3.15 ± 1.42
	controls	0.23 ± 0. 3	2.03 ± 1.95	4.68 ± 2.71
8 - 14	FD	0.25 ± 0.44	5.51 ± 6.06	6.35 ± 6.71
	controls	0.43 ± 0.44	3.17 ± 3.03	11.53 ± 11.55
> 14	FD	1.24 ± 1. 9	22.33 ± 27.57	6.74 ± 9.46
	controls	0.29 ± 0.23	2.54 ± 4.14	16.08 ± 22.58

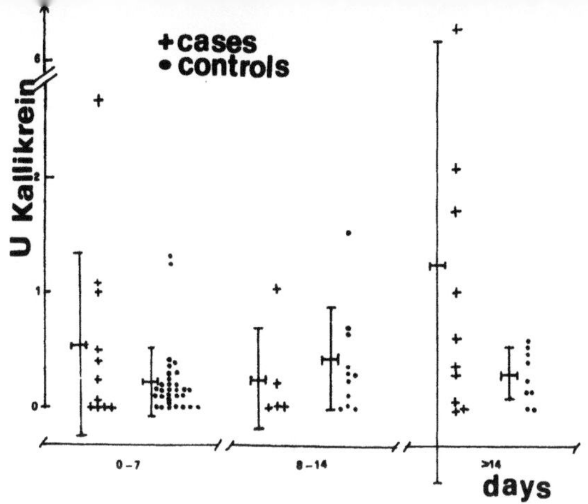

Fig.1. Urinary Kallikrein values of infants of drug
dependent mothers and controls at different ages.

Kallikrein was assayed with Morita et al. method; Kininase I and II were
determined according to Porcelli et al..Kallikrein and Kininase enzyme units
were reported in moles of substrate idrolized per minute of incubation, per
ml of urine and per mg of urinary creatinine[2,3].

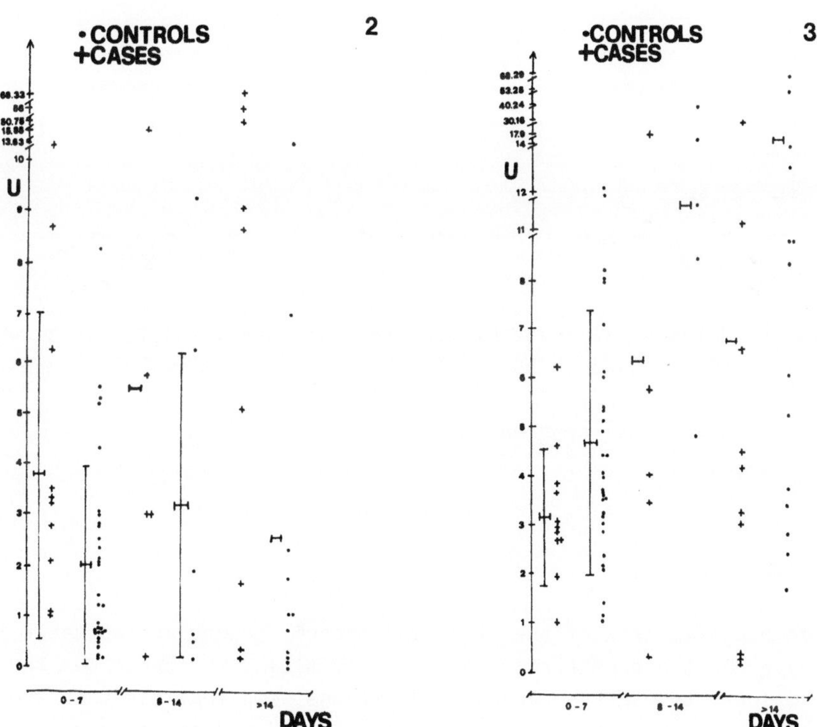

Fig. 2. Urinary Kininase I values of infants of drug dependent mothers and
controls at different ages.
Fig. 3. Urinary Kininase II values of infants of drug dependent mothers and
controls at different ages.

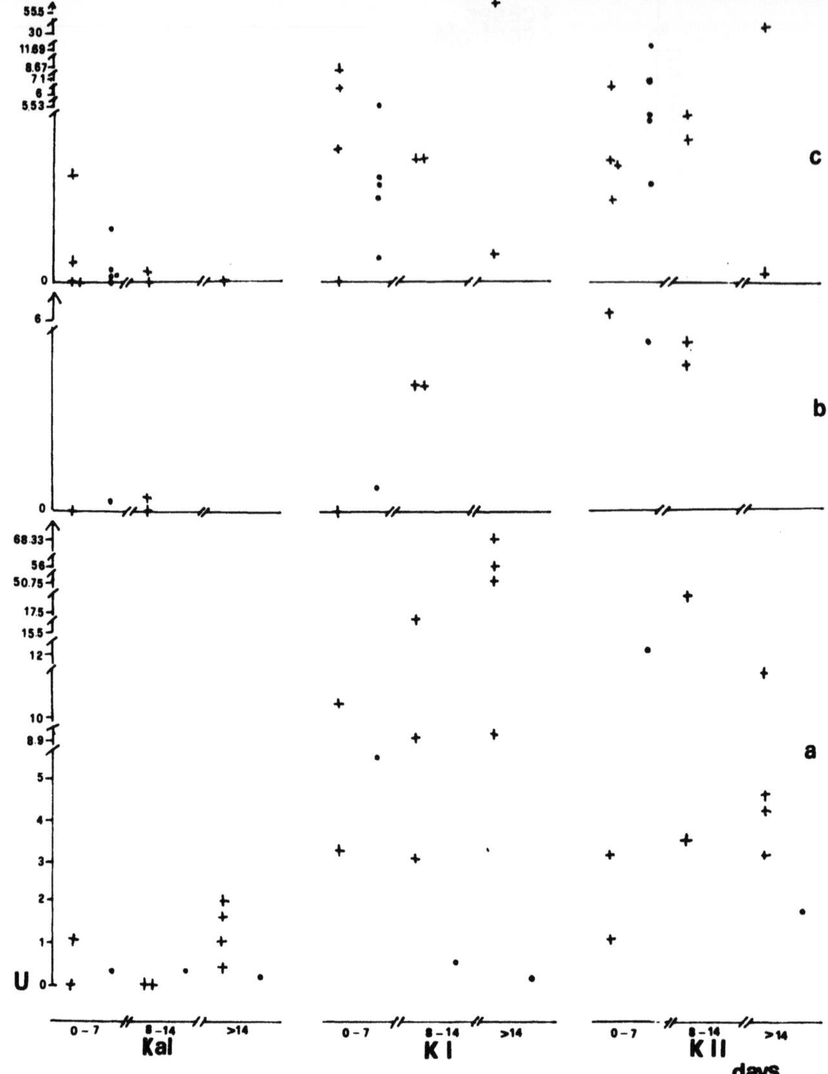

Fig. 4. Urinary values of Kallikrein, Kininase I and II, at different ages in babies (controls and cases) with: a) neonatal weight lower than 2500 gms; b) Apgar score lower than 7; c) cesarean section.

RESULTS AND DISCUSSION

Some neonatal data of the study and control groups are on table 1. In the study group the prematurity rate is only slightly greater but the birth weight is lower and the percentage of newborns weighing less than 2500 gms is noticeably higher than in the control group. Perinatal stress was much more frequent than in controls: cesarean section was performed in 35.3% cases to prevent or remove fetal suffering; in 35.3% meconium stained amniotic fluid was observed; the Apgar score was less than 7 in 17.6% of the babies; 23.5% of cases were affected by neonatal infections and 23.5% by metabolic disorders. 88.2% of "passively addicted" newborns had symptoms of withdrawal: 6

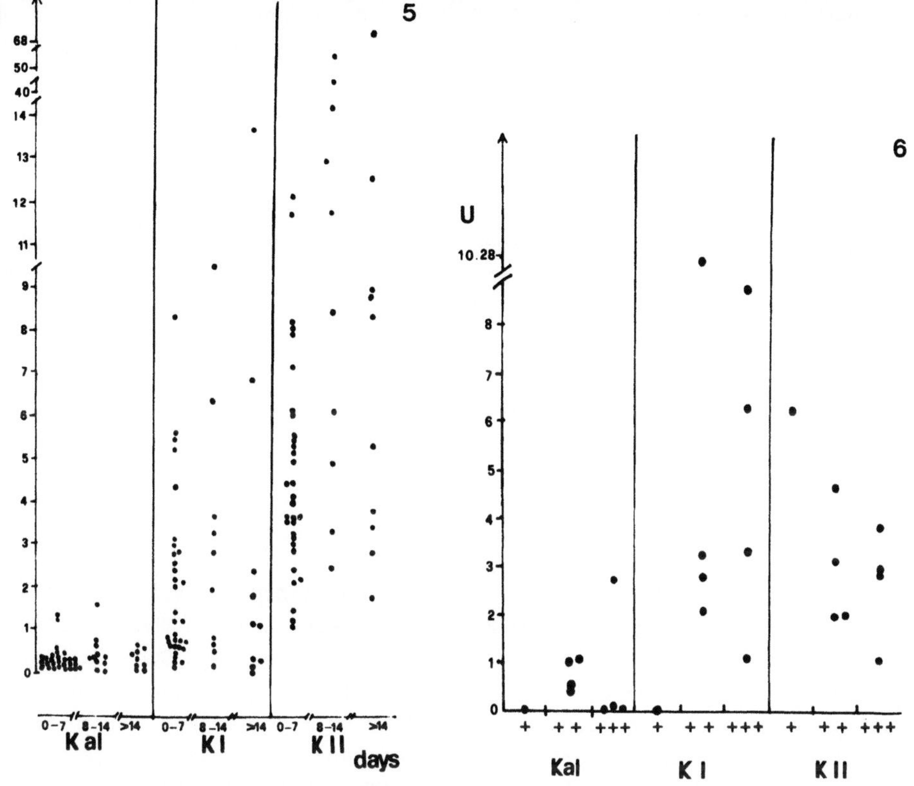

Fig. 5. Urinary values of Kallikrein, Kininase I and II of control infants
at different ages.
Fig. 6. Urinary values of Kallikrein, Kininase I and II of infants from drug
dependent mothers affected by neonatal withdrawal of different severity: + = mild; ++ = moderate; +++ = severe.

babies severe, 8 moderate, and 1 mild; all the babies had symptoms related
to the central nervous system, 9 had also autonomous nervous system signs and
12 gastroenteric symptomatology. In 14 cases pharmacologic treatment was necessary and methadone was administered at dosage of 0.1-0.36 mg/kg/die. The
evaluation of blood pressure revealed higher values in some newborns of drug
dependent mothers but the difference between the two groups of babies was not
relevant. Kallikrein and Kininase I and II urinary data of study group and
control group are illustrated in table 2, figures 1,2 and 3, divided in 3
groups for the day of urine collection. No urinary Kallikrein activity was
found in 36.3% of "passively addicted" newborns, versus 19.3% of controls
during the first week of life and in 40% versus 20% during the second week.
The data of the study group drew near to controls (22% vs 20.2%) after the
second week of life. The absolute values of Kallikrein, particularly in the
study group, varied in a wide range and an exact evaluation of our results
was impossible since we had few cases.

All samples but one had a greater or minor activity of Kininases I and
II. The evaluation of the excretion at different ages showed that Kininase I
increased in 40%, reduced in 40% and was unchanged in 20% of controls. In the
study group we observed a decrease in 1 case and an increase in 5. In 2 patient a noticeable decrease was evident after a second month of life. Mean
values of Kininase II were greater in controls, but the range was very large.
The follow-up of urinary excretion of this enzyme in 6 children of drug depen-

dent mothers showed a decrease in 2 of them and an increase in 4, during the
period of observation. In the control group the excretion increased in 55.5%,
decreased in 11.1% and had no variation in 33.3% during the second week.
Afterwards there was a decrease in 60% and an increase in 40%. Figure 4 shows
the data of two subgroups of newborns (drug addicted mothers and controls),
omogeneous regarding conditions of perinatal stress (weight 2500 gms, Apgar
index 7 and operative delivery) which alone can activate K-K system. They seem
to negate a direct correlation between drug addiction and activation of K-K
system, as no significative difference of urinary K-K leves was found. Even
perinatal stress related to neonatal drug withdrawal has no influence on K-K
system; data in fig. 5 and 6 show no significative difference in perinatal
urinary K-K levels between control group and newborns of drug addicted mothers who presented neonatal withdrawal. Moreover no correlations are found
with severity of symptomatology.

CONCLUSIONS

The evaluation of the urinary Kallikrein and Kininase excretion in a
group of newborns of drug dependent mothers suggests that in these babies
there is an activation of the system in the neonatal period. Such an activation seems to persist over a longer period of time in comparison with a group
of healthy newborns. We could hypothesize that this activation is correlated
to perinatal stress, and in particular to the rapid decrease of exogenous
opiates hematic level in neonatal blood and then to the symptomatology of
neonatal drug withdrawal. Nevertheless, it is necessary to extend the study
to a larger group of babies to achieve definitive conclusions.

REFERENCES

1. M. Mazzetti, G. Porcelli, C. Fundarò, M. Valente, A.R. Volpe, E. Salvaggio,
   1985, Kallikrein and Kininase activities excretion in newborns affected by
   jaundice, in "Abstracts Kinins 84", Savannah, Georgia, USA, page 87.
2. T. Morita, H. Kato, S. Iwanaga, 1977, Kallikrein activity determined by
   fluorimetric method, J. Biochem., 82: 1495.
3. G. Porcelli, M. Di Iorio, A.R. Volpe, 1987, Determination of Kininase II
   activities in human urine in high-performance liquid chromatography, J.
   Chromatography, 414: 423.
4. J.E. Robillard, et al., 1982, Development aspect of renal Kallikrein-like
   activity in fetal and newborns lambs, Kidney International, 22 : 594.
5. J.E. Robillard et al., 1985, Effects of aldosterone on urinary Kallikrein
   and sodium excretion during fetal life, Pediatrics Research, 10 : 1048.
6. G. Tortorolo, G. Porcelli, P. Curatolo, 1976, Urinary Kallikrein in pre-
   mature, small at term, normal newborns and in children. Chemistry and
   biology of the Kallikrein-Kinin system in health and disease, in "Fogarty
   International Center Proceedings", n.27, US Government Printing Office,
   433.
7. S. Zinner, H. Margolius, 1978, Stability of blood pressure rank and urinary Kallikrein concentration in childhood: an eight-year follow up,
   Circulation, 58.

PHYSIOLOGIC ROLE OF THE PERIPHERAL ENKEPHALINERGIC SYSTEM IN REGULATING CARDIOVASCULAR HOMEOSTASIS: EVIDENCE OF INTERACTIONS WITH THE RENIN--ANGIOTENSIN AND KALLIKREIN-KININ SYSTEMS

M. Carmignani[1,3], G. Porcelli[2], A.R. Volpe[1,2] and P. Preziosi[1]

Depts. of Pharmacology[1] and Chemistry[2], Center of Receptors Chemistry C.N.R.[2], Catholic University, School of Medicine Rome, Italy, and Dept. of Cell Biology and Physiology [3] University of L'Aquila, Italy

SUMMARY

On isolated heart preparation, it was found that Leu^5-Enkephalin (Leu^5-ENK) did not influence the cardiac function. On the other hand, Leu^5-ENK induced a specific dose - related inhibition, in the cardiac perfusate, of the activities of kininase II (KII) and angiotensin converting enzyme (ACE) (but not of kininase I-KI). Instead no detectable alterations of the above enzymatic activities with the used concentrations of Leu^5-ENK were observed in vitro.
This opioid also increased specifically the effects induced by some of the autacoids, related to both renin-angiotensin and kallikrein-kinin systems, on the KII and ACE activities. A specific correlation between these Leu^5--ENK -induced modifications and the functional responses of the heart to the same autacoids was observed.
Naloxone (NAL) and more significantly ICI 174864 (ICI) opposed or reversed the inhibitory effect of the used opioid whereas they had neither inhibitory nor synergic effect on both KII and ACE activity by themselves.
The possible physiologic role of the enkephalins in regulating cardiovascular function by acting peripherally on some humoral systems through modulatory mechanism was discussed.

INTRODUCTION

Opioid peptides such as leucine- and methionine- enkephalins have been reported to produce changes in systems blood pressure and heart rate[1,2,3,4,5,6].
Most of effects on cardiovascular response to these peptides are thought to involve actions mediated through the central nervous systems[1,3,5,6] or to result from stimulation of central opioid receptors[1,4,5,6]. In addition, opioid peptides appear to exert some direct actions on

peripheral tissues[2,7,8,10] and opiate receptors are distributed also in peripheral sites[2,9].
There are few reports of a direct cardiac action of these opioids[5]. But, enkephalins of sympathetic origin have been shown to be present in the heart[11]; moreover, these enkephalins may interact at the level of humoral systems, relevant for the cardiovascular regulation, characterized in cardiac tissue [12]. In this regard, various correlations seem to exist between enkephalinergic system and renin-angiotensin and kallikrein-kinin ones. There is evidence that ACE cleaves the Gly^3-Phe^4 amide bond of both (Leu/Met)^5-ENKs[13] although the physiologic specificity of this effect has been questioned[14].
KI cleaves (Arg/Lys)^6-ENKs most rapidly than all specific substrates, so modulating the action of these peptides which bind in native form k receptors while in des-(Arg/Lys)^6 form δ and μ ones [15,16]. Captopril, a specific inhibitor of ACE , also inhibits enkephalinase, a carboxypeptidase involved in the catabolism of endogenous opioids[17] and enhances the effects of the enkephalins in vivo[18]. Moreover, opioid peptides have been shown to influence the activity of brain and lung ACE[19].
On the whole, these data provided a tool to evaluate if the cardiovascular function may be regulated by peripheral actions of modulation of enkephalins on some humoral systems, mediated or not by opiate receptors.

MATERIALS AND METHODS

Perfusion   procedure

    Male Wistar rats of 250-300 g b.w. were stunned by a blow on the head and killed by cervical dislocation. The heart was removed, vertically mounted in a double walled chamber and perfused at 37° C from two reservoirs in a non-recirculating system at constant pressure (38 cm H_2O) according to the Langendorff technique. The perfusion medium, equilibrated with 95% O_2-5% CO_2, pH 7.40, was Krebs-Henselait buffer consisting of 120 mM NaCl, 20 mM $NaHCO_3$, 4.63 mM KCl, 1.17 mM KH_2PO_4, 2.5 mM $CaCl_2$, 1.20 mM $MgCl_2$ and 8 mM glucose. Myocardial contractility was measured by connecting the apex of the heart to an isometric transducer and a d.c. amplifier. Heart rate was obtained by a cardiotachometer coupler triggered by the R-peak of the Lead II epicardiogram. Coronary outflow was measured with a photoelectric drop counter connected to a Beckman type RM Dynograph recorder. The venous affluent was collected to determining the enzymatic activities according to experimental design (see Results). The tested substances were dissolved in the perfusion buffer and administered at a constant rate into the aortic cannula in a 0.2 ml-volume. In some experiments the perfusion medium contained Leu^5-ENK (10^{-8} M). Cumulative dose-responses curves for the various substances were obtained preliminarly in order to assess the concentration ranges to be used. All chemicals and drugs were of higher available purity.

Enzymatic assay

    Hip-Phe-Arg was synthetized from Hip-Phe (Serva, Heidelberger, F.R.G.) and Arg HCl (Merck, Darmastadt, F.R.G.)[20]. Hip-His-Leu was obtained from Serva, AG-50W-X8 from Bio-Rad Labs. (Richmond, CA, U.S.A.). Other chemicals were purchased from Fluka (Buchs, Switzerland).
Bio-Rad Model 1330 pump, a Rheodyne injection valve fitted with a 200-μl loop and a Bio-Rad Model 1306 UV monitor were used to perform

the analyses. An analitical column (25 x 0.4 cm I.D.) packed with 5-μm ODS2 (Violet, Rome, Italy) was employed with a mobil phase of acetonitrile-aqueous sulphuric acid (pH 3.0) (1/1, v/v) and a flow-rate of 1.5 ml/min. Chromatographic peaks were traced on a Leeds and Northrup Speedomax Recorder (C. Erba, Milan, Italy) (chart speed 12 cm/h).
Amounts of Bz-Gly and Hip-Phe were evaluated from the peak heights measured at 230 nm.
Enzymatic activities were determined according to Porcelli et al.[21]. The in vitro experiments were performed on the cardiac perfusate with Leu[5]-ENK added in medium either before or after dialysis. The unit of the activity was defined as that amount of KI, KII and ACE which hydrolized 1 μmole of Hip-Phe-Arg and Hip-His-Leu, respectively, per minute of incubation and per millilitre of perfusate.

RESULTS

Table I shows the results obtained with a representative concentration of the used substances. The different concentrations ($10^{-11}/10^{-3}$ M) of the Leu[5]-ENK brought about a dose-dependent decrease of KII activity and mostly of ACE one. No alterations of KI activity with the used concentrations of Leu[5]-ENK were observed. The above enzymatic activities were not inhibited in vitro by 10^{-6}, 10^{-5}, 10^{-4} M concentrations of Leu[5]-ENK in the medium.
The inhibitory effects of Leu[5]-ENK (10^{-8} M) appeared to be decreased not significantly by its combination with NAL ($10^{-7}/10^{-3}$ M). But ICI ($10^{-11}/10^{-5}$ M) completely antagonized the inhibition of Leu[5]-ENK (10^{-8} M). However, neither NAL nor ICI had effects on studied enzymatic activities by themselves.
Angiotensin I (AI; $10^{-12}/10^{-6}$ M) induced a more significant dose-related inhibition of ACE activity, increased by concomitant administration of Leu[5]-ENK (10^{-8} M).
So Bradykinin (BK; $10^{-12}/10^{-5}$ M) modified specifically the KII activity; further significant decrease of this activity was observed when Leu[5]-ENK (10^{-8} M) was given together.
Instead Angiotensin II (AII; $10^{-12}/10^{-6}$ M) influenced none of the studied enzymatic activities.
No significant changes of the cardiac functional indices were observed.

CONCLUSIONS

No significant changes of cardiac function were observed at physiological concentrations of Leu[5]-ENK. These data seem to support the possibility of an extracardiac mechanism in mediating the cardiovascular action of Leu[5]-ENK. But the considerable amount of (Leu/Met)[5]-ENKs present in the heart[11] suggests involvment of cardiac sites in the action of opioid peptides. Moreover, our findings demonstrate that the effects of Leu[5]-ENK on the heart may be brought about by its actions on some humoral systems through modulatory mechanism. The ACE activity appeared to be inhibited specifically and significantly by Leu[5]-ENK. But no detectable hydrolysis by ACE occured in vitro as long as the Leu[5]-ENK concentration was kept below 10^{-4} M so indicating that the partecipation of this enzyme to the physiological inactivation of endogenous enkephalins is unlike.This physiological specificity has just been questioned[14]. So Captopril could inhibit ACE through the observed inactivation of enkephalinase [17] and increase of the actions of enkephalins[18]. No alterations of KI activity

Table 1. Enzymatic and functional results obtained with a representative concentration of each tested substance.

	KININASE II (% change)[#]	AI-CONVERTING ENZYME (% change)[#]	MYOCARDIAL CONTRACTILITY (% change)[#]	CORONARIC OUTFLOW (% change)[#]	HEART RATE (% change)[#]
LEU^5-ENK(10^{-3} M)	-94.9±1.3	-97.1±0.7	-38.0±0.7	-57.5±5.8	+1.7±0.2
AI (10^{-6} M)	-12.3±1.1	-29.4±1.3	-12.2±4.6	-23.5±8.5	-5.2±2.3
LEU^5-ENK(10^{-8} M)	-39.8±1.0	-59.7±0.4	-14.5±5.1	-28.7±4.7	-3.5±0.9
AI + LEU^5-ENK	-58.6±7.3*	-94.8±0.8*	-58.7±7.3*	-43.5±3.5*	-5.0±1.0*
AII (10^{-6} M)	0.0	0.0	-21.2±5.6	-26.7±6.2	-6.5±2.1
LEU^5-ENK(10^{-8} M)	-42.0±3.4	-61.2±1.9	-12.5±0.7	-19.5±3.5	-4.2±1.3
AII + LEU^5-ENK	-43.5±3.6	-61.2±1.6	-30.4±4.7	-29.5±7.9	-12.5±5.5
BK (10^{-6} M)	-32.9±1.0	-13.1±0.4	-4.2±1.0	+2.2±1.7	+3.8±1.1
LEU^5-ENK(10^{-8} M)	-42.9±1.9	-60.7±0.6	-11.5±2.9	-20.6±4.2	-5.3±1.7
BK + LEU^5-ENK	-92.6±1.5*	-81.8±0.8*	-22.5±3.4*	-33.8±3.1*	+9.4±2.7*
NAL (10^{-3} M)	0.0	0.0	+3.7±1.8	+5.5±0.9	-2.9±1.9
LEU^5-ENK(10^{-8} M)	-41.1±1.3	-60.8±1.1	-2.4±1.1	-1.5±1.2	-1.1±0.6
NAL + LEU^5-ENK	-19.2±1.8*	-20.5±2.1*	+2.5±1.9*	+5.8±1.3*	-2.0±1.7*
ICI 174864 (10^{-5} M)	0.0	0.0	-7.9±2.9	-9.5±3.8	+2.1±1.8
LEU^5-ENK(10^{-8} M)	-41.3±0.8	-60.6±0.5	-21.7±4.8	-26.1±7.2	-2.7±2.1
ICI + LEU^5-ENK	-0.8±1.1*	0.0*	-6.0±1.4*	-9.6±3.2*	+3.3±0.8*

All values are mean ± S.D.
* P < 0.05 (NAL + LEU^5-ENK and ICI + LEU^5-ENK were compared with LEU^5-ENK)
# % change of the values preceding the drug administration

were observed.In fact,KI cleaves (Lys/Arg)^6-ENKs more rapidly than all specific substrates[15,16]. Many peptides hormones are now known to be synthetized as larger precursor molecule from which the mature peptide can be removed by a carboxypeptidase. KI could then act to remove C-terminal Arg or Lys so activing (Leu/Met)^5-ENKs. Besides, Leu^5-ENK increased the effects induced by AI and BK on the studied enzymatic activities. The specific correlation between these Leu^5-ENK-induced modifications and the functional responses of the heart to the same autacoids provided further evidence that the cardiovascular function may be regulate by action of modulation of enkephalins on some humoral systems. If these effects are mediated by opiate receptors is disputable. In fact, although NAL and more significantly ICI antagonized the inhibitory effects of Leu^5-ENK, they had no effects by themselves. Moreover, at the used physiological concentrations of Leu^5-ENK, it wasn't found a dose-related response of functional parameters.

REFERENCES

1. J. Floretz, A. Mediavilla. Brain Res.,138,585 (1977)
2. J. Hughes, H.W. Kosterlitz, T.W. Smith. Br. J. Pharmacol.,61,639 (1977)
3. M.A. Petty, W. De Jong. Eur.,J. Pharmacol.,81,449 (1982)
4. E.T. Wei, A. Lee, J.K. Chang. Life Sci.,26,1517 (1980)
5. S. Koyama, N. Terada, Y. Shiojima et al. Jpn. J. Physiol.,34,351 (1984)
6. K. Schaz, G. Stock, W. Simmon et al. Hypertension,2,397 (1980)
7. J. Knoll. Eur. J. Pharmacol.,39,403 (1976)
8. M. Benuck, M.J. Berg, N. Marks. Life Sci.,28,2643 (1981)
9. R. Simantov, S.R. Childers, S.H. Snyder. Mol. Pharmacol.,14,69 (1978)
10. S. Koyama, H. Hosomi. Am J. Physiol.,250,R973 (1986)
11. R.E. Lang, K. Hermann, R. Dietze et al. Life Sci.,32,399 (1983)
12. M.A. Cicilini, H. Caldo, J.D. Berti et al. Biochem. Pharmacol.,27,843 (1978)
13. E.G. Erdös, A.R. Johnson, N.T. Boyden. Biochem. Pharmacol.,27,843 (1978)
14. J. Schwartz, B. Malfroy, S. De La Baume. Life Sci.,29,1715 (1981)
15. A. Skidgel, A.R. Johnson, E.G. Erdös. Biochem. Pharmacol.,33,3471 (1984)
16. J. Magnan, J.S. Paterson, H.W. Kosterlitz. Life Sci.,31,1359 (1982)
17. A. Arregiu, C.M. Lee, P.C. Emson et al. Eur. J. Pharmacol.,59,141 (1979)
18. R. Di Nicolantonio, J.S. Hutchison, J.S. Takata et al. Br. J. Pharmacol.,80,405 (1983)
19. H. Koyuncuoglu, N. Enginar, I. Hatipoglu. Pharmacol. Res. Comm.,18,301, (1986)
20. G. Porcelli, M. Di Iorio M., M. Ranieri, A.R. Volpe. Il Farmaco,12,432 (1985)
21. G. Porcelli, M. Di Iorio, A.R. Volpe. J. Chromatogr.,414,427 (1987)

UTILIZATION OF KININASE ACTIVITIES AS INDICATORS OF MALIGNANT
DISEASE

A. Amato, L. De Giovanni, A.R. Volpe(*), A. Butti
and G. Porcelli(*)

Departments of Surgical Clinic and Chemistry (*)
Catholic University School of Medicine, Via P.
Sacchetti 664, 00168 Roma, Italy

Since many years, the plasmatic activities of the kininases
have been used to detect the onset or to monitor the evolution
of many diseases, both in the field of congenital errors of
metabolism, in inflamatory pathologies and in neoplasms.

Recently many researchers have underlined the role played by
the Kininase II (which is identical in structure to the
Angiotensin I Converting Enzyme) in the field of tumors. This
enzyme, in fact, has been significantly related to the presence
of malignancies as lymphomas and other white blood cell tumors,
lung primary carcinomas, liver and lung metastases from various
tumors, renal carcinomas (1-4). But, among the various neoplasms
analised, the gastric and colonic carcinomas were not still
included in this investigation, so this study was undertaken to
evaluate the role of the Kininase I (KI), Kininase II (KII) and
Phe-Arg Aminopeptidase (AP), which is an aspecific Kininase,
also for the most important gastrointestinal neoplasms. Twelve
patients with gastric and 16 patients with colonic carcinoma
(M/F ratio=1, stratified in different TNM classes) plus 20
normal subjects have been analised in this series. KI, KII and
AP activities have been tested on the citrated plasma obtained
from the sample population according to Porcelli's method (by
high performance liquid chromatography -5-). The blood samples
were obtained after 24 hours of absolute rest conditions and
then centrifuged. None of the patients had received drugs able
to modify the system reaction in the previous three weeks (4);
clinical and common laboratory findings were recorded for each
patient.

Statistical analysis included analysis of variance, T-test
for unpaired samples and linear/esponential regression test.

Our results showed no correlation among age, sex or common
lab values and the variables under investigation, and this is in
accordance with recently published series (2,4). The analysis of
variance has indicated that there is a lower mean KII level in
gastric and colonic carcinomas when compared to controls
(p<0.01, tab.1), present since the early stages of the diseases
(TNM stage I-II, p< 0.01, tab.2). No difference could be
detected between the two different tumors.

KI activity has showed statistically significant values only in advanced stages (T-test p<0.01, tab.2) and, like before, no difference between the gastric annd colonic tumors. AP has showed no significance at all, both in early and advanced stages.

tab.1

	Controls	Gastric Ca.	Colonic Ca.	F	p<
KII	13.2 ± 2.7	8.7 ± 2.6	6.8 ± 2.2	13.8	0.01

tab.2

	Controls	Patients	T	p<
KI (st.I-II)	9.6 ± 1.2	11.7 ± 3.5	1.44	N.S.
(st.III-IV)		12.5 ± 2.9	2.29	0.05
KII (st. I-II)	13.2 ± 2.1	6.7 ± 2.5	4.83	0.01
(st.III-IV)		8.8 ± 1.2	3.26	0.01

From this series it seems that KII activity has both an early and advanced imbalance in malignant intestinal diseases, therefore it can be used as a possible marker, besides the other commonly used ones. On the other hand, KI shows mostly a delayed activation, which is probably involved in its tissular activity related to the immune responses; hence its modifications could reveal the occurance of local or distant metastases and/or the presence of an infiltrating primary tumor.

Larger series are needed to further investigate the problem.

REFERENCES
- Scheweisfurth H., Brugger H., Mainwald L."The value of angiotensin I converting Enzyme in malignant and other diseases". Clin Physiol Biochem 3:184, 1985.
- Takada Y., Hiwada K. et Al."Angiotensin Converting enzyme: A possible histologic indicator for human renal cell carcinoma". Cancer 56:130, 1985.
- Mansfield C.M."Angiotensin I Converting Enzyme in cancer patients". J. Clin. Oncol. 2(5):452, 1984.
- Leuenberger P."Angiotensin Converting Enzyme in health and disease". Curr. Probl. Clin. Bioch. 13:99, 1983.
- Porcelli G. et Al."Preliminary study on Hypp-Phe-Arg substrate for human Kininase assay". Farmaco 40(12):432, 1985.

ROLE OF ENDOGENOUS VASODILATOR PROSTAGLANDINS IN THE PROLIFERATION OF
VASCULAR SMOOTH MUSCLE CELLS OF SPONTANEOUSLY HYPERTENSIVE RATS

Toshihiko Ishimitsu, Yoshio Uehara, [*]Masao Ishii and Tsuneaki Sugimoto

The 2nd Department of Internal Medicine, University of Tokyo Tokyo 113, Japan
[*]The 2nd Department of Internal Medicine, Yokohama City University, Yokohama 232, Japan

It is known that spontaneously hypertensive rats (SHR) exhibit a thickening of the vascular wall in the prehypertensive stage (1), and that the vascular smooth muscle cells (VSMC) have an increased proliferative activity (2) as compared to those of normotensive Wistar-Kyoto strain (WKY). Some humoral, neural, and mechanical factors are assumed to be responsible for the rapid VSMC growth. However, since the VSMC of SHR sustain an enhanced proliferative activiy even if they are cultured in an artificial medium, it is conceivable that the thickening of the vascular wall is related to alterations of the biological properties in VSMC.

On the other hand, the vascular wall is able to produce various prostaglandins (PG), e.g. prostacyclin (PGI_2), PGE_2 and $PGF_{2\alpha}$. Moreover, there is much evidence that exogenous PG exert an influence on the growth of VSMC (3). Thus, it seems possible that vascular PG system to some extent participates in the regulation of cell proliferation.

In this study, we investigated the roles of endogenously-produced vasodilator PG in the rapid proliferation of VSMC of SHR.

Firstly, we measured the production of PG by VSMC. VSMC were isolated from the aortas of 7-week-old SHR and WKY, and cultured according to the explant method of Ross (4). The cells were incubated in a Dulbecco's phosphate-buffered saline solution (pH 7.4) at 37°C for 1 hour with or without 10^{-6} M arachidonic acid (AA). The released PG were directly radioimmunoassayed (5).

The major metabolite of AA by VSMC was PGI_2. The basal PGI_2 production was increased in the VSMC of SHR as compared to those of WKY at the first (+43% , p<0.03) and the second passage (+34% , p<0.05). After the fourth passage, however, the VSMC of SHR generated a significantly lowered PGI_2 when compared to those of WKY (-23% for the fourth passage , p<0.025; -45% for the tenth passage , p<0.005). Similarly, when the cells were stimulated by 10^{-6}M AA, the productions of vasodilator PG by the VSMC of SHR were increased at the first passage as compared to those of WKY, whereas they were decreased at the sixth passage (Figure 1). These results suggest that the VSMC of SHR exhibit decreased productions of vasodilator PG after the fourth passage.

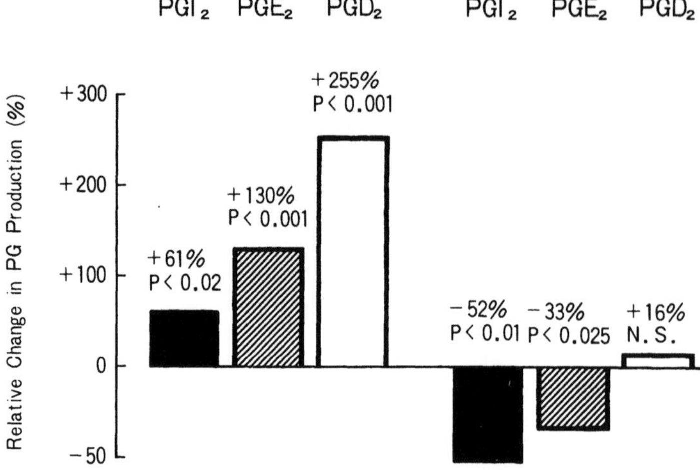

Figure 1. Production of vasodilator PGs potentiated by arachidonic acid (10^{-6}M) in cultured vascular smooth muscle cells of SHR when compared with those of WKY.

Secondly, we examined the proliferative activity of VSMC. The cell growth was evaluated by calculating the doubling time of cell number and measuring the incorporation of (^{3}H)thymidine into deoxyribonucleic acid (DNA). Although the doubling times of VSMC did not differ between the two strains at the second passage, the VSMC of SHR possessed a significantly shorter doubling time than those of WKY after the fourth passage (-24% for the fourth passage, p<0.002 ; -32% for the tenth passage, p<0.02). With regard to the synthesis of DNA, the VSMC of SHR incorporated a larger amount of (^{3}H)thymidine than those of WKY at the fifth (+56% , p<0.02) or the tenth (+24% , p<0.03) passage. Consequently, it is indicated that the VSMC of SHR possess a significantly enhanced proliferative activity as compared to WKY.

Next, to assess the roles of vasodilator PG in the proliferation of VSMC, we examined the effects of exogenous and endogenous vasodilator PG on the proliferation of VSMC of SHR and WKY. Vasodilator PG such as PGI_2 analog (OP-41483), PGE_2 and PGD_2 dose-dependently supressed the incorporation of (^{3}H)thymidine into the VSMC of both of the strains. Percent changes of thymidine uptake by the VSMC of SHR and WKY, when stimulated by 10^{-5}M vasodilator PG, are presented in Table 1.

When the endogenous production of PG were potentiated by 10^{-5}M AA), the (^{3}H)thymidine uptake by VSMC was significantly suppressed in WKY although it was not changed in SHR (Table 2). On the other hand, when the PG system was inhibited by 10^{-5}M indomethacin (IDM), the incorporation of (^{3}H)thymidine into DNA was enhanced in the VSMC of SHR while it was not altered in those of WKY. Our observations clearly demonstrate that vasodilator PG inhibit the proliferative activity of VSMC in culture, and that the VSMC of SHR is more likely to be influenced by the impaired vascular vasodilator PG system.

In this study we demonstrated that the VSMC of SHR possess an increased proliferative activity as compared to those of WKY, which is consistent with the previous work of Yamori et al (2). They related the

Table 1. Effects of vasodilator PG on the DNA synthesis of vascular smooth muscle cells (VSMC) in culture.

Vasodilator PG (10^{-5}M)	Changes in (^{3}H)Thymidine Uptake (%)*	
	VSMC of WKY	VSMC of SHR
PGI$_2$ (OP-41483)	-41% p<0.001	-23% p<0.003
PGE$_2$	-31% p<0.003	-29% p<0.02
PGD$_2$	-31% p<0.001	-28% p<0.005

* The values were compared to basal thymidine uptake by respective VSMC.

Table 2. Effects of arachidonic acid (AA) or indomethacin (IDM) on the DNA synthesis of vascular smooth muscle cells (VSMC) in culture.

	Changes in (^{3}H)Thymidine Uptake (%)*	
	VSMC of WKY	VSMC of SHR
AA (10^{-5}M)	-13% p<0.003	-3% n.s.
IDM (10^{-5}M)	+4% n.s.	+16% p<0.01

* The values are compared to basal thymidine uptake by respective VSMC. n.s. represents statistically not significant.

rapid proliferation of VSMC of SHR to the increased permeability of Na$^+$ through the cell membrane (6). However, the mechanism of rapid VSMC growth in SHR is still uncertain. In conjunction with this, our results provide evidence for a close relationship between the vascular vasodilator PG system and the regulatory mechanism for VSMC proliferation. It seems quite possible that the impaired generation of vasodilator PG in the vascular wall is at least partly responsible for the enhanced proliferative activity of VSMC of SHR.

There is some evidence that vascular vasodilator PG generation is increased in hypertensive models of rats (7,8). However, Uehara et al hence clearly demonstrated that the basal vascular PGI$_2$ generation is impaired in Dahl salt-sensitive rats (5). In this study, we also presented a possibility that the basal vasodilator PG generation in VSMC was decreased in SHR as well, and that the impairment might be veiled in vivo conditions. The enhanced generation of vascular vasodilator PG may be a sort of adaptation phenomenon to the elevation of blood pressure.

We summarize our results as follows: 1) Cultured VSMC of SHR exhibit decreased productions of vasodilator PG, and an enhanced proliferative activity after several passages. 2) Exogenous vasodilator PG suppress the proliferation of VSMC both in SHR and WKY. 3) Indomethacin, an inhibitor of endogenous PG synthesis, increases the thymidine uptake by the VSMC of SHR. Arachidonate, which stimulates PG synthesis, is able to suppress thymidine uptake by the VSMC of WKY, while it is unable to affect that of SHR.

Thus, it is concluded that the productions of vasodilator PG are decreased in the cultured VSMC of SHR, and that the alterations possibly participate in the rapid proliferation of the VSMC of SHR.

REFERENCES

1. G. Olivetti, M. Melissari, G. Marchetti and P. Anversa, Quantitative structual changes of the rat thoracic aorta in early spontaneous hypertension, <u>Circ Res</u>, 51:19 (1982).

2. Y. Yamori, T. Kanbe, T. Igawa, M. Kihara, Y. Nara and R. Horie, Electrolyte balance in cultured smooth muscle cells from the aorta of spontaneously hypertensive rats, <u>in</u>: "Hypertensive Mechanisms, The spontaneously hypertensive rat as a model to study human hypertension" W. Rascher, D. Clough, D. Ganten, eds., Schattauer, Stuttgart, pp281 (1982).

3. J.J. Huttner, E.T. Gwebu, R.V. Panganamala, G.E. Milo, D.G. Cornwell, H.M. Sharma and J.C. Geer, Fatty acids and their prostaglandin derivatives : Inhibitors of proliferation in aortic smooth muscle cells, <u>Science</u> 197:289 (1977).

4. R. Ross, The Smooth Muscle Cell : II. Growth of smooth muscle in culture and formation of elastic fibers, <u>J Cell Biol</u> 50:172 (1971).

5. Y. Uehara, L. Tobian, J. Iwai, M. Ishii and T. Sugimoto, Alterations of vascular prostacyclin and thromboxane A_2 in Dahl genetical strain susceptible to salt-induced hypertension, <u>Prostaglandins</u> 33:727 (1987).

6. Y. Yamori and Y. Nara, Electrolyte imbalance of cultured vascular smooth muscle cells from SHR, its cause and effect, <u>Klin Wochenschr</u> 63(Suppl III):33 (1985).

7. C.R. Pace-Asiak, M.C. Carrara, G. Rangaraj and K.C. Nicolaou, Enhanced formation of PGI_2, a potent hypotensive substance, by aortic rings and homogenates of the spontaneously hypertensive rat, <u>Prostaglandins</u> 15:1005 (1978).

8. L.A. Friedman, J. Webster, C.N. Hensby and P.J. Lewis, Prostacyclin production in arterial hypertension, <u>in</u>: "Clinical Pharmacology of Prostacyclin" P.J. Lewis, J. O'Grady, eds., Raven Press, New York, pp97 (1981).

ANGIOTENSIN CONVERTING ENZYME INHIBITORS, CAPTOPRIL AND
ENALAPRILAT, AUGMENT BRADYKININ-INDUCED PROSTACYCLIN
SYNTHESIS IN CULTURED RAT VASCULAR SMOOTH MUSCLE CELLS

Kazuhisa Takeuchi, Keishi Abe[*], Makito Sato
Minoru Yasujima, Ken Omata, Yutaka Kasai
Masayuki Kanazawa, Fang Shou-nan
and Kaoru Yoshinaga

Second Department of Internal Medicine, and
[*]Department of Clinical Biology and Hormonal
Regulation, Tohoku University, School of
Medicine, 1-1 Seiryo-cho, Sendai 980, Japan

INTRODUCTION

Angiotensin coverting enzyme (ACE) inhibitors have
been widely used as antihypertensive drugs. The
vasodepressor effect of these drugs is generally considered
to be due to inhibition of the conversion of angiotensin I
(AI) to A II. On the other hand, as ACE is thought to be
identical with kininase II which degrades vasodilatory
kinin, it has been postulated that inhibition of kininase
as well as ACE activity may participate in the
vasodepressor action of ACE inhibitors[1]. Bradykinin (BK)
has been shown to stimulate vasodilatory prostaglandin (PG)
synthesis[2,3] and ACE or kininase activity may exist in
vascular tissue[4,5]. Therefore, it is hypothesized that the
vasodepressor effect of ACE inhibitors may be partly
explained by the elevation of BK levels and subsequent
augmentation of BK-induced PG synthesis in vascular tissue.
To evaluate this hypothesis, we examined (1) the effect of
BK on prostacyclin synthesis (PGI_2), and (2) the effects of
ACE inhibitors, captopril and enalaprilat (MK 422), on
BK-induced PGI_2 synthesis, in cultured rat vascular smooth
muscle cells, which have been shown to have ACE activity[4].

METHODS

Cell Culture. Vascular smooth muscle cells (VSMC) were
prepared by enzymatic dispersion from rat mesenteric
artery, as previously reported[6]. Briefly, male Sprague-
Dawley rats weighing between 200-400 g were anesthetized by
nembutal, the superior mesenteric artery dissected out,
freed of surrounding tissue and incubated for 15-20 min. at
37 while being shaken in a modified Krebs-Ringer buffer
having the following composition (in mM) NaCl, 105; KCl,
5; KH_2PO_4, 1;HEPES, 25; $MgSO_4$, 1; glucose, 14; $CaCl_2$, 0.2;
$NaHCO_3$, 25. The media was further supplemented with
collagenase (360 U/ml), elastase (96 U/ml), DNase (56 U/ml)
and soybean trypsin inhibitor (1mg/ml). Cells which had

dissociated during the first 15 to 20 min were discarded because they were likely to be enriched in adventitial fibroblasts as well as endothelial cells. The remaining portion of blood vessel was incubated for another 30 to 90 min. Cells dissociated during this second incubation were cetrifuged and filtered through a 150 um nytex filter before they were allowed to attach to culture wells in the medium 199 lacking bovine serum. After 2 hours, most cells adhered to the bottom of the wells and were further cultured in medium 199 supplemented with 10% fetal bovine serum. Morphological examination revealed characteristic smooth muscle cells with criss-cross pattern and hills & valleys, and nodular structures in confluent culture with phase contrast micrography and myofilaments and dense bodies with electron microscopy. Cells were subcultured by treatment with 0.08% trypsin-EDTA. We have comfirmed that these cultured VSMC possessed some biochemical properties in response to vasorelaxants or vasoconstrictors, such as intracellular cyclic AMP accumulation induced by isoproterenol and cyclic GMP accumulation by atrial natriuretic peptide[6], or rises in cytosolic free calcuim induced specifically by vasoconstrictive hormones, vasopressin and angiotensin II[7].

Experiments and Assays. Confluent VSMC of the 5 to 8th passages were used in the experiments. One day before the experiments, the culture medium, medium 199 supplemented with 10% fetal bovine serum, was removed and replaced with the fresh medium, and 6 hours before the start of the experiments, the medium was replaced with serum-free medium 199. The former procedure was performed to greatly stimulate PG synthesis, and the latter to avoid the possible effects of ACE activity remaining in the serum contained by the culture medium and pre-occupation of BK-receptors by BK in the culture medium. Prior to the experiments, monolayers were incubated with MEM in the presence or absence of ACE inhibitors, captopril (Sankyo Pharmaceutical Company, Tokyo) and enalaprilat (Banyu Pharmaceutical Company, Tokyo), or acetylsalicylic acid (ASA) for 30 min. In the experiment, after gently washing cell monolayers two times with Eagle's minimum essential medium, they were incubated with the same medium containing graded doses of BK (Protein Research Institute, Osaka) in the presence or absence of ACE inhibitors or ASA, for 15 min at 37 in a atmosphere of 5% CO_2, 95% air. PGI_2 synthesis was estimated by radioimmunoassay as 6-keto-$PGF_{1\alpha}$ (6KF) found in the incubation media. Cell protein was determined by the method of Lowry et al[8].

RESULTS

As we have already reported that 6KF was the primary PG in VSMC, we measured 6KF in the following experiments[9]. We used cells in subculture the 4 to 8th passages, because 6KF production in response to such well known agonists as arachidonic acid, calcium ionophore A23187, and vasopressin decreased markedly after the 10 to 15th passages[9]. 6KF generation was rapidly increased and reached a plateau in 5 min of incubation. Therefore, we used a 15 min incubation period to fully detect 6KF production. As shown in Fig. 1a, the threshold dose of the stimulation

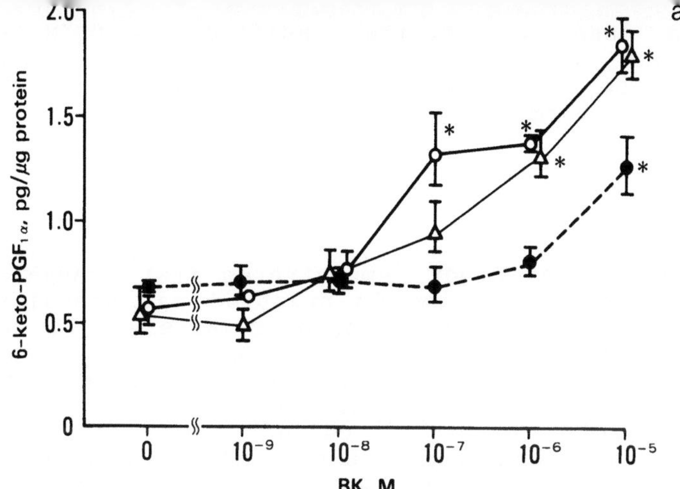

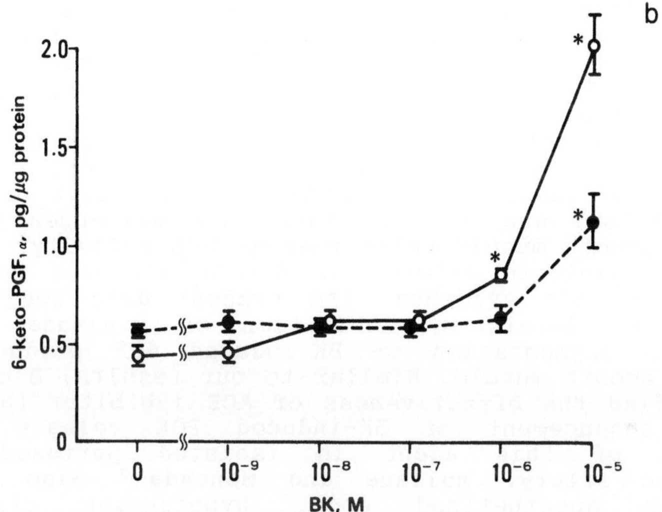

Fig. 1. Effects of angiotensin converting inhibitors, (a)
captopril (10^{-6}M, open triangle and 10^{-6}M, open
circle) and (b) enalaprilat (10^{-4}M, open circle),
on BK-induced 6-keto-PGF$_{1\alpha}$ production in cultured
rat vascular smooth muscle cells. Data are the
mean ± S.E.M. of 6 to 12 individual observations.
Asterisk indicates statistical significance at P <
.05 in comparison with control incubation (closed
circle).

of 6KF production in response to BK (10^{-9}-10^{-5}M) was 10^{-5}M.
The BK-induced 6KF production was almost completely
abolished by the treatment of acetylsalicylic acid, 3.3x
10^{-5}M. In the presence of captopril (10^{-6}M), the threshold
dose was shifted to 10^{-6}M and BK-induced 6KF production was
augmented, while captopril itself did not stimulated 6KF
production.

Furthermore, in the presence of captopril (10^{-4}M), the

threshold dose was further shifted to $10^{-7}M$ and the augmentation of BK-induced 6KF production was also observed. The same results were obtained by treatment of enalaprilat $(10^{-4}M)$ (Fig. 1b).

DISCUSSION

The present study demonstrates that bradykinin (BK) stimulates 6KF production in cultured rat vascular smooth muscle cells from the mesenteric artery. It has been reported that BK stimulates prostaglandin synthesis in a variety of cultured tissues including vascular endothelial cells[10], fibloblasts[11], renomedullary interstitial cells[12], renal glomerular mesangial cells[13], papillary collecting tubule cells[14] and human umbilical vein smooth muscle cells[15]. However, in cultured rat vascular smooth muscle cells from the mesenteric artery, BK-induced 6KF production has not been reported as yet. We could prove BK-induced 6KF production because we eliminated untoward effects of the serum contained by the culture medium as described in METHODS. Since both exogenous BK and PGI_2 dilate arteries, the effects of bradykinin on vascular contractility may be mediated, at least in part, by the stimulation of endogenous PG production within blood vessel walls, as concluded by Terragno et al[3].

Furthermore, in the present study, BK-induced 6KF production was augmented by an ACE inhibitor, captopril, and the same result was confirmed by treatment of another ACE inhibitor, enalaprilat. There are evidences that rat vascular smooth muscle cells possess ACE activity[4] and that the rat mesenteric artery has potent kininase activity[5]. Considering this evidence, the present data suggest that elevated BK levels by inhibition of kininase activity result in augmentation of BK-induced 6KF production in vascular smooth muscle. Similar to our results, Blumberg et al[2] verified the effectiveness of ACE inhibitor (SQ 20881) showing enhancement of BK-induced PGE release by the treatment of this agent in isolated perfused rabbit mesenteric artery. Mullane and Moncada[16] also reported that, in anesthetized dogs, hypotensive effect of bradykinin was potentiated by the treatment of captopril and that the potentiation of BK-induced hypotension was markedly attenuated by cyclo-oxygenase inhibition, which suggests that an increase in prostacyclin production by elevated kinin levels may contribute to the antihypertensive action of ACE inhibitor. Vinci et al[17] indicated that, in hyertensive patients, the fall in blood pressure produced by an ACE inhibitor correlated better with increased urinary kinin and plasma PG levels than with falls in plasma AII levels, suggesting that inhibition of kininase activity and subsequent response by BK accumulation may play a major role in the vasodepressor effect of ACE inhibitors. Our results support these observations. Moreover, Abe et al[18] previously hypothesized that captopril might lower blood pressure by elevated BK levels to stimulate prostacyclin generation in vascular wall via inhibition of kininase activity in human subjects with low renin hypertension. The present results in vascular smooth muscle would also support this hypothesis.

On the other hand, Nakagawa et al[19] failed to see any augmentation of BK-induced 6KF production by treatment with captopril in cultured endothelial cells from human

umbilical vein. The difference from our results may be due
to the difference in kind of tissue.

Finally, neither captopril nor enalaprilat increased
6KF production by itself. These results are compatible with
the observation in rat aorta by Sullivan et al[20].

In summary, in cultured rat vascular smooth muscle
cells from the mesenteric artery, bradykinin stimulated
prostacyclin synthesis, which was completely inhibited by
acetylsalicylic acid. Inhibition of angiotensin converting
enzyme with captopril and enalaprilat augmented the
bradykinin-induced prostacyclin synthesis. These data
support the hypothesis that angiotensin converting enzyme
inhibitors may potentiate its vasodilatory effect via the
augmentation of bradykinin-induced prostacyclin synthesis,
which is brought about by inhibition of kininase activity.

ACKNOWLEDGEMENTS

This study was supported in part by Grants-in-Aid
from the Ministry of Education, Science and Culture
(No.61132005 and No.62304041) and from the Ministry of
Health and Welfare (61-A-1). We wish to thank Dr. Michael
J. Dunn, Case Western Reserve University, Cleveland, OH,
for a generous gift of 6-keto-PGF$_{1\alpha}$ antibody. The technical
assistance of Miss Michiko Nakagawa is greatly appreciated.

REFERENCES

1. R. E. McCaa, J. E. Hall, S. S. McCaa, The effects of
   angiotensin I converting enzyme inhibitors on
   arterial blood pressure and urinary sodium
   excretion: Role of renin-angiotensin and kallikrein-
   kinin system. Circ. Res., 43 (Suppl 2): I-32 (1978)
2. A. Blumberg, S. E. Denny, G. R. Marshall, and P.
   Needleman, Blood vessel-hormone interaction:
   angiotensin, bradykinin, and prostaglandin. Am. J.
   Physiol., 232: H303 (1977)
3. D. A. Terragno, K. Crowshow, N. A. Terragno, and J. C.
   McGiff, Prostaglandin synthesis by bovine mesenteric
   arteries and veins. Circ. Res., 36 and 37 (Suppl I):
   I-76 (1975)
4. J. H. Resenthal, B. Pfeifle, M. L. Michailov, J. Pchorr,
   C.M. Jacob, and H. Dahlheim, Investigation of components of the renin-angiotensin system in rat vascular
   tissue. Hypertension, 6: 383 (1984)
5. L. M. Bendhack, C. L. Lindsey, and A. C. M. Paiva,
   Converting enzyme inhibitors decrease kininase but
   not converting activity in the rat mesenteric vascular bed. Hypertension, 8 (Suppl I): I-9 (1986)
6. M. Sato, K. Abe, K. Takeuchi, M. Yasujima, K. Omata, M.
   Hiwatari, Y. Kasai, M. Tanno, M. Kohzuki, K. Kudo,
   K. Yoshinaga, and T. Inagami, Atrial natriuretic
   factor and cyclic 3',5'-monophosphate in vascular
   smooth muscle. Hypertension, 8: 762 (1986)
7. K. Takeuchi, K. Abe, M. Sato, M. Yasujima, K. Omata, Y.
   Kasai, M. Kanazawa, and K. Yoshinaga, Effects of
   dihidropyridine calcium antagonists on agonist-
   induced rises in cytosolic free calcium in monolayers
   of cultured vascular smooth muscle cells. Proceedings
   of International Symposium: Calcium Signal and Cell
   Response, Biological and Clinical Aspects. K. Yagi
   et al. ed., (1988)

8. O. H. Lowry, N. J. Resebourg, A. L. Farr, and R. J. Randall, Protein measurement with the Folin Phenol regent. J. Biol. Chem. 193: 265 (1951)

9. K. Takeuchi, K. Abe, M. Sato, M. Yasujima, T. Hagino, S. Fang, and K. Yoshinaga, Effect of in vitro aging on prostaglandin synthesis in cultured rat vascular smooth muscle cells. Agents and Actions 22:49 (1987)

10. S. L. Hong, Effect of bradykinin and thrombin on prostacyclin synthesis in endothelial cells from pig aorta and human umbilical cord. Thromb. Res., 18: 787 (1980)

11. D. L. Bareis, V. C. Marganiella, F. Hirata, M. Vaughan, and J. Axelrod, Bradykinin stimulates phospholipid methylation, calcium influx, prostaglandin formation, and cAMP accumulation in human fibroblasts. J. Biol. Chem., 80: 2514 (1983)

12. R. A. Zusman and H. R. Keiser, Prostaglandin E_2 biosynthesis by rabbit renomedullary interstitial cells in tissue culture. J. Biol. Chem., 252: 2069 (1977)

13. A. Uglesity, J. I. Kreisberg, and L. Levine, Stimulation of arachidonic acid metabilism in rat kidney mesangial cells by bradykinin, antidiuretic hormone, and their analogue. Prostaglandin Leukot. Med., 10: 83 (1983)

14. F. C. Granier, T. E. Rollins, and W. Smith, Kinin-induced prostaglandin synthesis by renal papillary collecting tubule cells in culture. Am. J. Physiol., 241: F94 (1981)

15. R. W. Alexander and M. A. Gimbrone, Stimulation of prostaglandin E synthesis in cultured human umbilical vein smooth muscle cells. Proc. Natl. Acad. Sci. USA, 73: 1617 (1976)

16. K. M. Mullane and S. Moncada, Prostaglandin mediates the potentiated hypotensive effect of bradykinin following captopril treatmnt. Eur. J. Pharmacol., 66: 355 (1980)

17. J. M. Vinci, D. Horwitz, R. Zusman, J. J. Pisano, K. J. Catt, and H. R. Keiser, The effect of converting enzyme inhibition with SQ 20, 881 on plasma and urinary kinin, prostaglandin E, and angiotensin II in hypertensive man. Hypertension, 1: 416 (1979)

18. K. Abe, T. Ito, Y. Imai, M. Sato, T. Haruyama, Y. Sakurai, T. Goto, Y. Otsuka, and K. Yoshinaga, Implication of endogenous prostaglandin synthesis in antihypertensive effect of captopril, SQ 14225, in low renin hypertension. Jpn. Circ. J., 44: 422 (1980)

19. M. Nakagawa, S. Sawada, T. Toyoda, H. Takamatsu, H. Tsuji, and H Ichiji, Regulation of prostaglandin generation by angiotensin converting enzyme related substances in cultured human vascular endothelial cells. Clin. and Exper. Theory and Practice, A9(2&3): 405 (1987)

20. J. M. Sullivan and D. R. Patrick, Release of prostaglandin I_2-like activity from the rat aorta: effect of captopril, furosemide, and sodium. Prostaglandins, 22: 575 (1981)

RENAL FUNCTION AS AFFECTED BY INHIBITORS OF KININASE II AND OF NEUTRAL
ENDOPEPTIDASE 24.11 IN RATS WITH AND WITHOUT DESOXYCORTICOSTERONE
PRETREATMENT

Motoya Nakagawa and Alberto Nasjletti

Department of Pharmacology, University of Tennessee
Memphis, Tennessee and Department of Pharmacology
New York Medical College, Valhalla, New York, U.S.A.

INTRODUCTION

In the kidney, bradykinin and related peptides are degraded by three
or more enzymes (kininases) including kininase II (1), neutral
endopeptidase 24.11 (2), and a carboxypeptidase N-type enzyme (3). The
excretion rate of urinary kinins increases during treatment with
inhibitors of kininase II (4) or of neutral endopeptidase (5).
Additionally, inhibitors of kininase II and of neutral endopeptidase
elicit diuresis, natriuresis, and renal vasodilation (4,5), effects which
are attributable, at least in part, to increased renal kinin levels. If
so, the prevailing activity of the renal kallikrein-kinin system may
influence the renal functional response to treatment with inhibitors of
kinin degrading enzymes. Therefore, this study was designed to contrast
the effects of combined treatment with captopril and phosphoramidon-
inhibitors of kininase II and of neutral endopeptidase 24.11 (5),
respectively - on the renal function of normal rats and of rats pretreated
with desoxycorticosterone (DOC) to increase renal and urinary kallikrein
(6).

METHODS

Studies were conducted on twelve male Sprague-Dawley rats (Harlan
Industries, Indianapolis, IN). The animals were fed ad libitum a standard
chow (Purina 5001, Ralston-Purina, St. Louis, MO), had free access to tap
water, and received weekly injections of DOC (Percorten Pivalate, CIBA,
Summit, NJ; 25 mg/kg body weight, sc) or vehicle (0.15 M NaCl; 1 ml/kg).
On the 14th day after commencing treatment with DOC or vehicle, renal
function was examined before and during combined treatment with captopril
and phosphoramidon to inhibit kininase II and neutral endopeptidase,
respectively.
The rats,anesthetized by injection of Inactin (100 mg/kg, ip), were
placed on a thermostatically controlled board to maintain body temperature
at 36-37°C. After tracheostomy, cannulas were placed in the femoral
veins for infusion and administration of drugs, in the femoral artery for
measurement of blood pressure and blood sampling, and in the ureters for
collection of urine. An infusion of 0.15 M NaCl was started soon after
completion of the cannulation procedures. A saline load equal to 5% body

weight was given iv at a rate of 20 ml/h followed by a continuous
maintenance infusion at 6 ml/h; the maintenance infusion contained
^{3}H-inulin (1.5 µCi/h). Following a 60 min equilibration interval,
control urine samples were collected over a 40 min period. Captopril
(Squibb Institute, Princeton, NJ) and phosphoramidon (Sigma Chemical Co.,
St. Louis, MO) were then added to the maintenance infusion and
administered at 2 mg/kg/h and 330 µg/kg/h, respectively; 20 min later
urine was collected for an additional 40 min period. Blood samples (200
µl) were collected at the midpoint of urine collection periods for
measurement of plasma inulin concentration.

Glomerular filtration rate, as estimated by the clearance of tritiated
inulin, was derived from the concentrations of radioactive inulin in urine
and plasma. Urine samples for determination of kinins were collected in
pre-weighed polypropylene tubes, maintained at 4°C, containing pepstatin
(200 ng). The samples were tested for blood contamination and rats with
blood in the urine were excluded from the study. The concentration of
sodium in urine was determined by flame photometry. The concentration of
kinins in urine was measured by radioimmunoassay (7). The combined
activity of all urinary kininases (total kininase activity) was measured
as described by Ura et al. (5,8). One unit of kininase activity is
defined as the amount of enzyme that degrades 1 µg of synthetic
bradykinin per min of incubation under specific assay conditions (5,8).

Data are presented as mean $\pm$ SE. The data were analyzed by analyses
of variance followed by Newman-Keul's a posteriori test. The significance
of differences in kininase inhibitor-induced changes between rats with and
without DOC-pretreatment was determined by unpaired Student's t-test. The
null hypothesis was rejected when the p value was less than 0.05.

RESULTS

The combined administration of captopril and phosphoramidon reduced
($p < 0.05$) the urinary excretion of total kininase activity from 58.8±8.3 to
26.6±4.1 mU/min/100 g body weight (bw) in rats without DOC pretreatment,
and from 60.6±13.1 to 36.9±4.1 mU/min/100 g bw in rats pretreated with DOC
for 14 days. Associated with the kininase inhibitors-induced reduction in
urinary kininase activity, the urinary excretion of kinins increased
($p < 0.01$) from 9.7±2.5 to 15.6±1.5 pg/min/100 g bw in rats without DOC
pretreatment, and from 7.7±2.5 to 14.8±4.0 pg/min/100 g bw in rats
pretreated with DOC. Comparison of rats with and without DOC pretreatment
in terms of urinary kinin and kininase excretion values, before and after
the administration of captopril and phosphoramidon, revealed no
significant difference.

Shown in figure 1 are the values of blood pressure, glomerular
filtration rate, sodium excretion and urine volume in rats with and
without DOC pretreatment, before and after the administration of captopril
and phosphoramidon. The administration of the kininase inhibitors caused
in both groups of rats significant ($p < 0.05$) elevation of sodium excretion
and of glomerular filtration, without affecting urine volume or blood
pressure. Comparison of rats with and without DOC pretreatment in terms
of blood pressure, urine volume, glomerular filtration rate or urinary
sodium excretion, before and after the administration of captopril and
phosphoramidon, relealed no significant difference.

DISCUSSION

This study demonstrated that combined treatment with captopril and
phosphoramidon reduces urinary kininase activity and increases glomerular
filtration rate and the urinary excretion rates of kinins and sodium. Ura

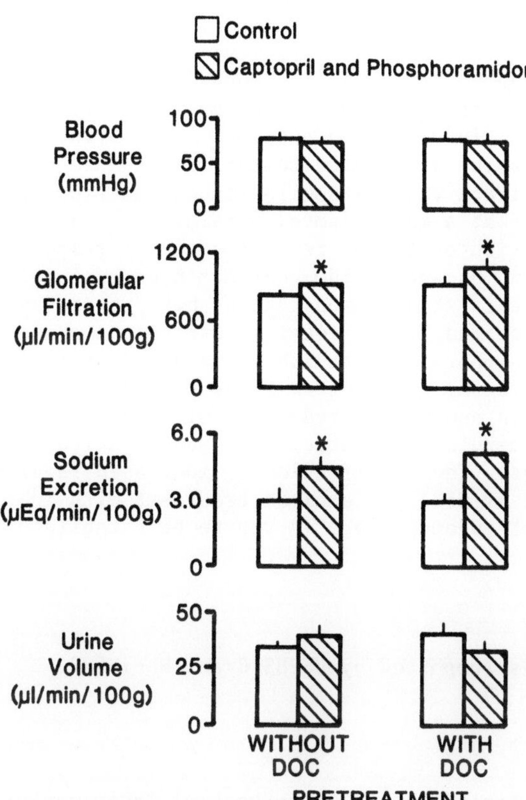

<u>Figure 1</u>. Effect of combined infusion of captopril (2 mg/kg/h) and phosphoramidon (330 µg/kg/h) on blood pressure and indices of renal function in rats with and without DOC-pretreatment (25 mg/kg/week) for two weeks. The asterisk denotes p<0.05 relative to control values before the infusion of captopril and phosphoramidon.

and co-workers (5) have already reported that phosphoramidon-induced
inhibition of neutral endopeptidase causes urinary kinins to increase,
and is accompanied by renal vasodilation and natriuresis. They also
reported that captopril-induced inhibition of kininase II in rats causes
slight elevation of urinary kinins without affecting renal function (5).

In the present study, the administration of captopril and
phosphoramidon produced similar increases of glomerular filtration rate
and of urinary sodium and kinin excretion rates in rats with and without
DOC-pretreatment. In addition, we found that the basal excretion rate of
urinary kinin was similar in rats with and without DOC-pretreatment. That
treatment with DOC increases urinary kallikrein is well established (6).
It would appear, then, that DOC-induced augmentation of urinary kallikrein
excretion does not result in elevation of urinary kinin excretion, a
presumed index of the level of activity of the renal kallikrein-kinin
system. Accordingly, it may be concluded that DOC-pretreatment does not
increase the level of activity of the renal kallikrein-kinin system.

The renal functional response to the administration of captopril and
phosphoramidon may be attributed to the increase in renal kinins, which
are thought to effect renal vasodilation and natriuresis (4,5). However,
the possibility that a mechanism(s) unrelated to inhibition of kinin
degradation contributes to the renal functional response to treatment
with captopril and phosphoramidon has not been excluded.

In summary, this study demonstrates that pretreatment with DOC for
two weeks does not modify the renal functional response to infusion of
captopril and phosphoramidon to inhibit kinin degradation. Rats with and
without DOC-pretreatment exhibited after the administration of captopril
and phosphoramidon equivalent reduction of urinary kininase activity and
increases of glomerular filtration rate and of urinary excretion rates of
sodium and kinins. The contribution of increased renal kinins to the
renal functional effects of combined treatment with inhibitors of kininase
II and of neutral endopeptidase is yet to be established.

ACKNOWLEDGEMENT

This work was supported by USPHS Grant HL-18579.

REFERENCES

1. E.G.Erdos. Kininases, in: Handbook of Experimental Pharmacology,
    Vol. 35, Suppl., ed. by E.G.Erdos, Springer-Verlag, pp. 427 (1979).
2. R.A.Skidgel, W.W.Schulz, L.T.Tam and E.G.Erdos. Human renal
    angiotensin I converting enzyme and its "helper enzyme". Kidney Int.
    (Suppl. 20), 31:S45 (1987).
3. R.A.Skidgel, R.M.Davis and E.G.Erdos. Purification of a human
    urinary kininase; a carboxypeptidase distinct from carboxypeptidase A,
    B, or N. Anal. Biochem., 140:520 (1984).
4. A.Nasjletti, J.Colina-Chourio and J.C.McGiff. Disappearance of
    bradykinin, the renal circulation of dogs: effects of kininase
    inhibition. Circ. Res., 37:59 (1975).
5. N.Ura, O.A.Carretero and E.G.Erdos. Role of renal endopeptidase
    24.11 in kinin metabolism in vitro and in vivo. Kidney Int., 32, 507
    (1987)
6. A.Nasjletti, J.C.McGiff and J.Colina-Chourio. Interrelations of the
    renal kallikrein-kinin system and renal prostaglandins in the
    conscious rat. Circ Res, 43:799 (1978).
7. K.Shimamoto, T.Ando, T.Nakao, M.Sakuma and M.Miyahara. A sensitive
    radioimmunoassay method for urinary kinin in man. J. Lab. Clin. Med.
    91:721 (1978).

8. N.Ura, K.Shimamoto, S.Tanaka, T.Nishimiya, T.Mita, M.Nakagawa, T.Maeda, Y.Yamaguchi and O.Iimura. Urinary excretions of kininase I and kininase II activities in essential hypertension. A sensitive and simple method for its kinin destroying capacity. J. Clin. Hypertens. 1:15 (1985).

8. N.Ura, K.Shimamoto, S.Tanaka, T.Nishimiya, T.Mita, M.Nakagawa, T.Maeda, Y.Yamaguchi and O.Iimura. Urinary excretions of kininase I and kininase II activities in essential hypertension. A sensitive and simple method for its kinin destroying capacity. J. Clin. Hypertens. 1:15 (1985).

PGE$_2$ SYNTHESIS IN CULTURED RENAL PAPILLARY COLLECTING TUBULE CELLS FROM

YOUNG AND AGED SPONTANEOUSLY HYPERTENSIVE RATS

Makito Sato, Keishi Abe*, Kazuhisa Takeuchi, Minoru
Yasujima, Masao Hiwatari, Ken Omata, Yutaka Kasai, Kei
Kudo, Masayuki Kanazawa, Kazunori Yoshida, Kazuo Tsunoda
and Kaoru Yoshinaga

Second Department of Internal Medicine, and *Dept of
Cinical Biology and Hormonal Regulation, Tohoku University
School of Medicine, 1-1, Seiryocho, Sendai 980, Japan
School of Medicine, 1-1, Seiryocho, Sendai 980, Japan

ABSTRACT

To investigate whether altered renal medullary prostaglandin (PG)
synthesis is involved in the development of hypertension in spontaneously
hypertensive rats (SHR), we compared the capacity of PGE$_2$ synthesis in
cultured renal papillary collecting tubule cells from young (4-week-old)
and aged (16-week-old) SHR and control Wistar-Kyoto rats(WKY). Basal
levels of PGE$_2$ synthesis were lower in young SHR cells than in WKY cells
(p < 0.001). Arachidonic acid-stimulated PGE$_2$ synthesis, however, had a
slight tendency to be higher in SHR cells than in WKY cells. Bradykinin-
and A23187-stimulated PGE$_2$ synthesis were similar in both strains. Basal
levels of cyclic AMP were also lower in young SHR cells than in WKY cells
(p < 0.001), but the cAMP response to exogenous PGE$_2$ was equall between
the strains. In papillary collecting tubule cells from aged rats, basal
levels of PGE$_2$ and cyclic AMP as corrected for cellular protein were
significantly lower than those in young rats, but there was no difference
between the strains. Urinary excretion of PGE$_2$ and thromboxane B$_2$ was
equall in aged SHR and WKY. These results suggest that papillary
collecting tubule of young SHR and WKY may differ in the metabolism of
PGE$_2$ and cyclic AMP. This difference may be attributed to the possible
defect in arachidonate availability in SHR.

INTRODUCTION

Prostaglandins (PGs) play an important role in renal hemodynamics and
sodium-water metabolism in the kidney (Dunn, 1983). Since PG may be
involved in the regulation of blood pressure, a lot of studies have been
focused on the possible alterations of renal PG synthesis or degradation
in genetic models of spontaneous hypertension. However, considerable
discrepancies exist between reports on the renal metabolism of PGs in
spontaneously hypertensive rats (SHR) (Dunn, 1983). It has been reported
that renal medullary microsomal PG cyclo-oxygenase activity was increased
in SHR (Dunn, 1976). In addition, the PG degradative enzyme 15-hydroxy-
dehydrogenase was decreased in whole renal homogenates of SHR (Pace-

Asciak, et al. 1976). However, renal medullary tissue levels of PGE_2
were similar in SHR and control Wistar-Kyoto rats (WKY) (Dunn, 1976).
Urinary excretion of PGE_2 in SHR has been controversially reported to be
similar (Dunn, 1978), increased (Herlitz et al., 1982) or decreased
(Martineau et al, 1984) compared with those in WKY. Since it has been
shown that renal inner medullary collecting tubule is a major site of PG
synthesis in the kidney, we cultured renal papillary collecting tubule
(RPCT) cells from young and aged SHR and WKY and compared synthetic rate
of PGE_2 in order to examine the hypothesis that altered PG metabolism is
involved in the development of hypertension in SHR.

MATERIAL AND METHODS

     <u>SHR and WKY</u>: Four-week-old rats (n = 24 each for SHR and WKY) and
16-week-old rats (n = 12 for each strain) were purchased from Charles
River Farm of Japan and housed in the Tohoku University Hospital,
experimental animal facility.   Blood pressures were obtained by tail cuff
pletysmography. Urine collections (24 hour) were made in metabolic cages
for 3 days.
     <u>Isolation and Culture of Cells</u>: RPCT cells were isolated from renal
papillae of SHR and WKY simultaneously according to methods previously
described (Sato and Dunn, 1984). The cells were initially cultured in a
1:1 mixture of Dulbecco's modified Eagle's medium (DMEM) and Ham's F12
medium supplemented with 10 % fetal bovine serum (all from Gibco Lab.).
After one day in culture, the media were changed to a fully defined K-1
media in order to favor epithelial rather than fibroblast overgrowth. The
RPCT cell cultures were used for experimentation on the 4th day (4-week-
old rats) or 7th day (16-week-old rats) after initiation of the culture
when the cells were confluent in Coaster 24-well dishes.
     <u>Experiments</u>: In all experiments, cells were incubated in 0.4 ml of
minimum essential medium made 900 mOsmol by the addition of NaCl and urea,
1:1 eqiosmolar ratio. Cells were incubated for 30 minutes in the presence
or absence of arachidonic acid (5 µg/ml, Sigma Chemicals), calcium
ionophore A23187 (2 µg/ml, Sigma Chemicals), bradykinin (10^{-5}M, Protein
Institute, Osaka) or kallikrein (30 µg/ml, Ono Pharmaceutical Co., Osaka)
to measure PGE_2, and for 5 minutes to measure intracellular cyclic AMP in
the presence of phosphodiesterase inhibitor isobutylmethylxanthine, 5 x
10^{-4}M. To measure cyclic AMP, experiments were terminated by the removal
of media immediately followed by the addition of 0.3 ml of 0.1 N HCl.
After cells were exposed into the HCl solution for 1 hour, intracellular
cyclic AMP was extracted into HCl fraction and part of the cellular
protein was precipitated and left on the bottom of the culture well (Sato
and Dunn, 1986). PGE_2 was measured by radioimmunoassay using antiserum
from Institut Pasteur and cyclic AMP also by radioimmunoassay after
succinylation (Yamasa Shoyu Co., Choshi, Japan). Cellular protein was
measured by the method of Lowry et al. (1951).   Urinary PGE_2 and TXB_2
were measured by radioimmunoassay after extraction and purification as
reported previously (Abe et al., 1977, Chiba et al., 1984).
     All results were expressed as mean ± SE. The statistical
significance was evaluated at the 95 % confidence level using Student's t-
test for unpaired observations.

RESULTS

     As summarized in the table, in cells from 4-week-old rats, basal
levels of PGE_2 synthesis were lower in SHR cells than in WKY cells (p <
0.001). PGE_2 synthesis was stimulated 9.8 folds in WKY cells and 15.3
folds in SHR cells by arachidonic acid, and 2.7 folds and 4.4 folds by
A23187, respectively (p < 0.001). However, there was no difference in AA-

stimulated and A23187-stimulated PGE_2 synthesis between the strains. Bradykinin also stimulated PGE_2 synthesis from 8.3 ± 1.7 to 12.6 ± 2.5 pg/µg protein/30 min in WKY cells and from 7.6 ± 0.5 to 14.6 ± 2.4 pg/µg protein/30 min in SHR cells (both $p < 0.05$), but there was no difference between the strains. Kallikrein failed to stimulate PGE_2 synthesis in these cells. Basal levels of PGE_2 in cells from 16-week-old rats were lower than those from 4-week-old rats ($P < 0.01$) and there was no difference between the strains. However, AA-stimulated PGE_2 synthesis was higher in cells from 16-week-old rats than those from 4-week-old rats ($p < 0.05$). There was a slight tendency that AA-stimulated PGE_2 synthesis was higher in SHR cells than in WKY cells. In cells from 16-week-old rats, bradykinin failed to stimulate PGE_2 synthesis.

Since the basal level of cyclic AMP is shown, at least partly, to depend on endogenous PGE_2 levels in papillary collecting tubule cells (Sato and Dunn, 1984), we then measured intracellular cyclic AMP levels. Basal levels of cyclic AMP were 57.5 ± 3.2 and 44.5 ± 2.9 fmol/µg protein in 4-week-old WKY cells and age-matched SHR cells, respectively, and 31.3 ± 5.8 and 39.3 ± 6.3 fmol/µg protein in 16-week-old WKY cells and SHR cells, respectively. Basal levels of cyclic AMP were lower in young SHR cells than in age-matched WKY cells ($p < 0.001$), and also lower in cells from 16-week-old rats than in 4-week-old rats ($p < 0.05$).

Table 1. Comparison of PGE_2 synthesis between SHR cells and WKY cells

	WKY		SHR	
	4-week-old	16-week-old	4-week-old	16-week-old
basal (n=48)	12.9 ± 0.8	$2.9 \pm 0.4^{*}$	$9.4 \pm 0.5^{\#}$	$3.6 \pm 0.4^{*}$
AA (n=18) -stimulated	126.4 ± 14.6	$327.4 \pm 55.1^{*}$	144.2 ± 15.4	$400.4 \pm 64.0^{*}$
A23187(n=18) -stimulated	34.3 ± 4.3	$13.4 \pm 3.3^{*}$	41.0 ± 5.1	$10.0 \pm 1.3^{*}$

PGE_2: pg/µg protein/30 minutes. Each value represents mean $\pm$ SE from 2 to 6 experiments. Numbers in parenthesis show the number of cultures. [#] $p < 0.001$ compared with 4-week-old WKY cells, [*] $p < 0.01$ with respective value in 4-week-old rat cells.

Table 2. Comparison of urinary PGE_2 and TXB_2 excretion between SHR and WKY

	WKY	SHR	
Systolic BP (mmHg)	153.7 ± 3.8	247.4 ± 3.1	$p < 0.001$
Urine Volume (ml/day)	9.0 ± 0.5	10.5 ± 1.8	n.s.
Urinary Na (µEq/day)	850 ± 54	843 ± 75	n.s.
Urinary K (µEq/day)	347 ± 23	323 ± 31	n.s.
Urinary creatinine (mg/day)	8.4 ± 0.4	8.5 ± 0.4	n.s.
PGE_2 (ng/day)	45.4 ± 8.4	47.0 ± 6.2	n.s.
TXB_2 (ng/day)	7.76 ± 0.62	7.37 ± 0.63	n.s.

n.s. : not significant

As urinary excretion of PGE_2 reflects most of renal medullary PGE_2 synthesis, urinary excretion of PGE_2 and TXB_2 were measured in 16-week-old WKY and SHR (each n = 7). As shown in Table 2, there was no difference in urinary PGE_2 and TXB_2 excretion between WKY and SHR.

<u>Discussion</u>

Although there are a lot of reports on the metabolism of PGs in SHR, the present study is the first report, as far as we know, on PG synthesis in inner medullary collecting ducts of SHR, which is shown by microdissection studies to be the major site of PGE_2 synthesis in the kidney (Farman et al., 1986, 1987). Previous studies have used many different approaches to evaluate PG synthesis in SHR including medullary microsomes (Dunn, 1976; Limas and Limas, 1977), renal slices (Limas and Limas, 1979; Stygles et al., 1978), renal venous plasma (Dunn, 1978), urinary excretion (Dunn, 1978; Ahnfelt-Ronne and Arrigoni-Martelli, 1977, Shibouta et al., 1982) and ex vivo perfusion of the kidney (Shibouta et al., 1981). These approches provide little information about PG synthesis in specific portions of the nephron, i.e. glomeruli, tubules, interstitial cells and arterioles. Konieczkowski et al. (1981) have reported that SHR glomeruli have increased synthesis of TXB_2, PGE_2, $PGF_{2\alpha}$ and 6-keto-$PGF_{1\alpha}$ in the presence of arachidonic acid or calcium ionophore A23187 but not in the basal condition.

The present study showed that PGE_2 synthesis is lower in cultured renal papillary collecting tubule cells from 4-week-old SHR than those from age-matched WKY. These results are consistent with the report by Sirosis and Gagnon (1974) in which PGE-like material was bioassayed in the papillae. These results are also supported by the present findings that the basal cyclic AMP level is lower in SHR cells than in WKY cells, since the level of basal cyclic AMP is partially dependent on the endogenous PGE_2 levels in RPCT cells (Sato and Dunn, 1984). Most of the previous studies, however, support the opposite hypothesis that PG synthesis is increased in SHR kidney. Dunn (1976) originally reported that medullary microsomes from SHR synthesized more PGE_2 and $PGF_{2\alpha}$ than age-matched normotensive WKY, although he could not find any differences in the medullary tissue content of PGE_2 between the strains and also not in renal venous and urinary PGE_2 and $PGF_{2\alpha}$ in subsequent studies (Dunn, 1979). Limas and Limas (1977,1979) confirmed increased PGE_2 and $PGF_{2\alpha}$ synthesis in medullary microsomes of SHR and also demonstrated the increased phospholipase A_2 and cyclo-oxygenase activity as well as enhanced PG biosynthesis in response to bradykinin and angiotensin II in medullary slices of SHR. Kawaguchi et al. (1986,1987) have recently observed that not only phospholipase A_2 but also phospholipase C and diglyceride lipase activities increased in the kidney of stroke prone SHR. In addition, the synthesis of TXA_2 and PGI_2 have been reported to be augumented in isolated perfused kidney or isolated glomeruli of SHR (Shibouta et al., 1979,1981; Konieczkowski et al., 1981). Although it is difficult to explain the discrepancies between the present results and previous studies, it may be related to the differences in experimental materials (whole kidney, slices, specific nephron or subcellular fraction), in vitro conditions for measurement of phospholipases and cyclo-oxygenase activity (cofactors, substrate concentration, etc.), preparations used, fresh cells or cultured cells, etc..

It is of note that in the presence of arachidonic acid or during stimulation with bradykinin or A23187, we could not find any difference in PGE_2 synthesis between the strains and it even tended to be higher in SHR cells than in WKY cells in these conditions. These results may suggest the possibility that a basic defect in arachidonic acid availability in SHR cells, which may induce the increases in enzyme activity such as phospholipases and cyclo-oxygenase. Such a dissociation between

phospholipase activity and actual PGE_2 synthesis in the kidney is already
found in previous reports. Although Kawaguchi et al. (1986, 1987) have
reported that the increased activity of phospholipase A_2 in the kidney of
SHR and of phospholipase C and diglyceride lipase in that of stroke-prone
SHR were age-dependent, renal venous and urinary PGE_2 and $PGF_{2\alpha}$ were shown
to decrease with age in SHR (Dunn, 1978). In the present study, basal
levels of PGE_2 were lower in cells from 16-week-old rats than those from
4-week-old rats in both strains. Arachidonic acid-stimulated PGE_2,
however, were higher in cells from aged rats than those from young rats.
These results may indicate the possibility that there is a common change
in arachidonic acid-availability during the process of aging and
spontaneous hypertension in the rat. Such a possibility of fundamental
disturbance of phospholipid metabolism has also been suggested in
vascular tissues of SHR (Dusting and Doyle, 1983). Although there are
conflicting reports on the renal activity of 15-hydroxy-dehydrogenase, a
major degradative enzyme for PGE_2 and $PGF_{2\alpha}$, it should not be taken into
account in the present study in cultured renal papillary collecting tubule
cells since the activity is shown to be localized only in proximal tubules
but not in inner medulla (Uchida et al., 1986).

In conclusion, renal papillary collecting tubule cells from 4-week-
old SHR showed lower basal levels of PGE_2 synthesis than those from age-
matched WKY, but the difference was not observed after stimulation with
arachidonic acid or A23187. These results may be attributed to the
possible defect in arachidonate availability in SHR.

ACKNOWLEDGMENT

This study was supported by a Grant-in Aid for Cardiovascular Disease
from the Ministry of Health and Welfare of Japan (61-A-1) and for
Scientific Research from the Ministry of Education, Science and Culture of
Japan (62870011).

REFERENCES

Abe, K., Yasujima, M., Chiba, S., Irokawa, N., Itoh, T., Yoshinaga, K.,
and Saito, T. 1977, Effect of furosemide on urinary rxcretion of
prostaglandin in normal volunteers and patients with essential
hypertension. Prostaglandins 14:513.

Ahnfelt-Ronne, I., and Arrigoni-Martelli, E. 1977, Renal prostaglandin
metabolism in spontaneously hypertensive rats. Biochem. Pharmacol.
26:485.

Chiba, S., Abe, K., Kudo, K., Omata, K., Yasujima, M., Sato, K., Seino,
M., Imai, Y., Sato, M., and Yoshinaga, K. 1984, Sex and age-related
differences in the urinary excretion of TXB_2 in normal human subjects: a
possible pathophysiological role of TXA_2 in the aged kidney. PG. LT. Med.
16:347.

Dunn, M.J. 1976, Renal prostaglandin synthesis in the spontaneously
hypertensive rat. J. Clin. Invest. 58:862.

Dunn, M.J. 1978, Renal prostaglandin production in the Japanese (Kyoto)
spontaneously hypertensive rat. Clin. Sci. Mol. Med. 55:191s.

Dunn, M.J. 1983, Renal prostaglandins, in "Renal Endocrinology" Dunn,
M.J. ed., Williams & Wilkins, Baltimore, p.1.

Dusting, G.J., and Doyle, A.E. 1985, Prostacyclin biosynthesis in experimental hypertension: A marker of a fundamental phospholipid disturbance that may contribute to increased vascular reactivity, in "Prostaglandins and cardiovascular diseases" Ozawa, T., Yamada, K., and Yamamoto, S. ed, Raven Press, New York, p.3.

Farman, N., Pradelles, P., and Bonvalet, J.P. 1986, Determination of prostaglandin E_2 synthesis along rabbit nephron by enzyme immunoassay. Am. J. Physiol. 251:F238.

Farman, N., Pradelles, P., and Bonvalet, J.P. 1987, PGE_2, $PGF_{2\alpha}$, 6-keto-$PGF_{1\alpha}$, and TXB_2 synthesis along the rabbit nephron. Am. J. Physiol. 252:F53.

Herlitz, H., Lundin, S., Henning, M., Aurell, M., Karlberg, B.E., Berglund, G. 1982, Hormonal pattern during development of hypertension in spontaneously hypertensive rat SHR. Clin. Exp. Hypertens. [A] 4:915.

Kawaguchi, H. and Yasuda, H. 1986, Increased phospholipase A_2 activity in the kidney of spontaneously hypertensive rats. Arch. Biochem. Biophys. 248:401.

Kawaguchi, H., Okamoto, H., Saito, H., and Yasuda, H. 1987, Renal phospholipase C and diglyceride lipase activity in spontaneously hypertensive rats. 10:100.

Konieczkowski, M., Dunn, M.J., Stork, J.E., and Hassid, A. 1983, Glomerular synthesis of prostaglandins and thromboxane in spontaneously hypertensive rats. 5:446.

Limas, C.J., and Limas, C. 1977, Prostaglandin metabolism in the kidney of spontaneously hypertensive rats. Am J. Physiol. 233:H87.

Limas, C., and Limas, C.J. 1979, Enhanced renomedullary prostaglandin synthesis in spontaneously hypertensive rats: Role of a phospholipase A_2. 5:H65.

Lowry, O.H., Rosenbrough, N.J., Farr, A.L., Randall, R.J. 1951, Protein measurement with the Folin phenol reagent. J. Biol. Chem. 193:265.

Martineau, A., Robillard, M., Falardeau, P. 1984, Defective synthesis of vasodilator prostaglandins in spontaneously hypertensive rats in vivo. Hypertension 6(Suppl. 1):161.

Pace-Asciak, C.R. 1976, Decreased renal prostaglandin catabolism precedes onset of hypertension in the developing spontaneously hypertensive rat. Nature 263:510.

Sato, M., and Dunn, M.J. 1984, Interactions of vasopressin, prostaglandins, cAMP in rat renal papillary collecting tubule cells in culture. Am. J. Physiol. 247:F423.

Sato, M., and Dunn, M.J. 1986, Osmolality, vasopressin-stimulated cAMP, and PGE_2 synthesis in rat collecting tubule cells. Am. J. Physiol. 250:F802.

Shibouta, Y., Inada, Y., Terashita, Z, Nishikawa, K., Kikuchi, S., Shimamoto, K. 1979, Angiotensin II-stimulated release of thromboxane A_2 and prostacyclin (PGI_2) in isplated, perfused kidneys of spontaneously hypertensive rats. Biochem. Pharmacol. 28:3601.

Shibouta, Y., Terashita Z.I., Inada, Y., Nishikawa, K., and Kikuchi, S. 1981, Enhanced thromboxane A_2 biosynthesis in the kidney of spontaneously hypertensive rats during development of hypertension. Eur. J. Phamacol. 70:247.

Shibouta, Y., Terashita, Z.I., Inada, Y., Kato, K., Nishikawa, K. 1982, Eur. J. Pharmacol. 85:51.

Sirosis, P., and Gagnon, R. 1974, Release of renomedullary prostaglandins in normal and hypertensive rats. Experientia 30:1418.

Stygles, V.G., Reinke, D.A., Rickert, D.E., and Hook, J.B. 1978, Increased blood pressure in the SHR is not related to a deficit in renomedullary PGE_2. Experientia 34:1025.

Uchida, S., Nonoguchi, H., and Endou, H. 1985, Localization and properties of NAD^+-dependent 15-hydroxyprostaglandin dehydrogenase activity in the rat kidney. Pflugers Arch. 404:278.

FACTOR XII LEVELS IN PATIENTS AFTER ABDOMINAL SURGERY

G. Fuhrer, M.J. Gallimore, M. Lambrecht,
and W. Heller

Department of Cardiovascular Surgery, University
of Tuebingen, 7400 Tuebingen, FRG

Introduction

Hageman factor (FXII) is thought to be an important component of the intrinsic fibrinolytic system. It might also
play an important role in the release of tPA via the activation of prekallikrein to kallikrein and liberation of
bradykinin from high molekular weight kininogen.
We have used a chromogenic substrate which detects both
alpha and beta FXIIa (S-2222) to develop a direct chromogenic
substrate assay for FXII.

Methods and materials

Citrated plasma was used for all assays.
FXII levels were determined in a clotting assay (Boehringer
Mannheim, FRG) according to the test instructions.
S-2222 was purchased from Deutsche KabiVitrum, Munich, FRG.
FXII antiserum was a generous gift from Dr. N. Heimburger,
Behringwerke AG, Marburg, FRG.
FXII activator, Kallikrein inhibitor, corn inhibitor and
standard plasma were obtained from Channel Diagnostics, Wal-
mer, Deal, Kent, U.K.
Sephadex G-150 fractionation of plasma was performed on a
column 85 x 2,5 cm. 3 ml fractions were collected.

Chromogenic Substrate Assay for FXII

Reagents.
Citrated plasma.
Standard plasma. Reconstitute with 1 ml distilled water.
FXII activator. Reconstitute with 5 ml distilled water.
S-2222. Dissolve 1 bottle (25 mg) in 16 ml distilled water.
Kallikrein inhibitor. Dissolve 1 bottle in 10 ml distilled
water. Label "stock solution" and store at +4°C.
Buffer A. Tris-HCl 0.05 mol/l pH 7.9, containing 0.15 M
methylamine, 3.36 g/l EDTA and 0.2 % albumin.
Buffer B. Tris-HCl 0.05 mol/l pH 7.9 plus kallikrein inhi-
bitor and albumin. 2 ml stock kallikrein inhibitor solution

plus 98 ml of Tris-HCl buffer 0.05 mol/l containing 0,2%
albumin.

Acetone treatment of plasma

600 μl standard plasma (300 μl test plasma) plus 200 μl acetone (100 μl for the test plasmas) are pipetted into siliconised glass test tubes (80 x 100), mixed well and left for
30 minutes at +4°C and then kept on ice.

Preparation of Standard Curve

The acetone treated plasma is diluted with buffer A as
follows:

standard %	plasma μl	buffer μl
200	200	200
150	150	250
100	100	300
75	75	325
50	50	350
25	25	375
0	use buffer only	

Dilute the test plasmas 100 μl acetone treated test plasma
plus 300 μl buffer A

Method

Have substrate and buffer B at 37°C
Into siliconised micro cuvettes, siliconised or plastic
tubes are pipetted

Plasma dilution or buffer A at 37°C	100 μl
plus	
FXII activator	100 μl
incubate at 37°C for exactly 10 min	
add	
Buffer B	300 μl
incubate for exactly 1 minute	
add	
S-2222	200 μl

Record ΔE_{405}/min (rate assay)
or incubate for exactly 10 min at 37°C
    add
Acetic acid (25%)   200 μl
read E_{405} (end point assay)

For the end point assay prepare blanks by adding the reagents in reverse order and substituting 300 μl buffer A for
the activator and substrate. Read E_{405} and substract the
values obtained from the test values.
Substract the 0% (buffer only values) from the other values
and plot the results as % standard plasma versus E_{405} and calculate the values for the test plasmas from this standard
curve.

<u>Results</u>

Typical standard curves for the rate and end point assays
are shown in figures 1 and 2.
Acetone treatment of plasma is essential to destroy inhibitors of alpha and beta FXIIa as shown in fig. 3.
The optimum pH in the activation stage of the assay was
found to be 7.9 as shown in fig. 4a, whilst that for the
reaction with the substrate was 8.3 (fig. 4b).
The optimum activation time for the assay was 10 minutes.
When fractions obtained by Sephadex G-150 gel filtration were
tested in the assay a peak of activity corresponding to
samples containing FXII antigen was found. The activity which
was generated in these samples was completely inhibited by
corn inhibitor.
When 25 normal plasmas were assayed for FXII in the chromogenic substrate and clotting assays a correlation between
the two assays of 0.81 was obtained.

100 patients before and after abdominal surgery were analysed for factor XII levels. Only 10% of patients showed
a preoperative value below 60% of normal. 3 days after surgery 40% of patients had factor XII levels below 60%
(table 1).

Table 1. Levels of FXII preoperative and 3 days after
operation

FXII levels in %

	60	60-80	81-100	101-120	121-140	140
preoperative	10	20	20	21	18	11
3 days after operation	40	26	17	11	4	2

<u>Discussion</u>

Routine studies on Hageman factor (FXII) have been hampered
by the lack of a simple, rapid assay for this important
central component of the plasma defence systems. Most of the
research work on this protein has involved clotting assays
with FXII-deficient plasma. We have used a new soluble activator of FXII together with a chromogenic peptide substrate
sensitive to alpha and beta FXIIa to develop a direct
chromogenic substrate assay for determing FXII levels in
plasma. Either rate or end point assays can be used. It has
been found that acetone treatment of plasma is essential to
destroy inhibitors of alpha and beta FXIIa. Without acetone
treatment very little enzyme activity was generated. The
optimum activation time in the assay was found to be 10 minutes. Initial plasma dilutions were performed in a buffer
containing methylamine to block the formation of enzyme-
$alpha_2$-macroglobulin complexes which might attack the substrate. Incubation with a kallikrein inhibitor containing
buffer was included to inhibit any plasma kallikrein activity. Gel filtration of plasma revealed that the assay detects

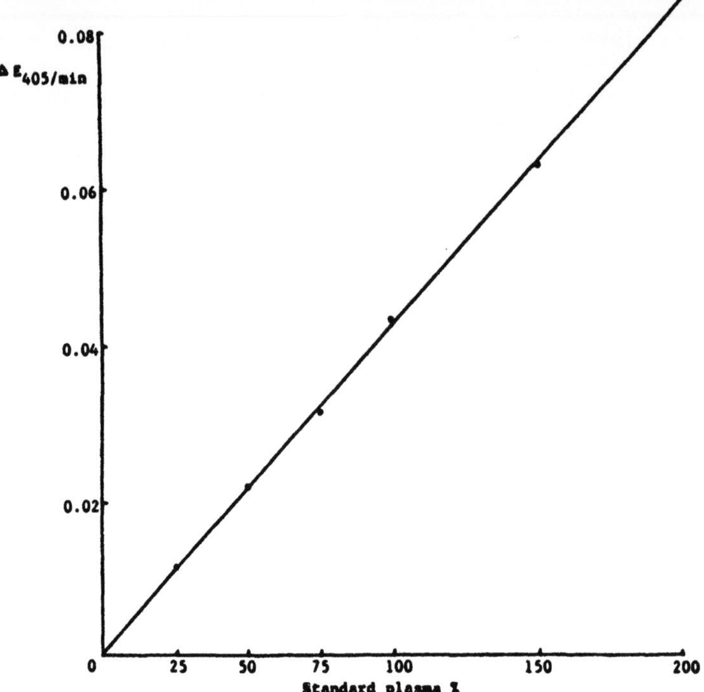

Fig. 1 Chromogenic substrate assay for FXII
Rate assay standard curve

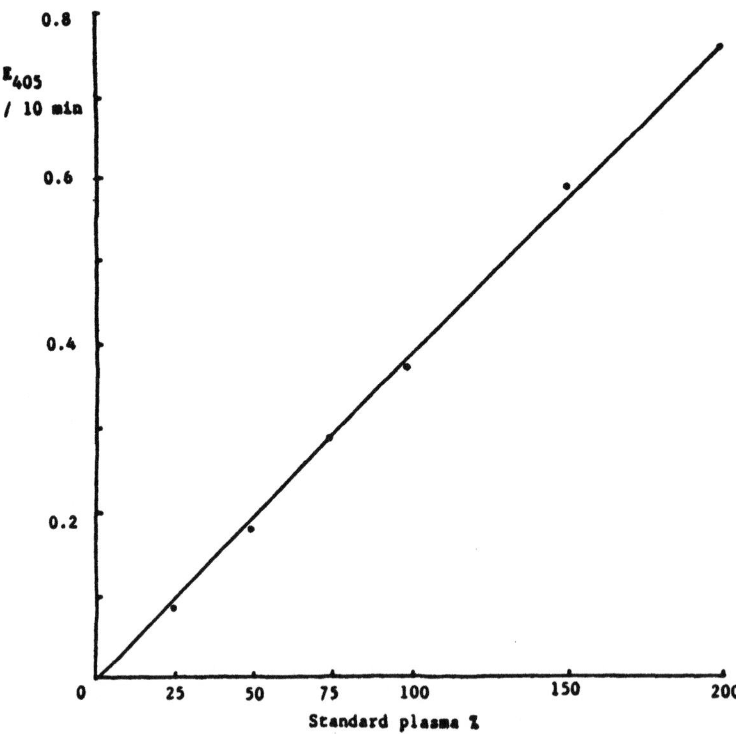

Fig. 2 Chromogenic substrate assay for FXII
End point assay standard curve

512

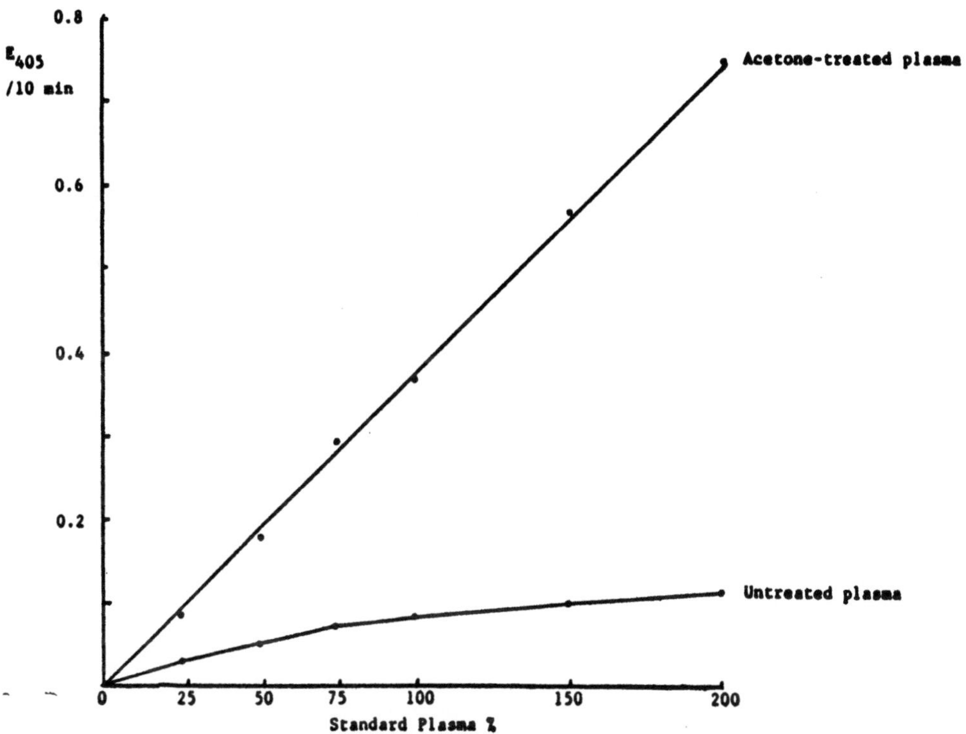

Fig. 3 Chromogenic substrate assay for FXII
Comparison between acetone-treated and
untreated plasma

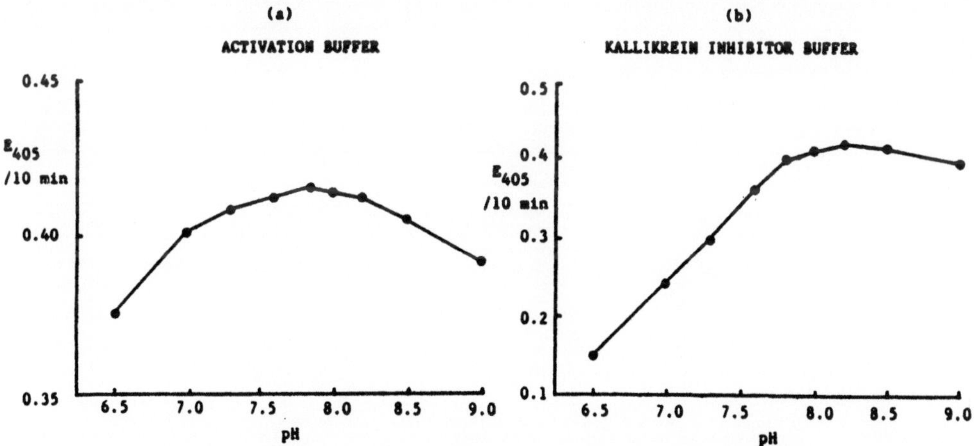

Fig. 4 Chromogenic substrate assay for FXII
Effects of the variation of pH of the
activation and kallikrein inhibition
buffers

FXII and that the activity generated can be inhibited by the
FXII enzyme inhibitor, corn inhibitor. Four FXII-deficient
plasma samples gave 0% FXII when tested in the assay. When
plasma samples from 25 normal healthy donors were assayed
for factor XII levels in the chromogenic substrate assay and
a clotting assay, a good correlation between the two assays
was obtained.

Furthermore, plasma samples from 100 patients before and after abdominal surgery were tested with this new assay. Factor XII levels were found to be below 60% of normal before
operation on 10%, whilst three days after operation 40% of
the patients had lower factor XII levels than 60%. Because
factor XII appears to play an important role for fibrinolysis, low levels of this protein together with reduced levels of inhibitors of coagulation could be a contributory
factor for thrombotic tendency seen following major abdominal surgery.

MECHANISM OF ACTIVATION OF THE KALLIKREIN-KININ SYSTEM IN PLASMA OF
PATIENTS WITH ATOPIC ALLERGIC DISEASES

V.L. Dotsenko, N.M. Nenasheva, E.A. Neshkova,
N.A. Morozova and G.A. Yarovaya

Central Institute for Post-Graduate Education of
Physicians, Moscow, USSR

INTRODUCTION

Changes in the activity of the kallikrein-kinin system (KKS) in patients with allergies may aggravate the course of the disease worsening
patients' state. The aggravation is mostly due to the increased content
in plasma of vasoactive peptides released from the specific substrate
kininogen by the activated kininogenase kallikrein (1.2). The mechanism of
such activation in atopic states upon contact with allergen is not yet
clear. Concept of the enzymic activation of XII blood-clotting factor
(Hageman factor) due to specific degranulation of basophil polymorphonuclear leukocytes upon their contact with allergen, put forward by Newball
et al. (3,4), seems to be in contradiction with the data of Hojima et al.
who consider the activation of Hageman factor as a result of contact interaction with negatively charged heparin molecules (5).

As the activation of KKS was observed in acute pollinose and urticaria, as well as in the period of hyposensibilizing treatment of these states (1), we made an attempt to study: 1. the initial stage of the activation of the system upon its contact with allergen, using the purified components of the system, Hageman factor and prekallikrein; 2. the role of
contact activation of Hageman factor as a possible initiator of kininogene-
sis; 3. changes in kallikrein activity and prekallikrein content just in
normal donor serum upon its incubation with the patients' leukocyte preparation in the presence of specific allergen. The absence of progressive
activation of Hageman factor upon its contact with "liberate" during prolonged incubation was also discussed. The data showing the inactivation
of the factor with "liberate" were presented.

METHODS

Leukocyte preparations enriched with basophils were obtained from
25 ml of blood of patients with pollinose. All the 18 patients were in
the remission period.

Leukocytes were obtained by sedimentation (6) or centrifugation in the
density gradient (7), then they were washed and resuspended in buffer solution containing Ca^{2+} and Mg^{2+} (3,4).

Effect of the "Liberate" on the Preparations of Hageman Factor and Prekallikrein

To study the effect of the "liberate" of the basophil-enriched mononuclear cells on Hageman factor (HF) and prekallikrein (PK), two modifications were used. In one series of experiments, 15-30 µl of specific allergen (water-salt extract of pollen from grass and trees) were mixed with 0.4-0.6 ml of leukocyte preparation (10^6-10^7 cells in 1 ml of the suspension) and incubated for 40-60 min. After the incubation and withdrawal of leukocytes, the supernate ("liberate") was studied for its ability to activate HF and PK. For that purpose, to 0.4 ml of the "liberate" were added 0.2 ml of HF or 0.4 ml of PK. The mixture was buffered with 0.05 ml of 0.5 M Tris buffer, pH 8.0, and incubated at 37°C; then the aliquote of 0.1-0.2 ml were collected and their activities assayed.

In the other series of experiments, cell suspension (0.4 ml-0.6 ml) was mixed with the same volume of HF, then 15 µl of specific allergen were added, and the mixture was incubated for definite time periods. The activity of HF was estimated in the supernate after the withdrawal of the cells.

As controls, in all modifications the allergen-free mixtures were used. Prior to the incubation with leukocytes or with the "liberate", the HF preparation was in some experiments thoroughly dialyzed against 0.05 M Tris buffer, pH 8.0, or against the buffer used for suspending leukocytes. In two experiments, beside HF, 0.1 ml (168 µg) of HMW-kininogen was introduced into the incubation mixture after the dialysis.

Preparation of Hageman Factor, Prekallikrein, and High-Molecular Weight Kininogen

__Hageman factor__ (XII factor of blood-clotting system) was obtained as a precursor from fresh serum in the course of 4 chromatographic steps using QAE-Sephadex, Sephadex G-200 and Sephadex G-150 procedures (8). The activity was estimated by the ability of the trypsin-treated HF to convert prekallikrein to the active enzyme. The HF activity was characterized by the augmentation of BAEE-esterase activity of prekallikrein per min. Used were the preparations having a specific activity of 1.5-1.8 E/min (0.5-0.6 E·min^{-1}·ml^{-1}).

__Prekallikrein__ was isolated on QAE- and KM-Sephadexes from fresh serum as described earlier (9). The studies were carried out using a preparation with a specific activity of 2-3 E (1.0-1.5 E·ml^{-1}). When using prekallikrein as substrate for the estimation of HF activity, the aliquot containing HF (0.1-0.2 ml) was mixed with 0.1 ml of 0.5 M Tris buffer, pH 8.0, and with 0.1 ml of prekallikrein. After the incubation of the mixture for 10-20 min at 37°C, its volume was brought to 2 ml with 0.05 M Tris buffer, pH 8.0, then 1 ml of 1.5×10^{-3} BAEE solution was added in the same buffer, and the BAEE-esterase activity of kallikrein estimated.

__High-Molecular-Weight Kininogen__ (HMW-kininogen) was isolated from plasma in two chromatographic steps by the method of Dittman et al. (12) with some modifications. The activity of the preparation was 2 mg-equiv. of bradykinin/mg protein.

Activation of the Kallikrein-Kinin System in Normal Serum

To study the KKS activation under the action of the "liberate" directly in normal serum, to 1 ml of serum was added 1 ml of the "liberate" obtained by incubation of the leukocyte preparation with specific allergen. The control sample contained a mixture of normal donor serum with the supernate of the leukocyte preparation without allergen. The incubation was carried out for 30 min at 37°C, after which the KKS activity and the activity of the serum antikallikrein potential were estimated by two different methods: a chromatographic method using DEAE-Sephadex A-50 (10) and a complex method with the use of the tripeptide chromogenic substrate S-2302 (11).

RESULTS AND DISCUSSION

Co-incubation of HF and PK with the supernate of the basophil-enriched leukocyte preparation upon its contact with specific allergen ("liberate") led to a more pronounced activation of the enzymes than the contact of their precursors with the allergen-free supernate. Fig. 1 (A) shows that progressive increase of HF activity occurs in the initial 1-2 h of incubation. Longer incubation periods did not essentially change the HF activity levels. The activation of PK under the same experimental conditions was more pronounced; however, in none of the 9 experiments the activity level surpassed 4% and 10% of potential activity of HF and PK, respectively.

Modification of the experiments, with the allergen being introduced directly into the incubation mixture containing the leukocyte preparation and HF, did not change the rate of proenzyme activation in the initial 2 h of the incubation. Longer incubation periods led to the levelling of HF activity in the experimental and control samples (Fig. 2).

For the evaluation of the possible role of contact activation of HF on the negatively charged heparin molecules released from basophil leukocytes upon contact with specific allergen, we changed the content of the incubation mixture by introducing into it equal volumes of the leukocyte preparation and of the polybrene-free HF. Incubation was carried out in plastic test-tubes in the presence of 80-160 µg/ml of HMW kininogen, the necessary cofactor of contact activation. The mixture was incubated for 1 h at 37°C, after which the leukocytes were withdrawn by centrifugation and HF activity estimated.

The results obtained (Fig. 3) show that there is no augmentation of the factor activity in the absence of polybrene. These data were interpreted as indicating the key role of enzymatic processes in the activation of HF by the "liberate" of the basophil-enriched leukocyte preparation upon its contact with specific allergens.

The retardation of HF activation or, in some cases, even the decrease of HF activity upon prolonged incubation with the "liberate", as will be seen in Fig. 3, prompted the study of the nature of this phenomenon. Selective assay for the nativity of HF (i.e. its ability to be activated by trypsin) upon its prolonged activation with the "liberate" showed that HF retained full potential activity only for the first half-hour, after which the activity was gradually decreased: within the first hour it fell to 80-90%, with subsequent fall at 4 h to 20% of the initial activity level. This finding may be accounted for by two processes: 1. slow inhibition of HF due to possible presence of some inhibitor in the "liberate"; 2. inactivation of HF and/or its precursors by the proteinases of the "liberate".

Modest activation of purified HF and prekallikrein by the "liberate" of the leukocyte preparation (only up to 4-10% of their potential activity), as well as the inhibition and/or inactivation of HF upon prolonged incubation, could possibly be due to the absence of optimal conditions for the

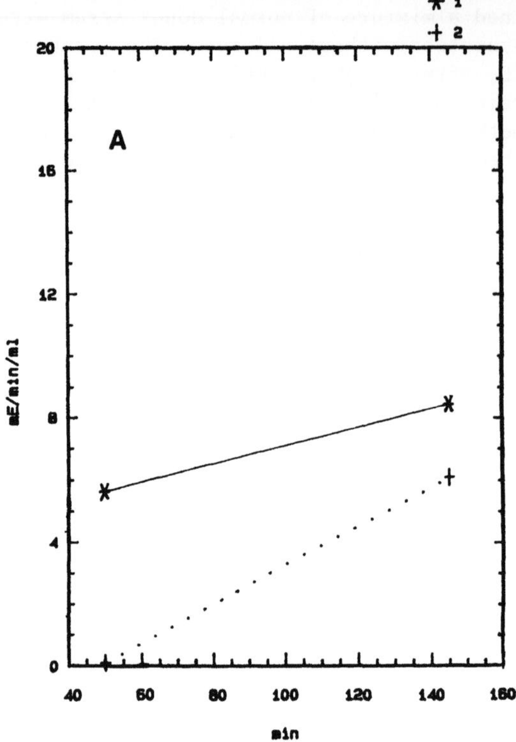

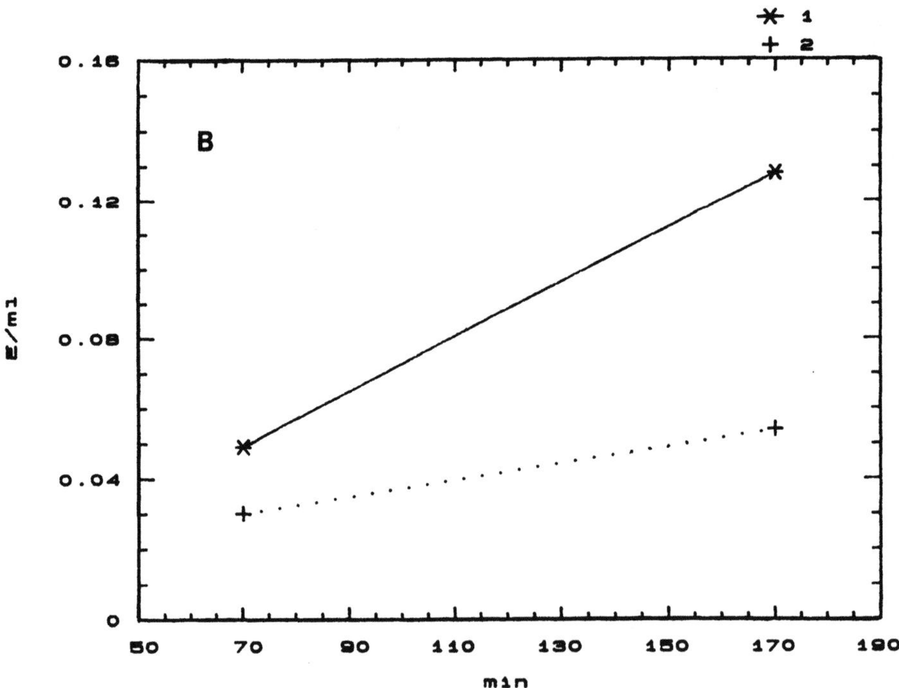

Fig. 1. Activation of Hageman factor (A) and prekallikrein (B) by the "liberate" of the sensibilized basophil-enriched leukocyte preparation obtained from a patient with pollinose and pre-incubated with specific allergen (curve 1). Control is the result of incubation under the same conditions but without allergen (curve 2).

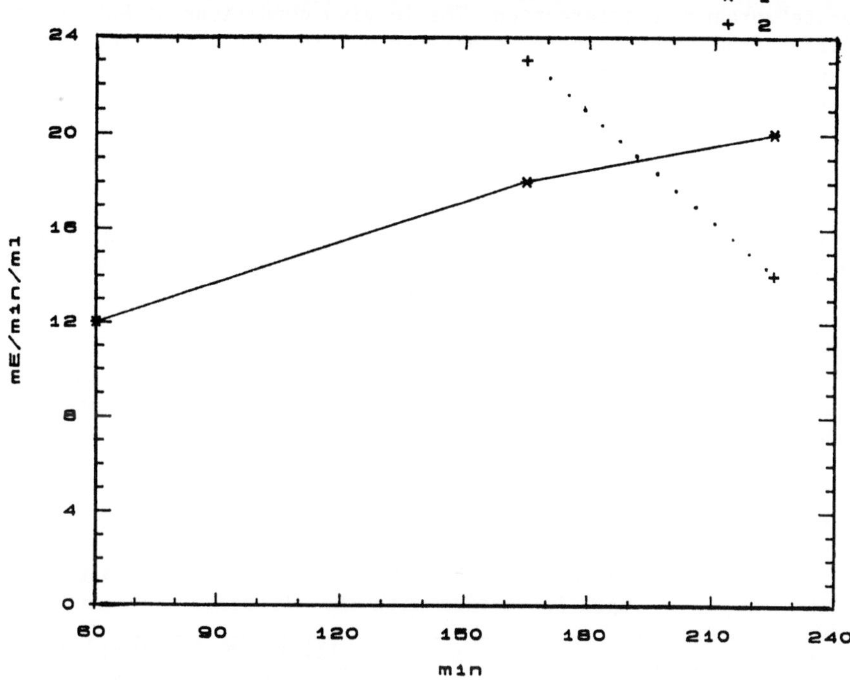

Fig. 2. Activation of Hageman factor in the presence of the sensibilized basophil-enriched leukocyte preparation and specific
allergen (curve 1). Control is the result of incubation
under the same conditions but without allergen (curve 2).

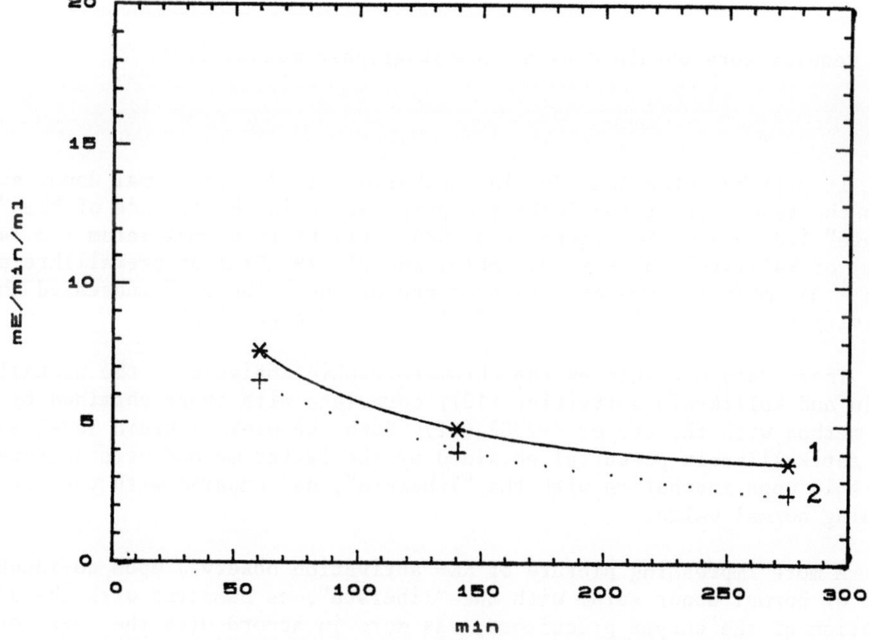

Fig. 3. Activation of Hageman factor after withdrawal of polybrene in
the presence of the sensibilized-basophil-enriched leukocyte
preparation, specific allergen, and high-molecular weight
kininogen (curve 1). Control is the result of incubation under
the same conditions but without allergen (curve 2).

"liberate"-proenzyme interaction. The in vivo conditions of KKS activation
may differ from those in model experiments: in vivo, both precursors (HF
and prekallikrein) occur in the medium simultaneously and may activate each
other under certain conditions; besides, in vivo activation of KKS components
upon specific degranulation of basophil and mast cells proceeds at high
plasma antiproteolytic potential inhibiting the non-specific degradation
of enzymes and their precursors.

Indeed, the interaction of the "liberate" of the patients' leukocyte
preparations directly with normal serum led to a sharp increase in kallikrein activity and decrease in precursor content.

Table 1 presents mean values of the kallikrein and prekallikrein activities obtained in experiments with the leukocyte preparations of 4 patients. In control assays, the activity of kallikrein and its precursor
was measured in the samples taken from the same normal donors as the experimental samples but incubated without the "liberate".

Table 1. Activation of Prekallikrein in Normal Donor Serum
upon Incubation with the "liberate"

Objects of studies	N	Kallikrein* (mE/ml)	Prekallikrein* (mE/ml)
Normal serum incubated without the "liberate" (control)	4	33.14±19.87	211.79±50.20
Normal serum incubated with the "liberate"	4	69.31±27.20	106.56±28.17

* Results were obtained by a chromatographic method (10).

It will be noted that 30 min incubation at 37°C of normal donor serum
with the supernate of the leukocyte preparation in the absence of the "liberate" led to a marked increase of KKS activity in normal serum (33.14
mE/ml of kallikrein at N = 3.4 mE/ml and 211.79 mE/ml of prekallikrein
at N = 340 mE/ml). However, the presence of the "liberate" increased this
activity still twice (69.31 and 106.56 mE/ml, respectively).

These data obtained by the chromatographic analysis of the prekallikrein and kallikrein activities (10), correlate with those obtained by
the method with the use of S-2302 (11). Both the prekallikrein level and
the antikallikrein potential obtained by the latter method were decreased
3-4-fold upon incubation with the "liberate", as compared with the corresponding normal values.

A more impressing picture of KKS activation observed upon co-incubation of normal donor serum with the "liberate", as compared with the activation of the enzyme precursors, was more in accord with the level of KKS
activation in patients with acute allergic diseases (1). The difference in
activation is apparently caused by two factors: the simultaneous presence
in the serum of 2 enzyme precursors (HF and prekallikrein) and the suppression of the "liberate"-induced non-specific proteolysis which leads to considerable inactivation of HF in the initial incubation period by serum
inhibitors.

REFERENCES

1. N. M. Nenasheva, V. L. Dotsenko, L. A. Goryachkina, and G. A. Yarovaya, Activity of the prekallikrein-kallikrein system and characteristic properties of its regulation in some allergic diseases, Vopr. Med. Chim., 32 (5): 106 (1986).
2. P. Norman, R. Naclerio, P. Creticos, A. Tobias, and L. Lichtenstein, Mediator release after allergic and physical nasal challenges, Inter. Archiv Aller. Appl. Immunol, 77: 57 (1985).
3. H. H. Newball, R. C. Talamo, and L. M. Lichtenstein, Anaphylactic release of a basophil kallikrein-like activity. II. A mediator of immediate hypersensitivity reactions. J. Clin. Invest., 64: 466 (1979).
4. H. H. Newball, H. L. Meier, and L. M. Lichtenstein, Basophil mediators and their release with emphasis on BK-A, J. Invest. Dermat., 74: 344 (1980).
5. Y. Hojima, C. G. Cochrane, R.C. Wiggins, K. F. Austen, and R. L. Steven, In vitro activation of the contact (Hageman factor) system of plasma by heparin and chondroitin sulfate E, Blood, 63: 1453 (1984).
6. L. M. Lichtenstein, and A. Osler, Studies on the mechanisms of hypersensitivity phenomena, J. Exper. Med., 12: 507 (1964).
7. S. P. Stahl, S. Nory, and B. Weeke, Basophil histamine release in patient with hay fever, Clin. Exper. Med., 27: 423 (1977).
8. V. L. Dotsenko, N. B. Serova, A. I. Logunov, N. P. Levkova, and G. A. Yarovaya, On the activation of kallikrein-kinin system in human blood plasma under conditions of gastroduodenal ulcer, Vopr. med. Chim., 33(4): 104 (1987).
9. J. Kawiak, M. Kawalec, V. L. Dotsenko, and G. A. Yarovaya, Purification of human serum prekallikrein, some properties of the purified proenzyme and its stability, Clin. Chim. Acta, 141: 287 (1984).
10. T. S. Paskhina, V. L. Dotsenko, and E. I. Blinnikova, Kallikreinogen in human blood serum; a method of estimation and some properties, Biokhimiya, 38: 420 (1973).
11. V. L. Dotsenko, G. A. Yarovaya, and E. A. Neshkova, Chromogenic peptide substrate assay for estimation of four indices of the kallikrein-kinin system activity, Vopr. Med. Chim. 34, in press (1988).
12. B. Dittman, A. Stager, R. Wimmer, H. Fritz, A convenient large-scale preparation of HMW-kininogen from human plasma, Hoppe-Seylers Z. physiol. Chem., 362: 919 (1981).

LOCALIZATION OF GLANDULAR KALLIKREIN IN NASAL MUCOSA OF ALLERGIC AND NONALLERGIC INDIVIDUALS

C.R. Baumgarten, R. Schwarting and G. Kunkel

Dept. of Clinical Immunology
Freie Universität Berlin
1000 Berlin 65, Germany

Introduction

The development of a reproducible, controlled model of
nasal challenge with allergen (1) has provided us with
a relatively noninvasive technique to study the
pathophysiology of allergic rhinitis. By using this model,
we have demonstrated that bradykinin and lysyl-bradykinin
are generated in nasal secretions during both the immediate
and late responses to antigen challenge (2,3 and 4). In
further studies we have begun trying to delineate the
mechanisms by which kinins are formed during the immediate
allergic response. Substrates for kinin-forming enzymes
are provided by a transudation of both high molecular weight
kininogen (HMWK) and low molecular weight kininogen (LMWK)
from plasma into nasal secretions (5), and we have recently
provided evidence that activation of plasma kallikrein
plays a significant role in kinin formation (6). Activation
of plasma kallikrein during the allergic response, however,
cannot explain generation of lysyl-bradykinin, because
this enzyme generates only bradykinin (7). We have shown,
however, that the concentrations of immunoreactive glandular
kallikrein in nasal secretions increase in response to
allergen challenge and have demonstrated that this material
represents predominantly authentic, active glandular
kallikrein which can generate lysyl-bradykinin from
kininogen (8). To our knowledge, this represents the first
demonstration that glandular kallikrein is present in
human nasal secretions. The source of the glandular
kallikrein in nasal secretions remains to be determined.
It is possible that it derives from the 100.000 small
serummucus glands or the 250 large anterior serous glands
in the lamina propria (9), or perhaps, in analogy to
the intestinal epithelium, from goblet cells (10). The
present study adresses this issue. To determine the source
of the glandular kallikrein in nasal secretions it was
visualized using a highly specific rabbit anti-serum
against highly purified HUK in the sensitive APAAP
(alkaline phosphatase antialkaline phosphatase)
immunohistochemical staining procedure (11) of nasal
tissue from the inferior turbinate of allergic and
nonallergic individuals.

<u>Materials and Methods</u>
<u>Subjects</u>

Allergic individuals (n=14) and nonallergic controls (n=15)
between the ages of 18 and 55 were recruited. All subjects
gave informed consent before being included in the study.
Allergic individuals were defined as having seasonal
symptoms to an antigen to which they had a positiv
intradermal skin reaction at a concentration of 10 protein
nitrogen units (PNU) per ml or less of crude antigen
extract and a RAST class $\geqslant$ 2. Nonallergic individuals
had no allergic history and a negativ skin test to allergen
extracts at a concentration of 100 PNU/ml and negativ
RAST tests. In each case nasal mucosa was optained from
the inferior turbinate in general anaesthesia.

<u>Rabbit-anti-HUK</u>

To visualize the glandular kallikrein highly purified
HUK was used to produce antisera in rabbits. The
monospecificity of the rabbit antiserum selected was
verified by immunodiffusion (12) against HUK and
concentrated human urine. An IgG fraction of this antiserum
was prepared by precipitation with 50 % ammonium sulfate
and chromatography on immobilized protein A. To ensure
that this IgG fraction was not contaminated with rabbit
plasma kallikrein, it was additionally purified by passage
over immobilized soybean trypsin inhibitor (SBTI). Finally,
the preparation was treated with diisopropylfluorophosphate
(DFP) and excess DFP was removed by extensive dialysis.
When used in binding studies this purified IgG fraction
showed good binding of ^{125}I-HUK but failed to bind
iodinated human plasma kallikrein. The IgG fraction was
also ineffective in inhibiting the generation of bradykinin
from HMWK by plasma kallikrein.

<u>Indirect immunoenzymatic Staining</u>

Indirect immunoperoxidase staining of tissue sections
was performed as previously described by Cordell et al.
(11). For immunoalkaline phosphatase staining, the fixed
tissue sections were incubated with the rabbit-anti-HUK
(1/2000 diluted) described above for 30 minutes, followed
by incubation with a rabbit-anti-mouse IgG and a complex
of alkaline phosphatase and monoclonal antialkaline
phosphatase (APAAP). To enhance the labeling, the
incubation with rabbit-anti-mouse-IgG and APAAP was
repeated once or twice. Between each incubation step,
the slices were briefly washed with 0.05 mol/l Tris-HCl,
pH 7.6. For visualization of the alkaline phosphatase
activity, the slides were incubated with the alkaline
substrate for 30 minutes with continual agitation. The
alkaline substrate was prepared as follows: 0.5 ml of
a 5 % solution of new fuchsin in 2N HCl was added to 1.25
ml of a freshly prepared 4 % solution of sodium nitrite.
After 60 seconds, this solution was added to 200 ml of
0.05 mol/l Tris-HCl (pH 8.7) containing 90 mg levamisole,
followed by the addition of 125 mg naphthol As-Bi-phosphate,
which had been freshly dissolved in dimethylformamide
at 10 mg/1.5 ml. This solution was then filtered and used
immediately. After the enzyme reaction, the slides were

washed in Tris-HCl (pH 7,6) and counterstained with
hemalum.

Results

Fig. 1 shows a light micrograph of human nasal mucosa
from the inferior turbinate illustrating the localisation
of tissue kallikrein (red staining) in one of the small
seromucus glands and in the apical portion of mucus
secreting cells in the epithelium. However it is not clear
whether the red-stained mucus - it is to say tissue
kallikrein content - was derived from the mucus secreting
cells in the epithelium itself or from different sources.
All smaller seromucus glands in each section were red
stained, without any exception in both the allergic and
nonallergic control group. In addition we could
demonstrate, that tissue kallikrein is present in the
larger ducts of human parotid and submandibular glands
if tissue sections of these glands were stained in preliminary studies (not shown).

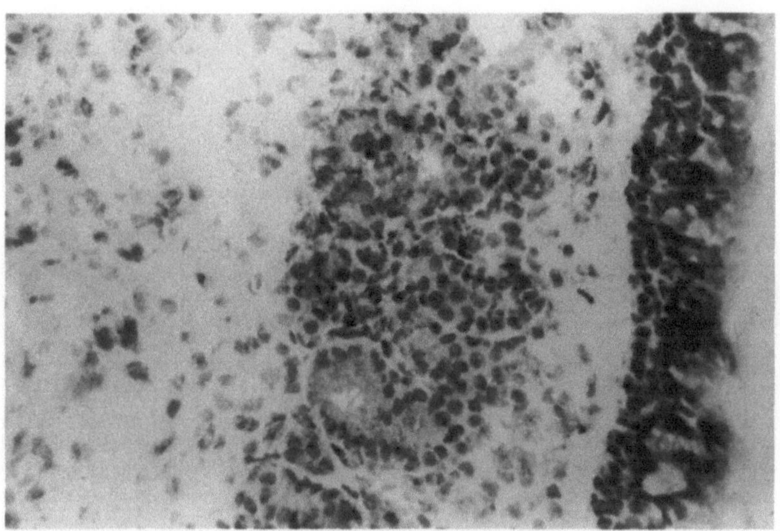

Fig. 1. Survey light micrograph of human nasal mucosa
from the inferior turbinate illustrating the localisation
of tissue kallikrein (red staining) in smaller seromucus
glands and in the mucus layer on the apical surface.

By contrast to the distribution of tissue kallikrein
in all smaller seromucus glands, there are only a few
sections of nasal mucosa, predominantly in those of
allergic individuals, containing red - stained cells,
see fig. 2 and table 1.

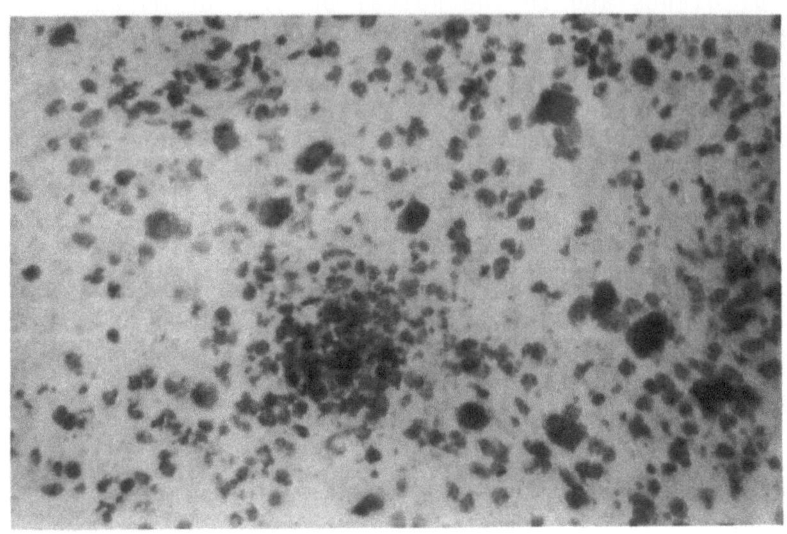

Fig. 2. Section of "allergic" human nasal mucosa with cells containing tissue kallikrein (red staining).

Tab. 1. Distribution of red-stained cells in allergic versus nonallergic controls.

| Pat.-No. | clinical evaluation | | | light microscopy stained | |
	History	skin test	RAST	seromucus glands	stroma cells
1-6	pos.	pos. $\geqslant$ 3 major allergens	4	all	+++
7-14	pos.	pos. $\geqslant$ 3 major allergens	1-3	all	++
15-20	neg.	pos. $\geqslant$ 3 major allergens	0	all	+
21-29	neg.	neg.	0	all	-

* semiquantitative estimations of the number of cells
  expressed as: - + ++ +++

Controls were performed in two ways:

1. by prior absorption of the antibody to tissue kallikrein
   with 20 microgramm per ml of purified human urinary
   kallikrein and
2. by staining of the tissue sections as
   a described without preincubation with the highly
   specific rabbit- anti-serum against human urinary
   kallikrein (fig.3).

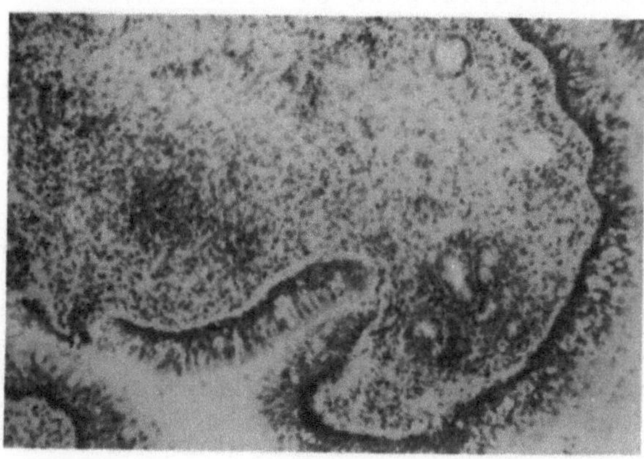

Fig. 3. Negative control: indirect immunoperoxydase-
staining of a tissue section without preincubation with
the highly specific rabbit-anti-HUK.

Discussion

These studies were prompted by our earlier observation
that immunoreactive human glandular kallikrein (iHGK)
is present in nasal secretions obtained by lavage and
that levels of iHGK increase after antigen challange of
allergic individuals (8). Furthermore, the demonstration
that iHGK in lavages has identical properties to authentic
HUK with its resistance to plasma inhibitors, with only
alpha$_1$-protease inhibitor having a weak and slow effect
(12), and its ability to generate kinin from both HMWK
and LMWK, so that available substrate is greater, makes
it to an important enzym of kinin generation.
We have demonstrated the localisation of glandular
kallikrein in the smaller seromucus glands of nasal mucosa
in 29 individuals with or without nasal allergy. In each
case sections of those glands in close proximity to the
nasal susrface were red-stained. Glandular kallikrein
is thus located in a position where it very well may
influence local blood flow. Interestingly, tissue
kallikrein has also recently been shown to increase in
bronchol alveolar lavage fluids from asthmatics after
bronchial challenge with allergen (13). Thus, tissue
kallikrein may be involved in local inflammatory events
in both the upper and lower airways.
In some cases we have identified a cell typ in sections
of nasal mucosa contanining red-stained tissue kallikrein
predominantly in allergic individuals. These cells have
to be characterized in further studies.

References

1. Naclerio, R.M., H.L. Meier, A. Kagey-Sobotka, N. F. Adkinson Jr., D. A. Meyers, P.S. Norman and L.M. Lichtenstein, 1983 Mediator release after nasal airway challange with allergen. Am. Rev. Respir. Dis. 128:597
2. Proud, D., A. Togias, R.M. Naclerio, S. A. Crush, P.S. Norman and L.M. Lichtenstein. 1983. Kinins are generated in vivo following nasal airway challenge of allergic individuals with allergen. J. Clin. Invest. 72:1678
3. Naclerio, R.M., D. Proud, A.G. Togias, N.F. Adkinson Jr., D.A. Meyers, A. Kagey-Sobotka, M. Plaut, P.S. Norman and L.M. Lichtenstein. 1985. Inflammatory mediators in late antigen-induced rhinitis. N. Engl. J. Med. 313:65.
4. D. Proud and C.R. Baumgarten: Kinins in nasal lavage fluid. 1987. In Allergicand vasomotor Rhinitis: Pathophysiological Aspects. N. Mygind and U. Pipkorn, ed. Munksgaard 198.
5. Baumgarten, C.R., A.G. Togias, R.M. Naclerio, L.M. Lichtenstein, P.S. Norman and D. Proud. 1985. Influx of kininogens into nasal secretions after antigen challenge of allergic individuals. J. Clin. Invest. 76:191.
6. Baumgarten, C.R., R.C. Nichols, R.M. Naclerio, L. M. Lichtenstein, P.S. Norman an D. Proud. 1986. Plasma kallikrein during experimentally induced allergic rhinitis: role in kinin formation and contribution to TAME-esterase activity in nasal secretions. J. Immunol. 137:977.
7. Webster, M.E. and J.V. Pierce. 1963. The nature of the kallidins released from human plasma by kallikreins and other enzymes. Ann. N.Y. Acad. Sci. 104:91.
8. C.R. Baumgarten, R.C. Nichols, R.M. Naclerio, D. Proud. 1986: Concentrations of glandular kallikrein in human nasal secretions increase during experimentally induced allergic rhinitis. J. Immunol. 137:1323.
9. Mygind, N. and A. Anggard. 1984. Anatomy and physiology of the nose-pathophysiologic alterations in allergic rhinitis. Clin. Rev. Allergy 2:173.
10. Schachter, M., M.W. Peret, A.G. Billing and G.D. Wheeler, 1983. Immunolocalization of the protease kallikrein in the colon. J. Histochem. Cytochem. 31:1255.
11. Cordell J, Falini B, Erber ON, Ghosh AK, Abdulaziz,Z. MacDonald S, Polford K, Stein H, Mason DY: Immunoenzymatic labeling of monoclonal antibodies using immune complexes of alkaline phosphatase and monoclonal anti-alkaline phosphatase (APAAP Complexes). J. Histochem. Cytochem. 32:219, 1984.
12. Ouchterlony, O. 1949, Antigen-antibody reactions in gels. Acta Pathol. Microbiol. Immunol. Scand 26:507.
13. S.C. Christiansen, D. Proud and C.G. Cochrane. 1987. Detection of tissue kallikrein in the bronchoalveolar lavage fluid of asthmatic subjects. J. Clin. Invest. 79, 188.

PARTICIPATION OF SUBSTANCE P IN INFLAMMATORY RESPONSES

Norifumi Yonehara, Yasuo Imai, Tooru Shibutani[*] and
Reizo Inoki

Departments of Pharmacology and [*]Anesthesiology, Faculty of
Dentistry, Osaka University, Suita 565, Osaka Japan

INTRODUCTION

The first description of efferential function in primary afferent
neurons was given by Goltz[1] and Stricker[2]. They observed that electrical
stimulation of the primary afferent neurons produced a flare phenomenon due
to vasodilatation of the skin of the hind limb on the same side. In 1927,
Lewis and Marvin[3] postulated that this inflammatory response in the skin
might be mediated by the release of substances at the peripheral endings of
cutaneous vasodilator nerve fibers. Many substances have subsequently been
suggested as mediators responsible for neurogenic inflammatory responses.
In 1953, Lembeck[4] proposed that substance P (SP) may be a primary afferent
neurotransmitter. Since then, evidence supporting that SP may be one of
the predominant mediators causing neurogenic inflammation in the cutaneous
tissue has accumulated in immunohistochemical[5] and pharmacological[6] fields.
In addition, recent pathophysiological[7] studies in laboratory animals and
human showed that sensory SP neurons might contribute to the pathogenesis
of polyarthritis, respiratory-tract irritation, migration, urticaria, etc..
These findings lead to the suggestion that the afferent impulses from nerve
terminals of the small-diameter afferent fibers generated by various kinds
of irritation to the tissue may induce the release of SP into the periphery,
which in turn may mediate several different inflammatory responses as a
local defence reaction to various kinds of irritation.

This study was, therefore, undertaken to clarify the participation of
SP released into the periphery in the inflammatory responses. For this
purpose, the volume of edema evoked by noxious heat stimulation was traced
in comparison with amount of SP.

MATERIALS AND METHODS

Double Coaxial Perfusion Technique and Radioimmunoassay of SP

Male Sprague-Dawley rats (120-180 g) were used. Rats were
anesthetized with urethane (780 mg/kg i.p.) and a double polyethylene tube
was introduced into the subcutaneous space according to the method of
Rocha e Silva and Antonio[8]. Using a peristaltic pump, perfusion was
carried out through the inner tube at a rate of 0.1 ml/min with saline
containing bestatin (3 mg/100 ml), an aminopeptidase inhibitor. Perfusates

were successively collected every 10 minutes in a test tube placed into an
ice bath. The samples were lyophilized and then immunoassayed for SP using
the corresponding antisera. For noxious stimulation, the paw on the
perfused side was immersed for 30 min in a water-bath (adjusted to 47°C)
one hour after the start of the perfusion, and then returned to room
temperature (25°C). In a parallel experiment, the volume of the paw was
measured to learn the extent of the edematous state evoked by the heat
stimulation.

Inflammatory Response

As an indicator of the inflammatory response induced by the noxious
heat stimulation, an edema of the hind paw was measured using a Volume
Meter (MK-550, Muromachi Kikai Co. LTD, Tokyo, Japan) at various time
intervals after the heat stimulation.

Treatment of Rats

Capsaicin pretreatment: Capsaicin at a dose of 40 mg/kg was injected
s.c. into a newborn rat within a week after birth as described by Jancsó et
al.[9]. Only the vehicle was administered to control rats. Two months after
the treatment with capsaicin, animals were used for experiments.

Chronic denervation: The saphenous and sciatic nerves were sectioned
unilaterally 7 days before the experiment. Control rats underwent sham
operations.

To examine the possible involvement of the bradykinin (BK) system in
the release of SP and the formation of edema, stem bromelain (10 mg/kg
i.v.) and emorfazone (50 mg/kg i.v.[9]) were given simultaneously 1 hr before
noxious heat stimulation. Des-Arg[9]-[Leu[8]]BK dissolved in saline was also
infused via an arterial cannula inserted into the contralateral iliac
artery to the perfused side at a rate of 0.1 ml/200 sec for a 40 min period
from 10 min before heating until the heat stimulation was terminated.

To examine the effect of steroidal compounds on the heat-induced SP
release, dexamethasone was given according to four different schedules.
The first and the second group of rats were injected intravenously at a
dose of 10 mg/kg 1 hr and 3 hr before noxious heat stimulation,
respectively. In the third group, dexamethasone at a dose of 10 mg/kg was
given three times; that is, the first and the second application were taken
subcutaneously at 10:00 a.m. and 5:00 p.m. the day before experiment, and
the third application was taken intravenously 3 hr before noxious heat
stimulation. The fourth group received simultaneously dexamethasone
(10 mg/kg i.v.) and actinomycin D (5 mg/kg s.c.) 3 hr after noxious heat
stimulation.

RESULTS

<u>Effects of Capsaicin and Denervation of the Hind Paw on the Release of</u>
<u>Immunoreactive SP (iSP) and Edema Induced by Heating in Rat Hind Paw</u>

A large release followed by a rapid decrease of iSP was detected
immediately after the start of the perfusion. Thirty minutes later,
spontaneous release of iSP was stabilized and this state lasted for 5 hr at
least. Immersion of the hind paw into hot water adjusted to 47°C for 30
min resulted in a marked increase of iSP release as compared with the non-
stimulated control (Fig. 1). The increase in volume of the hind paw
paralleled the amount of iSP release in the perfusate (Table 1). The
pretreatment with capsaicin in the newborn rat and cutting the sciatic and

saphenous nerves caused a marked decrease in the heat stimulus-evoked iSP release and formation of thermal edema (Table 1).

Effects of the Combination of Stem Bromelain with Emorfazone, and the Intraarterial Infusion of Des-Arg^9-[Leu^8]BK on the Heat Stimulus-evoked iSP Release and Edema

Pretreatment with stem bromelain (which causes a specific depletion of high molecular weight kininogens) together with emorfazone (a non-acidic anti-inflammatory drug that inhibits the release of BK into extravascular space) significantly decreased the heat stimulus-evoked iSP release (Fig. 2). The intraarterial infusion of Des-Arg^9-[Leu^8]BK (BK spedific inhibitor) also reduced the heat stimulus-evoked iSP release (Fig. 3).

Effects of Dexamethasone Alone or in Combination with Actinomycin D on the Heat Stimulus-evoked iSP Release

As shown in Fig. 4-I, when dexamethasone was given 3 hr or more before noxious heat stimulation, the heat stimulus-evoked iSP release was markedly reduced. However, this inhibitory effect was not apparent at 1 hr after administration. Thus, a time lag was requisite for manifestation of the inhibitory effect of the steroid. Based on this result, to test for the requirement for RNA and protein synthesis, actinomycin D (an inhibitor of RNA synthesis) was given in combination with dexamethasone 3 hr before the noxious heat stimulation. The effect of dexamethasone was blocked by the concomitant administration of actinomycin D (Fig. 4-II).

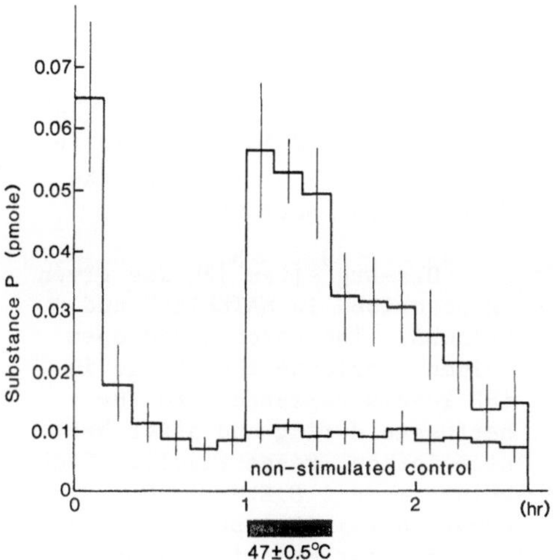

Fig. 1. Timewise observation of the release of iSP from rat hind paw.

One hour after the start of the experiment, the hind paw was immersed in hot water adjusted to 47°C for 30 min. As a result, a marked increase of iSP release was observed compared with the non-stimulated control.

Table 1. Effects of chronic denervation and pretreatment with capsaicin on the release of iSP into the subcutaneous perfusate and edema evoked by noxious heat stimulation (47°C)

		Control	Chronic denerv.	Capsaicin
Substance P	before ST.[a]	13.0(fmol)	18.9(fmol)	5.4(fmol)
	during ST.	48.8	18.9	9.6
	after ST.	27.8	15.4	11.7
Paw volume[b]		154.4(%)	128.5(%)	119.6(%)

(a) ST.: noxious heat stimulation (47°C)
(b) Paw volume indicates the swelling rate obtained immediately after ST..

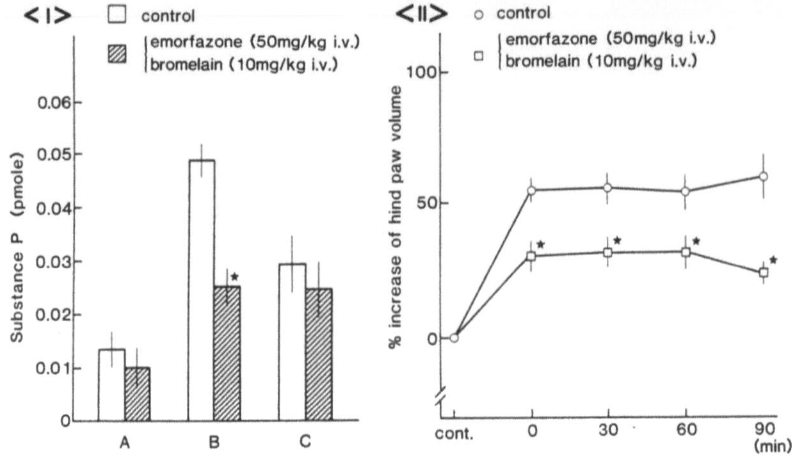

Fig. 2. Effect of pretreatment with stem bromelain (10 mg/kg i.v.) and emorfazone (50 mg/kg i.v.)

Drugs were given as described in MATERIALS and METHODS. <I> A, B and C indicate the mean value of iSP released in the 3 fractions obtained in the 30 min collection period before, during and after heat stimulation, respectively. * p < 0.05 when compared with the value of iSP release obtained in saline-treated animals (control) in Group B. <II> * p < 0.05 when compared with the swelling rate obtained in saline-treated animals (control) in each time measured.

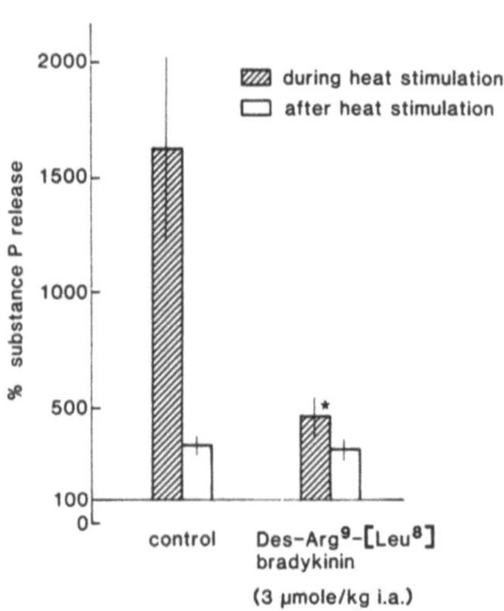

Fig. 3. Effect of Des-Arg^9-[Leu^8] BK administered intraarterially on the release of iSP into the subcutaneous perfusate

Des-Arg^9-[Leu^8]BK was given as described in MATERIALS and METHODS. The hatched and open columns indicate the change in iSP levels released into the perfusate during and after heat stimulation, respectively. Each value (mean ± S.E.M. of 6 experiments) is expressed as a % of the prestimulation value. * p < 0.05 when compared with the value for iSP release obtained in the saline-treated animals (control) during heat stimulation (47°C).

DISCUSSION

Recent immunohistochemical studies showed that SP was present in not only the central nervous system but also the nerve axons and terminals in most peripheral tissues such as visceral and sensory organs. Particularly in the skin, SP fiber was found in unmyelinated primary sensory neurons[5] terminating around the small blood vessels in the dermis and epithelium[5]. Furthermore, pharmacological studies[6] demonstrated that intradermal or intraarterial administration of SP caused the cutaneous vasodilatation and the plasma extravasation which were similar to the inflammatory responses observed after the stimulation of the small-diameter afferent fibers. In

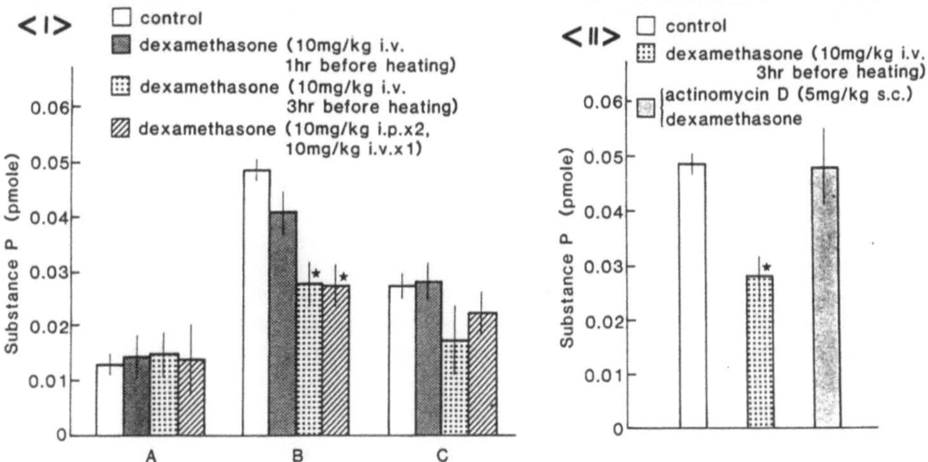

Fig. 4. Effects of dexamethasone alone ⟨I⟩ or in combination with actinomycin D ⟨II⟩ on the heat stimulus-evoked iSP release.

Dexamethasone and actinomycin D were given according to four different schedules as described in MATERIALS and METHODS. ⟨I⟩ A, B and C are described in a previous figure (Fig. 2). * p <0.05 when compared with the value of iSP release obtained in saline-treated animals (control) in Group B. ⟨II⟩ * p < 0.05 when compared with the value of iSP release obtained in saline-treated animals (control) in Group B.

the present experiments, the marked increase in iSP release and edema formation were observed after the heat stimulation at 47°C temperature equivalent to a critical temperature for pain sensation, and these phenomena were inhibited by neonatal pretreatment with capsaicin and by cutting the sciatic and saphenous nerves containing sensory afferent fibers in the hind paw. It has been known that pretreatment of newborn rat with capsaicin results in a selective and permanent degeneration of small-diameter afferent fibers with a significant decrease of iSP content[10]. Taking account of this observation, our results suggest that SP may be released from the peripheral endings of capsaicin sensitive, small-diameter afferent fibers, and that the released SP may be involved in the formation of thermal edema.

Concerning the mediators of thermal edema, Rocha e Silva and Antonio[8] showed that the release of BK predominantly took place in the paw perfusate when heat stimulation was performed at ca. 47°C, although histamine and serotonin could not be detected. In addition, Jancsó et al.[11] demonstrated that BK induced protein leakage in the skin, at least partly through activation of afferent C-fibers. These findings led us to examine the possible contribution of the BK system to both SP release and edema formation generated by heating. As shown in Figs. 2 and 3, the release of iSP and the edema formation induced at 47°C were inhibited significantly by the simultaneous pretreatment with stem bromelain and emorfazone, and by the intraarterial infusion of Des-Arg[9]-[Leu[8]]BK. This suggests that BK released into the extravascular space by noxious heat stimulation may activate capsaicin-sensitive afferent C-fibers to release SP from the peripheral endings through a mechanism such as axon-reflex arrangement.

It is known that BK can also stimulate the production and/or the release of prostaglandins[12], which modulate several biological actions of the kinins[13]. For example, Nasjletti and Malik[14] showed that anti-inflammatory drugs which block prostaglandin synthesis reduced biological

actions of the kinins. These findings suggest that not the BK, but also
the prostaglandin, system may be involved in the mechanism of SP release
from the peripheral sensory endings by the noxious heat stimulation.
Tsurufuji et al.[15] demonstrated that steroidal anti-inflammatory drugs such
as dexamethasone induced the biosynthesis of a phospholipase A_2 inhibitor
which prevents prostaglandin generation. We have therefore studied the
effect of dexamethasone on the release of SP induced by noxious heat
stimulation. As shown in Figs. 4-I and 4-II, dexamethasone inhibited the
heat-evoked iSP release, but a time lag preceded the manifestation of this
effect. Moreover, the inhibitory effect was abolished after the
simultaneous application of actinimycin D. Our present results indicate
that endogenous prostaglandins may modulate the release of SP from the
peripheral endings of the small-diameter afferent fibers through
cooperation with BK, and that the released SP may play an important role in
the thermal injury reactions.

REFERENCES

1. F. Goltz, Über gefäßerweiternde Nerven, Pflügers Arch. Ges. Physiol.
    9:174 (1874)
2. S. Stricker, Untersuchung über die Gefässerwurzeln des Ischiadeus,
    Sitz-Ber. Kaiserl. Acad. Wiss.(Wein) 3:173 (1876)
3. T. Lewis and H. M. Marvin, Observations relating to vasodilatation
    arising from antidromic impulses, to Herpes zoster and trophic
    effects, Heart 14:27 (1927)
4. F. Lembeck, Zur Frage der zentralen Übertragung afferenter Impulse.
    III. Mitteilung. Das Vorkommen und die Bedeutung der Substanz P in
    den dorsalen Wurzeln des Rückenmarks. Naunyn-Schmiedeberg's Arch.
    Exp. Path. Pharmakol. 219:197 (1953)
5. T. Hökfelt, J. O. Kellerth, G. Nilsson and B. Pernow, Experimental
    immunohistochemical studies on the localization and distribution of
    substance P in cat primary sensory neurons, Brain Res. 100:235
    (1975)
6. O. Hagermark, T. Hökfelt and B. Pernow, Flare and itch induced by
    substance P in human skin, J. Invest. Dermatol. 71:233 (1978)
7. F. Lembeck, Substance P and sensory neurones, in: "Substance P:
    Metabolism and Biological Actions" C. C. Jordan and P. Oehme, eds.,
    Taylor & Francis, London (1985)
8. M. Rocha e Silva and A. Antonio, Release of bradykinin and mechanisms
    of production of a thermic edema (45°C) in rat paw, Med. Exp. 3:371
    (1960)
9. N. Jancsó, A. Jancsó-Gábor and J. Szolcsányi, Direct evidence for
    neurogenic inflammation and its prevention by denervation and by
    pretreatment with capsaicin, Br. J. Pharmacol. Chemother. 31:138
    (1967)
10. G. Jancsó, E. Király and A. Jancsó-Gábor, Direct evidence for an axonal
    site of action of capsaicin, Naunyn-Schmiedeberg's Arch. Pharmacol.
    313:91 (1980)
11. G. Jancsó, E. Király and A. Jancsó-Gábor, Chemosensitive pain fibers
    and inflammation, Int. J. Tissue Reac. 11:57 (1980)
12. D. Regoli and J. Barabe, Pharmacology of bradykinin and related kinins,
    Pharmacol. Rev. 32:1 (1980)
13. K. Ikeda, K. Tanaka and M. Katori, Potentiation of bradykinin-induced
    vascular permeability increase by prostaglandin E_2 and arachidonic
    acid in rabbit skin, Prostaglandins 10:747 (1975)
14. A. Nasjletti and K. Malik, Relationships between the kallikrein-kinin
    and prostaglandin systems, Life Sci. 25:99 (1979)
15. S. Tsurufuji, K. Sugio and F. Takemasa, The role of glucocorticoid
    receptor and gene expression in the anti-inflammatory action of
    dexamethasone, Nature 280:408 (1979)

INTERACTION OF ENDOGENOUS KININS AND PROSTAGLANDINS IN THE PLASMA EXUDATION
OF KAOLIN-INDUCED PLEURISY IN RATS

Yozo Hori, Hirokuni Jyoyama, Katsutoshi Yamada, Hiroyasu
Kageyama, Atsushi Kurosawa, Katsumi Hirose and Makoto Katori*

Division of Pharmacology, Shionogi Research Laboratories
Shionogi & Co., Ltd., Fukushima-ku, Osaka 553 and *Department
of Pharmacology, Kitasato University School of Medicine
Sagamihara, Kanagawa 228, Japan

INTRODUCTION

Kaolin has long been used as a proinflammatory substance to induce
relatively long-lasting paw edema for the development of anti-inflammatory
drugs. Recently kaolin was shown to activate blood coagulating factor XII,
because of its negatively charged surface. We selected a kaolin-induced
pleurisy as a suitable inflammatory model for studying the involvement of
bradykinin in inflammation.[1] In the present experiments, we aimed to analyse
mediators involved in the plasma exudation of kaolin pleurisy by measuring
the levels of kinin, histamine and prostaglandin (PG) in the pleural exudate
and to demonstrate in vivo interaction of endogenously generated kinins and
PGs in the inflammatory sites.

MATERIALS AND METHODS

1. <u>Induction of pleurisy and measurement of plasma exudation</u>

Experimental pleurisy was induced by the intrapleural injection of 0.5
ml of 1 % kaolin saline solution into the right pleural cavity of male
Sprague-Dawley rats (8-10 weeks old). The plasma exudation at fixed time
was estimated by determination of the dye amounts exuded into the pleural
cavity of rats exsanguinated 20 min after the intravenous injection of
pontamine sky blue.[2]

2. <u>Enzyme immunoassay of kinins</u>

After the induction of pleurisy, rats were exsanguinated at various
time for sampling the pleural exudates. In order to inhibit artificial
breakdown and production of kinins during sample collection, 1 ml of ice
cold 60 mM Tris-HCl buffer containing ortho-phenanthroline (1 mg/ml),
captopril (0.2 mg/ml) and soybean trypsin inhibitor (1 mg/ml), was injected
into the pleural cavity immediately before the exsanguination. Samples were
immediately deproteinized by adding one fifth volume of 20 % TCA and centrifuged at 1500 g for 15 min at 4°C. The supernatants were diluted 1:1 in the
buffer (buffer B of the kit) and then kept -80°C. Kinins were estimated by
enzyme immunoassay without extraction, using a assay kit MARKIT-A-Bradykinin
(Dainippon Pharmaceuticals).[3]

3. <u>Radioimmunoassay of PGs and thromboxane (TX) B$_2$</u>

Another group of rats with kaolin pleurisy were exsanguinated for assay. To inhibit artificial biosyntheses of PGs and TXB$_2$ during harvesting the exudate, 4 ml of Ringer's solution containing 10 µg/ml of indomethacin was injected into the pleural cavity immediately after the exsanguination.[2] PGs and TXB$_2$ in the pleural exudate were extracted with Sep-pak C$_{18}$ cartridge and estimated by radioimmunoassay using ^{125}I-labeled PGE$_2$, 6-keto-PGF$_{1a}$ and TXB$_2$.[4]

4. <u>Assay of histamine</u>

After harvesting the exudate, the cavity was washed with 2 ml of HEPES (10 mM)-buffered Hanks' solution. Histamine in the cell pellet and supernatant were respectively extracted by the shore's method[5] and determined by high-performance liquid chromatography with fluorescence detection.

RESULTS AND DISCUSSION

1. <u>Pharmacological analyses of mediators involved in plasma exudation</u>

Figure 1 depicts the time course of plasma exudation in kaolin-induced pleurisy and the effect of captopril, a kininase II inhibitor. After intrapleural injection of 0.5 ml of 1 % kaolin, the volume of pleural fluid increased gradually from 1 to 5 hr (fig. 1, upper panel). The plasma exudation into the pleural cavity, however, showed two peaks at 20 min and 3-5 hr after kaolin injection, as indicated by large increase in the dye exudation at 20 min (55.1±11.6 µg), 3 hr (92.2±6.1 µg) and 5 hr (61.7±3.2 µg) (fig. 1, lower panel). An injection of 0.5 ml saline instead of kaolin hardly caused both the plasma exudation and the accumulation of pleural exudate.

Treatment of rats with captopril (3 mg/kg i.p.), a kininase II inhibitor, showed marked (350 % increase) and significant potentiation (73 %) of the exudation at 20 min and 5 hr, respectively, but the potentiation was not significant at 1, 2 and 3 hr (fig. 1, lower panel). The accumulation of pleural exudate was also significantly increased by captopril at 20 min (40 %) and this increase continued till 5 hr except 3 hr (fig. 1, upper panel).

The early phase (20 min) of the dye exudation was significantly inhibited by 65 % by combined treatment with a histamine antagonist, mepyramine (2.5 mg/kg i.v.), and a serotonin antagonist, methysergide (3 mg/kg i.v.), but the same treatment showed no significant inhibition (21 %) on the late phase (3 hr) of the exudation.

Pretreatment of rats with intravenous injection of bromelain(10 mg/kg), a thiolprotease known to deplete plasma prekallikrein and high molecular weight (HMW) kininogen through the activation of factor XII,[6] inhibited significantly the early phase of exudation by 61 % and the late phase by 36 %.

In contrast, indomethacin (10 and 30 mg/kg p.o.), a cyclooxygenase inhibitor known to suppress PG production, failed to inhibit the early phase (20 min) exudation, but it showed significant suppression at 3 hr (by 27 and 47 % with 10 and 30 mg/kg, respectively).

These results suggest that the early phase (20 min) of exudation was mediated mainly by kinins, histamine and serotonin, and the late phase (3 hr) by kinins and PGs.

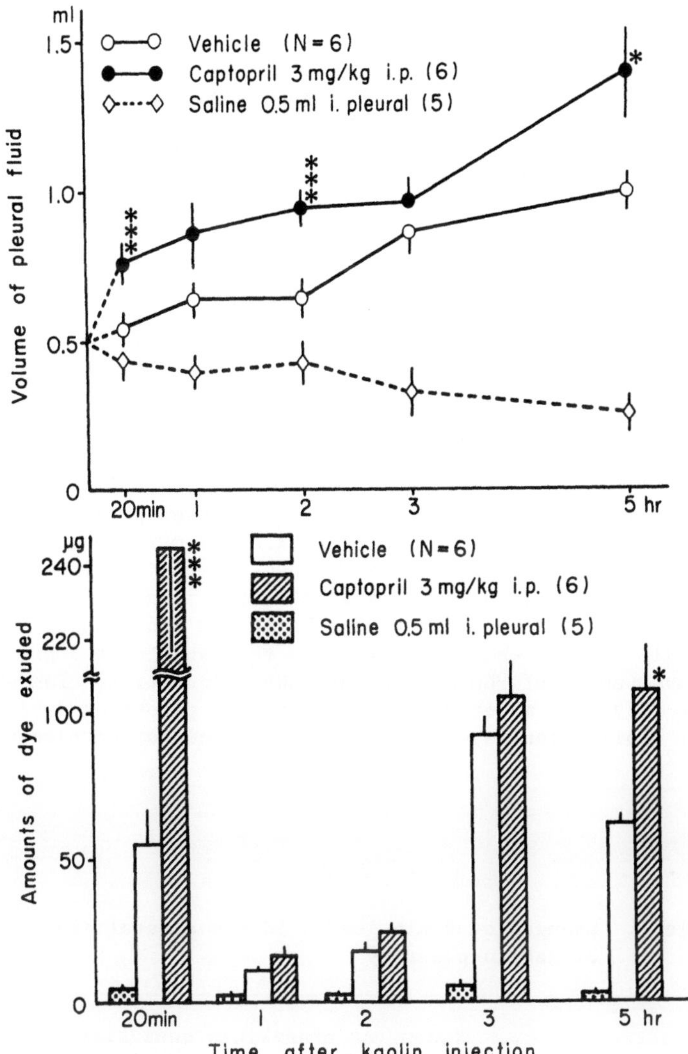

Figure 1. Time course of plasma exudation in kaolin-induced rat pleurisy and potentiating effect of captopril.

The volume of pleural exudate (upper panel) and the dye amounts exuded for 20 min periods at given time (lower panel) are shown. Vehicle or captopril (3 mg/kg i.p.) was administered 1 hr prior to dye injection for each period. Values indicate mean±S.E. *p<0.05, ***p<0.001 vs vehicle control. An intrapleural (i. pleural) injection of 0.5 ml of saline, instead of kaolin, hardly caused both plasma exudation and accumulation of pleural exudate.

2. <u>Changes of mediators in the pleural exudate of kaolin pleurisy</u>

To confirm the involvement of mediators mentioned above, we measured the levels of kinin, histamine and PGs in the pleural exudate.

As shown in table 1, the intrapleural injection of kaolin generated only the threshold levels of kinin in the pleural cavity from 20 min to 5 hr. on the other hand, captopril treatment (3 mg/kg i.p.) disclosed changes in the kinin levels in the course of the kaolin pleurisy. The levels of kinin peaked at 20 min and decreased with time thereafter. These results confirmed those of plasma exudation (fig. 1). Namely, kinins generated increased the dye exudation in the early phase and to a lesser degree in the late phase.

Histamine level in the pleural exudate at 20 min was measured. In the saline-injected group, about 98 % of histamine contents were present in the cell pellet. Twenty minutes after the intrapleural injection of kaolin, histamine contents in the cell pellet decreased markedly (from 14.6 ± 0.13 to 0.40 ± 0.13 µg/rat, n=5, p<0.01) and moved to the supernatant (from 0.25 ± 0.05 to 0.93 ± 0.17 µg/rat, n=5, p<0.01). This indicate occurrence of the degranulation of mast cells in the pleural cavity in the early phase of kaolin pleurisy.

The intrapleural injection of kaolin also caused production of PGs and TXB_2. The levels of 6-keto-PGF_{1a} and TXB_2 reached maximum at 20 min (12.7 ± 4.3 and 4.3 ± 1.7 ng/rat, respectively) and decreased with time thereafter. In contrast, PGE_2 was gradually but significantly increased from 20 min to 5 hr (0.62 ± 0.08 ng/rat at 5 hr). Indomethacin (10 and 30 mg/kg p.o.) suppressed markedly the PGs and TXB_2 levels in the exudate at 3 hr, which confirmed the involvement of PGs in the late phase exudation. These results indicate that PGE_2 is a major effective PG in the plasma exudation of the late phase of kaolin pleurisy, as has been reported for carrageenin-induced rat pleurisy.[2]

Table 1. Changes of kinin levels in the pleural exudate of kaolin pleurisy

Time after kaolin	Kinin (ng bradykinin equivalent/rat)	
	Saline (n = 3)	Captopril (3 mg/kg i.p.) (n = 5-6)
0 min	N.D.	N.D.
20 min	1.2 ± 0.3	8.4 ± 0.7***
1 hr	1.4 ± 0.3	3.7 ± 0.5*
3 hr	0.8 ± 0.4	2.0 ± 0.5
5 hr	1.3 ± 0.7	1.8 ± 0.5

N.D.: not detected. Captopril or saline was administered 40 min before the exsanguination at each time. Values indicate mean±S.E. *p<0.05, ***p<0.001 vs saline control.

3. <u>Interaction of kinins and PGs in the plasma exudation of early phase</u>

The early phase (20 min) of plasma exudation was markedly poetnetiated
by captopril (fig. 1 and fig. 2-panel A). To examine the interaction of
kinins and PGs in this phase, captopril-treated rats were further treated
with bromelain and indomethacin. As shown in figure 2-A, the potentiating
effect of captopril was completely diminished by the simultaneous treatment
with bromelain (10 mg/kg i.v.). It should be noted, however, that potentiation by captopril was also potently inhibited by simultaneous treatment with
indomethacin (5 mg/kg i.v.)(fig. 2-panel B).

These results suggest that the potentiation by captopril was dependent
on plasma kallikrein-kinin system because bromelain is known to deplete
plasma prekallikrein and HMW-kininogen in plasma,[6] and consequently inhibit
the generation of kinins. However, the potent inhibitory effect of indomethacin implies the involvement of PGs in addition to kinins in this potentiation by captopril.

It is supposed that the increase in kinin levels by captopril, already
shown in table 1, might stimulate the production of PGs in the early phase
of kaolin pleurisy. However, captopril (3 mg/kg i.p.) failed to affect the
PGs (6-keto-PGF_{1a} and PGE_2) and TXB_2 levels in the pleural exudate at 20 min

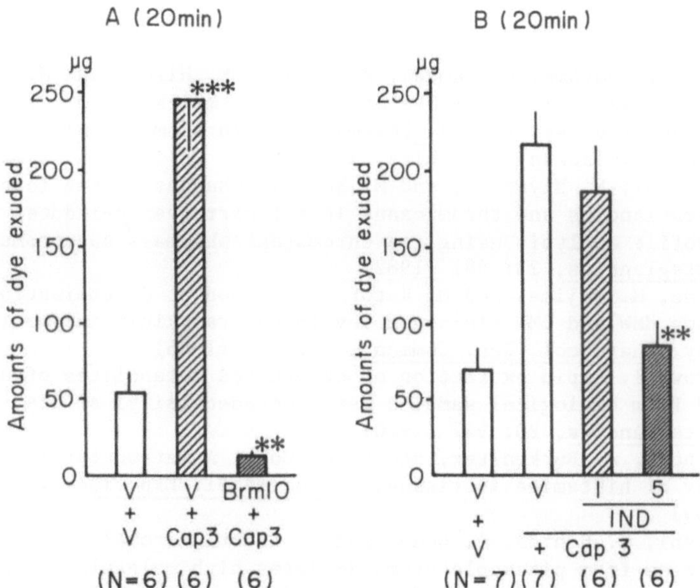

Figure 2. Effect of bromelain and indomethacin on captopril-induced potentiation of the early phase (20 min) exudation in kaolin pleurisy.

Captopril (Cap, 3 mg/kg i.p.) and bromelain (Brm, 10 mg/kg i.v.)
were administered 1 hr before kaolin injection. Indomethacin
(IND, 1 and 5 mg/kg i.v.) was given 30 min before kaolin. Values
indicate mean±S.E. **$p<0.01$, ***$p<0.001$ vs vehicle (V) + vehicle
(V) group for panel A, and vs vehicle (V) + captopril (Cap) group
for panel B.

after kaolin. In the captopril-treated rat, indomethacin (5 mg/kg i.v.)
markedly suppressed PGs and TXB_2 levels, and significantly reduced kinin
levels in the exudate at 20 min after kaolin (from 5.2 ± 1.0 to 2.7 ± 0.3 ng
bradykinin equivalent/rat, n=5 to 6, $p<0.05$), in which the reduction of
kinin levels by indomethacin was in good accordance with that of plasma exudation by indomethacin (fig. 2-B).

These results indicate that kinins and PGs might be generated independently for each other, but these mediators could come to interact when they
coexist in the pleural cavity.

In conclusion, the kaolin-induced rat pleurisy is a kinin-related inflammatory model, and histamine, serotonin and PGs are also involved in the
plasma exudation into the pleural cavity. Kinins and PGs seem to be generated independently for each other. However, these mediators could come to
interact when the increase of kinin levels was superimposed on the presence
of PGs in the pleural cavity. Kaolin pleurisy was accordingly proved to be
a excellent inflammatory model for studying in vivo interaction of kallikrein-kinin system and PGs.

ACKNOWLEDGEMENTS

We wish to thank Mrs. S. Noda and Miss M. Akao for their skillful
technical assistance.

REFERENCES

1. Y. Hori, H. Jyoyama, K. Yamada, M. Takagi, K. Hirose,and M. Katori,
    Time course analyses of mediators in plasma exudation of rat kaolin-
    induced pleurisy, Eur. J. Pharmacol., (in submission)
2. Y. Harada, K. Tanaka, Y. Uchida, A. Ueno, S. Oh-ishi, K. Yamashita, M.
    Ishibashi, H. Miyazaki, and M. Katori, Changes in the levels of
    prostaglandins and thromboxane in rat carrageenin-induced pleurisy---
    A profile analysis using gas chromatography-mass spectrometry,
    Prostaglandins, 23: 881 (1982)
3. Y. Uchida, M. Majima, and M. Katori, A method of determination of human
    plasma HMW and LMW kininogen levels by bradykinin enzyme immuno-
    assay, Pharmacol. Res. Commun., 18: 831 (1986)
4. W. S. Powell, Rapid extraction of oxygenated metabolites of arachidonic
    acid from biological samples using octadecylsilyl silica,
    Prostaglandins, 20: 947 (1980)
5. P. A. Shore, A. Burkhalter, and V. N. Cohn, A method for fluorometric
    assay of histamine in tissue, J. Pharmacol. Exp. Ther., 127: 182
    (1959)
6. S. Oh-ishi, Y. Uchida, A. Ueno, and M. Katori, Bromelain, a thiol-
    protease from pineapple stem, depletes high molecular weight
    kininogen by activation of Hageman factor (factor XII),
    Thromb. Res., 14: 665 (1979)

ROLE OF BRADYKININ GENERATING AND DEGRADING SYSTEMS IN THE VASCULAR
PERMEABILITY RESPONSE INDUCED WITH KAOLIN IN RATS

Seiichiro Kumakura, Izumi Kamo and Susumu Tsurufuji

Department of Biochemistry, Faculty of Pharmaceutical
Sciences, Tohoku University
Aoba, Aramaki, Sendai 980, Japan

INTRODUCTION

In order to elucidate mechanisms for inflammatory processes from
the viewpoint of biochemistry, it is important to know about balancing
between the generation and disappearance of a putative chemical mediator
such as bradykinin in the extracellular fluid or exudate in inflammatory
sites. However, there has been no reliable data in the literature on the
correlation of time changes between bradykinin level and increased
vascular permeability at the site of inflammation. The present
experiments were designed, therefore, to analize the role of bradykinin
in increased vascular permeability in kaolin-induced inflammation of air
pouch type in rats. The experimental model of inflammation of air pouch
type that we have employed have been proved to be highly efficient for
the determination of chemical mediators at the site of inflammation
(Hirasawa et al., 1986. Ohuchi et al., 1985. Tsurufuji et al., 1984).
Kaolin was used in an attempt to cause bradykinin generation in the air
pouch preformed on the back of rats, as activation with kaolin of plasma
kallikrein system has been described extensively in the literature
(Heimerk et al., 1980).

MATERIALS AND METHODS

Animals. Male rats of the sprague-dawley strain (specific pathogen-free)
were purchased from Charles River Japan, Inc. (Kanagawa, Japan).

Kaolin-induced inflammation in the air pouch. Rats were injected under
light ether anesthesia with 7 ml of air s.c. on the back to make an air
pouch in the shape of an ellipsoid or oval. After 24 hr 4 ml of a kaolin
suspension (10mg/ml) in 0.8% (w/v) solution of CMC-Na in 0.9% NaCl was
injected into the air pouch to provoke an inflammatory reaction.

Measurement of plasma exudation. Plasma exudation into the pouch tissues
was measured as described elsewhere (Watanabe et al., 1984) using F-BSA
as a tracer.

Extraction of bradykinin from the pouch fluid. Collection of pouch fluid
for the extraction and determination of bradykinin was done according to
a novel method (Minami et al., 1983) with slight modification (Kumakura

et al., 1987). Briefly, 1 ml of the fluid in the pouch was drawn into a plastic syringe holding 0.2 ml of an inhibitor solution consisting of a phosphate-buffered saline-ethanol (80:1) containing SBTI (62.5 µg), aprotinin (12.5 µg), polybrene (17.5 µg), disodium EDTA (75 µg) and o-phenanthrolin (42.5 µg). Immediately after drawing pouch fluid, 2 ml of ethanol was added to the sample and mixed well. After standing 0°C for 1 hr, the mixture was centrifuged. The pellet was removed and the supernatant was evaporated. The dried sample was dissolved in 200 µl of 0.05 M Tris-acetate buffer (pH 8.5) containing gelatin at 0.1% (w/v), Tween 20 at 0.05% (w/v) and NaN$_3$ at 0.02% (w/v). Fifty µl of 1,1,2-trichloro-1,2,2,-trifluoroethane was added to remove lipids. To the aqueous portion, 40 µl of 20% (w/v) trichloroacetic acid aqueous solution was added and mixed. The mixture was centrifuged and supernatant was used as a sample solution.

<u>Enzyme immunoassay for bradykinin</u>. Bradykinin in the above sample solution was assayed according to the method of Ueno et al. (1981) with modifucations (Kumakura et al., 1987).

RESULTS AND DISCUSSION

The present model of inflammation of the air pouch type provides a method by which extracellular fluid can be collected through a syringe. In this respect we took precautions against the possibilities of artifactual generation of bradykinin via activation of the kallikrein system as well as degradation of bradykinin by kinin degrading enzymes during and after drawing the sample fluid from the pouch. The addition of the inhibitor solution (See materials and method) at the time of drawing of the pouch fluid was able to maintain bradykinin level without

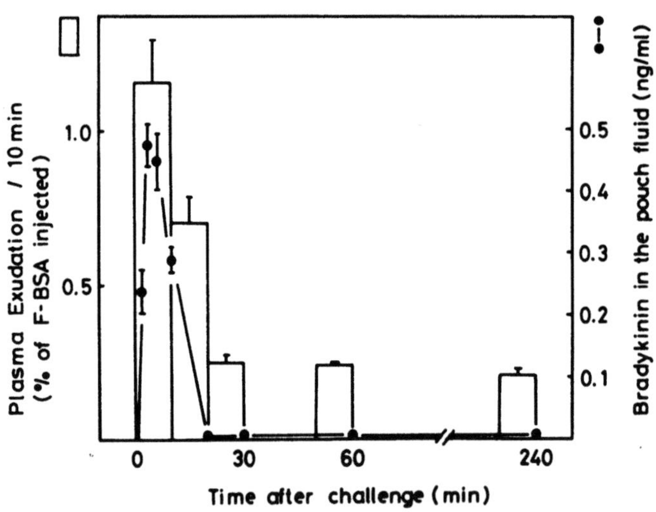

Fig.1 Time course of the vascular permeability (plasma exudation) and bradykinin levels during the first 4 hr following the challenge with kaolin in the air pouch. ☐ and ●——● indicate plasma exudation and bradykinin levels in the pouch fluids, respectively, with the standard errors of mean indicated by vertical bars. The column hight indicates the leakage of F-BSA into the pouch fluid per 10 minutes.

any detectable change over 30 min after its drawing (data not shown).

In kaolin-induced inflammation, the time change of vascular permeability was well correlated with the time change of bradykinin level in the pouch fluid (fig. 1). The bradykinin level began to rise immediately after the challenge and reached a maximum about 4 to 6 min later. And then by 20 min after the challenge it declined down to a range lower than the assay limit of 0.07 ng/ml. A maximum response of the exudation of F-BSA was observed in the first 10 min period. Such a close correlation of the time changes between the bradykinin level and vascular permeability response supports a concept that bradykinin is responsible for the vascular permeability response observed immediately after the infusion of the kaolin suspension into a preformed air pouch.

Quick decline of the bradykinin level in the period from 6 to 20 min (fig. 1) suggests rapid appearance of some kininase activities in the inflammatory sites. Therefore, we examined bradykinin-degrading activity in the pouch fluid. Three fold dilutions of the pouch fluids were centrifuged at 2,500xg for 15 min. The supernatant was collected and preincubated for 10 min at 37°C. Five nanograms of bradykinin were then dissolved in 0.1 ml of 0.9% NaCl and added to 1 ml of the supernatant. After incubation at 37°C, bradykinin was extracted and measured by the enzyme immunoassay method. As shown in figure 2, a rapid degradation of bradykinin was observed with the pouch fluid colleced as early as 10 min after the infusion of the kaolin suspension while there was no kininase activity in the air pouch before the challenge, as the washing fluid (PBS) collected from the pouch on dead animals was inactive. In the 4 hr pouch fluid, bradykinin was degraded much more quickly.

A possible correlation between changes in vascular permeability and bradykinin levels was examined with the aid of inhibitors of kininase I and II as well as an inhibitor of the plasma kallikrein system. DL-2-mercaptomethyl-3-guanidinoethylthiopropanoic acid (MGTPA), an inhibitor of kininase I (Plummer and Ryan, 1981), captopril, an inhibitor of

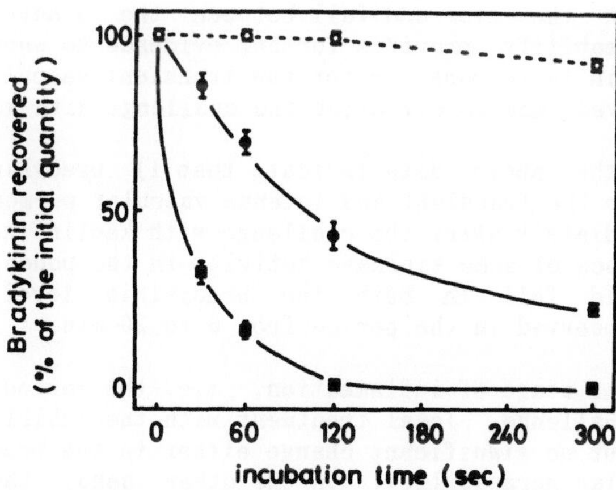

Fig.2 Bradykinin degrading activity in the pouch fluid collected at 10 min (●) and at 4 hr (■) after challenging with kaolin. (O) indicates the bradykinin degrading activity in the washing fluid (PBS) placed in the pouch before the challenge.

Table 1 Effects of inhibitors of kininase I and II and of plasma kallikrein on vascular permeability response and bradykinin levels in the initial stage (0-10 min) of the kaolin-induced inflammation.
MGTPA at a dose of 0.1 mg/pouch, captopril at a dose of 0.2 mg/pouch and SBTI at a dose of 8.4 mg/pouch were injected at time 0 into the pouch, dissolved singly or in combination in 0.2 ml of 0.9% NaCl. F-BSA was injected i.v. at time 0. Rats were sacrificed 10 min later and bradykinin and F-BSA in the pouch fluid were determined. Values represent the mean ± S.E.M.

Treatment	Plasma exudation (% of F-BSA injected)	Bradykinin (ng/ml)
None	1.18 ± 0.11	0.22 ± 0.04
MGTPA	$1.55 \pm 0.15^{*}$	$0.98 \pm 0.10^{***}$
captopril	$1.72 \pm 0.13^{**}$	$2.07 \pm 0.58^{***}$
MGTPA + captopril	$1.63 \pm 0.19^{*}$	$3.93 \pm 0.37^{***}$
SBTI	$0.23 \pm 0.04^{***}$	$< 0.07^{***}$
MGTPA + captopril + SBTI	$0.17 \pm 0.02^{***}$	$< 0.07^{***}$

$^{*}p < 0.05$, $^{**}p < 0.01$, $^{***}p < 0.001$.

kininase II (Ondetti et al., 1977) and soybean trypsin inhibitor (SBTI), an inhibitor of plasma kallikrein system (Garcia Leme, 1978) were selected for this purpose. In the initial stage from time 0 to 10 min of kaolin-induced inflammation, the kininase I inhibitor, the kininase II inhibitor as well as the combination all caused significant rises both in bradykinin levels and exudation of F-BSA. In contrast, SBTI caused a significant fall not only in the bradykinin levels but also in the exudation of F-BSA. In the presence of SBTI, the combination of the two kininase inhibitors was unable to reverse the effect of SBTI either on the bradykinin levels or on the exudation of F-BSA (Tabe 1). The parallelism in the rise and fall between the bradykinin level and vascular permeability provides further evidence to support a concept that bradykinin is responsible for the transient vascular permeability response observed immediately after the challenge with kaolin.

All of the above data indicate that 1) bradykinin was mainly responsible for the transient and intense vascular permeability response observed immediately after the challenge with kaolin in the air pouch and 2) appearance of some kininase activity in the pouch are responsible for the rapid fall in both the bradykinin level and vascular permeability observed in the period from 6 to 20 min.

In the 4-hr stage of inflammation, i.e. the period from 3.5 to 4.0 hr after the challenge, local treatment with the inhibitors of kininase I brought about no significant change either in the bradykinin level or in the vascular permeability. On the other hand, the inhibitor of kininase II caused considerable enhancement of the vascular permeability response accompanied by marked elevation of bradykinin levels in the pouch (Table 2). It is evident, therefore, that in the late stage of kaolin-induced inflammation in rats kininase II was mainly responsible for the degradation of bradykinin in the inflammatory locus.

Table 2 Effects of inhibitors of kininase I and II and of plasma
kallikrein on vascular permeability response and bradykinin
levels in the 4-hr stage (3.5-4 hr) of the kaolin-induced
inflammation.

The doses of inhibitors used were the same as in table 1. They
were applied at 3.5 hr into the pouch. F-BSA was injected i.v.
at time 3.5 hr. Rats were sacrificed at 4 hr. Bradykinin and F-
BSA in the pouch fluid were determined. Values represent the
mean ± S.E.M.

Treatment	Plasma exudation (% of F-BSA injected)	Bradykinin (ng/ml)
None	0.76 ± 0.13	< 0.07
MGTPA	1.11 ± 0.11	< 0.07
captopril	2.71 ± 0.39***	1.97 ± 0.83***
MGTPA + captopril	2.42 ± 0.02***	2.33 ± 0.14***
SBTI	0.71 ± 0.07	< 0.07
MGTPA + captopril + SBTI	0.90 ± 0.05	< 0.07

*** $p < 0.001$.

As the results of experiments performed with the aid of the
kininase inhibitors disclosed that bradykinin was generated still
actively in the late stage, the effects of SBTI in this stage were
investigated and it was demonstrated that SBTI decreased markedly both
bradykinin and the vascular permeability in the group treated with the
kininase inhibitors (Table 2). In fact, the vascular permeability and
bradykinin levels fell down to levels comparable to those in the
untreated control group. In contrast, SBTI did not exert any significant
lowing effect on the vascular permeability in animals not treated with
any of the kininase inhibitors, although bradykinin generation is
thought to be inhibited in a similar way as in the group treated with
the kininase inhibitors (Table 2) as well as in experiments for the
early stage (Table 1). These data indicate that in the untreated control
group bradykinin was so quickly degraded by the action of kininase that
the concentration of bradykinin could not reach a level of significant
to provoke a vascular permeability response.

In conclusion, regardless of the source of the kinin degrading
enzymes in the inflammatory locus, whether they originate from
translocation of the blood-born enzymes or from release of the tissue
enzyme into inflammatory exudates, the kinin degrading enzyme is
considered to protect tissue from the proinflammatory action of
bradykinin when bradykinin is generated activity in the site of
inflammation.

ACKOWLEDGEMENT

We are grateful to Dr. S. Kurooka and Dr. N. Sunahara, Dainippon
Pharmaceutical Co. Ltd., Osaka, Japan, for the generous supply of
MRAKIT-BK (enzyme immunoassay kit for bradykinin).

REFERENCES

Garcia Leme, J., 1978, The bradykinin system. Handbook. Exp. Pharmacol.,
    50:464.
Heimerk, R. L., Kurachi, K., Fujikawa, K. and Davie, E. W., 1980,
    Surface activation of blood coagulation, fibrinolysis and kinin
    formation. Nature (Lond)., 286:456.
Hirasawa, N., Ohuchi, k., Sugio, K., Tsurufuji, S., Watanabe., M. and
    Yoshino, S., 1986, Vascular permeability response and the role of
    prostagrandin E_2 in an experimental allergic inflammation of air
    pouch type in rats. Br. J. Pharmacol., 87:751.
Kumakura, S., Tsurufuji, S., Kurooka, S. and Sunahara, N., 1987, Role of
    bradykinin generating and degrading systems in the vascualr
    permeability response induced with kaolin in rats. J. Pharmacol.
    Exp. Ther., in press.
Minami, M., Togashi, H., Sano, M., Endoh, T., Saito, H., Hashimoto,
    F., Fujita, K., Yasuda, H., Kuriyamoto, Y. and Nishino, T.,
    Plasma bradykinin concentration in patients with essential
    hypertention, effect angina and other cardiac disease. Folia
    Pharmacol. Jpn., 82:195.
Ohuchi, K., Hirasawa, N., Watanabe, M. and Tsurufuji, S., 1985,
    Pharmacological analysis of the vascular permeability in the
    anaphylactic phase of allergic inflammation in rats. Eur. J.
    Pharmacol., 117:337.
Ondetti, M. A., Rubin, B. and Cushman, D. W., 1977, Design of specific
    inhibitors of angiotensin converting enzyme. Science., 196:441.
Plummer, Jr. T. H. and Ryan, T. J., 1981, A potent mercapto bi-product
    analogue inhibitor for human carboxypeptidase N. Biochem.
    Biophys. Reserch. Commun., 98:448.
Tsurufuji, S., Kurihara, A., Kiso, S., Suzuki, Y. and Ohuchi, K., 1984,
    Dexamethasone inhibits generation in inflamatory sites of the
    chemotactic activity attributable to leukotriene B_4. Biochem.
    Biophys. Reserch. Commun., 119:884.
Ueno, A., Ohishi, S., Kitagawa, T. and Katari, M., 1981, Enzyme
    immunoassay of bradykinin using β-D-galactosidase as a labeling
    enzyme. Biochm. Pharmacol., 30:1659.
Watanabe, K., Nakagawa, H. and Tsurufuji, S., 1984, A new sensitive
    fluoroometric method for measurement of vascular permeability. J.
    Pharmacol. Method., 11:167.

ENDOTOXIN SHOCK, KININ SYSTEM AND PAF-acether IN THE RAT

J. Damas, G. Remacle-Volon, A. Adam and V. Bourdon

Department of Human Physiology
University of Liège, Clinical Biology
Sainte-Ode, Belgium

INTRODUCTION

The activation of Hageman factor and the consumption of the
kallikrein-kinin system have been observed during endotoxin shock in some
animal species (1, 2). Thus the kinin system has been proposed as a
major factor involved in the development of this kind of shock. However,
the role of the kinins in the cardiovascular changes following endotoxin
injection has not been delineated precisely. In order to evaluate this
role, we compared the blood pressure changes and the accumulation of
^{125}I-labelled albumin in the digestive tract obtained in response to
endotoxin infusion in normal Wistar rats and in kininogen-deficient Brown
Norway rats (3, 4).

Recently, several observations have demonstrated that PAF-acether
participates to the development of endotoxin shock in rats (5, 6, 7, 8).
Thus we examined also the relationship between PAF-acether and the kinin
system.

MATERIALS AND METHODS

We used Wistar rats and Brown Norway rats (BN/May Pfd f) from the
animal farm of the Catholic University of Leuven (Belgium). The plasma
of the Brown Norway rats contains T-kininogen only and is deficient in
the two usual rat kininogens (3, 4).

The animals were anaesthetized with sodium pentobarbital (35 mg/Kg).
A tracheostomy was performed and a jugular vein and a carotid artery were
cannulated. The mean systemic blood pressure was measured with a Harvard
50-8952 transducer connected to a Harvard Universal Oscillograph. The
animals were not heparinised. ^{125}I-labelled serum bovine albumin (25 uC)
was administered intravenously and after five min, an infusion of
lipopolysaccharide (0.6 mg/Kg.min) or of PAF-acether (0.2 or
0.5 ug/Kg.min) or of solvent was performed for ten min. Ten min after,
blood was taken by cardiac puncture and additioned with sodium citrate
(3.8%; 1/9, vol/vol). The stomach was removed, the fundus separated from
the antrum. Pieces of 4 cm in length of proximal duodenum and of terminal ileum were removed. Tissues were rinsed with physiological saline,
blotted dry, weighed and placed directly in counting tubes. The blood

was centrifuged (10 min, 5000 g) and a 0.2 ml aliquot of the plasma was
transferred to a counting tube.

In other experiments in Wistar rats, we did not use labelled albumin
in order to measure blood platelet content by contrast phase microscopy,
plasma prekallikrein with S2302 (Kabi) as substrate, plasma high
molecular weight kininogen (HMWK) either by bioassay using ellagic acid
as prekallikrein activator, or by its procoagulant activity.

We used lipopolysaccharide and bradykinin triacetate from Sigma,
PAF-acether from Bachem, ellagic acid from Janssen Chimica, ^{125}I-labelled
serum albumin from New England Nuclear, BN-52021 and BN-52020 from
Institut Henri Beaufour, SDZ 63-675 from Sandoz. Ellagic acid was
dissolved in Tris HCl (0.15 M; pH 7.4), BN-52021 and BN-52020 were
dissolved in DMSO and diluted in hot physiological saline. We used also
C.K. Prest (Diagnostica Stago) for the coagulation assay. The other
drugs were dissolved in saline.

Results were expressed as mean $\pm$ SEM. Unpaired Student's t test was
used for statistical evaluation of the results. Statistical significance
was set at $p < 0.05$.

RESULTS

1. Blood Pressure Response

The mean blood pressure was similar in both strains before the
infusion of lipopolysaccharide (LP) : 109 $\pm$ 3 mmHg in Wistar rats and 102
$\pm$ 6 mmHg in Brown Norway rats. Five min after LP infusion, the blood
pressure was decreased in both strains similarly and reached 53 $\pm$ 7 mmHg
in Wistar rats and 53 $\pm$ 4 mmHg in Brown Norway rats. At the end of the
infusion, the blood pressure level was 45 $\pm$ 6 mmHg in Wistar rats and
49 $\pm$ 6 mmHg in Brown Norway rats. Ten min after this infusion, it was
47 $\pm$ 6 mmHg in the former (n = 9) and 38 $\pm$ 7 mmHg in the latter (n = 6).
The evolution of the endotoxin shock was thus identical in both strains.

2. Leakage of Plasma in the Digestive Tract

Opening the abdominal wall showed marked hyperemia of the small
intestine in LP-treated rats. The duodenum appeared the most affected
region. LP induced an increase of weight for the duodenum of Wistar rats
from 239 $\pm$ 9 mg/100 g body weight to 292 $\pm$ 9 mg/100 g body weight
($p < 0.005$; n = 9), while in Brown Norway rats, a decrease of the weight
of the antrum was observed: from 479 $\pm$ 20 mg/100 g body weight to 394 $\pm$ 25 mg.
/100 g body weight ($p < 0.05$; n = 6). The wet weight of the other organs
(fundus, ileum) did not vary significantly. The leakage of plasma was
observed in the duodenum of Wistar rats and in the duodenum and ileum of
the Brown Norway rats (Table 1).

3. Blood Parameters

In Wistar rats, the blood platelet level was greatly decreased after
LP infusion : 414 $\pm$ 29.10^3 against 913 $\pm$ 82.10^3 platelets/ul in control
rats (n = 6; $p < 0.001$). The hematocrit was not significantly increased
: 41.8 $\pm$ 0.9% (n = 6) against 37.2 $\pm$ 0.9% in rats treated with the
solvent. Plasma prekallikrein, 0.510 $\pm$ 0.034 U/ml (n = 9) and HMWK

measured by bioassay : 525 $\pm$ 40 ng bradykinin equivalent/ml (n = 6) were not significantly modified as the respective values in control rats were 0.562 $\pm$ 0.056 U/ml and 560 $\pm$ 80 ng bradykinin equivalent/ml (n = 6). The procoagulant activity of HMWK after LP was 96 $\pm$ 11% (n = 6) of control values.

4. Effects of PAF-acether Antagonists on Endotoxin Shock

The hypotensive response to LP was significantly diminished by BN-52021 and by BN-52020, two PAF-acether antagonists (9). Mean blood pressure was respectively 114 $\pm$ 9 mmHg (n = 4) and 102 $\pm$ 5 mmHg (n = 4) before LP, in the two groups, not significantly different from control level. The maximum decrease was observed twenty min after the start of LP infusion and reached : 83 $\pm$ 4 mmHg in BN-52021 treated rats (p < 0.01) and 76 $\pm$ 6 mmHg in BN-52020 treated rats (p < 0.02). DMSO had no influence on the effects of LP.

Table 1. Interstitial leakage of ^{125}I-labelled albumin in the digestive tract of Wistar and Brown Norway rats

	Fundus	Antrum	Duodenum	Ileum
Wistar rats				
NaCl	12.2 $\pm$ 1.8	15.8 $\pm$ 3.0	10.5 $\pm$ 0.7	6.6 $\pm$ 0.6
LP	10.8 $\pm$ 0.9	10.8 $\pm$ 0.9	19.0 $\pm$ 2.4 p < 0.005	9.2 $\pm$ 1.6
LP + BN 52021			11.3 $\pm$ 0.9	
LP + BN 52020			12.9 $\pm$ 1.1	
Brown Norway rat				
NaCl	13.4 $\pm$ 4.0	23.2 $\pm$ 4.2	10.3 $\pm$ 0.5	6.9 $\pm$ 0.7
LP	13.2 $\pm$ 1.5	17.0 $\pm$ 0.9	23.8 $\pm$ 0.9 p < 0.001	13.0 $\pm$ 1.4 p < 0.01

Results are expressed as the mean $\pm$ SEM of microlitres of plasma present per 100 mg of tissue (wet weight). Each group of observations contained 4 to 9 animals.

These inhibitors suppressed the accumulation of ^{125}I-labelled albumin in the duodenum wall (Table 1). In another series of experiments, the same inhibitory effect was observed with another PAF-acether antagonist, SDZ 63-675 (1 mg/Kg) (10). The leakage of plasma was 11.34 $\pm$ 0.8 µl/100 mg of tissue in SDZ 63-675 treated rats (n = 6; p < 0.001) against 19.43 $\pm$ 1.36 µl/100 mg of tissue in control animals (n = 8).

5. Effect of PAF-acether

Infusion of PAF-acether (0.2 µg/Kg.min) in Wistar rats induced a nearly identical decrease of the blood pressure like the one recorded during LP infusion. That decrease was accompanied by an interstitial leakage of plasma - the hematocrit was increased to $51.4 \pm 0.9\%$ - and by an hyperemia in the small intestine. The weights of the duodenum and of the ileum were increased from 239 ± 9 mg/100 g body weight to 281 ± 12 mg/100 g body weight (n = 10; p<0.02) and from 184 ± 11 mg/100 g body weight to 217 ± 9 mg/100 g body weight (n = 10; p < 0.05) respectively. A significant accumulation of ^{125}I-labelled serum albumin was observed in duodenum : 15.7 ± 1.1 ul plasma/100 mg of tissue (n = 10; p < 0.005). No significant accumulation of this tracer was observed in fundus, antrum and ileum. All these effects of PAF-acether were blocked by BN-52021 and by SDZ 63675.

PAF-acether infusion did not change the blood platelet content : 869 ± 97.10^3 platelets/µl (n = 8) but decreased the level of HMWK (n = 9) : 418 ± 35 ng bradykinin equivalent /ml (p < 0.05) and $54 \pm 4\%$ of the procoagulant activity of control plasma (p < 0.01). For this dose of PAF-acether, plasma prekallikrein was not significantly decreased : 0.457 ± 0.033 U/ml (n = 10, NS) but for 0.5 µg/Kg.min, this decrease was significant : 0.255 ± 0.024 U/ml (n = 6; p < 0.005).

DISCUSSION

Following LP infusion in Wistar rats, we observed a vascular collapse with plasma extravasation in the digestive tract. These are typical features of the endotoxin shock in rats (5, 6). However, we did not observe any significant consumption of prekallikrein and HMWK. Previously, Latour et al. (11) have noted a partial depletion of prekallikrein in hyperlipemic rats two hours after LP injection. The activation of the kinin system in rats following LP would be seen at the plasma level under special circumstances only. Anyway, the kinins are not essential for endotoxin shock, because the vascular changes after LP were nearly similar in normal rats and in kininogen-deficient Brown Norway rats. Moreover, the activation of Hageman factor with ellagic acid in rats induced specific vascular lesions which were not observed after LP injection (12). However we noted a small difference between Wistar and Brown Norway rats : in the former, LP induced an increase in the weight of the duodenum while, in Brown Norway rats, LP provoked a decrease of the weight of the antrum but no changes in the duodenum. This difference might indicate that kinins are locally formed in Wistar rats and participate to the vasodilatation and increase in vascular permeability affecting the digestive wall. This local activation would not be sufficient to affect plasma levels.

This local activation of the kinin system could be indirect. Indeed, the vascular collapse and the plasma leakage induced by LP were inhibited by PAF-acether antagonists. These results agree with other observations (5, 6, 7, 8) indicating a major role for PAF-acether in endotoxin reactions in rats. That agent mimicked the main features of the vascular changes following LP, except for the platelet stimulation which was absent. In PAF-acether treated rats, plasma prekallikrein and HMWK were reduced. This reduction could result from a real activation or from the plasma leakage. Reduction in the plasma level of the kallikrein-kinin system has been previously reported following injection of other agents that increase vascular permeability such as histamine (13, 14).

We can conclude that the kinin system is not essential for the development of endotoxin shock in rats. However, our results suggest that
kinins could be activated locally in the digestive wall and participate
to the vascular changes in that region. PAF-acether plays a major role
in the induction of endotoxin shock in rats, in part by activation of the
kinin system.

REFERENCES

1. J.G. Latour, Modulation of disseminated intravascular coagulation
(DIC) by steroidal and non-steroidal anti-inflammatory drugs, Agents and
Actions 13: 487-495 (1983).

2. H.Z. Movat and C.E. Burrowes, The local Shwartzman reaction :
endotoxin-mediated inflammatory and thrombo-hemorrhagic lesions, in:
"Handbook of Endotoxin", vol. 3, 260-302, L.J. Berry, ed. Elsevier
Science Publishers, Amsterdam (1985).

3. J. Damas and A. Adam, The relationship between kininogens and
kallikreins in deficient Brown Norway rat, Mol. Physiol., 8, 307-316
(1985).

4. I. Hayashi, S. Oh-ishi, H. Kato, K. Enjoyi, S. Iwanaga and T. Nakano,
Identification of T-kininogen in high and low molecular weight kininogens
deficient rat (Brown Norway Katholiek strain), Thrombos. Res., 39, 313-
321 (1985).

5. T.W. Doebber, M.S. Wu, J.C. Robinson, B.M. Chang and T.Y. Chen,
Platelet activating factor (PAF) involvement in endotoxin-induced hypo-
tension in rats. Studies with PAF-receptor antagonist kadsurenone,
Biochem. Biophys. Res. Commun., 127, 799-808 (1985).

6. Z. Terashita, Y. Imura, K. Nishikawa and S. Sumida, Is platelet activating factor (PAF) a mediator of endotoxin shock? Eur. J. Pharmacol.,
109, 257-261 (1985).

7. J.L. Wallace and B.J.R. Whittle, Prevention of endotoxin-induced
gastrointestinal damage by CV-3988, an antagonist of platelet-activating
factor, Eur. J. Pharmacol, 124, 209-210 (1986).

8. J.L. Wallace, G. Steel and B.J.R. Whittle, Gastrointestinal plasma
leakage in endotoxin shock. Inhibition by prostaglandin E_2 and by a
platelet-activating factor antagonist, Can. J. Physiol. Pharmacol., 65,
1428-1432 (1987).

9. P.G. Braquet, T.Y. Shen, L. Touqui and B.B. Vargaftig, Perspectives
in platelet activating factor research, Pharmac. Rev., 39, 97-145 (1987).

10. D.A. Handley, R.G. Van Valen, C.M. Winslow, J.C. Tomesch and R.N.
Saunders, In vitro and in vivo pharmacological profiles of the PAF receptor antagonist SRI 63-675, Thromb. Haemostas., 57, 187-190 (1987).

11. J.G. Latour, C. Groulx and C. Leger-Gauthier, Activation of the
Hageman factor-prekallikrein system in the pathogenesis of the generalized Shwartzman reaction and of hepatic vein thrombosis phenomenon in
the rat. Lab. Invest., 41, 237-246 (1979).

12. J. Damas, BN-52021 : PAF-acether and ellagic acid in rats, Methods
and Findinns, in press (1987).

13. G.P. Lewis, Plasma kinins and other vasoactive compounds in acute inflammation, <u>Ann. N.Y. Acad. Sci.</u>, 116, 847-854 (1964).

14. J. Damas and J. Lecomte, Kininogènes plasmatiques chez le rat intoxiqué par l'histamine ou la 5-hydroxytryptamine, <u>C.R. Soc. Biol.</u>, 163, 1983-1985 (1969).

ESTIMATION OF PLASMA KALLIKREIN IN SICKLE-CELL ANEMIA, AND ITS RELATION

TO THE COAGULATION AND FIBRINOLYTIC SYSTEMS

Dayse Lourenço, Misako U. Sampaio, Jose Kerbauy and
Claudio A. M. Sampaio

Departamento de Bioquimica e Departamento de Medicina
Escola Paulista de Medicina
Caixa Postal 20372, CEP 04034 S.Paulo, SP, Brasil

INTRODUCTION

Sickle cell anemia, a disease due to the replacement of one single amino acid residue in the primary structure of haemoglobin molecule, exhibits two major clinical manifestations, haemolysis and vascular occlusion,caused by sickled erythrocytes. This occlusion causes ischemia and endothelium injury, that can lead to platelet activation and blood clotting [1].

Plasma kallikrein, a serine proteinase involved in the contact phase of blood clotting , occurs in plasma as prokallikrein, and its activation is dependent upon a negative surface, Factor XII and high-molecular weight kininogen [2]. C1-inactivator is the major inhibitor involved in the physiological inactivation of plasma kallikrein[3].

Blood clotting in sickle cell anemia is probably an intravascular event, and since its activation proceeds via plasma kallikrein activation, kallikrein level would seemingly be decreased in patients during crisis or even steady-state[4].

Fibrinolysis plays an important role in fibrin degradation formed in the microcirculation, following vascular occlusion in sickle cell anemia A decrease of the fibrinolytic activity has been observed during infections or crisis [5].

The aim of this communication is to estimate the levels of prokallikrein of a group of sickle cell anemia patients during remission, and verify possible changes in fibrinolysis.

MATERIAL AND METHODS

Blood level of plasma prokallikrein was measured after its activation to kallikrein, by hydrolysis of the chromogenic substrate[6] Ac-Phe-Arg-pNA, kindly provided by Dr. Luis Juliano, from the Departamento de Biofisica, Escola Paulista de Medicina [7]. Blood was collected with 0.4% sodium citrate, and following its centrifugation the obtained plasma was kept at -20°C up to it use. Activation of 0.1 mL plasma kallikrein was performed with 0.05 mL dextran sulfate (1.0 mg/mL in 70% v/v acetone) at $0^{\circ}C$, for 15 minutes. The reaction was stopped by the addition of 0.4 mL 0.05 M tris-HCl, pH 8.0. Plasma kallikrein activity was followed at $37^{\circ}C$, by the hydrolysis of 1.0 mL 1.0 mM Ac-Phe-Arg-p-NA, in 0.05 mM tris-HCl, pH 8.0, and formed p-nitroaniline was measured spectro-photometrically at 405 nm. One unit of plasma kallikrein is defined as the quantity of enzyme that hydrolyzes one umol substrate per min, under these assay conditions.

Prothrombin time (PT) was performed with citrated plasma, and human brain thromboplastin[8] ; activated partial prothromboplastin time (APTT) was measured with kaolin and human brain cephalin[9] . Fibrinogen, Factor VIII and Factor V were measured by a described procedure[10,12,13] . The evalution of fibrinolysis was performed by euglobulin lysis time[13] , and by fibrin lysis on fibrin plates[14], prior to and after a sphygmo-manometric venous occlusion kept at the mean arterial blood pressure for 5 minutes. C1-inactivator, anti-thrombin III, and plasminogen were measured by radial immunodiffusion[15] in commercial agarose plates (Boehringer).

The studies were performed with 15 homozigous patients aged 14 to 64 years old, during the remission periods without apparent infectious process, and lacking recent blood transfusion; ten apparently healthy voluntiers, aged 20 to 41 years old were the control group.

Table 1

CONCENTRATION OF PROKALLIKREIN AND C1-INACTIVATOR

SICKLE CELL ANEMIA IN PATIENTS

	Control	Patients
Prokallikrein (mUnits/mL)	1.63 (0.36)	1.05 (0.36)*
C1-Inactivator (mg/mL)	0.29 (0.04)	0.23 (0.04)*

Mean (S.E.M)   *Siginificantly different p 0.05

RESULTS

Plasma prokallikrein level was lower (67%) in the sickle cell anemia patients group when compared to the control group (100%) (Table 1). This difference was significant at p 0.05 in t-test. No significant levels of free active kallikrein was found in plasma of both patient and control groups, and no significant differences were found between males and females in both groups.

Table 2

BLOOD CLOTTTING FACTORS IN SICKLE CELL

PATIENTS AND CONTROL GROUP

Test	Control	Patients
PT (%)	102	99
APTT (%)	101	101
Factor V (%)	92	91
Factor VIII-C (%)	98	126 *
Fibrinogen (mg/mL)	2.73	3.03
Plasminogen (ug/mL)	67	60
1-Antitrypsin (ug/mL)	55	57
2-Macroglobulin (ug/mL)	123	149
Antithtombin III (mg/mL)	0.30	0.27

* Level significantly different of a p   0.05

C1-Inactivator was also decreased in sickle cell anemia patients when compared to the control group (Table 2). Blood clotting factors were not significantly changed except for Factor VIII-C, that is increased in patients group (Table 2).

Plasminogen level in patients was not significantly different from the control group, and measurements of prokallikrein prior to and following venous occlusion did not differ significantly both in patients and controls. Lysis of fibrin plates was larger for patient samples than for control group, and although no significant differences were detected after venous occlusion for both groups, ratio between fibrin lysis after and before venous occlusion was lower for the patient (table 3).

DISCUSSION

Patients were studied during remission periods, uneventful with regard to infectious diseases, to avoid conditions which could, per se, alter both clotting and fibrinolytic systems.

The lower level of prokallikrein (67%) in plasma of sickle cell anemia patients can be attributed to consumption, since activation of the contact phase is triggered by the exposition of subendothelial structures that follows the ischemic lesion of the endothelium, subsequent to microcirculation occlusion by sickle cells. C1-inactivator, the major kallikrein inhibitor in plasma[3] , is decreased parallelly to kallikrein, when the diminished levels of this enzyme reflect its consumptiom in the contact phase activation. So, the observed reduced levels of C1-inactivator indicated that kallikrein is being consumed in sickle cell anemia patients. The finding of lower kallikrein levels during the crisis may be related to more complex physiopathology[16].

As no siginificant variaton of blood clotting factors was observed, but for Factor VIII-C, presumably no major alteration takes place in the common pathways of coagulation. The increased spontaneous fibrinolysis, observed in sickle cell disease patients, could be due to kallikrein ability to activate plasminogen, as it has been seen "in vitro"[2]. Neverthless, no correlation between kallikrein level, and fibrin lysis, has been found. It has been reported that vascular oclusion may release endothelial plasminogen activator[1], and an indication that such a phenomenon may be occurring in sickle cell anemia is the decreased ability to stimulate fibrinolysis shown by patients, in response to vascular occlusion.

Table 3

EUGLOBULIN AND FIBRIN PLATES LYSIS IN SICKLE CELL DISEASE

	Control	Patients
Euglobulin lysis (min) (before occlusion)	208	166
Euglobulin lysis (min) (after occlusion)	144	129
Fibrin lysis (mm2) (before occlusion)	114	181
Fibrin lysis (mm2) (after occlusion)	206	264

Fibrinolytic tests were performed before and after a experimental venous occlusion as described in Methods

REFERENCES

1 - L.W.Diggs, Sickle cell crisis, Am. J.Clin. Pathol. 44:1 (1965)
2 - J.J.Pisano, Chemistry and biology of the kallikrein kininin system, in Proteases and Biological Control, E.Reich, D.B. Rifikin and E.Shaw, eds., p.199, Cold Spring Harbor Laboratory, Cold Spring Harbor (1975).
3 - J. Travis and G.G. Salvesen, Human plasma protease inhibitors, Ann. Rev. Biochem. 41:655 (1983).
4 - R.W. Colman and P.Y. Wong, Paticipation of Hageman factor dependent pathways in human diseases states, Thromb. Haemost. 38:251 (1977).
5 - D. Green, H.C. Kwaan and G. Ruiz, Impaired fibrinolysis in sickle-cell disease - Thromb. Diath. Haemorr. 24:10 (1970).

6 - M.L.V. Oliva, D.Grisolia, M.U. Sampaio and C.A.M. Sampaio, Properties of a highly purified human plasma kallikrein, <u>Agents Actions</u> 9:52 (1982)

7 - M.A.Juliano and L.Juliano, Synthesis and kinetic parameters of hydrolysis by trypsin of some acyl-arginyl-p-nitroanilides and peptides containing arginyl-p-nitroanilide, <u>Brazilian J.Med.Biol. Res.</u> 18:435 (1985).

8 - A.J. Quick, The prothrombin in haemophilia and obstructive jaundice, <u>J.Biol. Chem</u>. 109:73 (1935)

9 - P.R. Proctor and S.I. Rappaport, The partial thromboplastin time with kaolin, <u>Am. J. Clin. Pathol</u>. 36:212 (1961)

10- O.D. Ratnoff and C. Menzie, A new method for the determination of fibrinogen in small samples of plasma, <u>J.Lab.Clin Med</u>. 62:1005 (1955).

11- C.F.Abildgaard, J.V. Simone, I. Schulman, Factor VIII activity in sickle cell anemia, <u>Brit J. Haemotol</u>. 13:19, (1967).

12- A.J. Quick, The assay and properties of labile factor V , <u>J. Clin Pathol</u>. 13:457 (1960).

13- <u>European Concerted Action on Thrombosis</u>, Bulletin 2r. 2, Assay Procedures (1985).

14- T.Astrup, Fibrinolysis in the the organism, <u>Blood</u> 11:781 (1956).

15- G.Mancini, A.O. Carbonara and J.F. Heremans, Immunochemical quantification of antigens by single radial immunodiffusion, <u>Immunochemistry</u> 2:235 (1965).

16- R.L. Miller, P.S. Verma and R.G. Adams, Studies of the kallikrein kinin system in patients with sickle cell anemia, <u>J. Nat. Med. Assoc.</u> 75: 551 (1974).

STUDIES ON COAGULATION-FIBRINOLYSIS AND KALLIKREIN-KININ SYSTEMS AND
KININASE ACTIVITY AND KININASE II QUANTITY IN AMNIOTIC FLUID

S. Mutoh[1], Y. Yaoi[1], A. Teh[1], M. Saito[1], N. Aoki[2], T. Abe[3],
Y. Ohno[4], and N. Itoh[5]

Dept. of Obst. and Gyn.[1] and the First Dept. of Internal
Med.[2], Tokyo Medical and Dental University School of Medicine
Japan Woman's University[3], SRL[4] and TEIJIN[5], Tokyo

INTRODUCTION

Amniotic fluid embolism associated with disseminated intravascular
coagulation is a well-known complication especialy occuring in full term
of pregnancy and labor.

The kallikrein-kinin system and kininase in amniotic fluid has been
postulated to play a role in the regulation of vascular dilatation and
constriction, permeability in uteroplacental circulation, and uterine
muscular dilatation and constriction, however multifactor's informations
of coagulable-fibrinolytic and kallikrein-kinin systems, kininase activity
and kininase II quantity in amniotic fluid based on stage dependent
analysis have not been reported until now.

The purpose of this study is to investigate the clinical significance
of coagulable-fibrinolytic and kallikrein-kinin systems, and kininase in
amniotic fluid.

Material and Method

The amniotic fluid was collected by trans-abdominal and vaginal
amniocentesis from 72 heathy women in 17-20 weeks of gestation as a
control group, full term pregnancy before and during labor.

After extraction, the samples were preserved in ice until -4°C
centrifugation at 3,000 r.p.m for 10 minutes as soon as possible, and
stored -70 - -80°C until to use.

Specific assays were performed for fibrinopeptide A, fibrin-derived
peptide Bß15-42, plasminogen activator (urokinase, tissue plasminogen
activator), α_2-plasmin inhibitor (TD-80), α_2PI-plasmin-complex
(TD80C), D-dimer, glandular kallikrein activity and quantity (anti-human
urinary kallikrein antibody), kallikrein inhibitor, high and low molecular
weight-kininogen, kinin, kininase activity and kininase II quantity.

Table 1. Method for measurement

FPA (ng/ml)	RIA (PEG separation)	IMCO Co., Ltd., Sweden.　1), 2), 3)
Bβ15-42 (ng/ml)	RIA (PEG separation)	IMCO Co., Ltd., Sweden.　1), 2), 3)
U K (ng/ml)	RIA (secondary antibody separation)	4), 5)
t-PA (ng/ml)	ELISA assay	AMERICAN DIAGNOSTICA Co., Ltd., America.
α_2-PI (μg/ml)	TD-80	Teijin Co., Ltd., Japan.　6)
α_2PI-Pm-Complex (ng/ml)	TD-80C	Teijin Co., Ltd., Japan.　6)
D-dimer (ng/ml)	ELISA assay	MAbCO Co., Ltd., Australia.
Kall. activity (pg/min/ml)	RIA (PEG separation)	
Kall. quantity (ng/ml)	RIA (PEG separation)	
Kall. inhibitor (%)	S-2302	AB Kabi diagnotica Co., Ltd., Sweden.
LMW-kg. (ngBKeq/ml)	enzym immunoassy (MARKIT Bradykinin) by M.Katori's method	Dainippon pharmaceutical Co., Ltd., Japan.
HMW-kg (%)	APTT (Fitzgerald factor's deficient plasma)	7)
kinin (pg/ml)	RIA (PEG separation)	8)
Kininase activity (pg/min/ml)	RIA (PEG separation)	9)
Kininase II quantity (IU/I/37°C)	Kasahara's method	

<u>Results</u>

1.   <u>The coagulable and fibrinolysis system in amniotic fluid</u>

1) Levels of FPA were slightly increased in the full term pregnancy before onset of labor (1.3 ± 0.8 ng/ml, n=24, M ± SE) when compared to 17-20 weeks of gestation as a control group (0.9 ± 0.12 ng/ml, n=24, M ± SE), but were not significantly.

Levels of FPA were significantly increased during labor (55.6 ± 7.08 ng/ml, n=24, M ± SE, p<0.001) as compared to a control group and in the full term pregnancy before onset of labor (Table 2, Fig. 1).

2) Levels of Bß15-42 were markedly decreased in full term pregnancy before onset of labor (10.9 ± 1.02 ng/ml, n=24, M ± SE, p<0.01) when compared to a control group (13.9 ± 0.47 ng/ml, n=24, M ± SE).

Levels of Bß15-42 were significantly increased during labor (22.9 ± 2.7 ng/ml, n=24, M ± SE, p<0.01) as compared to a control group and in the full term pregnancy before onset of labor (Table 2, Fig. 1).

3) plasminogen activator.

1 Levels of urokinase were markedly increased in a control group (3.4 ± 0.28 ng/ml, n=24, M ± SE, p<0.01) when compared to in the full term pregnancy before onset of labor (2.3 ± 0.31 ng/ml, n=24, M ± SE).

Levels of urokinase were significantly increased during labor (6.5 ± 0.55 ng/ml, n=24, M ± SE, p<0.001) as compared to a control group and in the full term pregnancy (Table 2, Fig. 2).

2   Levels of tissue-plasminogen activator in a control group
(12.3 $\pm$ 4.41 ng/ml, n=24, M $\pm$ SE) increased significantly to in the full
term before onset of labor (482.3 $\pm$ 121.15 ng/ml, n=24, M $\pm$ SE, p<0.001)
and during labor (639.1 $\pm$ 110.65, n=24, M $\pm$ SE, p<0.001).
During labor, levels of t-PA were gradually increased more
than in the full term pregnancy before onset of labor, but were no
significantly (Table 2, Fig. 2).

4)   Levels of α_2-plasmin inhibitor during pregnancy (1.04 $\pm$ 0.21
μg/ml, n=24, M $\pm$ SE) were unchanged in the full term pregnancy before
onset of labor (1.01 $\pm$ 0.18 g/ml, n=24, M $\pm$ SE), α_2-PI during labor
(0.93 $\pm$ 0.11 g/ml, n=24, M $\pm$ SE) slightly decreased but there was no
significant change as compared with a control group (Table 2, Fig. 3).

5)   Levels of α_2PI-plasmin-complex in the full term pregnancy before
onset of labor (26.9 $\pm$ 5.87 ng/ml, n=24, M $\pm$ SE) gradually decreased but
there was no significantly change as compared with a control group (33.3 $\pm$
6.21 ng/ml, n=24, M $\pm$ SE).
During labor (77.2 $\pm$ 11.54 ng/ml, n=24, M $\pm$ SE, p<0.01), levels of
α_2PI-Pm-C were markedly increased when compared to a control group and
in the full term pregnancy before onset of labor (Table 2, Fig. 3).

6)   Levels of D-dimer in a control group (179.6 $\pm$ 20.31 ng/ml, n=24, M
$\pm$ SE) markedly decreased in the full term pregnancy before onset of labor
(56.7 $\pm$ 7.41, n=24, M $\pm$ SE, p<0.01).
Levels of D-dimer during labor (174.4 $\pm$ 38.81 ng/ml, n=24, M $\pm$ SE,
p<0.05) were markedly increased when compared to in full term pregnancy
before onset of labor (Table 2, Fig. 4).

2.   <u>The kallikrein-kinin system and kininase in amniotic fluid</u>

7)   glandular kallikrein.
1   Levels of kallikrein activity during labor (121.0 $\pm$ 22.0
pg/min/ml, n=24, M $\pm$ SE) were slightly increased but there was no
significant change as compared with a control group (93.8 $\pm$ 18.3
pg/min/ml, n=24, M $\pm$ SE) and in full term pregnancy before onset of labor
(82.8 $\pm$ 23.7 pg/min/ml, n=24, M $\pm$ SE) (Table 2, Fig. 5).

2   Levels of kallikrein quantity during pregnancy (4.0 $\rightarrow$ $\downarrow$ ng/ml,
n=24, M $\pm$ SE) markedly increased in full term pregnancy before onset of
labor (20.85 $\pm$ 4.89, n=24, M $\pm$ SE, p<0.01), and significantly increased
during labor (32.24 $\pm$ 5.75 ng/ml, n=24, M $\pm$ SE, p<0.01) (Table 2, Fig. 5).

8)   Levels of kallikrein inhibitor during pregnancy (41.7 $\pm$ 7.20%,
n=24, M $\pm$ SE) significantly decreased in the full term pregnancy before
onset of labor (0.2 $\pm$ 0.14%, n=24, M $\pm$ SE, p<0.001) and during labor (0.3
$\pm$ 0.30%, n=24, M $\pm$ SE, p<0.001) (Table 2, Fig. 6).

9)   high and low molecular weight-kininogen.
1   Levels of HMW-kg during pregnancy (29.6 $\pm$ 1.75%, n=24, M $\pm$
SE) gradually decreased in the full term pregnancy before onset of labor
(15.0 $\pm$ 1.00%, n=24, M $\pm$ SE. p<0.001), but although markedly increased
during labor (39.0 $\pm$ 3.16%, n=24, M $\pm$ SE, p<0.01).
The levels of HMW-kg in the full term pregnancy were
significantly increased when compared to the levels during labor (Table 2,
Fig. 7).

2   Levels of LMW-kg during pregnancy (70 $\pm$ 6.1 ng BK eq/ml,
n=24, M $\pm$ SE) were slightly decreased but there was no significant change

as compared with in the full term pregnancy before onset of labor (60 +
6.1 ng BK eq/ml, n=24, M + SE). Levels of LMW-kg during labor (40 + 2.0
ng BK eq/ml, n=24, M + SE, p<0.001) were significantly decreased when
compared to a control group and in the full term pregnancy before onset of
labor (Table 2, Fig. 7).

10) Levels of kinin during pregnancy (17.6 + 2.7 pg/ml, n=24, M + SE)
markedly increased in the full term pregnancy before onset of labor (68.3
+ 4.4 pg/ml, n=24, M + SE, p<0.001) and significantly increased during
labor (342.3 + 38.2 pg/ml, n=24, M + SE, p<0.001).
Levels of kinin during labor were significantly increased when
compared to in the full term pregnancy before onset of labor (Table 2,
Fig. 8).

11) Kininase activity and kininase II quantity.
1   Levels of kininase activity in a control group (2099.5 +
265.9 pg/min/ml, n=24, M + SE) significantly decreased in the full term
pregnancy before onset of labor (592.8 + 103.1 pg/min/ml, n=24, M + SE,
p<0.001) and during labor (637.5 + 163.9 pg/min/ml, n=24, M + SE, p<0.001)
(Table 2, Fig. 9).

2   Levels of kininase II quantity in a control group (8.2 +
0.63 IU/1/37°C, n=24, M + SE) significantly decreased in the full term
pregnancy before onset of labor (1.2 + 0.08 IU/1/37°C, n=24, M + SE,
p<0.001) and during labor (1.1 + 0.05 IU/1/37°C, n=24, M + SE, p<0.001)
(Table 2, Fig. 9)

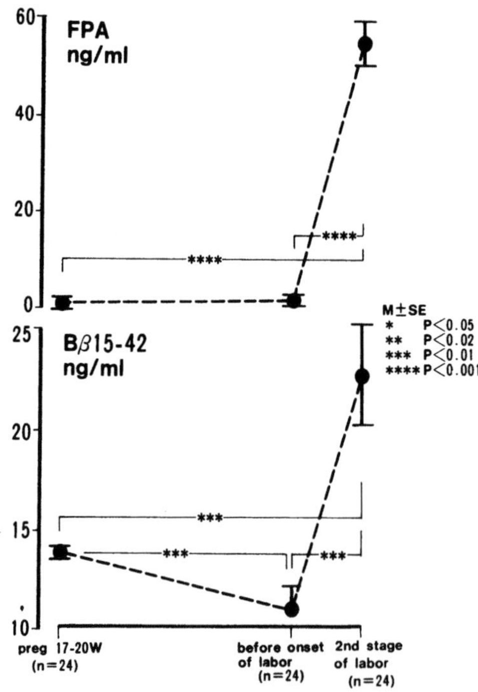

Fig. 1. Comparison of the levels of fibrinopeptide A and fibrin-derived
        peptide Bβ15-42 in amniotic fluid in mid pregnancy, and before and
        during labor in full term pregnancy

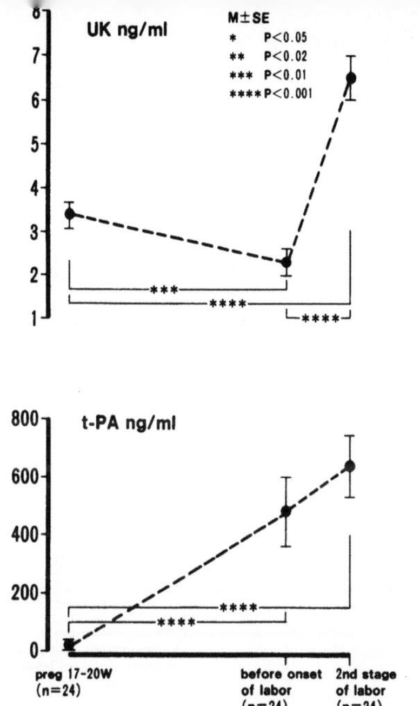

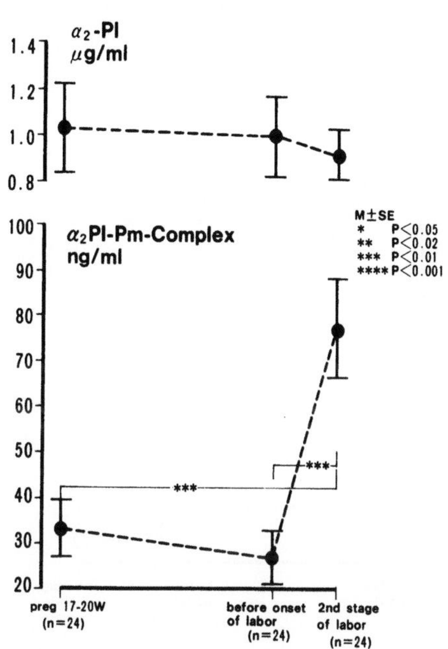

Fig. 2. Comparison of the levels of urokinase quantity and tissue plasminogen activator in amniotic fluid in mid pregnancy, and before and during labor in full term pregnancy.

Fig. 3. Comparison of the levels of α_2-plasmin inhibitor and α_2PI-plasmin-complex in amniotic fluid in mid pregnancy and before and during labor in full term pregnancy.

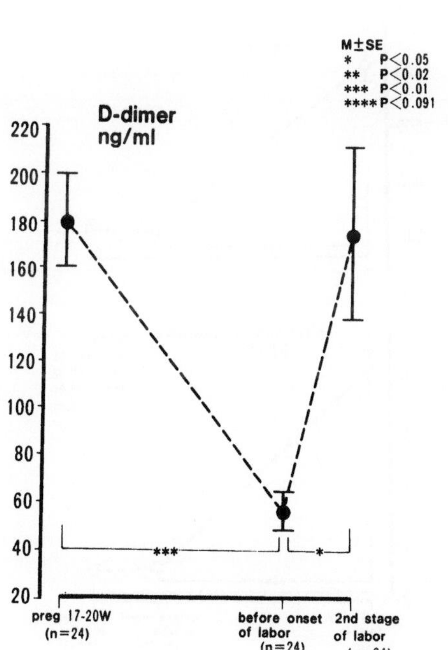

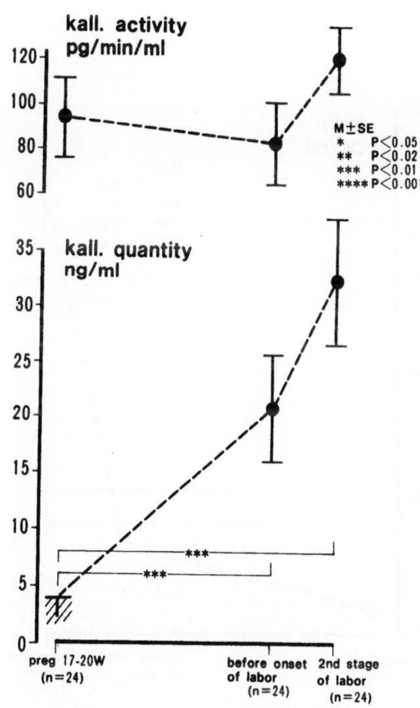

Fig. 4. Comparison of the levels of D-dimer in amniotic fluid in mid pregnancy, and before and during labor in full term pregnancy.

Fig. 5. Comparison of the levels of Kallikrein activity and Kallikrein quantity in amniotic fluid in mid pregnancy, and before and during labor in full term pregnancy.

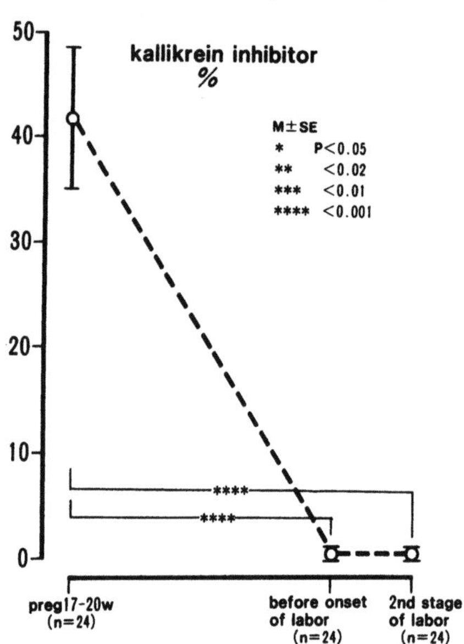

Fig. 6 Comparison of the levels of kallikrein inhibition in amniotic fluid in mid pregnancy, and before and during labor in full term pregnancy.

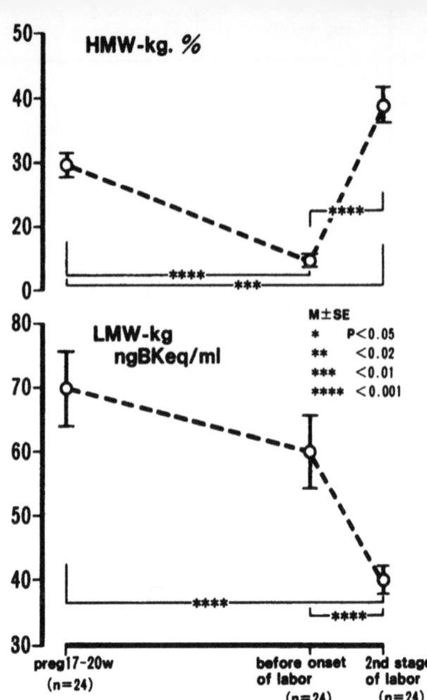

Fig. 7. Comparison of the levels of high molecular weight-kininogen(HMW-kg.) and low molecular weight-kininogen(LMW-kg.) in amniotic fluid in mid pregnancy, and before and during labor in full term pregnancy.

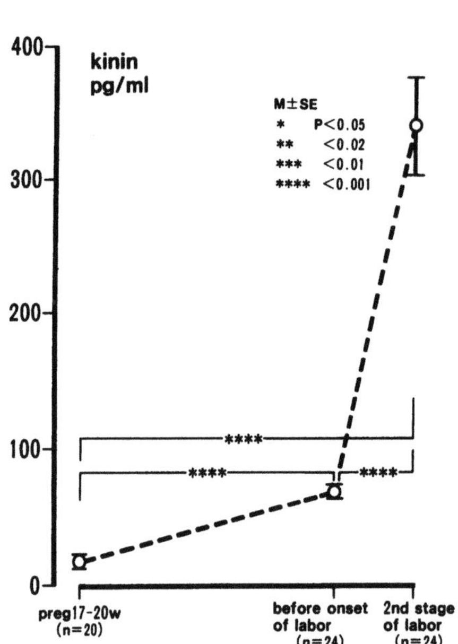

Fig. 8. Comparison of the levels of kinin in amniotic fluid in mid pregnancy, and before and during labor in full term pregnancy.

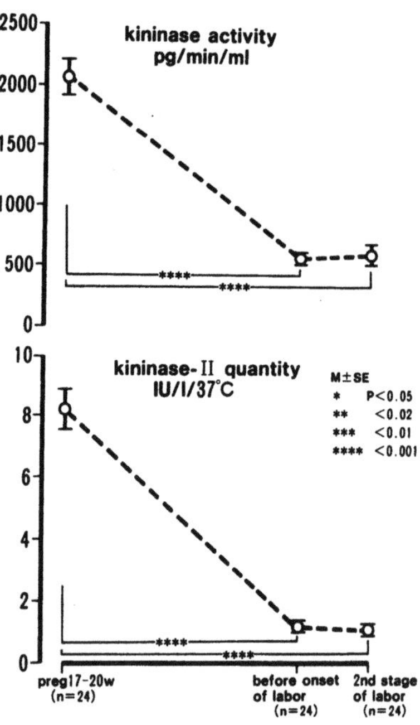

Fig. 9. Comparison of the levels of kininase activity and kininase-II quantity in amniotic fluid in mid pregnancy and before and during labor in full term pregnancy.

Table 2. Comparison of these factors in amniotic fluid in mid pregnancy and before and during labor in full term pregnancy.

	preg. 17-20 weeks (n=24)	before onset of labor (n=24)	onset of labor (1st and/or 2nd stage) (n=24)
FPA (ng/ml)	0.9 ± 0.12	1.3 ± 0.18	55.6 ± 7.08 ****
$B\beta15$-42 (ng/ml)	13.9 ± 0.47	10.9 ± 1.02 ***	22.9 ± 2.7 ***
U K (ng/ml)	3.4 ± 0.28	2.3 ± 0.31 ***	6.5 ± 0.55 ****
t-PA (ng/ml)	12.3 ± 4.41	482.3 ± 121.15 ****	639.1 ± 110.65 ****
α_2-PI (μg/ml)	1.04 ± 0.21	1.01 ± 0.18	0.93 ± 0.11
α_2PI-Pm-Complex (ng/ml)	33.3 ± 6.21	26.9 ± 5.87	77.2 ± 11.54 ***
D-dimer (ng/ml)	179.6 ± 20.31	56.7 ± 7.41 ***	174.4 ± 38.81
Kall. activity (pg/min/ml)	93.8 ± 18.3	82.8 ± 23.7	121.0 ± 22.0
Kall. quantity (ng/ml)	$4.0\ (\rightarrow,\downarrow)$	20.85 ± 4.89 ***	32.34 ± 5.75 ***
Kall. inhibitor (%)	41.7 ± 7.20	0.2 ± 0.14 ****	0.3 ± 0.30 ****
HMW-kininogen (%)	29.6 ± 1.75	15.0 ± 1.00 ****	39.0 ± 3.16 ***
LMW-kininogen (ngBKeq/ml)	70 ± 6.1	60 ± 6.1	40 ± 2.0 ****
Kinin (pg/ml)	17.6 ± 2.7	68.3 ± 4.4 ****	342.3 ± 38.2 ****
Kininase activity (pg/min/ml)	2099.5 ± 265.9	592.8 ± 103.1 ****	637.5 ± 163.9 ****
Kininase II quantity IU/l/37°C	8.2 ± 0.63	1.2 ± 0.08 ****	1.1 ± 0.05 ****

M±SE

*   P < 0.05
**   P < 0.02
***   P < 0.01
****   P < 0.001

Discussion

In previously, we have reported that the changes of blood coagulation-fibrinolysis and kallikrein-kinin systems in the utero-placental circulation (10). The blood sample from the uterin artery (UA), uterine vein (UV) and the peripheral vein (PV) were collected and the changes of FPA, Bß15-42, HMW-, LMW-kg and kinin during pregnancy and labor.

The levels of FPA in UV increased significantly during onset of labor as compared to the increase in UA and PV and although the UV level of Bß15-42 also showed the same as that of FPA pattern of increase during labor but the increasing slope was not so sharp. Levels of HMW-, LMW-kg gradually decreased during onset of labor but significant differences among UV, UA and PV were not found. Level of kinin in PV increased signficantly during labor but remained unchanged in UV.

These findings suggested that with the increased consumption of HMW-, LMW-kg and kinin during labor, the uteroplacental circulation exhibited a state of hypercoagulability with secondary hyperactivity of plasmin.

In amniotic fluid, we tried to find out the changes of the coagulation-fibrinolysis and kallikrein-kinin systems and kininase.

1. <u>The coagulation-fibrinolysis system in amniotic fluid</u>.
Thromboplastic activity of amniotic fluid was measured by Quick's one-stage method for prothrombin time (H. Yaff, MD, et al)[13] and by a two-stage assay (I.H.Omsjɸ, et al)[14], but until the amounts of thromboplastin was not able to be measured.

There is a gradual increase of thromboplastic activity of amniotic fluid from 16 to 34 weeks of gestation followed by a more abrupt increase from 34 weeks to term.

In the full term preg., amniotic fluid contains the massive thromboplastic material, however thromboplastin is not activated until then.

During labor, thromboplastin is significantly activated.

The levels of α_2-PI was high (1.04 ± 0.21 µg/ml, M $\pm$ SE) and unchanged during preg., but slightly decreased during labor (0.93 ± 0.11 µg/ml, M $\pm$ SE). This finding indicated the fibrinolysis system was depressed on the whole, while the homeostatic plasmin activity in amniotic fulid was exhibited by multifactorial analysis.

1) In the control group; the levels of FPA were depressed. The levels of urokinase, α_2PI-Pm-C and Bß15-42 were slightly increased, and D-dimer increased significantly as compared to the full term pregnancy. These findings suggested that the secondary fibrinolytic activity was markedly increased after the hypercoagulable state.

2) In the full term preg.; the levels of FPA were depressed. The low levels of urokinase, α_2PI-Pm-C, Bß15-42 and D-dimer showed that the coagulable and fibrinolytic system was depressed. The high levels of the t-PA (482.3 ± 121.15 ng/ml, M $\pm$ SE) in amniotic fluid were thought to be the result of the cross reaction with the t-PA antigen to the thromboplastin.

3) During labor; the levels of FPA were significantly increased. The levels of urokinase, t-PA, Bß15-42, α_2PI-Pm-C and D-dimer were significantly increased and α_2PI was slightly decreased. These pattern suggested the hypercoagulability with secondary hyperfibrinolytic activity.

2. <u>In the kallikrein-kinin system and kininase in amniotic fluid</u>; the levels of kallikrein activity were unchanged during normal pregnancy, but slightly increased during labor, and kallikrein quantity were markedly

increased in full term pregnancy (20.85 + 4.89 ng/ml, M + SE) and
significantly increased during labor (32.34 + 5.75 ng/ml, M + SE) as
compared to the control group (≦4.0 ng/ml). The levels of HMW-kg were
significantly decreased in full term pregnancy, but markedly increase
during labor. During labor, the high levels of HMW-kg were thought to be
the result of the vascular permeability in utero-placental circulation and
the cross reaction with the method for measurement of HMW-kg to the
hyperactivity of thromboplastin, because HMW-kg activity was measured by
the activity partial thromboplastin time using of Fitzgerald factor's
deficient plasma[7]. The levels of LMW-kg were slightly decreased
inhibitor, kininase activity and kininase II quantity were signficantly
decreased in full term pregnancy before and during labor (Kall. inhibitor
0.2 + 0.1%, kininase activity 592.8 + 103.1 pg/min/ml, kininase II
quantity 1.1 + 0.05 IU/1/37°C, M + SE) as compared to the control group
(kall, inhibitor 41.7 + 7.20%, kininase activity 2099.5 + 265.9 pg/min/ml,
kininase II quantity 8.2 + 0.63 IU/1/37°C, M + SE).

These findings suggested that with the significantly increase kall.
quantity, marked decreased kininogen and decreased a consumption of kall.
inhibitor, kininase activity and kininase II quantity during labor
exhibited the hyperproduction of kinin.

REFERENCES

1) Nossel, H.L., Younger. L.R et al: Proc. Nat. Acad. Sci. SA.,
   68:2350-2353, 1971.
2) Kudryk. B., Robinson. D., et al: Thromb., Res., 25:277-291, 1982.
3) Ohno. Y., Itabashi, et al: Thromb. Haemostas., 50:300, 1983.
4) Humer. K., Kirchheimer. J., et al: J. Lab. Clin. Med. 103:684-694,
   1984.
5) Kirchheimer. J., Binder. B.R., et al: Thromb. Research. 36:643-646,
   1984.
6) Mimuro. J., Koike. J., et al: Blood, 69:446-453, 1987.
7) Saito. H., Goldsmith. G., et al: Blood, 48:941-947, 1976.
8) Takanashi. N., Ohno. Y., et al: Thromb, Haemostas., 50:230, 1983.
9) Porcelli. G., Die Jorio. M., et al: V. National Congress of Soc.
   Ital of Clinical Biochemistry. October. 18-22. Rome , 1978.
10) Mutoh. S., Teh. A., et al: Blood & Vessel. 17:51-58, 1986.
11) Mutoh. S., Teh. A., et al: KININ IV. Part B:41-44, Edited by Lowell.
    M., Greenbaum and Harry S. Margolis (Plenum Publishing Corporation,
    1986).
12) Mutoh. S., Teh. A., et al: KININ IV. Part B:35-40, Edited by Lowell.
    M., Greenbaum and Harry S. Margolis (Plenum Publishing Corporation,
    1986)
13) Yaff. H. MD., Eldor. A., et al: Obst & Gyne. 50:454-456, 1977.
14) Omsjφ. I.M., φian. P., et al: Gynecol. Obstet. Invest. 19:1-5, 1985.
15) Aznar. J., Gilabert. J., et al: Thromb. Haemost. 43:182, 1980.

STUDIES ON URINARY COAGULATION-FIBRINOLYSIS AND KALLIKREIN-KININ SYSTEMS

AND KININASE IN NORMAL PREGNANCY, LABOR AND PUERPREIUM

S. Mutoh[1], Y. Yaoi[1], A. Teh[1], M. Saito[1], N. Aoki[2],
T. Abe[3], Y. Ohno[4] and N. Itoh[5]

Dept. of Obst. and Gynecology[1] and the First Dept. of Internal
Med.[2], Tokyo Medical and Dental University School of Medicine
Japan Woman's University[3], SRL[4] and TEIJIN[5], Tokyo

INTRODUCTION

In previously, we have reported the changes of blood
coagulation-fibrinolysis and kallikrein-kinin systems during normal
pregnancy, labor and in puerperium, and in cases of Caesarean section
(KININ IV. Part B: 35-40 and 41-44. 1986. Blood & Vessel. 15:186-189,
1984).
These findings suggested that hypercoagulable state with secondary
homeostatic activity of plasmin appeared during pregnancy and labor.
HMW-kininogen was consumed and hyperproduction of kinin was seen during
false labor. In puerperium and in cases of Caesarean section during and
after operation, levels of FPA was seen with its peak at 15 minutes and
Bß15-42 was at 3 hours. The prekallikrein-kinin system showed the
consumption of prekallikrein and kallikrein inhibitor with slight
decrease of HMW-kg. A tendency of increase in kinin production was seen
from 3 hours to 12 hours after operation. Systemic information of
urinary coagulation-fibrinolysis and kallikrein-kinin systems, kininase
activity and kininase II quantity based on stage dependent
multifactorial analysis have not been reported until now.
In this study, we tried to find out the changes of urinary
coagulation-fibrinolysis and kallikrein-kinin systems, and kininase
during normal pregnancy, labor and in puerperium. To understand the
roles of these systems and kininase in the kidney, it is necessary all
components of the system and localization to be considered.

Material and Method

In 30 non-pregnant women who were chosen as control and 206 cases
of normal gravida from early stage to term pregnancy together with 17
cases of transvaginal delivery.
The urinary flesh samples were collected at 9°am-10°am, and
preserved in ice at -4°C centrifugation at 3,000 r.p.m as soon as
possible, and stored at -70° - -80°C until to use.
Specific assys were performed for urinary fibrinopeptid A, fibrin-
derived peptide Bß15-42, urokinase, α_2-plasmin inhibitor, α_2PI-plasmin-
complex, D-dimer, urinary kallikrein activity and quantity (anti-human
urinary kallikrein antibody), kinin, kininase activity, kininase II
quantity and creatinine.

Table 1. Method for measurement

u-FPA/CRE-index (ng/mg)	RIA (PEG separation)	IMCO Co., Ltd., Sweden. [1,2,3]
u-Bβ15-42/CRE-index (ng/mg)	RIA (PEG separation)	IMCO Co., Ltd., Sweden. [1,2,3]
u-Kallikrein activity/CRE-index (ng/min/mg)	RIA (PEG separation)	
u-Kallikrein activity/CRE-index (ng/mg)	RIA (PEG separation)	
u-Kininase activity/CRE-index (pg/min/mg)	RIA (PEG separation)	[9]
u-Kininase II quantity/CRE-index ($\times 10^{-3}$ IU/min/mg)	Kasahara's method	
u-Kinin/CRE-index (ng/mg)	RIA (PEG separation)	[8]
u-Urokinase/CRE-index (ng/mg)	RIA (secondary-antibody separation)	[4,5]
u-α_2-plasmin inhibitor/CRE-index (ng/mg)	TD-80	Teijin Co., Ltd., Japan [6]
u-α_2PI-plasmin-Complex/CRE-index (ng/mg)	TD-80C	Teijin Co., Ltd., Japan [6]
u-D-dimer (ng/ml)	ELISA assay	MAbCO Co., Ltd., Australia

The ratio of these factors to creatinine (CRE) were showed as the index.

Results

1. The urinary coagulation-fibrinolysis system

1) Levels of u-FPA/CRE (M+SD) during pregnancy gradually increased from mid-term preg., (A = 0.90 + 0.69 ng/mg. p<0.001) and increased significantly in the third trimester (A = 0.99 + 0.43 ng/mg, p<0.001) and significantly increased in full term preg., (A = 0.82 + 0.35 ng/mg, p<0.001) as compared to a control group (A = 0.44 + 0.20 ng/mg), but slightly decreased in full term preg., when compared with the third trimester and in 2nd stage of labor, it was significantly increased (A = 1.18 + 0.71 ng/mg. p<0.001) as compared to full term preg.,. In puerperium, levels of u-FPA/CRE gradually decreased when compared with 2nd stage of labor (Fig. 1).

2) Levels of u-Bβ15-42/CRE (M + SD) during pregnancy gradually increased from first-term preg., (B = 7.76 + 3.31 ng/mg, p<0.001) and significantly increased in full term preg., (B = 12.24 + 3.5 ng/mg. p<0.001). Levels of u-Bβ15-42/CRE in 2nd stage of labor (B = 23.1 + 15.61 ng/mg, p<0.01) markedly increased as compared to full term preg.,. In puerperium, levels of u-Bβ15-42/CRE significantly increased when compared with full term preg., and a control group (Fig. 1).

3) Levels of u-urokinase/CRE (M + SD) were slightly depressed in 4-7 weeks of gestation (5.02 + 2.31 ng/mg), slightly increased from 8-11 weeks to 20-23 weeks as compared to a control group, but were not significant. Levels of u-UK/CRE were markedly increased in 24-27 weeks (8.83 + 4.20 ng/mg, p<0.05) as compared to a control group, but were significantly decreased ih 32-35 weeks (5.53 + 1.65 ng/mg, p<0.02) when compared with 24-27 weeks. Levels of u-UK/CRE were markedly increased in full term preg., (9.03 + 3.80 ng/mg, p<0.01) and significantly increased

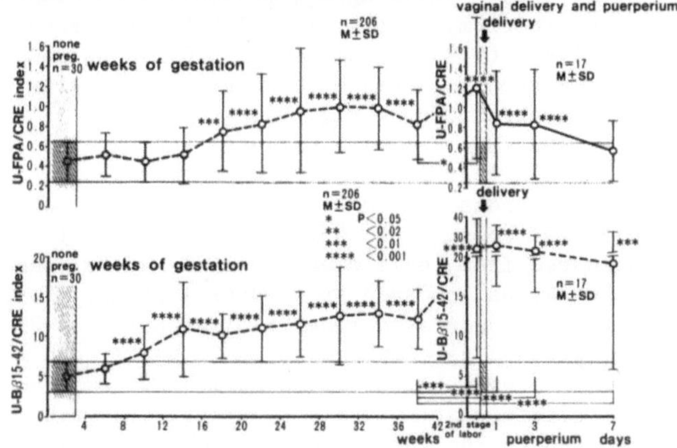

Fig. 1. Fluctuation of urine fibrinopeptide A(FPA)/CRE and fibrin-derived peptide Bβ15-42(Bβ15-42)/CRE index during pregnancy, labor and puerperium.

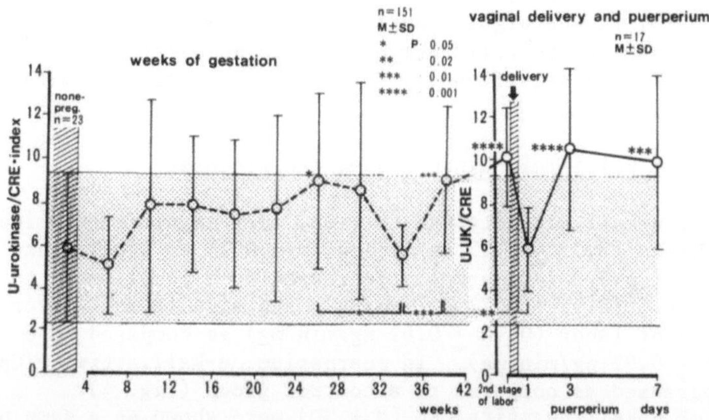

Fig. 2. Fluctuation of urine urokinase (UK)/CRE index during pregnancy, labor and puerperium.

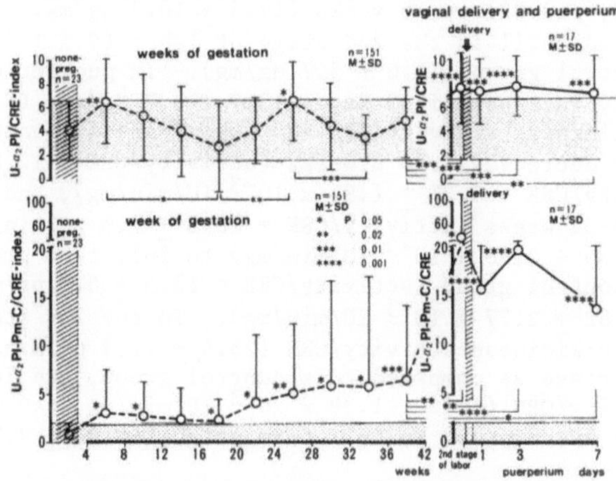

Fig. 3. Fluctuation of urine α2-plasmin inhibitor (TD-80)/CRE and α2PL-plasmin-complex (TD-80C)/CRE index during pregnancy, labor and puerperium.

in 2nd stage of labor (9.40 $\pm$ 2.55 ng/mg, p<0.001) when compared with a
control group. In puerperium, levels of u-UK/CRE were markedly decreased
in 1st day after delivery (5.95 $\pm$ 1.91 ng/mg, p<0.02) as compared to full
term preg., and were markedly increased during 3-7 days after delivery
when compared with a control group (Fig. 2).
4)   Levels of u-α_2PI/CRE (M $\pm$ SD) were markedly increased in 4-7 weeks
(6.66 $\pm$ 3.46 ng/mg. p<0.02) as compared to a control group (4.4 $\pm$ 2.56
ng/mg), and gradually decreased from 8-11 weeks to 16-19 weeks (2.66 $\pm$
3.73 ng/mg, p<0.01) when compared to 4-7 weeks. Levels of u-α_2PI/CRE
were gradually increased from 16-19 weeks to 24-27 weeks, and sligthly
increased in 20-23 weeks as compared to a control group. Levels of
u-α_2PI/CRE were gradually decreased from 28-31 weeks to 32-35 weeks
(3.43 $\pm$ 1.81 ng/mg, p<0.02) as compared to 20-23 weeks, and slightly
increased in full term preg., (4.78 $\pm$ 2.68 ng/mg) as compared to 32-35
weeks, but were not significant. Levels of u-α_2PI/CRE were
significantly increased in the 2nd stage of labour (6.77 $\pm$ 2.63 ng/mg,
p<0.01 --- 0.001) and in puerperium when compared to full term preg., and
a control group (Fig. 3).
5)   Levels of u-α_2PI-Pm-C/CRE (M $\pm$ SD) were gradually increased from
first-trimester (2.67 $\pm$ 1.34 ng/mg, p<0.01) and markedly increased in
full term preg., (6.86 $\pm$ 8.01 ng/mg, p<0.001) as compared to a control
group (0.28 $\pm$ 1.37 ng/mg), and in the 2nd stage of labor (40.88 $\pm$ 74.82
ng/mg, p<0.001), it was significantly increased when compared with a
control group and in the full term preg.. In puerperium, levels of
u-α_2PI-Pm-C/CRE were significantly increased when compared with full
term preg., (Fig. 3).

2.   The urinary kallikrein-kinin system and kininase

6)   Levels of u-kall.activity/CRE (M $\pm$ SD) were significantly increased
from 12-15 weeks (2.33 $\pm$ 1.17 ng/min/mg, p<0.001) to 24-27 weeks (2.29 $\pm$
0.86 ng/min/mg, p<0.001), markedly decreased from 28-31 weeks to in the
full term preg., (0.95 $\pm$ 0.72 ng/min/mg), and significantly decreased in
the 2nd stage of labor (0.70 $\pm$ 0.62 ng/min/mg) as compared to a control
group (1.28 $\pm$ 0.92 ng/min/mg). In puerperium, u-kall.activity/CRE
markedly decreased as compared to a control group (Fig. 4).
7)   Levels of u-kall.quantity/CRE (M $\pm$ SD) were shown as a same pattern
of u-kall.quantity/CRE, but markedly decreased in full term preg., (160.3
$\pm$ 125.7 ng/mg, p<0.001) as compared to a control group (228.2 $\pm$ 132.1
ng/mg). In puerperium, levels of u-kall.quantity/CRE were shown as a
same pattern of u-kall.quantity/CRE (Fig. 4).
8)   Levels of u-kinin/CRE (M $\pm$ SD) were markedly increased from 8 weeks
(16.3 $\pm$ 8.6 ng/mg, p<0.02) to 15 weeks (17.5 $\pm$ 10.3 ng/mg, p<0.01), and
gradually decreased until in the 2nd stage of labor (9.5 $\pm$ 7.5 ng/mg)as
compared to a control group (11.0 $\pm$ 5.7 ng/mg). In puerperium, levels of
kinin/CRE slightly increased in 3 days (13.7 $\pm$ 6.7 ng/mg) (Fig. 5).
9)   Levels of u-kininase activity/CRE and u-kininase II quantity/CRE (M $\pm$
SD) were slightly decreased from 8 weeks (activity/CRE = 12.8 $\pm$ 4.9
pg/min/mg, quantity/CRE = 5.21 $\pm$ 1.94 x 10^{-3} IU/min/mg), and slightly
increased from 28-31 weeks (activity/CRE = 18.2 $\pm$ 7.6 pg/min/mg,
quantity/CRE = 6.36 $\pm$ 2.88 x 10^{-3} IU/min/mg) to full term preg., when
compared with a control group (activity/CRE = 13.5 $\pm$ 6.8 pg/min/mg,
quantity/CRE = 5.82 $\pm$ 2.77 x 10^{-3} IU/min/mg). In the 2nd stage of
labor, levels of u-kininase activity/CRE (23.4 $\pm$ 12.7 pg/min/mg, p<0.01)
significantly increase as compared to a control group, and levels of
kininase II quantity/CRE (4.42 $\pm$ 1.39 x 10^{-3} IU/min/mg, p<0.02)
markedly decrease as compared to full term preg., (6.31 $\pm$ 2.92 IU/min/mg)
(Fig. 6).
10)   Levels of u-D-dimer during preg., were unable to be measured for
ELISA assy's method, because there were under 30 ng/ml.

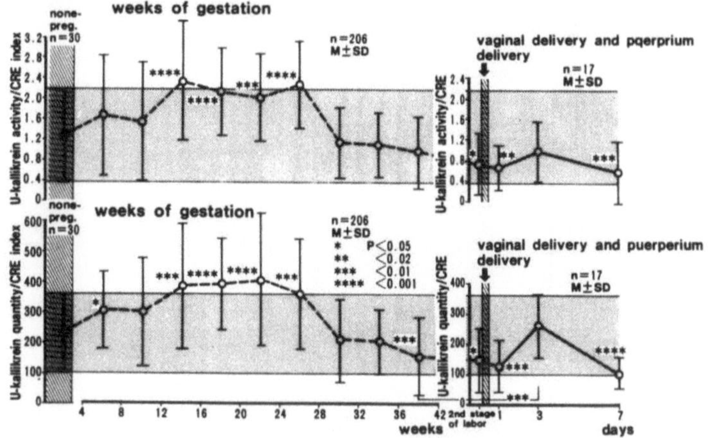

Fig. 4. Fluctuation of urine kallikrein activity/CRE and kallikrein quantity/CRE index during pregnancy, labor and puerperium.

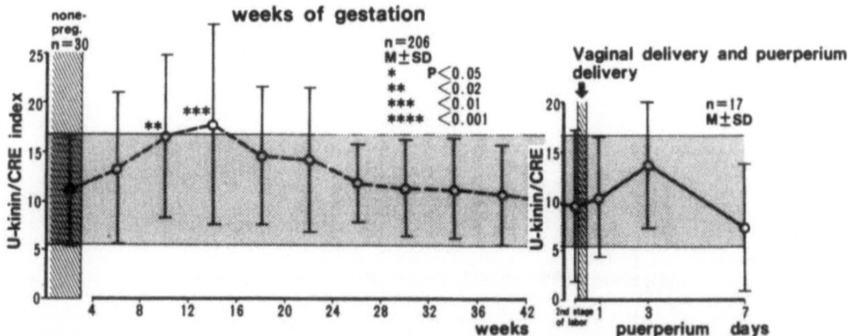

Fig. 5. Fluctuation of urine kinin/CRE index during pregnancy, labor and puerperium.

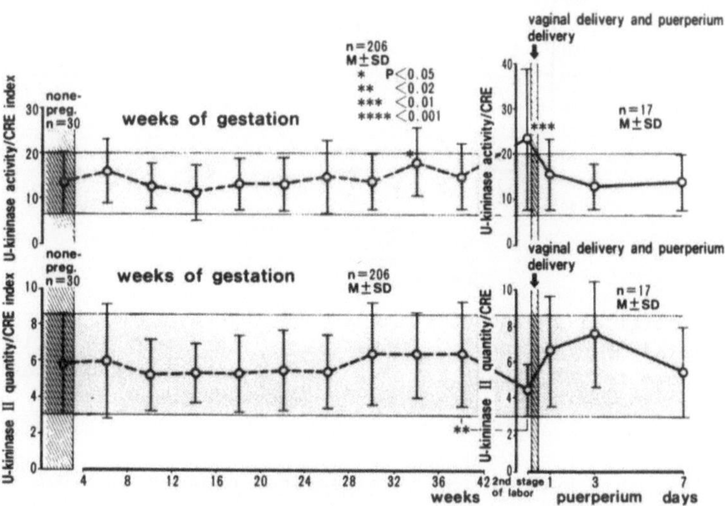

Fig. 6. Fluctuation of urine kininase activity/CRE and kininase II quantity x 10^{-3}/CRE index during pregnancy, labor and puerperium.

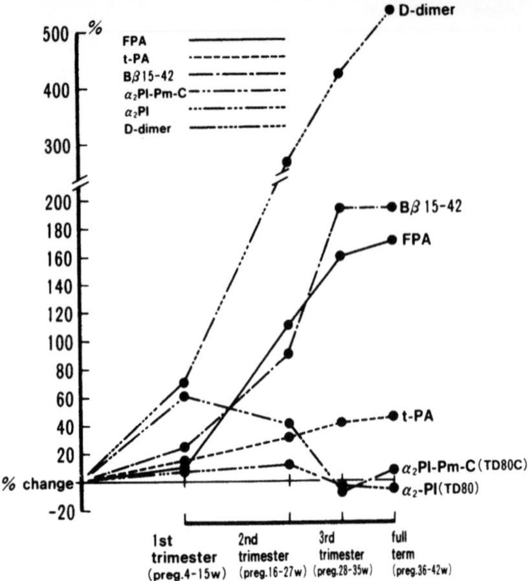

Fig. 7. Physiological changes of blood induced by pregnancy (non-pregnant (NP) to 42 weeks of pregnancy). Increment and decrement in various parameters are shown in % term with reference to non-pregnant baseline.

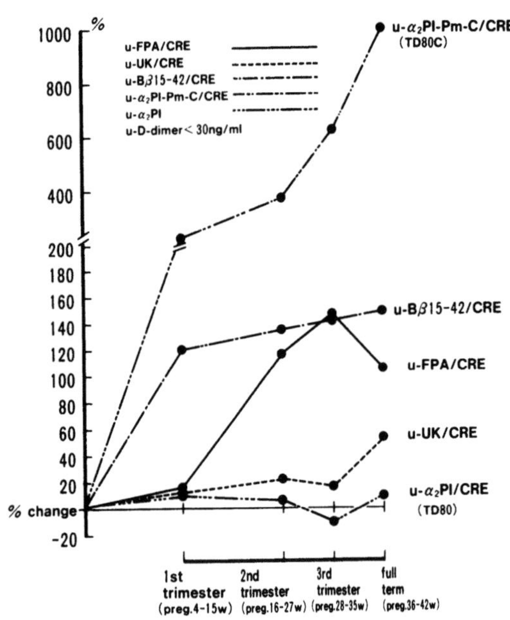

Fig. 8. Physioligical change of urine induced by pregnancy (non-pregnant (NP) to 42 weeks of pregnancy). Increment and decrement in various parameters are shown in percentage term with reference to non-pregnant baseline.

3. The relationship between the physiological changes of blood and urinary coagulation-fibrinolysis induced by pregnancy (non-pregnant (N.P.) to 42 weeks of pregnancy. Increment and decrement in various parameters were shown in percentage term with reference to non-pregnant baseline (Fig. 7,8, Table 2.3).

Table 2. Fluctuation of blood-fibrinopeptide A(FPA), fibrin-derived peptide Bβ15-42(Bβ15-42), tissue plasminogen activator(t-PA), α_2Pl-Plasmin-Complex (α_2Pl-Pm-C), α_2-plasmin inhibitor(α_2-Pl), and D-dimer during normal pregnancy.

	non-pregnancy (coptrol)	during pregnancy			
		1st trimester (preg. 4−15w)	2nd trimeser (preg. 16−27w)	3rd trimester (preg. 28−35w)	full term preg. (preg. 36−42w)
FPA ng/ml	1.0±0.09 (n=30)	1.1±0.09 (n=30) 10%	**** 2.1±0.16 (n=30) 110%	**** 2.6±0.18 (n=36) 160%	**** 2.7±0.17 (n=56) 170%
t-PA ng/ml	2.6±0.18 (n=23)	3.0±0.25 (n=23) 16%	*** 3.4±0.22 (n=21) 31%	*** 3.7±0.29 (n=18) 42%	*** 3.8±0.32 (n=20) 46%
Bβ15−42 ng/ml	3.3±0.33 (n=30)	**** 4.1±0.38 (n=30) 24%	**** 6.3±0.62 (n=30) 91%	**** 9.7±0.76 (n=36) 194%	**** 9.7±0.66 (n=56) 194%
α_2Pl-Pm-C(TD80C) μg/ml	0.29±0.07 (n=10)	* 0.47±0.05 (n=22) 62%	0.41±0.06 (n=22) 41%	0.27±0.04 (n=20) −7%	0.31± 0.05 (n=20) 7%
α_2-Pl (TD80) μg/ml	47.4± 3.0 (n=10)	51.5± 1.9 (n=22) 9%	53.1± 3.1 (n=22) 12%	45.7± 2.5 (n=20) −4%	44.9± 3.3 (n=20) −5%
D-dimer ng/ml	50.7±7.35 (n=23)	**** 86.8±14.38 (n=18) 71%	**** 185.3±21.81 (n=18) 266%	**** 264.9±27.15 (n=18) 423%	**** 318.8±36.65 (n=19) 529%

(In the α_2Pl-Pm-C row, a *** bracket spans the 1st–3rd trimester values and a * bracket spans the 1st trimester–full term preg. values.)

M±SE
* P<0.05
** <0.02
*** <0.01
**** <0.001

Table 3. Fluctuation of urinary-fibrinopeptide A(FPA)/CRE, urokinase(UK)/CRE, fibrin-derived peptide Bβ15-42(Bβ15-42)/CRE, α_2Pl-plasmin-complex(α_2Pl-Pm-C)/CRE, α_2-plasmin inhibitor(α_2-Pl)/CRE · index and D-dimer (ng/ml) during normal pregnancy.

	non-pregnakcy (control)	during pregnancy			
		1st trimester (preg. 4−15w)	2pd trimester (preg. 16−27w)	3rd trimester (preg. 28−35w)	full term preg. (preg. 36−42w)
u-FPA/CRE index ng/mg	0.44±0.04 (n=30)	0.48±0.04 (n=51) 15%	**** 0.90±0.09 (n=64) 116%	**** 0.99±0.06 (n=50) 146%	**** 0.82±0.05 (n=42) 105%
u-UK/CRE index ng/mg	5.93±0.67 (n=24)	6.73±0.73 (n=30) 14%	7.21±0.61 (n=47) 22%	6.86±0.58 (n=38) 16%	*** 9.03±0.75 (n=26) 52%
u-Bβ15-42/CRE index ng/mg	4.91±0.32 (n=39)	**** 7.76±0.50 (n=51) 120%	**** 10.51±0.47 (n=64) 135%	**** 11.97±0.54 (n=50) 144%	**** 12.24±0.62 (n=42) 149%
u-α_2Pl-Pm-C(TD80C)/CRE·index ng/mg	0.76±0.28 (n=24)	* 2.67±0.68 (n=30) 242%	* 3.68±0.84 (n=50) 372%	* 5.82±1.63 (n=48) 647%	**** 6.86±1.46 (n=30) 999%
u-α_2Pl(TD80)/CRE· index ng/mg	4.4±0.53 (n=23)	4.93±0.68 (k=30) 12%	4.67±0.74 (n=50) 6 %	3.94±0.42 (n=48) −10%	4.78±0.51 (n=30) 8 %
u-D-dimer ng/ml	<30	<30	<30	<30	<30

M±SE
* P<0.05
** <0.02
*** <0.01
**** <0.001

575

1) The blood changes of these factor's during pregnancy were shown as
compared to non-pregnant values that were induced slightly and/or
markedly in the first trimester (blood-FPA at about 10%, t-PA: 16%,
Bß15-42: 24%, p<0.001, α_2PI-Pm-C: 62%, p<0.05, α_2-PI: 9% and
D-dimer: 71%, p<0.001) and significantly increased from the second
trimester to full term preg., (blood-FPA at about 170%, p<0.001, t-PA:
46%, p<0.01, Bß15-42: 194%, p<0.001 and D-dimer: 529%, p<0.001), but
although levels of blood-α_2PI-Pm-C gradually decreased to about 41%
from the second trimester and markedly decreased to about -7% in the
third trimester and slightly increased to about 7% in the full term
preg.,. Compared with in the first trimester, levels of α_2PI-Pm-C
markedly decreased in the third trimester (p<0.01) and slightly decreased
in the full term preg., (p<0.05). The levels of blood-α_2PI increased
furthermore to about 12% in the second trimester and slightly decreased
by approximately -4% – -5% from the third trimester to the full term
preg., but were not significant (Fig. 7, Table 2).

2) In previously, the changes of urinary coagulation-fibrinolysis system
based on various stages of pregnancy, labor and puerperium followingv
multifactor's analysis have been reported (Fig. 1, 2, 3). These results
of the patterens were shown as in percentage with reference to
non-pregnant baseline (Fig. 8, Table 3).

<u>Discussion</u>

In the renal function during pregnancy[13], calculation of
incremental changes from non-pregnant values suggested that ERPF
increased by approximately 80 per cent during pregnancy, whereas GFR
increased by approximately 50 per cent and plasma volume increased by
approximately 5 per cent at this time and plasma volume significantly
increased by approximately 40 per cent in third trimester. At 36 weeks
of pregnancy, however, ERPF had decreased to a levels of approximately 60
per cent higher than the value in the non-pregnant mean, whereas GFR had
not changed from the values of early pregnancy. These findings indicated
that hyper-renal function was appeared during pregnancy, labor and in
puerperium.

<u>1. Analysis of urinary coagulation-fibrinolytic factors during pregnancy</u>

1) Levels of blood-FPA were significantly increased from the second
trimester, and levels of blood-Bß15-42 were significantly increased from
the first trimester to the full term preg., (Fig. 7, Table 2). Levels of
urinary FPA and Bß15-42 were shown as same as the pattern in the levels
of blood-FPA and Bß15-42 (Fig. 7, 8, Table 2, 3).
The high levels of urinary FPA is rapidly cleared from the high
levels of blood-FPA by glomerular Over-filtration and hypermetabolism in
part in the proximal tubule of the kidney[14], and also the high levels
of urinary Bß15-42 is rapidly the hyper-renal catabolism played an
important role in their hyper-clearance from the circulation[15].
2) The levels of urinary-UK were depressed, the levels of u-α_2PI were
markedly increased and the levels of u-α_2PI-Pm-C were slightly increased
in 4-7 weeks (Fig. 2, 3). These findings suggested that the coagulant
dominant with hypofibrinolytic state was appeared in 4-7 weeks.
3) The levels of urinary-UK and α_2PI-Pm-C were slightly increased as
compared to non-preg., but although compared with 4-8 weeks, the levels
of u-α_2PI were slightly decreased from 8-11 weeks to 16-19 weeks (Fig.
2, 3). These findings suggested that the changes of urinary fibrinolysis
were appeared a tendency to slightly increase from 8-11 weeks to 16-19
weeks.
4) The levels of urinary-UK, α_2-PI and α_2PI-Pm-C were slightly
and/or markedly increased from 20-23 weeks to 28-31 weeks, especially

these factors were shown at peak in 24-27 weeks (Fig. 2, 3). These findings suggested that changes of urinary fibrinolysis were appeared a tendency to markedly increased in 24-27 weeks.

5) The levels of urinary-UK and α_2-PI were deep-depressed in 32-35 weeks when compared with in 24-28 weeks and in the full term preg., (Fig. 2, 3). The levels of u-α_2PI-Pm were markedly increased in 32-35 weeks (Fig. 2, 3). These findings suggested that urinary-hypofibrinolytic state was appeared in 32-35 weeks.

6) The levels of urinary-UK and α_2PI-Pm-C were markedly increased and the levels of u-α_2PI were unchanged in the full term (Fig. 2, 3). These findings suggested that urinary-hyperfibrinolytic state was appeared in the full term preg.,.

The relationship between the physiological changes of blood and urinary α_2PI-Pm-C induced by pregnancy. The levels of blood-α_2PI-Pm-C were markedly increased in the first trimester, but although the levels of blood-α_2PI-Pm-C gradually decreased from mid-term. Compared with the first trimester, markedly decreased in third trimester and slightly decreased in the full term (Fig. 7, Table 2).

The levels of u-α_2PI-Pm-C were significantly increased from the first trimester to full term preg., (Fig. 3, 8, Table 3).

For this reason, the high levels of urinary α_2PI-Pm-C during pregnancy, labor and in puerperium were suggested rapidly cleared from circulation for the effect of glomerular selective Over-filtration and add to their metabolism by the hyper-activation of the reticuloendotherial system from mid term preg., to the full term preg.,[16],[17].

2. Analysis of urinary kallikrein-kinin system and kininase during pregnancy, labor and in puerperium

1) The levels of u-kall.activity and quantity gradually increased from 4-7 weeks and significantly increased from 12-15 weeks to mid-term preg., but gradually decreased to the full term preg., and furthermore in the 2nd stage of labor and in 1st day after vaginal delivery (Fig. 4).

2) The levels of u-kinin during pregnancy markedly increased in 12-15 weeks and gradually decreased from mid-term to the full term preg., (Fig. 5).

3) The levels of u-kininase activity and kininase II quantity slightly increased in 4-7 weeks, but slightly decreased from 8-11 weeks to mid-term, and slightly and/or markedly increased from third trimester. In the 2nd stage of labor, the levels of u-kininase activity were markedly increased as compared to non-preg., and kininase II quantity were markedly decreased when compared with the full term preg., (Fig. 6).

These findings suggested that availability of renal kallikrein activity and quantity, and kininase activity and kininase II quantity during pregnancy, labor and in puerperium were major determinants of levels of kinin in the kidney.

Reference

1) Nossel, H.L., Younger, L.R., et al: Proc. Nat. Acad. Sci. SA., 68:2350-2353, 1971.

2) Kudryk, B., Robinson, D., et al: Thromb., Res., 25:277-291, 1982.

3) Ohno, Y., Itabashi, M., et al: Thromb, Haemostas., 50:300, 1983.

4) Humer, K., Kirchheimer, J., et al: J. Lab. Clin. Med. 103:684-694, 1984.

5) Kirchheimer, J., Binder, B.R., et al: Thromb, Reserach, 36:643-646, 1984.

6) Mimuro, J., Koike, J., et al: Blood, 69:446-453, 1987.

7) Saito, H., Goldsmitth, G., et al: Blood, 48:941-947, 1976.

8) Takanashi, N., Ohno, Y., et al: Thromb, Haemostas., 50:230, 1983.

9) Porcelli, G., Die Jorio, M., et al: V. National congress of Soc. Ital of clinical Biochemistry. October. 18-22. Rome. 1978.

10) Mutoh, S., Teh, A., et al: Blood & Vessel. 15:186-189, 1984.

11) Mutoh, S., Teh, A., et al: KININ IV, Part B:41-44, Edited by Lowell. M., Greenbaum and Harry S. Marglolius (Plenum Publishing Corporation, 1986).

12) Mutoh, S., Teh, A., et al: KININ IV, Part B:35-40, Edited by Lowell. M., Greenbaum and Harry S. Margolis (Plenum Publishing Corporation, 1986)

13) Davison, J.M.: Sand, J. Clin. Lab. Invest (Suppl). 169:15-27, 1984.

14) Harenberg, J., Stehle, G., et al: Thrombosis Research 32:1-13, 1983.

15) Lane, D.A., Markwick, J., et al: Thrombosis Research 33:571-581, 1984.

16) Horie, N., Wada, Y., et al: Blood & Vessel. 18:No.6, 1988.

17) Umesaki, N., Kawabata, M., et al: Acta Obst Gynaec Jpn. 39:387-394, 1987.

ELASTASE RELEASE IN PLASMA WITH INCREASED C1-INHIBITION

CAPACITY DURING RECIRCULATION OF BLOOD

W. Heller, G. Fuhrer, A. Philapitsch, and
H.-E. Hoffmeister

Dept. of Cardiovascular Surgery, University of
Tuebingen, D-7400 Tuebingen, FRG

Introduction

It has been reported by Philapitsch et al. that infusion of
C1-inhibitor concentrates during extracorporeal circulation
result in a reduced release of elastase (determined by
measuring elastase-α_1-proteinase-complexes).
No effects were seen on the consumption of factor XII , factor XI and prekallikrein in this investigation (1).
In our former studies significant changes were detected in
kallikrein like activity, prekallikrein and high molecular
weight kininogen in plasma shortly after the onset of extracorporeal circulation. Furthermore, levels of C1-inhibitor
decreased in plasma of these patients undergoing open-heart
surgery (2). This activation of the contact phase system
could also be demonstrated in experiments using stored blood
for recirculation in a heart-lung machine for infants (3).
Since C1-inhibitor is an important inhibitor of the kalli-
krein-kinin- and complement system another series of experiments were performed to test the influence of increased
C1-inhibitor levels on these defense systems in our in vitro
model.
Therefore 1500 plasma units of C1-inhibitor were added to
the prime volume of the heart-lung machine prior to recirculation. Changes in plasma levels of different enzymes and
inhibitors were compared to a series without administration
of C1-inhibitor.

Material and methods

The reservoir of the heart-lung machine was filled up with
500 ml of stored blood, 100 ml Ringer's solution, 50 ml glucose 5 % and 10 ml sodium bicarbonate. Because stored blood
contains ACD, a calcium solution was added to the blood
after anticoagulation with heparin. During the experiments
the temperature of the recirculating volume was kept at 28°C,
the pressure in this system was regulated to have 60 mmHg.
1500 plasma units of C1-inhibitor were added to the prime
volume of the heart-lung machine in ten of eighteen experiments.

Blood was taken according to the following schedule:
1) From stored blood
2) From the prime volume
3) After addition of C1-inhibitor
4) 15 minutes after recirculation
5) 30 minutes after recirculation
6) 45 minutes after recirculation
7) 60 minutes after recirculation
8) 90 minutes after recirculation
9) 120 minutes after recirculation

Prekallikrein, kallikrein like activity and kallikrein inhibition levels were determined using reagents supplied by
Deutsche KabiVitrum, Munich, FRG, according to the methods
of Gallimore and Friberger (4).
Antithrombin III activities, heparin levels and ß-FXIIa-inhibition were measured by means of the chromogenic substrate
S-2222 (Deutsche KabiVitrum, Munich, FRG und Channel Diagnostic, Walmer, Deal Kent, U.K)
C1-esterase-inhibitor levels were determined by reagents
supplied by Immuno AG, Heidelberg, FRG.
Elastase-α_1-proteinase-inhibitor-complexes were measured
by an enzyme immunoassay (Merck AG, Darmstadt, FRG).

Results

Kallikrein like activity levels were not significantly
different in both groups. In the series with C1-inhibitor
the initial levels were higher, but during recirculation
KK-activities increased up to 240 % of initial values in
both groups. No significant differences in prekallikrein
levels were observed in both groups (fig. 1).
The kallikrein inhibition capacitiy was significantly enhanced by C1-inhibitor (500 % of normal), whereas in the
group without C1-inhibitor a continous fall in kallikrein
inhibition was seen.
The ß-FXIIa-inhibition capacity was elevated by the addition
of C1-inhibitor. No significant changes occurred in the
group without increased C1-inhibitor plasma levels (fig.2).
In both groups plasma levels of antithrombin III fell from
82 % to 69 % of normal after recirculation of blood (fig. 3).
Before recirculation C1-esterase-inhibitor levels were low
in both groups. After the addition of C1-INH, levels of 642%
were determined and fell to 610 % during the observation
period (fig. 4).
In the group without administration of C1-INH, levels below
normal (68 %) were seen after recirculation (fig. 5).
A continous increase of elastase-α_1-proteinase-inhibitor-
complexes could be detected during recirculation of blood.
No significant differences were seen in both groups (fig. 6).

Discussion

Recirculation of blood within the heart-lung machine resulted in an activation of the kallikrein-kinin system. This
could be demonstrated by a slight decrease in prekallikrein
plasma levels and an increase in kallikrein like activity.
Kallikrein inhibition fell in the series with and without
the addition of C1-inhibitor to the prime volume.
Furthermore, elastase-α_1-proteinase-inhibitor-complexes (E-
α_1-PI) increased during the recirculation period indepen-

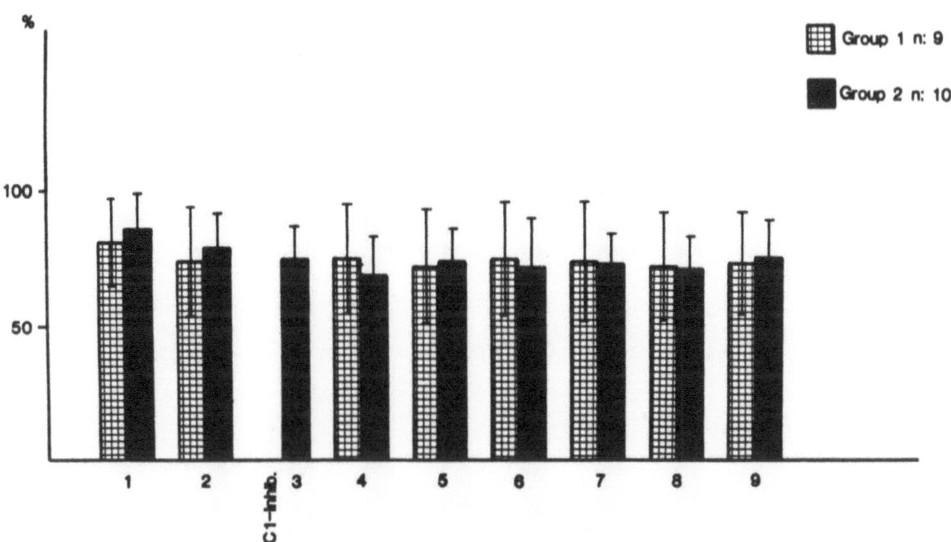

Fig. 1   Prekallikrein

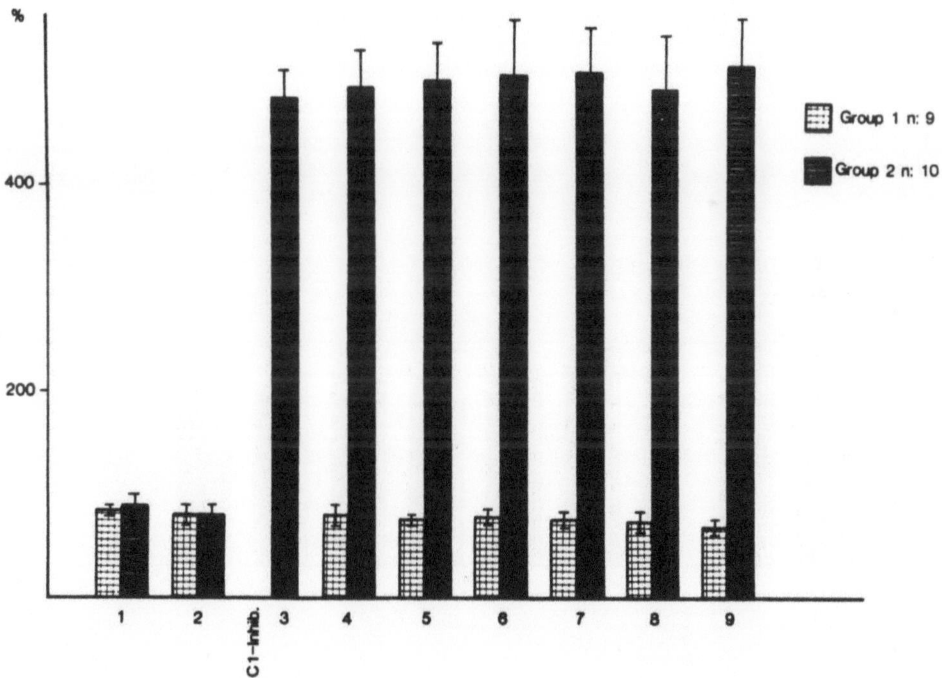

Fig. 2   Kallikrein inhibition

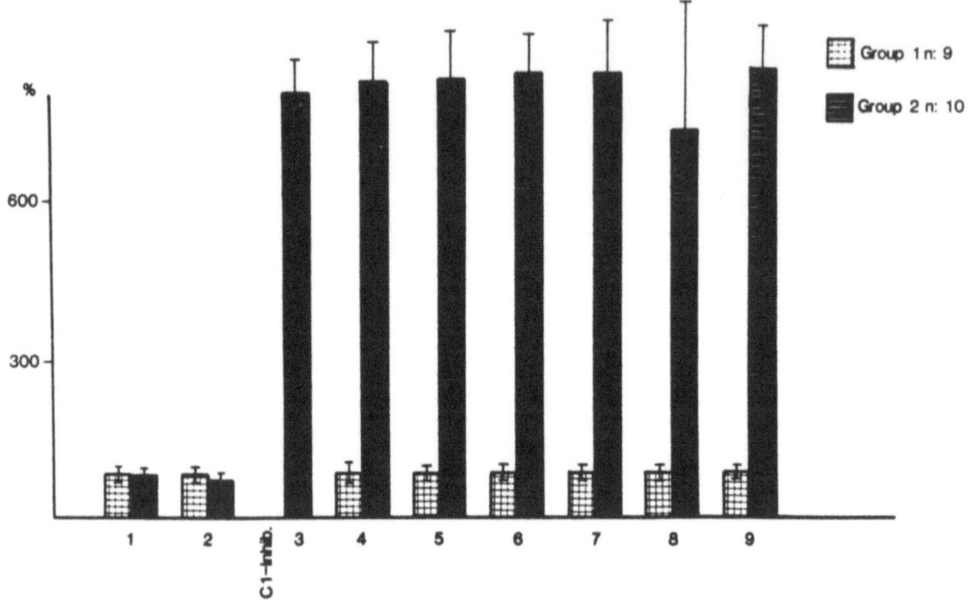

Fig. 3   ß-FXIIa-inhibition

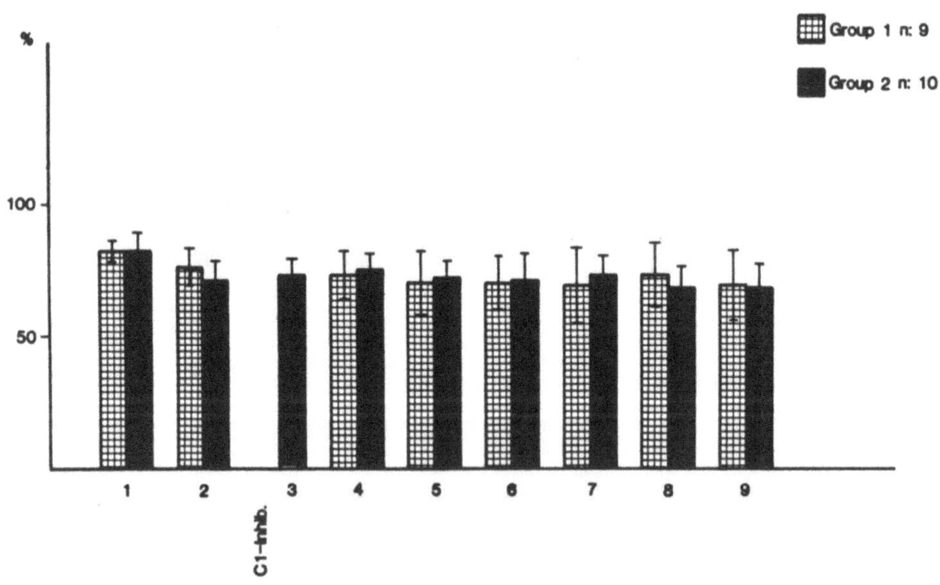

Fig. 4   Antithrombin III

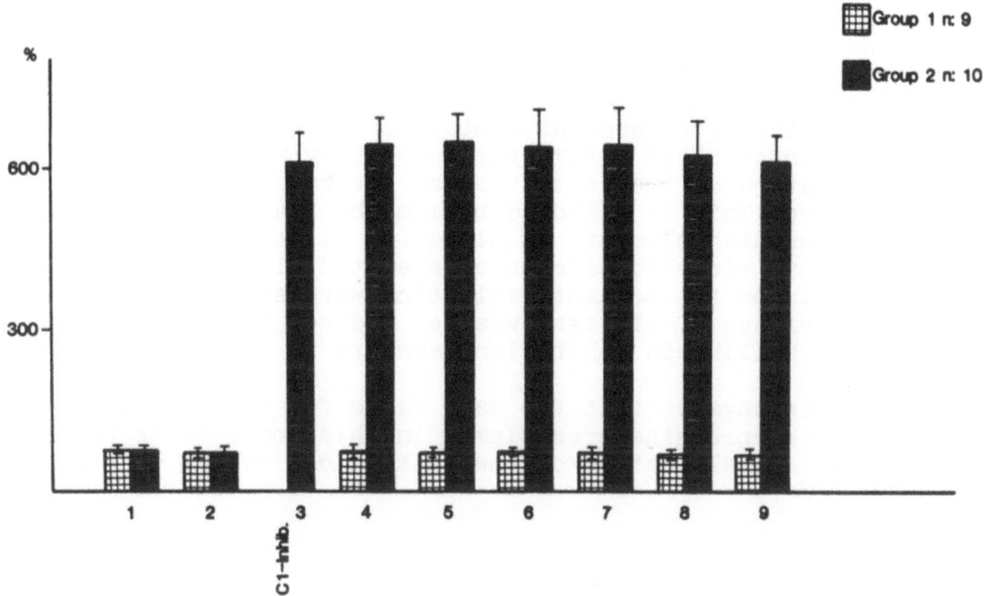

Fig. 5   C1-esterase-inhibitor

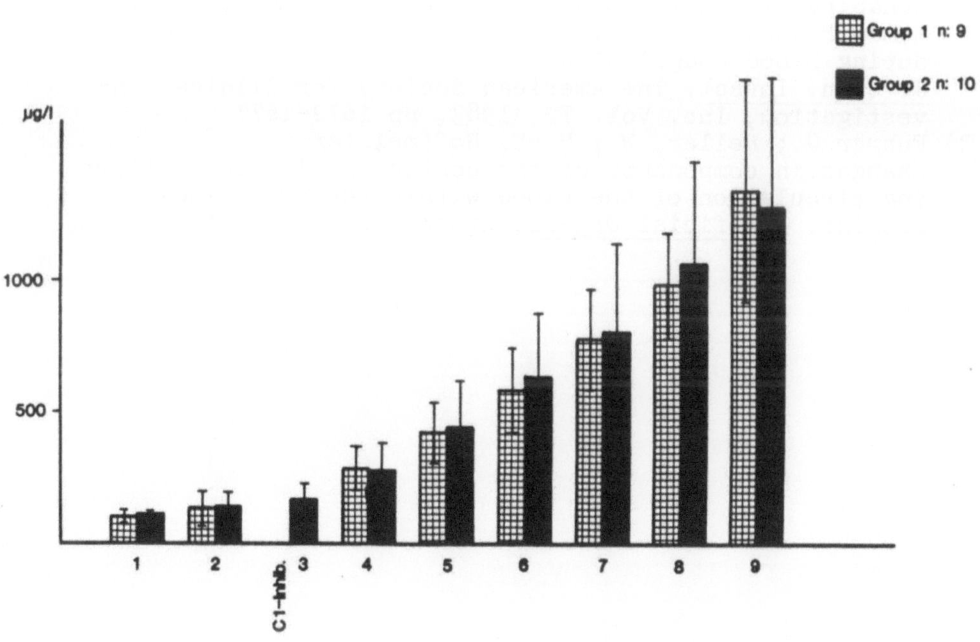

Fig. 6   Elastase-α_1-proteinase-inhibitor complexes

dently from Cl-inhibitor plasma activities.
Elastase is released from human neutrophils during the early
events of blood coagulation. Human plasma kallikrein has
been shown to stimulate neutrophil aggregation and chemo-
taxis, and is followed by the release of elastase from neutrophils.
Antithrombin III levels were not significantly changed during the observation period indicating that the used heparin
dose is sufficient to prevent clotting.
Recirculation of blood within the heart-lung machine leads
to an activation of the contact phase system during the
first minutes. This is followed by a mechanical destruction
of all corpuscular elements in blood (by filters, oxygenator
etc.). In this study no effects of elevated Cl-inhibitor
plasma levels on the contact activation were seen. Furthermore, the release of elastase was not reduced by augmentation of the kallikrein inhibition capacity up to 500 % of
normal.
These results suggest that the main cause for the increase
of elastase-α_1-proteinase-complexes in this model seems to
be a mechanical alteration of the white blood cells.

References

1) Philapitsch, A.; Popov-Cenic, S.; Murday, H.; Jochum, M,;
   Anderle, K.. Inhibition of contact phase activation and
   fibrinolytic activity in a placebo-aprotinin-Cl INH
   study. Xth International congress Thrombosis and Haemostasis, San Diego, 1985
2) Wachtfogel, Y.; Kucich, U.; James, H.L.; Scott, C.F.
   Schapira, M.; Zimmerman, M.; Cohen, A.B.; Colman, R.W..
   Human Plasma Kallikrein Releases Neutrophil Elastase
   during Blood Coagulation.
   J. Clin. Invest. The American Society for Clinical Investigation, Inc. Vol. 72, 1983, pp 1672-1677
3) Fuhrer G.; Heller, W.; H.-E. Hoffmeister.
   Changes in components of the contact activation following circulation of the blood within the heart-lung
   machine. Artificial Organs, Athens, 1985, in press

CHANGES IN COMPLEMENT COMPONENTS AFTER
INTRAVASCULAR APPLICATION OF CONTRAST MEDIA

H. M. Hoffmeister*, G. Fuhrer**,
H. P. Platten**, and W. Heller**

* Department of Internal Medicine III
** Department of Thoracic and Cardiovascular
Surgery, University of Tübingen
D-7400 Tübingen, Fed. Rep. of Germany

INTRODUCTION

A risk of adverse reactions is associated with the intravascular application of radiographic contrast agents. An
activation of the complement cascade by contrast media
either via the classical or via the alternative pathway was
supposed after in vitro studies by some authors (1,7).
However, there are only few data (2) available up to now
from in vivo studies on a possible complement activation .
It was therefore the aim of our study i) to examine the
effect of intravascular contrast media on components of the
complement system and ii) to investigate whether there are
differences in the side effects between ionic and non-ionic
contrast agents.

METHODS

Venous blood samples were obtained before, at the end and
20 minutes after a diagnostic urography. In 22 patients 250
ml of the conventional ionic contrast medium sodium-/
meglumine-amidotrizoate (Urovison R Schering) and in 24
patients 100 ml of the non-ionic contrast agent iohexol
(Omnipaque R Schering) were infused. The duration of the
infusion was 10 minutes. The blood samples - mixed with
citrate - were quickly centrifugated. The supernatant was
thereafter rapidly deep frozen (liquid nitrogen). Laser-
nephelometry was used for determination of the components of
the complement system. Factor VIII was measured using a
clotting method. The values were corrected for hematocrit.
All data were expressed as mean +/- SD in % of the preinfusion values. For statistical evaluation a p<0.05 was defined as level of significance (paired Wilcoxon test).

The infusion of contrast agents for a diagnostic urography had significant effects on the complement system. The values at the end of infusion for C3, C1q and C1-inhibitor are illustrated in fig. 1 demonstrating the reduction of C3 and C1-inhibition levels by the ionic contrast medium. 20 minutes after the infusion the data showed a trend to renormalization of C3 and C1-inhibitor (fig. 2).

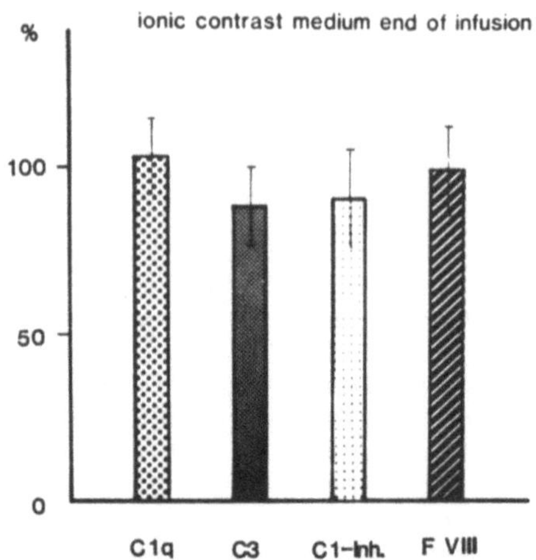

Fig. 1   Effect of infusion of sodium-/meglumine-amidotrizoate on components of the complement system and on factor VIII. Values at the end of infusion in % of preinfusion control. Mean +SD, *p<0.05, **p<0.01.

The nonionic contrast agent iohexol also influenced the complement system. Figure 3 illustrates the decrease of C3 and C1-inhibitor. Additionally, we found a significant reduction of C1q . The effects of the non-ionic contrast medium iohexol were only transient as shown on figure 4. The trend of a normalization included the recovery of the decreased C1q levels.
In both groups the factor VIII levels were not altered, neither directly at the end of infusion nor 20 minutes later.

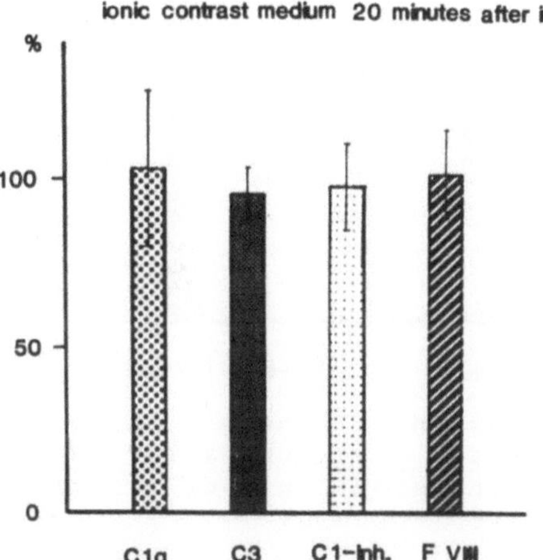

Fig. 2   Effect of infusion of sodium-/meglumine-amidotrizoate
         on components of the complement system and factor VIII.
         Values   20 minutes after infusion in % of preinfusion
         control. Mean +SD, *p<0.05, ** p<0.01.

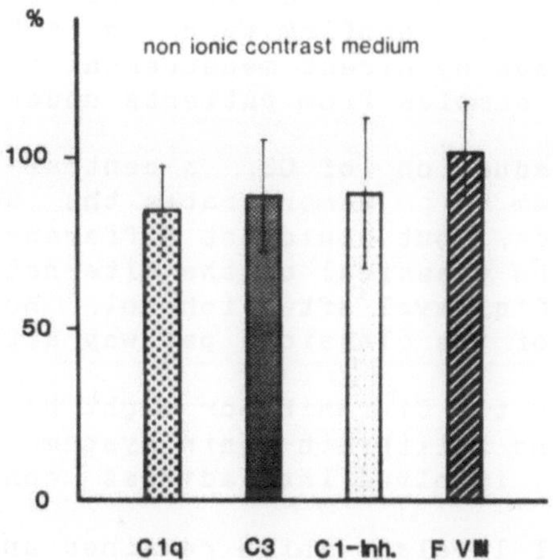

Fig. 3   Effect of infusion of iohexol on components of the
         complement system and on factor VIII. Values at the
         end of infusion in % of preinfusion control.
         Mean +SD, *p<0.05, **p<0.01.

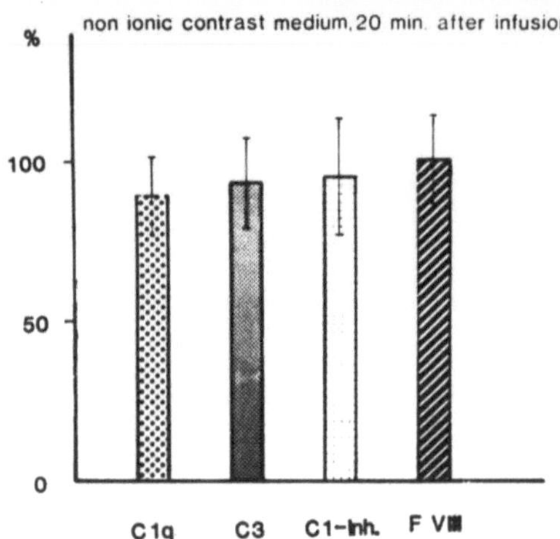

Fig. 4   Effect of infusion of iohexol   on components of   the
complement   system   and   on factor   VIII.   Values   20
minutes after infusion   in % of preinfusion   control.
Mean +SD, p<0. 05, **p<0. 01

DISCUSSION

An involvement   of the complement system in   the   patho-
mechanism   of adverse reactions against contrast agents   was
supposed   by some authors after in vitro studies (1, 7).   Our
present   study   could   confirm such   an   activation   of   the
complement   cascade by direct measurement of complement components in blood samples from patients undergoing an   intravenous urography.
The   observed   reduction   of C3,   a central protein   of   the
complement   system (6),   demonstrates the   activation of the
complement cascade,   but could not differenciate between   an
activation via the classical or the alternative pathway. The
decrease of the C1q-level after iohexol,   however, indicates
an   involvement of the classical pathway after injection   of
this agent.
The   reduction of the C1-inhibitor might be indicative for a
connection   to the kallikrein-kinin system,   which   is   also
supposed   to   be   involved into adverse   contrast   reactions
(4, 5).
The   factor   VIII levels,   which remained unchanged in   both
groups,   demonstrate that the reduction of the level of some
proteins was not caused by dilution.
The   observed   changes   of the complement system   were   only
transient.   Despite of the limited extent of the alterations
it must be taken into account,   that the changes were   found
after   a clinically well tolerated contrast medium   infusion.
After a certain predisposition (3) a more extensive   activation of the complement cascade might be possible. This could
be   of importance for the pathogenesis of adverse   reactions
against contrast agents.

REFERENCES

1
Dawson, P., Turner, M. W:, Bradshaw, A., Westaby, S.
Complement activation and generation of C3a anaphylatoxin by
radiological contrast agents
British Journal of Radiology 56: 447-448 (1983)

2
Freyria, A. M., Pinet, A., Belleville, J., Eloy, R., Traeger, J.
Effects of different contrast agents on serum complement and
calcium levels after excretory urography
J. Allergy Clin. Immunol. 69: 397-403 (1982)

3
Lasser, E. C., Lang, J. H., Lyon, S. G., Hamblin, A. E.
Complement and contrast material reactors
J of Allergy and Clinical Immunology 64: 105-112 (1979)

4
Lasser, E. C., Lang, J. H., Lyon, S. G., Hamblin, A. E., Howard,
M. M.
Activation systems in contrast idiosyncrasy
Invest. Radiology 15: 2-5 (1980)

5
Lasser, E. C.
Adverse   reactions   to   intravascular   administration   of
contrast media
Allergy 36: 369-373 (1981)

6
Mayer, M. M.
Complement. Historical perspectives and some current issues
Complement 1: 2-26 (1984)

7
Neoh, S. H., Sage, M. R., Willis, R. B., Roberts-Thomson, P.,
Bradley, J.
The in vivo activation of complement by radiologic contrast
materials and its inhibition with e-Aminocaproic acid
Invest. Radiology 16: 152-158 (1981)

PLASMA KALLIKREIN CLEARANCE BY THE LIVER OF NORMAL AND INJURED RATS

Carlos F. Toledo*, Maria Kouyoumdjian**, and Durval Rosa
Borges*

Departments of Medicine* and Biochemistry**, Escola Paulista
de Medicina
D.R. Borges - Caixa Postal 20239 04034 São Paulo, Brasil

SUMMARY

We report the clearance of rat plasma kallikrein (RPK) by the perfused
livers of normal rats and from others at 2 and 4 days after subcutaneous
injection of turpentine oil. RPK removal from the perfusate follows a logarithmic curve (y = a+b lnx) and from this equation its half-life of removal can be calculated. RPK clearance rate followed the potential equation
y = ax^b. Both the half-life of RPK removal and RPK clearance rates were
similar in the 3 groups of perfused livers. We conclude that, at the initial
concentration of RPK used (approximately 3 nM), its liver clearance is not
affected during the acute-phase response to inflammation.

INTRODUCTION

The plasmatic coagulation-kinin pathway seems to be related to the
pathogenesis of inflammatory reactions as well as to the local control of
blood flow and perhaps control of blood pressure (1). Aside from the role
of bradykinin in inflammation, several changes in proteins of the kallikrein-kinin system have been observed during the acute-phase response to
inflammation. In rats, plasma kininogen behaves as an acute-phase protein
(2) and it was demonstrated that the "acute-phase kininogen" represented
in fact, both T kininogens, I and II (3). Livers from rats at 2-3 days after
subcutaneous injection of turpentine, when perfused, synthesized prokallikrein 3 times faster than did livers from normal rats (4). On the other
hand, the liver is the main organ to clear plasma kallikrein in vivo (5) and
the perfused rat liver clears native plasma kallikrein efficiently (6).
Although some other native acute-phase plasma proteins (α_2-macroglobulin,
α_1-acid-glycoprotein and α_1-protease-inhibitor) are not cleared by the perfused rat liver (7) it was described that the liver uptake of asialo-α_1-glyco-
protein decreases during the acute-phase response to inflammation (9). This
means that one of the liver systems for receptor-mediated endocytosis
of glycoproteins, may be deficient during an inflammatory process. We now
report the clearance of rat plasma kallikrein (RPK) by the livers of normal
rats and rats after 2 and 4 days of an inflammatory stimulus.

MATERIALS AND METHODS

Rat plasma kallikrein (RPK) was purified to a specific activity of 107 U/mg (S2302 Kabi Vitrum, Stockholm, as substrate) or 34 U/mg (benzoil-Pro--Phe-Arg-p-nitroanilide, "Bz", Department of Biophysics, Escola Paulista de Medicina, São Paulo, as substrate). RPK is a 87 kDa neutral serine proteinase glycoprotein with residues of galactose, N-acetyl-glucosamine, mannose, glucose and fucose (9)

Certain of the rats received 0.5 ml turpentine oil subcutaneously at each of two sites on either side of the abdomen.

Isolated and exsanguinated livers of normal 250-300 g male Wistar albino rats or of rats after 2 or 4 days of the inflammatory stimulus were perfused (6) with 30 ml of a BSA-saline solution saturated with 5% CO_2 in oxygen at $37^{\circ}C$, and containing 0.3 BzU of RPK (approximately 3 nM). The RPK clearance was followed by serial determinations of the amidolytic activity of the perfusate using "Bz" as substrate (6).

During the surgical procedure a citrated blood sample was collected in order to measure plasma concentrations of fibrinogen, rat α_1-acute-phase globulin and rat α_2-macroglobulin (2).

RESULTS

1. Acute-phase response: the inflammatory stimulus used was efficient, as demonstrated by the significant increase in plasma concentrations of three acute-phase proteins (Table 1).

TABLE 1 - Mean plasma levels (±SE) of fibrinogen (mg/dl), rat α_1-acute--phase globulin (arbitrary units) and rat α_2-macroglobulin (arbitrary units).

GROUP	FIBRINOGEN	α_1-ACUTE-PHASE GLOBULIN	α_2-MACROGLOBULIN
Control (n=6)	177±22	34±6	Not determined
2 days ex-turpentine (n=4)	755±102	60±7	61±8
4 days ex-turpentine (n=4)	305±37	72±5	26±7

2. RPK liver clearance: the percentual clearance of RPK (Table 2) follows a logarithmic curve (r^2 = 1.000), in the 3 groups; from the equation y = a+b lnx the half-life of RPK removal from the perfusate can be calculated; the analysis of variance indicates that there was no difference (p>0.05) in RPK half-life of removal by the 3 groups of perfused livers.

TABLE 2 - Mean (±SE) RPK activity at different perfusion times and its half-
-life of removal by the 3 groups of perfused livers.

GROUP	0	2	10	20	40	CALCULATED HALF-LIFE (min)
			PERFUSION TIME (min)			
		(percentual RPK activity)				
Control	100	64±5	45±4	36±3	28±4	7.7±1.8
2 days ex-turpentine	100	58±10	37±3	28±2	20±3	4.8±2.1
4 days ex-turpentine	100	62±8	43±5	38±4	30±4	8.3±3.6

3. RPK clearance rate: RPK liver clearance is a 2 phase phenomenon (where an initial rapid clearance is succeeded by a slow phase) which can be expressed ($r^2 = 0.999$) by the potential equation $y = ax^b$. Using this equation one can calculate RPK clearance rate at any chosen time. Table 3 compares the experimental data obtained with the calculated clearance rates: the experimental and the calculated data are similar/equal and there are no difference among the 3 groups.

TABLE 3 - Mean experimental (exp) and calculated (calc) RPK clearance rates
(mU/min .g liver) at different perfusion times.

GROUP	2 exp	2 calc	10 exp	10 calc	20 exp	20 calc	40 exp	40 calc
Control	3.4	3.4	1.0	1.0	0.6	0.6	0.3	0.3
2 days ex-turpentine	3.6	3.6	1.1	1.1	0.6	0.6	0.4	0.4
4 days ex-turpentine	3.5	3.6	1.0	1.0	0.6	0.6	0.3	0.3

DISCUSSION

We have previously shown that RPK clearance rate by the perfused rat liver depends on the initial concentration of the enzyme in the perfusate (6). With the RPK initial concentration (approximately 3 nM) used in the present set of experiments, its clearance rate was sub-maximal; this initial concentration corresponds to approximately 1% of plasma prokallikrein concentration. In this circumstances we verified that there are no differences among the 3 groups of perfused livers and conclude that RPK liver clearance is not affected by the acute-phase response to inflammation.

Once in its active form, plasma kallikrein can act on its physiological substrates, and this action may be limited by inhibition and/or liver clearance. The liver may thus clear either free kallikrein or the complex kallikrein-plasma inhibitor. Since some, if not all, natural inhibitors are not cleared by the perfused liver (7) one can postulate that such a complex will be recognized by hepatocytes, through its RPK moiety. The existence of binding sites of hepatocytes for complexes such as α_2-macroglobulin-thrombin, α_2-macroglobulin-plasmin, antithrombin III-thrombin (10) and α_2-macroglobulin-trypsin (11) have indeed been demonstrated.

Our present results show that liver RPK clearance capacity is preserved during the acute-phase response to inflammation. In agreement with our previous finding of a reduced bradykinin release in the rat-paw thermic oedema model during an inflammatory process (4), this information suggests that, during the acute-phase response to inflammation, the mechanisms which control the kallikrein-kinin system activities are not impaired.

REFERENCES

1. A.P. Kaplan and M. Silverberg, The coagulation-kinin pathway of human plasma. Blood 70:1-5 (1987).
2. D.R. Borges and A.H. Gordon, Kininogen and kininogenase synthesis by the liver of normal and injured rats. J. Pharm. Pharmac. 28:44-48 (1976).
3. R. Kageyama, N. Kitamura, H. Ohkubo and S. Nakanishi, Differential expression of the multiple forms of rat prekininogen mRNAs after acute inflammation. J. Biol. Chem. 260:12060-12064 (1985).
4. E.A. Limãos, D.R. Borges, J.C. Souza-Pinto, A.H. Gordon and J.L. Prado, Acute turpentine inflammation and kinin release in rat-paw thermic oedema. Br. J. exp. Path. 62:591-594 (1981).
5. D.R. Borges, C.A.M. Sampaio, P. Llosa and J.L. Prado, The liver is the main organ to clear plasma and tissue kallikreins from rat plasma, in vivo, in: "Kinins IV", Part A, L.M. Greenbaum and H.S. Margolius, eds., Plenum Publishing Corporation, p. 229-233 (1986).
6. D.R. Borges, A.H. Gordon, J.A. Guimarães and J.L. Prado, Rat plasma kallikrein clearance by perfused rat liver. Brazilian J. Med. Biol. Res. 18:187-194 (1985).
7. K. Steube, V. Gross, D. Haüssinger, T. Thran-Thi, K. Decker, W. Gerok and P.C. Heinrich, Clearance of acute-phase proteins with no, high- -mannose-hybrid, or complex type oligosaccharide side chains by the isolated perfused rat liver. Biochem. Biophys. Res. Commun 141:949- -955 (1986).
8. M.W.C. Wong and J.C. Jamieson, Evidence for reduced uptake of asialo- -α_1-glycoprotein during the acute phase response to inflammation. Life Sci. 25:827-834 (1979).
9. M. Kouyoumdjian, D.R. Borges, Y.M. Michelacci, J.A. Guimarães, C.A.M. Sampaio and J.L. Prado, Purification and characterization of the alpha form of rat plasma kallikrein. Brazilian J. Med. Biol. Res. 20: (In press, 1987).
10. Z. Spolaricz, J. Mandl, R. Machovich, P. Lambin, T. Garzó, F. Antoni and I. Horváth, Association of α_2-macroglobulin-thrombin and α_2- -macroglobulin-plasmin complexes with isolated hepatocytes. Biochim. Biophys. Acta 845: 389-395 (1985).
11. J. Gliemann and O. Davidsen, Characterization of receptors for α_2-macroglobulin-trypsin complex in rat hepatocytes. Biochim. Biophys. Acta 885:49-57 (1986).

STUDIES ON THE MECHANISM OF THE SEDATIONAL STATE; "TRANQUILIZATION"

EVOKED BY BRADYKININ OR KALLIKREIN IN RATS

K. Yazaki

Department of Pharmacology
Tokyo Dental College
1-2-2 Masago, Chiba 260, Japan

SUMMARY

The mechanism of the sedative state "tranquilization" evoked by
bradykinin(BK) or kallikrein(Kal), was studied. The drugs were injected
intracerebroventricularly(icv) into the lateral ventricle, according to
Yaksh's procedure. The behavior of a rat was estimated comparatively by
the spontaneous movement. Two groups of animals were examined; one group
was pretreated with prostaglandin(PG)-synthesis inhibitors, and the
other group was not pretreated. The tranquilization was observed at the
period of 12 to 16min after BK or Kal injection. Almost of the PG-synthesis inhibitors reduced the tranquilization. On the contrary, eugenol
or guaiacol, elongated the tranquilization. The levels of monoamines and
PGs in the rat brain at the tranquilization, 15min after BK injection
detected with HPLC (high performance liquid chromatography). The levels
of almost monoamines in the rat brain were decreased, however, PGE_2 was
increased considerably. Those results suggest that PGs is greatly
involved in tranquilization evoked by BK or Kal.

INTRODUCTION

Lambert and Land(1) showed the icv injection of BK evoked a 2-phase
alternation of behavior. The first phase was excitement immediately
after BK icv injection and the second phase was a sedative state, tranquilization, appeared later than excitement. But the mechanism of the
induction of the tranquilization in a brain by BK or Kal, is not clear.
Many worker demonstrated that endorphines took part in the sedative or
depressive state. In a brain Kal localized in hypothalamus or third
ventricle(2), and kininogen was contained in cerebellum and brainstem
(3). In the peripheral, meanwhile, the injection of BK released PGs.(4)
So, in the brain, Kal clearly synthesizes BK from kininogen, and BK
makes free of PGs, clearly. Moreover, the sedative effect is, the
characteristic property of PGE induced BK.
    Thus, it was suggested that PGs was released by BK and concerned in
the tranquilization evoked by BK. And in order to make clear of the
mechanism of tranquilization, these experiments were carried out.

MATERIALS AND METHODS

Animals and Drugs

Adult male Wistar-SD rats weighing 200-220g, fed a pallet diet at 23-25°C, 60% humidity for one week, were used. A intracerebroventricular cannula assembly was stereotaxically implanted into the lateral ventricle of a rat, according to Yaksh(5). After 1-week post-operative recovery period, the drugs were injected using a microsyringe. As drugs, BK, Kal, prostaglandin Es(PGEs) were dissolved in Hartmann's solution and prepared to be 10μl. As the control animal, 10μl of Hartmann's solution was single icv injected. When the drugs were injected, the spontaneous movement was estimated. The inhibitors of PG-synthesis; indomethacin, quinacrine, eugenol or guaiacol was icv injected in 10μl, 60min before BK or Kal icv injection.

The Detecting Methods

The separation of a rat brain according to the procedure of Glowinski(6), and taken from the rat brain, the hypothalamus was frozen. Monoamine were extracted according to the procedure of our department of Pharmacology (7), and detected with HPLC using electro chemical detector.

The whole brain of the rat was taken from the rat body and frozen immidiately. The method of extraction method of PGs was the procedure as illustrated in the following illustration(8). The PGs were detected with HPLC by fluorescence monitor detector, using ADAM as a fluorescence indicator of PGs.

The condition of HPLC(ECD)

solvent:0.1M phosphate buffer
(pH 3.0)including 8%MeOH
flow rate:600μl/min
applied volt:300mV
column:ODS 4.0x250mm
temperature:25°C

The condition of HPLC(PGEs)

solvent:10mM phosphate buffer
(pH 3.0)including 65%MeOH
flow rate:1200μl/min
column:ODS-H 4.0x250mm
temperature:46°C

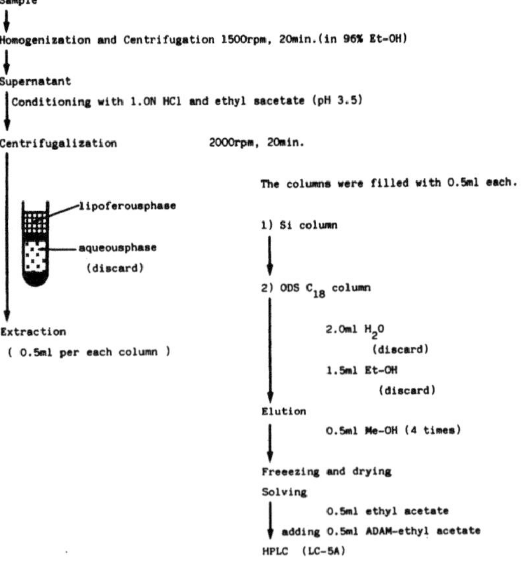

Fig. 1. The procedures of extraction or detection of PGs.

I. Behavioral Effects

I.1 Effects of BK, Kal,or PGs on the Spontaneous Movement and Behavior of a Rat

BK and Kal, icv injected 10µg/10µl or 8KIU /10µl respectively, induced 2-phase alternation in spotaneous movement: a great increase at 0
to 6 or 8min and a small increase at 24 to 30min; a marked decrease, at
the "tranquilization", the sedative period induced BK, accompanied with
piloelection, at 12 to 16min after BK injection. The control, injected
with the 10µl of Hartmann's solution, was observed more or less the excitement. In comparison to the control animal, the first great increase
of the spontaneous movement was observed at first, after BK injection,
but the second increase was not so marked. However, the decrease was,
much more significant than the control. At the excitement, as BK icv injected, the animal was observed grooming, jumping, rearing, struggling,
exploration, etc and the restlessness rapid moving, too. At the
tranquilization, it was observed that the animal crouched at another
site of a cage, with piloelection and ptosis of the eyelids. When 8KIU/
10µl of Kal was injected icv, the same alternation of behavior was observed. However there were a few
minutes of time-lag; the
time-lag between BK- and
Kal-injection was 2 or
4min on the average.

As the dose of 10ng/
10µl PGE was icv injected,
the rat-spontaneous move-
ment increased markedly,
immediately after injection.
However, on the cotrary to
the case of BK or Kal,
the excitement at 0 to 4min
was not followed by the
excitement, but only followed by the sedative state,
at which the spontaneous
movement significantly decreased. And at this sedative
period, a rat was observed the
sedative or depressive state
considerably, as if it had been
injected sedatives. Compared to
the tranquilization, evoked by
BK or Kal icv injection, this
sedative period was not accompanied with the piloelection, but with
most of the subjects which were observed at the tranquilization.

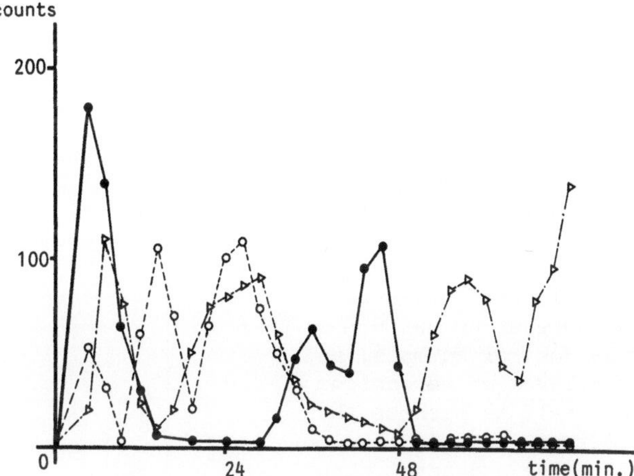

Fig 2. The alternation of spontaneous
movement induced by BK or Kal.
(●) showes BK, (▷) showes Kal,
(O) showes Hartmann's solution
respectively.

I.2 Effects of PG-Synthesis Inhibitor on the Behavior evoked by BK of a Rat

The difference of PG-synthesis inhibitors showed two different
alternation of spontaneous movement. One of the inhibitor of PGs;
indomethacin and quinacrine, showed this way: the dose of 100µg/ 10µl of
indomethacin and the dose of 10µM/10µl quinacrine, complately inhibited
PG-synthesis, the first excitment was reinforced and prolonged remarkably, twice as much as BK single injection, and reduced the tranquilization considerably, half as long as BK single injection.

The other PG-synthesis inhibitors, such as phenol derivatives, are well known to
inhibit the PG synthesis
partially, and especially to
inhibit the synthesis of
prostacycline. While eugenol
or guaiacol 10µg/10µl was
pretreated, the first excitement was equal with BK single
injection, however tranquilization was elongated markedly,
twice as long as BK single
injected. The second excitement was however reduced
markedly, two-thirds as long
as BK single injected,
the spontaneous movement at
this period was increased
slightly. The characteristic
behaviors evoked by BK or
Kal, was observed, when
PGE-synthesis inhibitor
was injected.

II. The Level of the Mono-
amines in the Rat Brain
at the "Tranquilization"

The monoamine level
at the tranquilization
in the hypothalamus of
the rat, BK injected icv,
as follows: the level of
noradrenaline was 95% of
the control animals, and
the level of adrenaline
was half as much as the
control, and the level of
dopamine and serotonine
in the hypothalamus, was
three quarters of the
control, respectively.

III. The Level of PG
in the Rat Brain at
the "Tranquilization"

The level of PG in the
rat brain at the tranquilization, evoked by BK,
increased considerably.
Especially, PGE_2 in the rat
whole brain at the sedative
period, tranquilization,
15min after BK 10µg/10µl
injection, was increased
28% over the control animal,
injected vehicle.

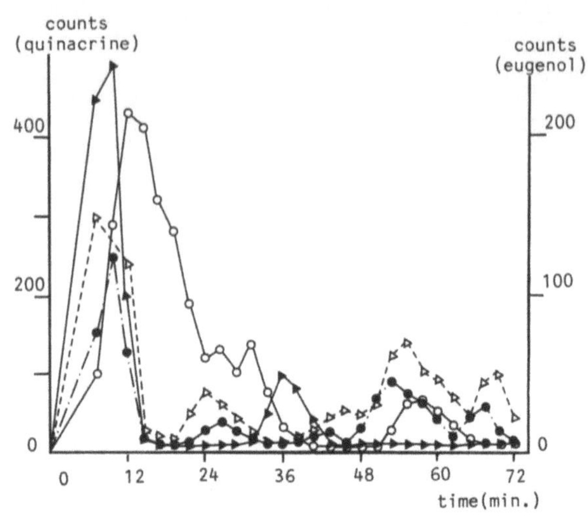

Fig 3. Alternation of spontaneous movement when Kal and PG-synthesis inhibitor icv co-administrated;
(●) as Kal, (O) as quinacrine,
(▶) as eugenol and (▷) as Kal,
respectively.

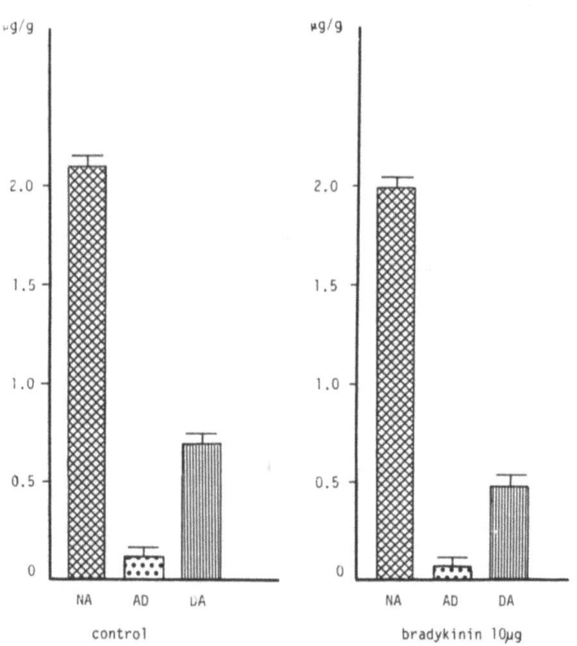

Fig 4. The levels of catecholamines at
the tranquilization induced by BK.

DISCUSSION

BK icv injection evokes the excitement, followed by the sedative state; tranquilization, has been studied many authors, such as Sicuteri, Lambert and Land(1).
But, as Roche e Silva said that BK icv injection evoked only the sedative state. Many reports shown by Iwata, Graff,Kaneko, or Kariya, on the BK induced-sedative state. Reported by Iwata(9), the activity of the kininase in the cerebrum, was increased at the excitement and decreased at the sedative state evoked by BK. He concluded that BK did not evoke the sedative state, but the metabolite of the BK evoked it. Kariya(10), on the other hand, demonstrated BK and Kal evoked the 2-phase alternation of behavior of a rat, and the sedative state was accompanied with piloelection. Furthermore, he detected level of BK in the rat brain, when Kal icv injected and found that level of BK was dependent upon the dose of Kal. Through the fact, it was suggested that there were kinin-synthesis systems in a brain, and might be some factor of physiological actions in the central nervous system(CNS). In this experiments, the same alternation of the behavior evoked by BK or Kal icv-injection was observed. Although the tranquilization induced by BK or Kal observed by many workers, the mechanism of tranquilization is not clear. As Inoki(11) announced, recent reports suggested that endorphines might be a key of the sedative and analgesic effects of BK or Kal on the CNS.

BK is well known to act on the phospholipase A_2 and to synthesize PGs(12). PGE_1 or PGE_2 among PGEs, has the characteristic sedative effect on the CNS. And the sedative state evoked by PGE, might be mediated by endorphines. The findings of this study, the tranquilization was negatively influenced by PG-synthesis inhibitors, and BK markedly increased the level of PGE. Thus, the tranquilization evoked by BK or Kal, may be induced by the increase of PGE. Furthermore, on the relationship between the levels of monoamines and BK was investigated, BK made a decrease of the levels of monoamines; 5HT, NA, DA and AD. This result supported many studies that reported the reduction of levels of monoamines by BK in the rat whole brain(13)(14). On the other hand, the relationship between PGEs and monoamines is well known that PGE makes reduction the levels of monoamines in the brain(15)(16). Through the facts as mentioned above, in the present study, those results suggest that in the CNS BK released and synthesized PGs, and evoked the characteristic sedative or depressive state; tranquilization.

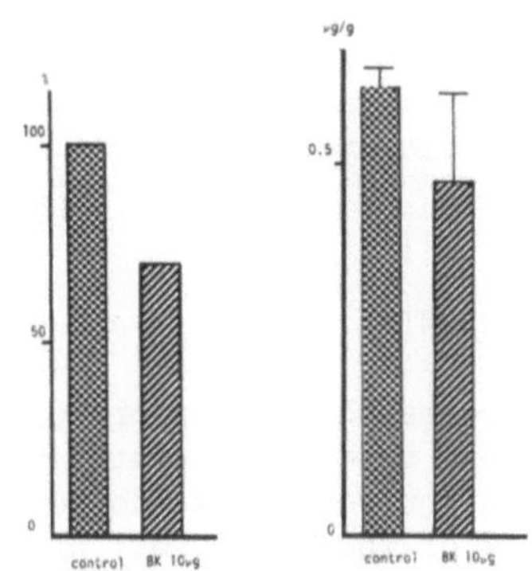

Fig 5. The level of 5-HT in the hypothalamus of a rat at the tranquization evoked by BK. a column of showes control and showes BK 10ug/10ul icv injected.

Table 1. PG-levels in the rat whole brain at the tranquilization by BK.

items	PGE_2 (ng/brain)
basal level	1.436±0.0634
BK 10μg icv	1.832±0.0383 *

* : $p < 0.01$ vs basal level.
means±SD (n=5)

CONCLUSION

        The results in the present study suggested as followed:
1) Kal acted on the kininogen in the central nervous system, and synthesized
   kinins.
2) At the sedative state, tranquilization, the levels of monoamines were
   reduced by BK or Kal.
3) The tranquilization evoked by BK or Kal, was induced by the increase of
   PGs, especially PGEs.

ACKNOWLEDGEMENTS

        This research was supported financially in part by the scientific
research fund from the Ministry of Education (1983).
        The author would like to acknowledge the helpful, continuous guidance
and support of the late Prof. Dr. S. Tsutsumi; the former director of Dept.
of Pharmacology: and to thank the director, Co-Prof. Dr. M. Kawaguchi for
helpful advice.

REFERENCES

1) Lambert, G.A. and Lang, W.J. Eur. J. Pharmacol. 9, 383 (1970)
2) Simson, J.A.V. J. Histochem. Cytochem. 33, 951 (1985)
3) Shikimi, T. Biochem. Pharmacol. 22, 567 (1973)
4) Ferreira, S.H. Br. J. Pharmacol. 49, 86 (1973)
5) Myers, R.D. and Yaksh, T.L. J. Appl. Physiol. 30, 589 (1971)
6) Glowinski, J. Neurochem. 13, 655 (1966)
7) Kawano, T. and Tsutsumi, S. Shikwa Gakuho 84, 203 (1984)
8) Yazaki, K. Shikwa Gakuho 85, 1575 (1985)
9) Iwata, H. Biochem. Pharmacol. 18, 119 (1969)
10) Kariya, K. Neuropharmacol. 20, 1221 (1982)
11) Inoki, R. and Kudo, T. Recent Progress on Kinins 270, (1982)
12) Damas, J. and Deby, C. Arch. Int. Physiol. Biochem. 84, 293 (1976)
13) Moniuszko-Jakoniuk, J. Pol. J. Pharmacol. Pharm. 29, 301 (1977)
14) Moniuszko-Jaconiuk, J. Psychopharmacology 50, 181 (1976)
15) Capek, R. Pharmacology 2, 161 (1969)
16) Kariya, K. Neuropharmacol. 21, 267 (1982)

DOES KALLIKREIN IMPROVE THE BRAIN FUNCTION IN DEMENTIA?

Yoshikazu Ishizuka, Hitoshi Fukuzawa,
Takashi Asada, and Tetuhiko Kariya

Department of Psychiatry
Yamanashi Medical College
Tamaho, Yamanashi 409-38, Japan

SUMMARY

Forty biological units of Kallikrein were administered intra-muscularly to nine persons suffering from multi-infarct dementia. With automatic analysis equipment, the wave-form recognition method was used to analyze EEG before injection, immediately after injection, and 30, 60, 90, and 120 minutes after injection. The results of analysis done the five times after injection were then compared with the analysis results before injection. With the passage of time after injection, delta and theta waves showed a gradually decreasing tendency, while alpha and beta waves showed a gradual increase. It was inferred that these changes in the EEG were caused by an increase in the flow of cerebral blood, which in turn was the effect of the dilatation of cerebral blood vessels resulting from the action of the Kallikrein.

INTRODUCTION

The substance Kallikrein, an enzyme that exists in a wide variety of organisms, has been known about for a relatively long time. Kallikrein produces bradykinin and kallidin, which are both types of kinin that have a pharmaceutical effect, from kininogen. One of the various known pharmaceutical effects of Kallikrein is a strong one in which the blood vessels of the internal organs, the extremities and the brain are greatly dilated and blood circulation is markedly increased[8]. This effect has been used clinically in almost every field.

Even though cerebral blood flow increases due to this effect, unexpectedly, there are few reports on changes in the brain functions from that effect.

Kugler has recorded the electro-encephalogram(EEG) of healthy peoples for a 40-minute period after administering kallikrein intramuscularly[9]. He compared this with the response of subjects to doses of a physiological saline solution.

The results indicated that, after doses of a saline solution, and with the passage of time, the subjects' EEG showed a pattern of light sleep. On the other hand, the response to the doses of Kallikrein was one of continued arousal in which the subjects would not enter into a condi-

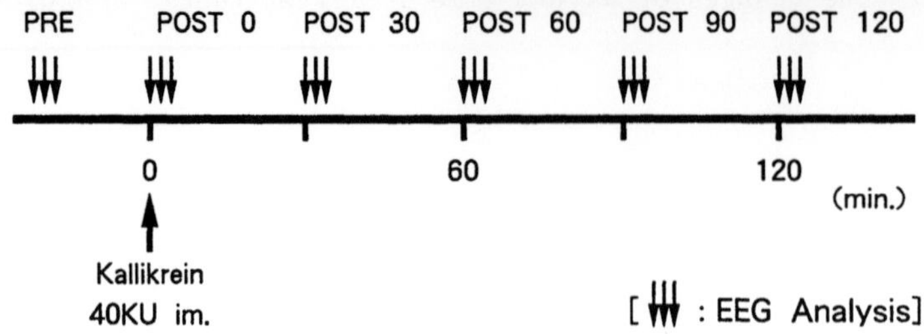

Figure 1. The design of our experiment. The abbreviations are explained in the text.

tion of sleep. He considered these results to be a possible indication that Kallikrein has the effect of maintaining peoples' vigilance.

Another researcher, Held, experimentally compared subjects in a state of hypoxia when they had been administered Kallikrein and when they had not[4]. He reported a slight reduction of the slowing of EEG due to hypoxia with Kallikrein administration.

There was no report, however, about variations in the subjects' EEG in each frequency, with the passage of time, after they received dosages of Kallikrein. In addition, there was no report of observations of the effect of Kallikrein on the EEG of multi-infarct dementia patients whose condition is associated with reduced cerebral blood flow.

We, therefore, decided to administer Kallikrein intramuscularly to multi-infarct dementia patients to observe changes in EEG with the passage of time. The observations we made, which may be of interest, are reported in the following pages.

SUBJECT AND METHOD

Subjects

Nine multi-infarct dementia patients were clinically examined. The purpose of the research was explained to the subjects and their families, and their consent was obtained. The ages of the subjects were from 53 to 82; average age was 72. The extent of dementia was measured in accordance with the Hasegawa Brief Dementia Scale in which "subnormal" and below were employed. The average score of the subjects was 18.6.

Method (see Figure One)

Referential derivations of EEG were obtained for Fp. C. O. T. At the same time, electrodes were attached to the both outer canthus to record an electro-oculogram.

After recording EEG at times of rest and wakefulness, 40 biological units of Kallikrein were injected into muscle tissue of subjects. At six different time points -- before injection, immediately after injection, then 30, 60, 90, 120 minutes after -- the subjects eyes were opened and shut in order to maintain a wakefulness. Immediately after each time, three epochs in which slow eye movements were not observed were selected to conduct quantitative EEG analysis using the computerized wave-form recognition method. In figure 1, PRE represents pre-injection, then Post 0, 30, 60, 90, and 120 each indicate the number of minutes after injection when recordings were conducted.

Regarding the results of C3 lead EEG analysis, five conditions after injection were compared with the pre-injection period, and statistical verification was done using the two-way ANOVA with repetition.

Regarding the method used to conduct quantitative EEG analysis, EEG was analyzed by computerized wave-form recognition method. The procedure for this method is similar to the method of wave-reading in the usual

Table 1. The changes of wave % time of delta, theta, alpha, and beta waves by Kallikrein administration. The abbreviations are as same as figure 1.

	PRE	POST 0	POST 30	POST 60	POST 90	POST 120
% Time δ	4.0 (5.3)	3.8 (3.8)	3.9 (5.5)	3.8 (5.6)	3.3 (4.7)	2.7 (3.5)**
% Time θ	37.9 (16.5)	38.1 (18.2)	37.3 (18.7)	36.3 (17.8)	35.5 (19.7)*	35.4 (19.7)*
% Time α	44.9 (14.3)	45.7 (14.5)	47.3 (16.7)	49.9 (15.5)***	50.9 (16.3)***	49.6 (15.3)***
% Time β	17.9 (12.8)	16.8 (11.3)	18.1 (12.3)	16.5 (11.2)	18.8 (11.2)	21.0 (13.7)***

*:p < 0.05, **:p < 0.01, ***:p < 0.005, compared with "PRE" Mean (SD)

inspective assessment of EEG, and that the results obtained by this method [10,11] can be utilized as the clinical EEG diagnosis of today. In this system the following categories of frequencies were (Hz) used: 0.5 < delta < 4.0; 4.0 < theta < 8.0; 8.0 < alpha < 13.0; 13.0 < beta < 30.0.

RESULTS (see Table one; Figure 2)

The amount of delta waves appearing showed a tendency to decrease after 60 minutes from the time of injection. At 120 minutes after injection, a significant decrease had occurred compared with the pre-injection recording.

The amount of theta waves appearing began to show a tendency to decrease 30 minutes after injection. Compared to the recording before injection, at 90 minutes and at 120 minutes after injection, the number of theta waves had significantly decreased.

The amount of alpha waves appearing slowly increased after injection. At 60 minutes after and at 90 minutes after, the amount of alpha waves showed a sharp increase over the amount registered in the pre-injection recording. Although a tendency toward a slight decrease began to appear at 120 minutes after injection, the increase was still significant.

The amount of beta waves appearing began to increase slightly at 90 minutes after injection. At 120 minutes after, there was a significant increase over the pre-injection amount.

A point worthy of our attention here is that immediately after injection, there was not much of a change in EEG, but about 60 minutes later clear changes were apparent: delta and theta waves had decreased slightly, while alpha and beta waves had increased slightly.

DISCUSSION

Earlier reports indicated that, among the persons suffering from dementia, multi-infarct dementia patients showed decreased cerebral blood flow compared to healthy persons[2]. In addition, it was a well-known fact that persons suffering from dementia have much slow wave of EEG[3]. It had also been reported that the effect of Kallikrein on human cerebral arteries was to dilate them. And experiments with animals had proven that increased cerebral blood flow had been caused by the same substance[8].

However, research conducted Kugler and Held had been conducted with healthy subjects, and there had been no report on the effects of Kallikrein on the EEG characteristics of dementia patients with reduced cerebral blood flow.

We, therefore, decided to study the changes that occur with time in the EEG of persons administered Kallikrein.

There were no changes in the EEG before and immediately after the injection. From this we understood that there had been no effect on EEG

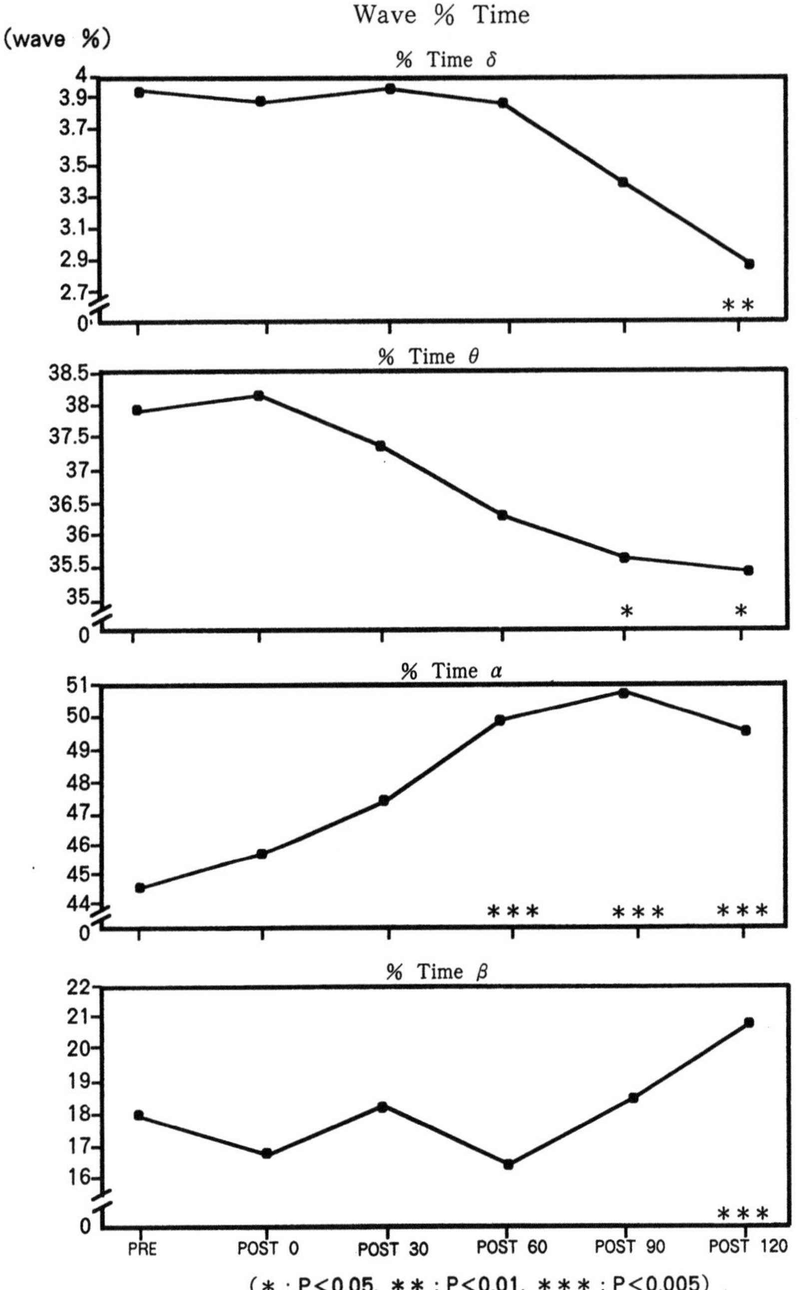

Figure 2. With the passage of time after Kallikrein injection, delta and theta waves showed gradually decreasing tendency, while alpha and beta waves showed a gradual increase.

caused by any physical pain stimulation associated with the injection.

Then after 60 minutes had elapsed, changes in EEG began to appear. From this we could surmise that Kallikrein had some type of pharmaceutical effect that was producing changes in EEG.

Hollwich had measured the diameter of the arteries in the retinas of healthy subjects that had received injections of Kallikrein intramuscularly[5]. He reported that dilation began to be observed 45-60 minutes after injection and that the dilation peaked about three hours after injection.

The specific points in elapsed time at which effects were observed in our study, closely resembled the time points at which effects were observed in Hollwich's study. From this we can infer that the changes in EEG observed in our study accompanied an increased cerebral blood flow, and that these changes were caused by enlargement of the diameter of cerebral arteries .

The decrease in slow waves and the increase in alpha waves that we observed could be viewed in terms of the action of a so-called "anti-dementia drug" or as a "nootropic" ("noo"=thought or reason; and "trepo"=turn or change). A nootropic is characterized as a drug which selectively affects the higher cerebral functions[1].

Itil reported that there were significant positive correlation between increased alpha activity caused by a nootropic and overall clinical improvement of dementia[6,7]. Considering Itil's report along with the results of our study, one can infer that a connection could possibly be made between Kallikrein acting to improve EEG and Kallikrein acting to improve the condition of patients with the clinical symptoms of dementia.

REFERENCES

1) C. Giurgea, The "Nootropic" Approach to the Pharmacology of the Integrative Activity of the Brain. Cond. Reflex, 8:108 (1973).
2) V.C. Hachinski, L. Iliff, E. Zilhka, G.H. Du Boulay, V. McAllister, J. Marshall, R.W. Ross Russel, and L. Syman, Cerebral Blood Flow in Dementia. Arch. Neurol., 32:632 (1975).
3) B. Harvald, EEG in Old Age. Acta Psychiat. Neurol. Scand., 33:193 (1958).
4) K. Held, Effect of Kallikrein on Cerebral Capacity and EEG-Activity of Man during Hypoxia. in: Kininogenases-Kallikrein 4. B.L. Haberlan, J.W. Rohen, and T. Suzuki ed., F.K. Schattauer Verlag, Stuttgart-New York (1977).
5) F. Hollwich und A. Wethmar, Gefasserweiternder Einfluss korpereigener und korperfremder Stoffe auf die Arterien der Netzhaut, in: Leistungen und Ergebnisse der neuzeitligen Chirurgei. Emil. K. Fren zum 70. Geburtstag, Georg Thieme Verlag, Stuttgart-New York (1958).
6) T.M. Itil, Nootropics:Status and Prospects. Biological Psychiatry, 18:521 (1983).
7) T.M. Itil, G.N. Menon, A. Songar, and K.Z. Itil, CNS Pharmacology and Clinical Therapeutic Effects of Oxiracetam, Clinical Neuropharmacology, 9:S70 (1986).
8) S. Kazda, Influence of Kallikrein on the Cerebral Flow in the Dog. in: Kininogenases-Kallikrein 3. G.L. Haberlan, J.W. Rohen, G. Blumel, and P. Huber ed., F.K. Schattauer Verlag, Stuttgart-New York (1975).
9) J. Kugler, R. Schichtl, and J. Empt, The Influence of Kallikrein on the Vigilance in the EEG. in: Kininogenases-Kallikrein 3. G.L. Haberlan, J.W. Rohen, G.Blumel, and P. Huber ed., F.K. Schattauer Verlag, Stuttgart-New York (1975).
10) K. Yamamoto, N. Nakamura, Y. Shimazono, M. Miyasaka, and H. Fukuzawa, The System Construction on a Newly Developed Automatic EEG Diagnosing System-with Special Regard to the Wave-form Recognition Method-, Psychiat. Neurol. Jap., 77:127 (1975).

11) K. Yamamoto, Basic Activity of The Healthy Adult EEGs by The
Computerized Wave-Form Recognition Method, in: Recent Advances in EEG Data
Processing, N. Yamaguchi and K. Fujisawa, ed., Elsevier/North-Holland
Biomedical Press, Amsterdam, New York, Oxford (1981).

CIRCULATORY EFFECT OF KALLIKREIN;

WITH SPECIAL REFERENCE TO CEREBRAL CIRCULATION

Manabu Miyazaki

Department of Internal Medicine
Bell-land Hospital, Sakai City
Osaka, Japan

INTRODUCTION

The effects of kallikrein on the cerebral circulation in humans have
been demonstrated by N_2O method[1] and cerebral angiography[2]. The agent
is known to improve cerebral circulation by increasing kinin release, and
its promotive effect on prostacyclin (PGI_2) release has been noted
recently as an important part of its action mechanism.

Kallikrein is often administered at oral doses of 2-3 tablets t.i.d
(6-9 tablets per day), but a comparative study on its clinical effects
demonstrated that 9 tablets is more effective than 6 tablets[3].

In this study, the effects of kallikrein on the cerebral circulation
were examined by Doppler ultrasonography[4] along with its effects on the
blood pressure and heart rate as well as its side effects.

SUBJECTS AND METHODS

Fifteen outpatients with ischemic cerebrovascular disorders
(cerebral arteriosclerosis and sequelae of stroke) participated in this
study.

Three kallikrein tablets were administered t.i.d. daily for 4 weeks,
and changes in the cerebral blood flow (percent changes in the flow in
the internal carotid and vertebral arteries) were examined by Doppler
ultrasonography before and after the administration.

Changes in the blood pressure and heart rate as well as side effects
were also evaluated.

RESULTS

1. <u>Blood flow in internal carotid and vertebral arteries</u> (Fig. 1)

The blood flow increased in 11 (73.3%) of the 15 patients. Of these
11 patients, the increase in the blood flow was to a similar degree in

both arteries in 5 patients (Fig. 2), more notable in the internal
caroted artery in 2 (Fig. 3), and more notable in the vertebral artery in
4 (Fig. 4).

The mean percent increase in the blood flow was 20.3 ± 14.9% in the
internal carotid artery and 24.7 ± 24.4% in the vertebral artery, with
no significant difference between the two values.

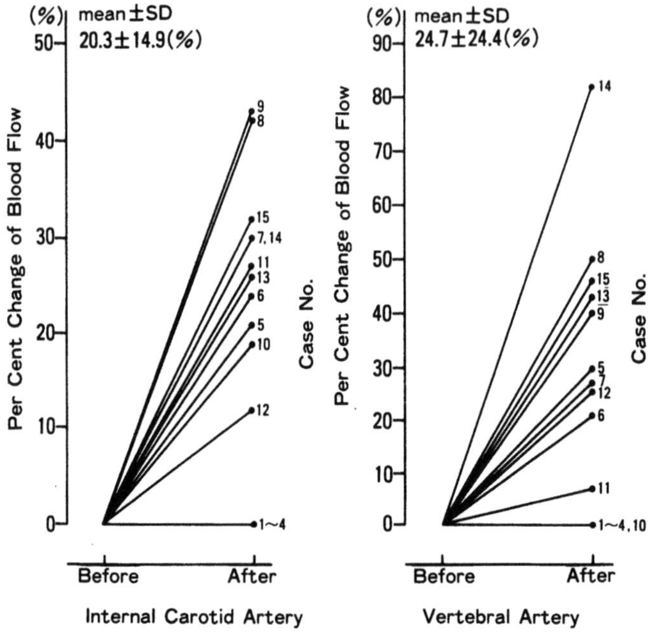

Fig.1 Change of blood flow in internal carotid and vertebral
arteries after repeated administration of kallikrein

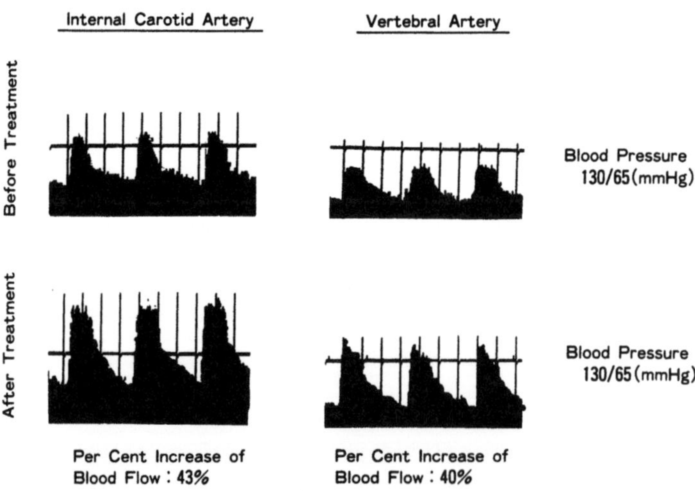

Fig. 2 Effect of kallikrein on cerebral circulation (internal carotid and
vertebral arteries) in an 80-year-old patient with
cerebral arteriosclerosis.

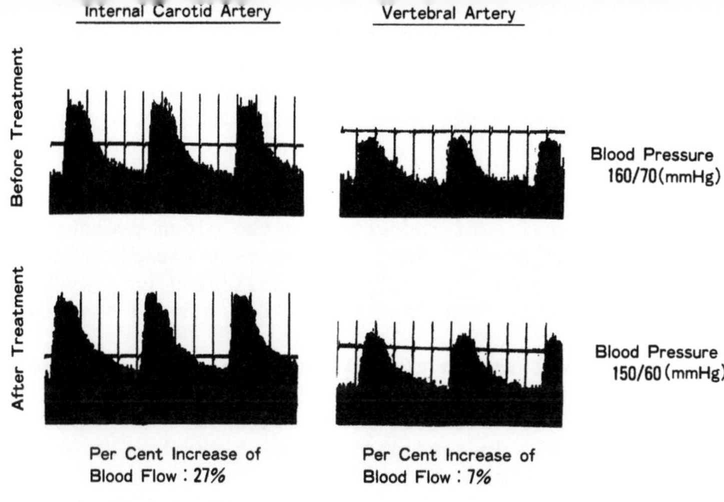

Fig. 3 Effect of kallikrein on cerebral circulation (internal carotid and vertebral arteries) in an 83-year-old patient with sequelae of cerebral stroke

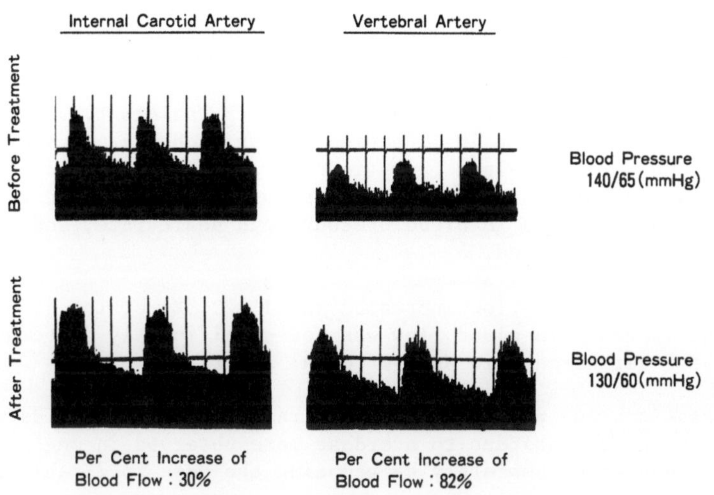

Fig. 4 Effect of kallikrein on cerebral circulation (internal carotid and vertebral arteries) in an 71-year-old patient with cerebral arteriosclerosis.

2. Blood pressure, heart rate, and side effects

Changes in the blood pressure and heart rate were very small. As for side effects, one patient complained of headache and dizziness, which disappeared completely after reducing the dose to 2 tablets t.i.d. (6 tablets per day). No other side effects were observed.

DISCUSSION

Cerebral circulatory drugs and cerebral metabolism activators are the most important ones in the treatment of cerebrovascular disorders. The following three criteria are important in the selection of these drugs[5-7]: 1) High organ-specificity to the cerebral vessels and tissues, 2) long duration of effects, 2) absence of marked secondary effects on the heart and other major organs.

These criteria become all the more important because most of the
patients who receive these drugs are aged individuals, in whom multiple
diseases are present and interact with each other, and secondary effects
of such drugs may trigger a sequence of events leading to deterioration
of the condition.

Kallikrein is generally considered to have mild antihypertensive
effect[8-9], but no significant reduction in the blood pressure was
observed in the present study. Therefore, direct vasodilating effects of
kinin or PGI_2 on the cerebral vessels are considered to play the primary
role in the increase in the cerebral blood flow induced by this drug.

As shown above, kallikrein clearly increases cerebral blood flow but
exerts no major effect on the blood pressure or heart rate and is
considered to generally fulfill the above criteria. This drug may,
therefore, be used safely in aged patients with cerebrovascular disorders
complicated by severe ischemic heart diseases.

The overdosing observed in one patient administered 3 tablets t.i.d.
indicates the importance of carefully adjusting the dose in individual
patients.

CONCLUSION

Kallikrein was administered at a dose of 3 tablets t.i.d. (9 tablets
per day) daily for 4 weeks in 15 patients with ischemic cerebrovascular
disorders, and cerebral blood flow (internal carotid and vertebral
arteries) was evaluated by Doppler ultrasonography before and after the
administration. Changes in blood pressure and heart rate, and side
effects were also observed.

The cerebral blood flow increased in 11 (73.3%) of the 15 patients.
The percent increase in blood flow was not significantly different
between the internal carotid and vertebral arteries.

Changes in blood pressure and heart rate were small. Side effects
(headache and dizziness) due to overdose were observed in one patient,
but they disappeared completely by reducing the dose to 2 tablets t.i.d.
(6 tablets per day).

These results suggest that kallikrein is useful for improving
cerebral circulation in aged patients with ischemic cerebrovascular
disorders.

REFERENCES

1) Goto, Y.: Active peptides in the vascular system and proteinase
    inhibitors, International Symposium (1975), p.81
2) Azuma, K. et al.: J. New Remedies & Clinics 16: 127 (1967)
3) Ogino, H. et al.: Otol. Fukuoka 32: 275 (1986)
4) Miyazaki, M.: Impaired cerebral circulation and correlation with
    organs studied by ultrasonic doppler flowmetry, Iyaku Journal, Tokyo
    (1981)
5) Miyazaki, M.: Gendai Iryo (Tokyo) 2: 529 (1970)
6) Miyazaki, M.: Medicina 10: 75 (1973)
7) Miyazaki, M.: J. Clin. Sci. (Osaka) 14: 28 (1978)
8) Kataoka, K.: Jpn. Pharmacol. Ther. (Tokyo) 5: 59 (1977)
9) Tsutsui, S. et al.: Clin. Report 11: 216 (1977)

SERIAL MEASUREMENT OF BRADYKININ AND FIBRINOPEPTIDE A OF CEREBROSPINAL

FLUID AND PLASMA IN PATIENTS WITH SUBARACHNOID HEMORRHAGE

Hidetoshi Kasuya, Takashi Shimizu, Takaharu Okada,
Kenji Takahashi, Taeko Summerville, and Koichi Kitamura

Department of Neurosurgery, Neurological Institute
Tokyo Women's Medical College
8-1 Kawada-cho, Shinjuku-ku, Tokyo 162, Japan

INTRODUCTION

The pathogenesis of late cerebral vasospasm following subarachnoid hemorrhage (SAH) has not been clarified. It is important to understand the coagulation, fibrinolytic, and kinin systems in the subarachnoid space in determining the pathogenesis of delayed cerebral vasospasm. In this study we measured BK and FPA serially in cerebrospinal fluid (CSF) and plasma in patients with SAH following an aneurysmal rupture. In this discussion, particular emphasis is placed on the relationship between the activation of the coagulation system and the production of BK in the subarachnoid space.

METHODS AND MATERIAL

1. Twenty-seven patients with SAH were studied. There were 14 females and 13 males, with a mean age of 60.3 years (range 30 to 85 years). CSF samples were obtained by lumbar puncture or ventricular drainage. Some samples were also obtained at the time of the operation. BK in the plasma from seven patients with SAH in whom BK was detected in the CSF was measured serially. One ml of CSF and 5 ml of blood were obtained in a precooled siliconized vacuum tube containing 2 ml of 6000 K.I.U. of aprotinin, as well as 0.5 mg of soybean trypsin inhibitor (kallikrein inhibitor), 20 mg of ethylenediaminetetraacetic acid disodium salt, and 5 mg of protamine sulfate (kininase inhibitor). After centrifugation at 1500 g at 4°C for 5 min, supernatant fluid from CSF samples and plasma from blood samples were obtained. These samples were stored at -20°C until measurement. After defatting with petroleum ether and precipitation with isopropyl alcohol, BK was measured by RIA as described (1).

2. Twenty-five patients with SAH were studied. There were 12 females and 13 males, with a mean age of 57.3 years (range 30 to 72 years). Serially collected, 28 plasma samples and 40 CSF samples were obtained from these patients from onset to 14 days after onset. Each specimen (1.6 ml) was allowed to run directly into a plastic tube containing 0.4 ml of an anticoagulant solution containing of heparin (200 I.U.) and aprotinin

(4000 K.I.U.). The tube was centrifuged at 1500 g at 4°C for 5 min, then
the supernatant was frozen and stored until assay. After fibrinogen was
removed with ethanol, FPA was measured by RIA using BF (binding and free)
separation by PEG (polyethyleneglycol). FPA samples of CSF and plasma
were divided into four groups according to the day of sampling, that is,
those obtained between days 0 and 1, days 2 and 4, days 5 and 7, and days
8 and 14 (day 0 was defined as the day of hemorrhage).

RESULTS

1. Figure 1 shows the time course of CSF-BK levels after SAH: 122.7 ± 22.7 pg/ml (mean $\pm$ standard error) on day 0, 38.6 ± 6.9 pg/ml on day 1, 22.7 ± 6.3 pg/ml on day 2, and 17.1 ± 3.0 pg/ml or less thereafter. CSF-BK levels averaging 8.0 ± 3.3 pg/ml (mean $\pm$ standard deviation n=10) were obtained in the control group.

2. The mean plasma BK level was 19.0 ± 6.0 pg/ml (mean $\pm$ standard deviation, n=20) in the control group. The time course of plasma BK levels in seven patients with SAH did not show statistically significant change over time.

3. Figure 2 shows the transition of FPA in CSF. The mean FPA levels were extremely high between days 0 and 1, at a level of 1253 ± 269 ng/ml (mean $\pm$ standard error). The level fell rapidly to 11.3 ± 3.9 ng/ml between days 2 and 4, and gradually decreased (10.7 ± 5.9 ng/ml on days 5-7, 6.3 ± 1.5 ng/ml on days 8-14, Control: 1.2 ± 0.9 ng/ml, mean $\pm$ standard deviation).

4. Plasma FPA levels in patients with SAH showed no statistically significant changes with time (Control: 1.0 ± 0.8 ng/ml, mean $\pm$ standard deviation).

DISCUSSION

The first reports to on the role of the kallikrein-kinin system in
the central nervous system were those by Sicteri et al. (2, 3). These
authors mentioned that BK is a vasoneuroactive substance. They stated
that the intrathecal injection of BK by lumbar puncture into healthy men
causes nuchal stiffness and followed by headache. Thus, it was concluded
that BK might be responsible for headache and nuchal stiffness after SAH,
and also for brain edema after intracerebral hemorrhage. Since first
publication of these reports, there have been no other reports on the role
of BK in SAH, although in some papers the relationship between brain edema
and the kallikrein-kinin system was discussed (4, 5, 6). Measurement of
the plasma BK level has been difficult until now, because the kininase in
1 ml of plasma can destroy 100 ng of BK, and 2000 ng of BK can be formed
from 1 ml of plasma. Recently, however, kallikrein and kininase inhibitors
were mixed with the samples immediately, and thereafter BK was then
measured quantitatively by RIA (1).

The average CSF-BK level in the control group was 8.0 ± 3.3 pg/ml
(mean $\pm$ standard deviation). CSF-BK levels in patients with SAH were extremely high on day 0 and day 1, and decreased immediately over the next
2 or 3 days. The transition of BK in CSF in patients with SAH closely
resembled that of FPA. CSF-BK levels were much higher than plasma BK
levels in patients with SAH. This phenomenon suggests that CSF-BK might
be formed in the subarachnoid space and the BK level might be much higher
at the bleeding point.

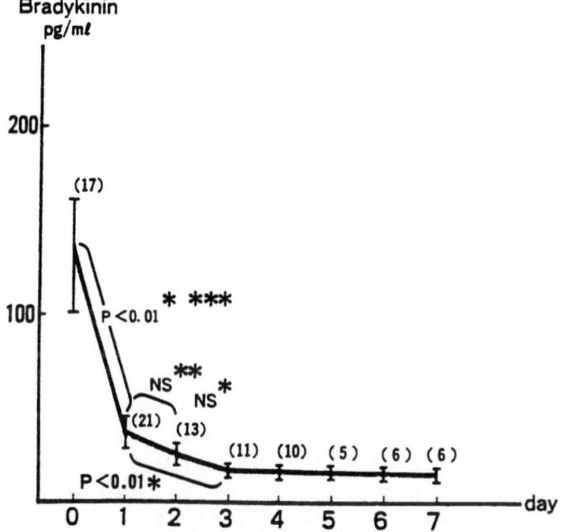

Fig. 1. Transition of BK in CSF in patients with SAH
(mean ± standard error).
(BK: bradykinin   *: Welch t test   **: Student t test
***: Wilcoxon rank sum test   NS: not significant)
( ): number of cases

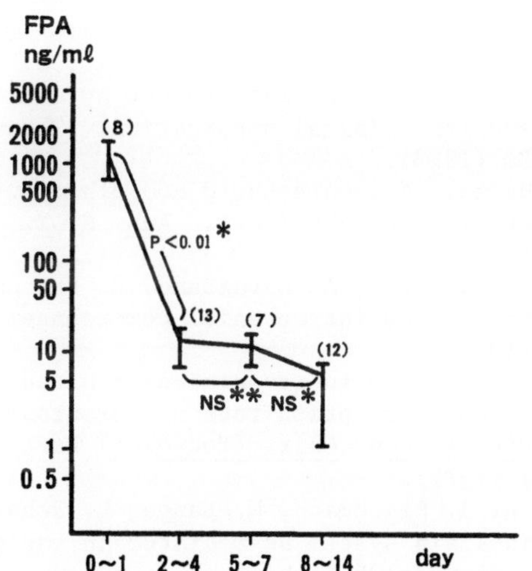

Fig. 2. Transition of FPA in CSF in patients with SAH
(mean ± standard error).
(0 is day of hemorrhage   FPA: fibrinopeptide A
CSF: cerebrospinal fluid   SAH: subarachnoid hemorrhage
*: Welch t test   **: Student t test   NS: not significant)
( ): number of cases

Kariya et al. (7) reported an experimental study on the half-life of
BK after intraventricular injection into rats in which they found that the
half-life of BK was 26.6 ± 3.6 min after the inactivation of kininase by
microwave irradiation. CSF-BK in the ventricle was washed out immediately.
Kininase is present in the CSF as well as the brain tissue (4, 8). Therefore, when SAH develops, plasma kininase also spreads in the subarachnoid
space. CSF-BK is destroyed immediately by these kininases.

We showed that the coagulation system in CSF is strongly activated
in the early stage of SAH by measuring FPA as an indicator of thrombin
activity. There are two types of factors in the coagulation system: intrinsic and extrinsic. We also showed SAH formed BK in the subarachnoid
space in the initial stage. The formation of BK in the subarachnoid space
after SAH is thought to be due to activation of the Hageman factor (intrinsic factor) in the subarachnoid space by negatively charged surfaces (9).

Contact activation is caused by collagen (10), platelets, uric acid,
chondroitin sulfuric acid, and others. It can be assumed that the possible factor responsible for contact activation in the subarachnoid space
is the collagen bundles of the trabecula (11). The authors suggest that
at onset of SAH the arterial blood spreads rapidly into the subarachnoid
space and touches the trabecula, which forms a network surrounding the
vessels that originates in the arachnoid membrane and pial-glial membrane.
At this point Hageman factor as well as prekallikrein and kininogen are
activated, thereby generating a large amount of BK in the subarachnoid
space. Trabecula could be considered to play a role in activating the
Hageman factor when bleeding occurs, in addition to its well known role
in supporting the central nervous system.

REFERENCES

1. N. Takanashi, Y. Ohno, M. Aoyama, I. Maruyama, A. Okada, K. Shinmyozu
    and A. Igata, Plasma kinins measurement by sensitive kinin radio-
    immunoassay and its clinical application. _Thrombosis_ _and_ _Haemo-_
    stasis 50 : 230 (1983).
2. F. Sicteri, Treatment of subarachnoid and other intracranial hemor-
    rhages with proteinase inhibitors. _Ann._ _N._ _Y._ _Acad._ _Sci._ 146 :
    682–700 (1968).
3. F. Sicteri, M. Fanciullaci, A. Bavazzano, G. Franchi and P. L.
    Del Bianco, Kinins and intracranial hemorrhages. _Angiology_
    21 : 193–210 (1970).
4. T. Asai, The effect of the intraventricular blood component on both
    the production and absorption rate of cerebrospinal fluid in dog
    (Part II). _Neurol._ _Med._ _Chir._ _(Tokyo)_ 17 Part II : 493–498,
    (in Japanese) (1977).
5. K. Maier-Hauff, A. J. Beathmann, M. Lange, L. Schurer and A. Unterberg,
    The kallikrein-kinin system as mediator in vasogenic brain edema.
    _J._ _Neurosurg._ 61 : 97–106 (1984).
6. A. Unterberg, C. Dautermann, A. Beathmann and W. Müller-Esteri, The
    kallikrein-kinin system as mediator in vasogenic brain, edema,
    Part 3: Inhibition of the kallikrein-kinin system in traumatic
    brain swelling. _J._ _Neurosurg._ 64 : 269–276 (1986).
7. K. Kariya, A. Yamauchi, S. Hattori, Y. Tsuda and Y. Okada, The dis-
    appearance rate of intraventricular bradykinin in the brain of
    the conscious rat. _Biochem._ _Biophys._ _Res._ _Commun._ 107 : 1461–1466
    (1982).
8. K. Kariya, R. Kawauchi and H. Okamoto, Regional distribution of
    kininase in rat brain. _J._ _Neurochem._ 36 : 2086–2088 (1981).

9. M. Nakahara, Binding and dissociation of Hageman factor, prekalli-
    krein and high molecular weight kininogen in human plasma during
    contact activation. Biochem. Pharmacol. 29 : 1247-1254 (1980).
10. P. C. Harpel, Studies on the interaction between collagen and a
    plasma kallikrein-like activity. J. Clin. Invest. 51 : 1813-1822
    (1972).
11. C. A. S. Lopes and W. G. P. Mair, Ultrastructure of arachnoid
    membrane in man. Acta. Neuropath. (Berlin) 28 : 167-173 (1974).

EFFECTS OF THE KALLIKREIN-KININ SYSTEM ON PHASIC CORONARY VASOSPASM

IN DOGS

H. Ohde, K. Morimoto, T. Kitao, K. Terada, H. Kohara,
H. Tai, M. Fujimoto, T. Ogihara* and Y. Kumahara*

Research Laboratory of Fujimoto Pharmaceutical Corp.
Matsubara-shi, Osaka 580 and *Department of Medicine and
Geriatric, Osaka University Medical School, Fukushima-ku
Osaka 553, Japan

SUMMARY

It is well known that kinins are liberated from kininogen in blood
during angina attack to maintain blood flow in coronary artery. We
examined the effects of bradykinin, one of kinins, on the coronary artery
other than vasodilation.
The isolated canine coronary artery ring was suspended in gassed (95%
O_2, 5% CO_2) Krebs-Henseleit buffer at 37°C in vitro.   The experimental
phasic contraction of coronary artery was induced by 6×10^{-4}M of 3,4-di-
aminopyridine which decreases K conductance (Y. Uchida, Jpn. Circ. J : 49,
128, 1985). The effect of bradykinin and other substances on the cycle
length of contraction(CL), the peak tension of contraction phase(PT)
and the tension during relaxation phase(RT) were observed.
The phasic contraction was eliminated by 10^{-7}M nifedipine and 10^{-6}M
diltiazem which block voltage dependent Ca channels. These Ca blockers
reduced PT, but slightly increased CL, and weakly reduced RT. The phasic
contraction was also eliminated by 10^{-6}M bradykinin. However,
bradykinin, unlike Ca blockers, did not reduce PT, but markedly prolonged
CL and decreased RT significantly. This inhibition mode was very similar
to those of nicorandil which increases K conductance.
These data suggest that bradykinin plays a protective role in coronary
vasospasm, and this antivasospasm effect may be mediated through the
increase in K conductance.

INTRODUCTION

The kallikrein-kinin system is present in various peripheral tissues
and has been demonstrated to be involved in the inflammation and induction
of pain and vasodilation. Kallikrein as well as kinin appears to dilate
the coronary vessels in vivo and in vitro. However, effects of kinin in
the spasm of coronary artery are still unclear.
Recently, the evaluation method of antivasospasm drugs has been
developed using 3,4-diaminopyridine which decreases K conductance of
vascular cell membrane.[1]
In the present study, we have found that bradykinin produces potent,
and concentration-dependent reduction in the experimental vasospasm of
canine coronary artery.

MATERIALS AND METHODS

Seven mongrel dogs of either sex weighing between 7.5 and 10kg were anesthetized with pentobarbital sodium (30mg/kg) administered intravenously. The chest was opened by the fourth intercostal thoracotomy of the left side, and the heart was quickly excised and placed in cold saline. The circumflex branch of the left coronary artery was carefully dissected free from the heart, cleaned of adhering connective and fatty tissue and cut into 3mm wide rings. The rings were suspended in an organ bath, which contained 10ml of the Krebs-Henseleite buffer of the following composition (in mmole/1) : NaCl 118, KCl 4.0, $CaCl_2$ 1.5, $MgSO_4$ 1.2, NaH_2PO_4 1.2, $NaHCO_3$ 25, glucose 5. The buffer was aerated with a gas mixture of 95% O_2 and 5% CO_2 and maintained at 37°C(see Fig. 1).

Contractile responses of the preperation were determined by an isometric transducer (TB 612T, Nihon koden) and tension developments were recorded on polygraph recorder (RM-85, Nihon koden).

The preperation was equilibrated under 1-2g resting tension for 40 min. prior to initiation of experimental procedures. The drugs used were: bradykinin (Peptide Institute, Osaka), nifedipine (LEK Pharm. Co., Yugoslavia), diltiazem (Abic Pharm. Co., Israel), nicorandil (2-nicotinamidoethyl nitrate, Chugai Pharm.Co., Tokyo).

Bradykinin was dissolved in saline, nifedipine was diluted in distilled water after dissolving in ethanol. Diltiazem and nicorandil were dissolved in distilled water.

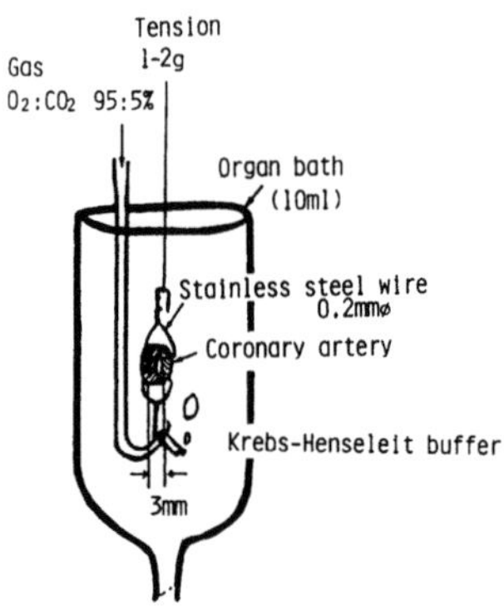

Fig.1 Scheme of the experiment

The experimental phasic contraction of coronary artery was induced by 6×10^{-4}M of 3,4-diaminopyridine (3,4-DAP). Effects of drugs on the cycle length of contraction (CL), the peak tension of contraction phase (PT) and the tension during relaxation phase (RT) were observed.

Values are given in terms of means ± s.e. The statistical difference of values were analysed by Student's t-test and judged to be significant when p values were less than 0.05.

RESULTS

Figure 2 shows the phasic contraction induced by 6×10^{-4}M of 3,4-DAP in canine coronary arteries, and the effects of each drug.

The phasic contraction was eliminated by 10^{-6}M of bradykinin. Cyclic length was prolonged by 10^{-8}M or over of bradykinin and the tension during relaxation phase was decreased markedly by 10^{-9}M or over of bradykinin, however tension of phasic contraction not change by 10^{-7}M or below of bradykinin (Fig. 3). Nifedipine and diltiazem decreased tension of phasic contraction, and weak decreased tension of relaxation phase, however no effect or slightly increase on frequency of cycle length of phasic contraction were observed (Fig. 4,5). 10^{-5}M or over of nicorandil prolonged cycle length like bradykinin, but the effective dose of nicorandil was much more than that of bradykinin (Fig. 6).

Table 1. Effects of bradykinin, nifedipine, diltiazem and nicorandil on phasic contraction of canine coronary arteries.

Final conc.	Items	Bradykinin	Nifedipine	Diltiazem	Nicorandil
Control	CL	27.0±23.4min (100%)	27.5±14.9 (100%)	26.7±10.6 (100%)	37.9± 8.7 (100%)
	PT	4.12± 1.04g (100%)	4.52± 1.48 (100%)	4.32± 0.68 (100%)	5.02± 0.78 (100%)
	RT	2.23± 0.58g (100%)	2.47± 0.26 (100%)	2.10± 0.20 (100%)	2.20± 0.28 (100%)
	n	12	6	6	4
10^{-10}M	CL	137.3±22.7%	91.4±12.1	94.8±10.6	
	PT	105.7± 4.0%	86.0± 6.1	97.0± 3.8	
	RT	87.4± 7.1% *	107.3± 3.2	95.2± 6.7	
	n	12	6	6	
10^{-9} M	CL	151.6±19.8**	89.2±13.1	112.8±15.1	104.8± 6.1
	PT	104.6± 4.1	77.4± 6.6*	97.5± 5.0	100.0± 3.5
	RT	78.9± 9.9**	103.2± 5.7	87.6± 9.5	104.5± 6.4
	n	12	6	6	4
10^{-8} M	CL	374.1±43.4**	78.1±20.0	116.3±10.0	96.0± 0.0
	PT	104.6± 9.5	57.2±11.9**	95.6± 5.1	101.8± 2.0
	RT	27.4±25.1**	100.8±11.3	84.8± 12.4	97.3± 6.4
	n	10	6	6	4
10^{-7} M	CL	>750	>500	113.0±14.0	98.0± 5.8
	PT	167.5± 9.5	88.0±38.0	74.9± 7.6*	105.3± 6.6
	RT	·17.0±24.2**	·77.3±14.6*	89.5±13.3	94.5± 9.1
	n	2(10·)	2(6·)	6	4
10^{-6} M	CL	1350		377.0±483	121.8±12.7
	PT	160		42.3±29.0	101.5± 6.1
	RT	-12.1		·84.8±19.0	83.6± 7.2*
	n	1		2(6·)	4
10^{-5} M	CL				287.5±59.4
	PT				91.5±12.0
	RT				·62.7±13.6*
	n				2(4·)
10^{-4} M	CL				593.0±16.0
	PT				72.0± 6.0
	RT				·56.4±11.8*
	n				2(4·)

CL: cycle length(% change from control), PT: peak tension(% change from control), RT: relaxatin g tension(% change from control), Each value is shown in mean ±s.e. significant differnce from control ∗ : p<0.05, ∗∗ : p<0.01

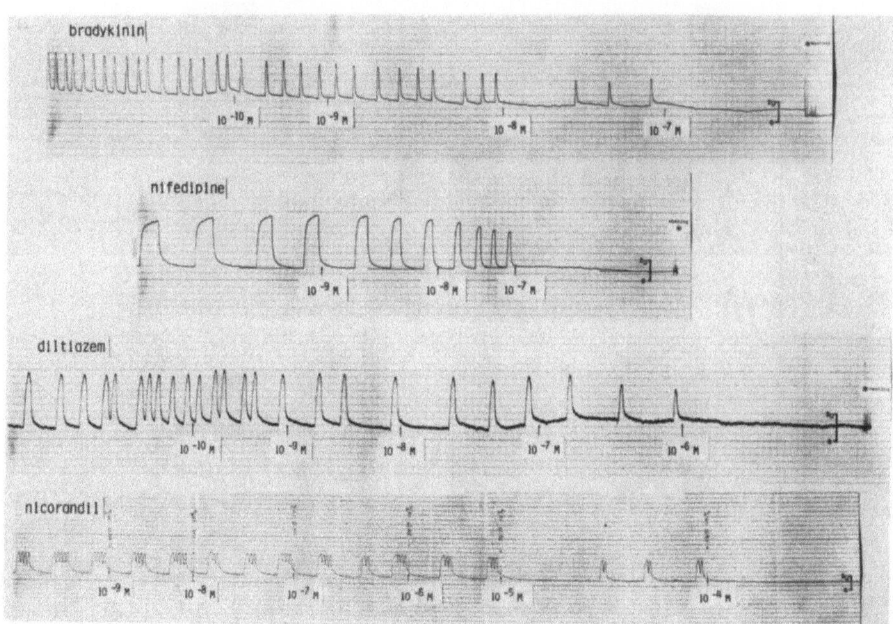

Fig. 2. Effects of bradykinin, nifedipine, diltiazem and nicorandil on phasic contraction of canine coronry arteries.

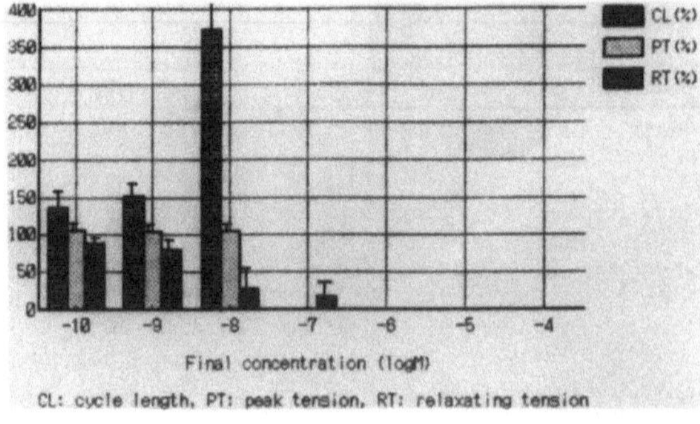

Fig. 3. Effect of bradykinin on phasic contraction

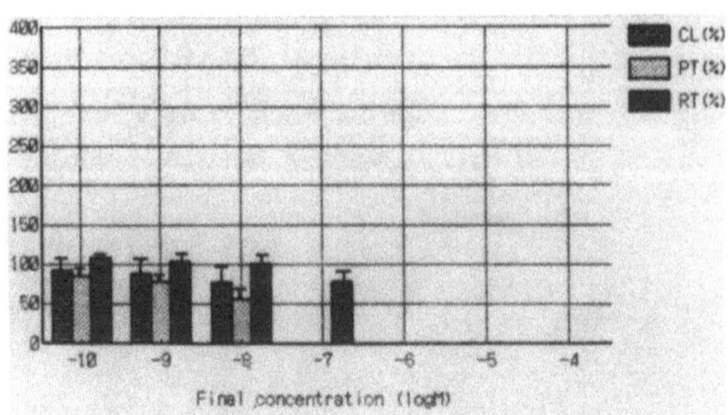

Fig. 4. Effect of nifedipine on phasic contraction

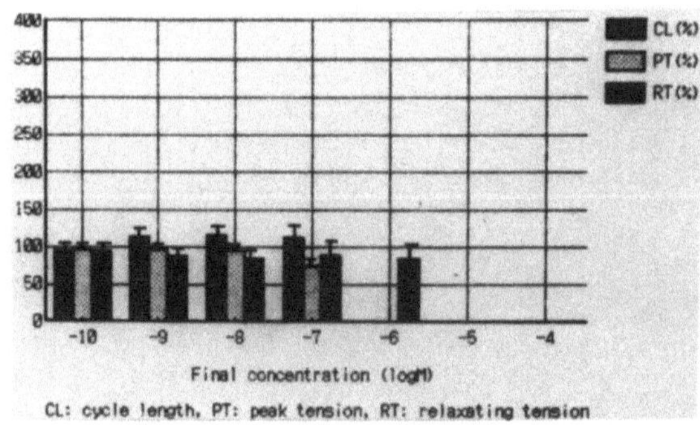

Fig. 5. Effect of diltiazem on phasic contraction

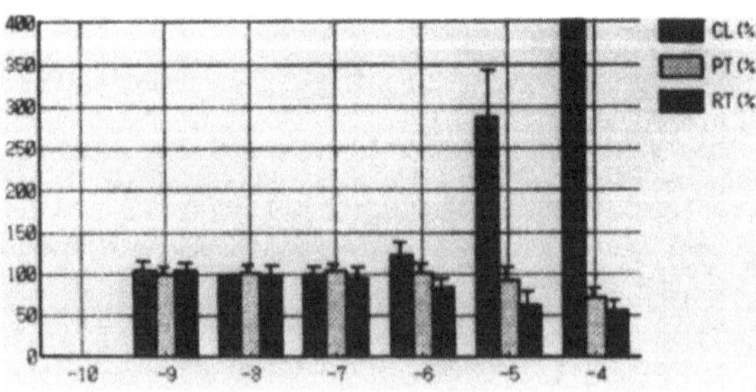

Fig. 6. Effect of nicorandil on phasic contraction

Clinically, the mechanism of coronary spasm is unclear. Experimentally, it has been known that coronary spasm was induced by ergonovine (methylergometrine malate) in vivo[2,3]. On the other hand, phasic contraction was induced by 3,4-DAP, 4-aminopyridine and tetraethylammonium chloride which decrease K conductance of isolated artery in vitro[1].

Uchida et al[4] reported that these experimental phasic contraction were not mediated by α-receptor and cholinergic receptor. 3,4-DAP causes reduction in K conductance, which in turn depolarizes the cell membrane resulting in the opening of a voltage dependent Ca channel, and accordingly in contracts smooth muscles.

Nicorandil has been reported that it causes increase in K conductance[5], resulting in hyperpolarized cell membrane, accordingly nicorandil probably inhibited to reduction of K conductance induced by 3,4-DAP.

In this study, both Ca channel blockers and nicorandil, a drug which increase K conductance reduced phasic contraction induced by 3,4-DAP, however modes of these actions were different, and bradykinin was very similar to nicorandil in terms of action mode. And it is especially noteworthy that bradykinin was more potent than nicorandil. Our results of nicorandil and nifedipine were in agreement with the findings of Uchida[1,2]. Three possibilities may be considered as the mechanism of bradykinin action, the first is increase in K conductance, the second is increase in cyclic AMP and the thrid is increase in cyclic GMP mediated through endothelium derived relaxant factor(EDRF) on endothelial cells. Becaue, bradykinin enhanced cyclic AMP[6,7] and cyclic GMP in neural cells[8] and in muscle cells[9], and these cyclic nucleotids play as second messenger in muscle relaxation.

Recently, Endoh and Taira reported[10] that nicorandil increases cyclic GMP level in the isolated canine mesentric artery, and the level of cyclic GMP and relaxation of artery correlated well. However, it does not clear that phasic contraction is inhibited by the effect of relaxant induced by increase in cyclic GMP in smooth muscle. In our preliminary experiment, we have obtained that increase in cyclic AMP or cyclic GMP did not inhibit the phasic contraction(unpublished data). Accordingly, these suggest that mechanism of bradykinin on reduction of phasic contraction is probably depend on increase in K conductance.

It is well known that bradykinin which is vasoactive polypeptide, is liberated from kininogen by kallikrein due to maintain blood flow during heart attack and ischaemia. In the present study, we found a new effect of bradykinin which may play a protective role in coronary vasospasm, directly.

CONCLUSIONS

(1) Bradykinin markedly reduced experimental coronary vaspspasm induced by 3,4-diaminopyridine which decreases K conductance.

(2) The action mode of bradykinin differed from that of nifedipine, Ca channel blockers, and was very similar to that of nicorandil which increases K conductance.

(3) It is suggested that bradykinin play a protective role in coronary vasospasm.

REFFERNCES

1. Y. Uchida and T. Sugimoto, Phasic contraction of coronary smooth muscles induced by 3,4-diaminopyridine, J. Jpn. Coll. Angiol., 24: 133 (1984).

2. P.R. Ciprian, D.F. Guthaner, A.E. Orlick, D.R. Ricci, L. Wexler and J.F. Silverman, The effects of ergonovine malate on coronary artery size, Circ., 59: 82 (1979).

3. J.S. Schroeder, J.L. Bolen and R.A. Quint, Provocation of coronary spasm with ergonovine malate, Am. J. Cardiol., 40: 487 (1977).

4. Y. Uchida, Decreasing potassium coductance – A possible mechanism of phasic coronary vasospasm –, Jpn. Circ. J., 49: 128 (1984).

5. T. Yanagisawa and N. Taira, Effect of 2-nicotinamidoethyl nitrate (SG-75) on the membrané potential of left atrial muscle of the dog, Naunyn-Schmiedeberg's Arch. Pharmacol., 312: 69 (1980).

6. T.V. Zenser, N.S. Rapp, L.A. Spry and B.B. Davis, Independent effects of bradykinin on adenosine 3',5'-monophosphate and prostaglandin E_2 metabolism by rabbit renal medulla, Endocrinol., 114: 541 (1984).

7. D.L. Bareis, Bradykinin receptor stimulation of cyclic AMP involves phospholipid sequation calcium flex phospholipases A_2 activation and prostaglandin formation, Fed. Pro., 40: 367 (1984).

8. G. Reiser, U. Walter and B. Hamprecht, Bradykinin regulated the level of guanosin-3',5'-cyclic monophosphate(cyclic GMP) in neural cell line, Brain Res., 290: 367 (1983).

9. H. Frucht, G. Lilling and R. Beitner, Influence of bradykinin on glucose 1,6-bisphosphate and cyclic GMP levels and on the activities of glucose 1,6-bisphosphatase, phosphofructkinase and phosphoglucomutase in muscle, Int. J. Biochem., 16: 397 (1984).

10. M. Endoh and N. Taira, Relationship between relaxation and cyclic GMP formation caused by nicorandil in canine mesentric artery, Naunyn-Schmiedeberg's Arch. Pharmacol., 322: 319 (1983).

THE ROLE OF BRADYKININ ON THE EFFECT OF PLASMA KALLIKREIN ON PLATELET

AGGREGATION

Nair Y. Maeda*, Celia M.F. Cassaro*, M.U. Sampaio,
Dalton A.F. Chamone* and C.A.M. Sampaio

Departamento de Bioquimica, Escola Paulista de Medicina
Caixa Postal 20372, CEP 04034, S.Paulo, SP - Brazil
*INCOR, Faculdade de Medicina, USP

INTRODUCTION

Plasma kallikrein participates in early steps of the activation
of blood clotting contact phase, through the amplification of the signal
for activation of Factor XII [1] . Platelet aggregation is also an early
event in the process of haemostasia and the hypothesis that activated
platelets could provide the negative surface for the development of the
intrinsic pathway of clotting was raised [2] . The role of plasma
kallikrein as a modulator of platelet aggregation, induced by different
aggregating agents, has been recently described [3] . The enzyme, by
itself, does not induce aggregation, but in small concentration increases
the rate of aggregation induced by ADP, collagen and adrenalin in platelet
rich plasma (PRP), and inhibits aggregation induced by arachidonic acid
and phospholipids in PRP, as well aggregation induced by all the agents
tested, when used in high concentration; kallikrein also inhibits
aggregation in blood in all conditions [3] , and was also shown to decrease
cAMP content of platelets [4] .

Plasma kallikrein releases bradykinin from high-molecular weight
kininogen [5] , and this vasoactive peptide could be involved in the action
of kallikrein on platelets. The objective of this communication is to
describe some of the effects of bradykinin on induced aggregation, in
comparison to the effects of plasma kallikrein and a tissue kallikrein,
porcine pancreatic kallikrein.

MATERIAL AND METHODS

Plasma kallikrein was prepared by a described procedure, and only
α-kallikrein, as seen on SDS-polyacrilamide gel electrophoresis, was used
in all experiments. Porcine pancreatic kallikrein was a kind gift from
Bayer. Thrombin was from Roche (USA). Bradykinin, a kind gift of Dr.
A.C.M. Paiva, from the Departamento de Biofisica of Escola Paulista de
Medicina, was further purified on SP-Sephadex chromatography [6] . ADP and
arachidonic acid were from Sigma (USA), collagen from Hormon Chemie
(Germany) and adrenalin was a product from Clinical Hospital Pharmacy.

Platelet rich plasma (PRP) was prepared from blood of healthy donors, by centrifugation at 250 x g, for 4 minutes. Washed platelets were prepared from PRP, as indicated previously [3]. Aggregation was measured in plasma and washed platelets, by the rate of decrease of transmittance [7], and in whole blood by differences in impedance [8]. Concentration of plasma kallikrein, pancreatic kallikrein and bradykinin are indicated in the tables, and the concentration ranges of the aggregating agents were 10-5 to 10-6 M ADP, 0.1-2.0 ug/mL collagen, 90-300 ug/mL sodium arachidonic acid, 10-7-10-8 M adrenalin, 0.022 NIH Units thrombin, 0.01-1.0 ug/mL PAF.

Statistical analysis was performed with a t-paired test and the results are expressed in percentage of control (induced aggregation in absence of kallikrein or bradykinin).

TABLE 1

EFFECT OF PLASMA KALLIKREIN ON THE INDUCED PLATELET AGGREGATION

	PRP	WHOLE BLOOD	WASHED PLATELET
ADP	1.69*	0.69*	–
COLLAGEN	1.68*	–	–
ARACHIDONIC ACID	0.44*	–	–
PAF	0.97	0.66*	–
THROMBIN	0.94	–	0.61*

Aggregation rate is expressed relatively to the same sample, in absence of kallikrein. Plasma kallikrein (1.0 ug/mL). * difference significant at $p < 0.05$.

RESULTS

Plasma kallikrein (1.0 ug/mL) increases the rate of platelet aggregation induced by ADP and collagen, but causes inhibition of aggregation induced by arachidonic acid in PRP; in whole blood the enzyme inhibits the rate of aggregation both for ADP and PAF, in washed platelets plasma kallikrein inhibits the aggregation induced by thrombin; on the other hand the enzyme alone does not cause aggregation even in concentration as high as 30.0 ug/mL (table 1).

Bradykinin does not affect the aggregation induced by ADP and PAF in PRP and by thrombin washed platelets, but it decreases the rate of aggregation induced by thrombin in PRP and by ADP and PAF in whole blood. The effect of porcine kallikrein was also restricted to the inhibition of the aggregation induced by PAF on whole blood and by thrombin in PRP (table 2)

Bradykinin does not seem to mediate the effects of HuPK on platelet aggregation, in PRP and washed platelets, since in the presence of HuPK the effects observed on aggregation are quite different from those observed for bradykinin. Pancreatic kallikrein effect was similar to the effect of bradykinin, on platelet agregation, both in PRP and washed platelets. This could be an evidence that a kallikrein released kinin would not be the agent responsible for the effect on platelet aggregation.

TABLE 2

EFFECT OF PORCINE PANCREATIC KALLIKREIN AND BRADYKININ
ON INDUCED PLATELET AGGREGATION

Inducing agent	Pancreatic kallikrein			Bradykinin		
	PRP	Whole blood	Washed platelets	PRP	Whole blood	Washed platelets
ADP	1.04	1.00	–	1.06	0.61*	–
PAF	0.92	0.70*	–	0.90	0.17*	–
Thrombin	0.80*	–.	0.80	0.78*	–	1.01

Aggregation rate is expressed relatively to the same sample in absence of kallikrein or bradykinin. Porcine pancreatic kallikrein (2 ug/mL), bradykinin (20 pg/mL).
*– difference significant at $p < 0.05$

Inhibition caused by the presence of bradykinin, on the thrombin induced aggregation in PRP, could be due to plasma factors, since no inhibition was observed on washed platelets thrombin induced aggregation. The observation that HuPK does not affect thrombin induced aggregation, in PRP, may be explained by specific plasma inhibitors, which inactivate HuPK but not pancreatic kallikrein. Furthermore, minute amounts of slowly HuPK released bradykinin would be inactivated by kininases, much before reaching an effective concentration on platelets.

In whole blood, HuPK and bradykinin exhibited the same effect on platelet aggregation. The same was true for pancreatic kallikrein that, at 20 ug/mL concentration inhibited ADP induced aggregation (results not shown). Thus, enzimatically released bradykinin would be ultimately involved in whole blood platelet aggregation. Bradykinin mediation may be dependent on blood cells interaction since aggregation induced by PAF and ADPP was not affected by bradykinin.

REFERENCES

1 - S. Nagasawa, H. Takahashi, M. Koido and T. Suzuki, Partial purification of bovine plasma kallikreingen. Its activation by the Hageman factor, <u>Biochem. Biophys. Res. Commun</u>. 32, 644-649 (1968).

2 - N. Walsh, The role of platelets in the contact phase of blood, <u>Brit. J. Haematol</u>., 22: 237 (1972).

3 - C.M.F. Cassaro, M.U. Sampaio, N.Y. Maeda, D.F. Chamone and C.A.M. Sampaio, Human plasma kallikrein: effect on the induced platelet aggregation, <u>Thromb. Res</u>., 48: 81 (1987).

4 - H. Ohde, T. Mozai, Hase M., J. Kitakogi, F. Ninomiya; Y.H. Chung and M. Fujimoto, Effects of kallikrein on human platelets aggregation, <u>Adv. Exp. Med. Biol</u>., 156 (pt B): 741 (1983).

5 - J.J. Pisano, Chemistry and biology of the kallikrein-kinin system, in <u>Proteases and biological control</u>, E. Reich, D.B. Rifkin and E. Shaw, eds.,p 199, Cold Spring Harbor Laboratory, Cold Spring Harbor (1975).

6 - M.U.Sampaio, M.L. Reis, E.Fink, A.C.M. Camargo and L.J. Greene, SP-Sephadex equilibrium chromatography of bradykinin and related peptides: application to trypsin-treated plasma, <u>Anal. Biochem</u>.,81:369 (1977).

7 - G.U.R. Born and M.J. Cross, The aggregation of blood platelets, <u>J. Physiol</u>., 168: 178 (1963).

8 - P.C. Cardinal and R.J. Flower, The eletronic aggregometer: a novel device for assessing platelet behvior in blood, <u>J. Pharmacol. Meth</u>.,3: 158 (1980).

ACTIVATION OF CALCIUM ION-DEPENDENT PROTEINASES BY BRADYKININ

IN DENTAL PULP OF THE RAT

Teruo Kudo, Er-Qin Wei and Reizo Inoki

Department of Pharmacology
Osaka University Faculty of Dentistry
1-8, Yamadaoka, Suita, Osaka 565, Japan

SUMMARY

The present study was aimed to examine whether BANA-degrading enzyme
activities could be enhanced by bradykinin(BK) in dental pulp of the rat
in vitro. The results showed that BK(0.1-10 µM) dose-dependently enhanced
BANA-degrading enzyme activity at pH 7.4. The effects of BK(1 µM) were
found to be most effective at both pH 7 and 8, with enhancement of the
enzyme activities at a wide range of pH. The BK effects at both the pH were
not inhibited by FOY-305(0.1 µM), an inhibitor of trypsin-like enzymes,
differing from that at pH 6 in adrenal medulla of the rat. On the other
hand, the effects of BK at both the pH were remarkably inhibited by EGTA
(2 mM), followed by reversal with calcium ion(2.42 mM). These results
suggested as follows: 1) there might be two kinds of BANA-degrading enzymes
activated by BK in the pulp. 2) it was conceivable that BANA-degrading
enzymes activated by BK were quite different from serine proteinases and
were interfered with them in the pulp. 3) calcium ion might play a role in
BK-induced enhancement of BANA-degrading enzyme activities which were
regarded as met-enkephalin(ME) processing enzyme activities in the pulp.

INTRODUCTION

It has been known that ME-like peptides were contained within granules
of the pulp cells of the dog canine tooth and the rat incisor[1,2,3].
Furthermore, it has been also reported that production of ME-like peptides
from the precursor protein which co-existed in the pulp cells of the rat
incisor could be induced by noxious stimuli to the pulp, such as cavity
formation in the tooth[4] and infusion of BK, a pain producing substance, into
the pulp cavity[5] in vivo experiments as well as addition of BK into the
incubation medium of the pulp in vitro experiment[6]. These findings suggested that processing enzyme of ME-like peptides might be activated by BK[7].
Since it was considered that the processing enzymes might be primarily
trypsin-like enzymes[8] and carboxypeptidase B-like enzymes[9] in adrenal medulla, it was designed to examine, in the present study, whether degradation of
BANA, a synthetic substrate for trypsin-like enzymes, could be increased by
BK in an in vitro experimental system using whole pulp of the rat incisor.

Animals used were male rats(Sprague-Dawley strain) weighing 200-250 g. The animals were anesthetized with urethane. Both mandibular and maxillary incisors were extirpated and the pulps were isolated from them on ice. The isolated pulps were washed in ice-cold Hanks solution at pH 7.4 and then quickly weighed after wiping with filter papers. Hanks solution as incubation medium was usually contained 20 μM of bestatin and 1 μM of captopril. Two pulps, weighing 20-30 mg, consisted of each pulps from mandibular and maxillary incisors at one side, were preincubated in 3 ml of Hanks solution at a variety of pH at 37°C for 5 min and then were incubated with various agents including BK for 30 min.

Measurement for BANA-degrading Enzyme Activity. Two μM of Nα-benzoyl-arginine-β-naphthylamide(BANA), a synthetic substrate for trypsin-like enzymes, was added to the incubation medium 2 min before incubation of pulps with BK. After the incubation, the reaction was finished by heating at 90°C for 4 min. After removing the tissues from the medium, the medium was rapidly cooled to 0°C on ice. The cooled medium was subjected to measure BANA-degrading enzyme activity by fluorophotometry(ex. 338 nm, em. 410 nm)[10] using a spectrofluorophotometer(Shimadzu RF-540). Agents used were BK, FOY-305([N,N-dimethylcarbamoyl-4-(4-guanidinobenzoyloxy)-phenyl acetate] methanesulfonate)[11], an inhibitor of serine proteinases, EGTA and $CaCl_2$. TPCK(p-tosyl-L-phenylalanine chloromethyl ketone)-treated trypsin from bovine pancreas was used as standard enzyme in Hanks solution at pH 7.4. The values obtained were expressed as activity equivalent to trypsin(μg/ g tissue).

Statistical Analysis. The data obtained were analyzed using Student's t-test or Mann-Whitney's U-test, in order to examine the significant difference.

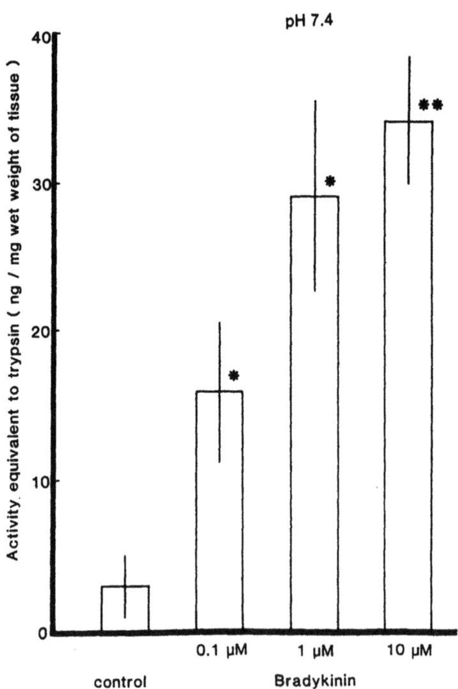

Fig. 1. Effect of BK on BANA-degrading enzyme activity in dental pulp at pH 7.4. Each value represents the mean ± SEM. *p<0.05 and **p<0.01, in comparison with the control.

RESULTS AND DISCUSSION

As shown in Fig. 1, it was clear that BK(0.1-10 μM) enhanced BANA-
degrading enzyme activity of the pulp at pH 7.4 in a dose-dependent manner
and in addition, the effects of BK in a dose of 1 μM on BANA-degrading enzyme activities were most effective at both pH 7 and 8 with enhancement of
the enzyme activities at a wide range of pH(data not shown), suggesting that
there were, at least, two kinds of BANA-degrading enzymes activated by BK in
the pulp. These results appeared to support our previous findings[6] that BK
dose-dependently increased production of ME-like peptides in the pulp at
pH 7.4. The BK-effect was also found in pulp homogenate, of which the membrane and lysosomal fractions and the supernatant showed the enhancement of
BANA-degrading enzyme activity by BK at pH 7.4, but not the mitochondrial
and microsomal fractions(data to be published elsewhere). These facts suggested that BANA-degrading enzymes activated by BK were localized at a few
subcellular component. In the present study, further examinations on influences of various agents on BK-induced enhancement of the enzyme activities
were performed in a dose of 1 μM of BK at both pH 7 and 8.

Firstly, influence of FOY-305(0.1 μM), a specific inhibitor of serine
proteinases, on BK-induced enhancement of BANA-degrading enzyme activities
in the pulp was examined at both pH 7 and 8, in order to certify whether
BANA-degrading enzymes activated by BK were trypsin-like enzymes or not.
FOY-305 was added to the incubation medium 3 min before incubation of the
pulp with BANA. BK was added to the medium 2 min after addition of BANA.
As shown in Fig. 2, at both the pH, BANA-degrading enzyme activities were
remarkably enhanced by FOY-305, regardless of presence or absence of BK,
differing from the results[12] which were found at pH 6 in adrenal medulla of

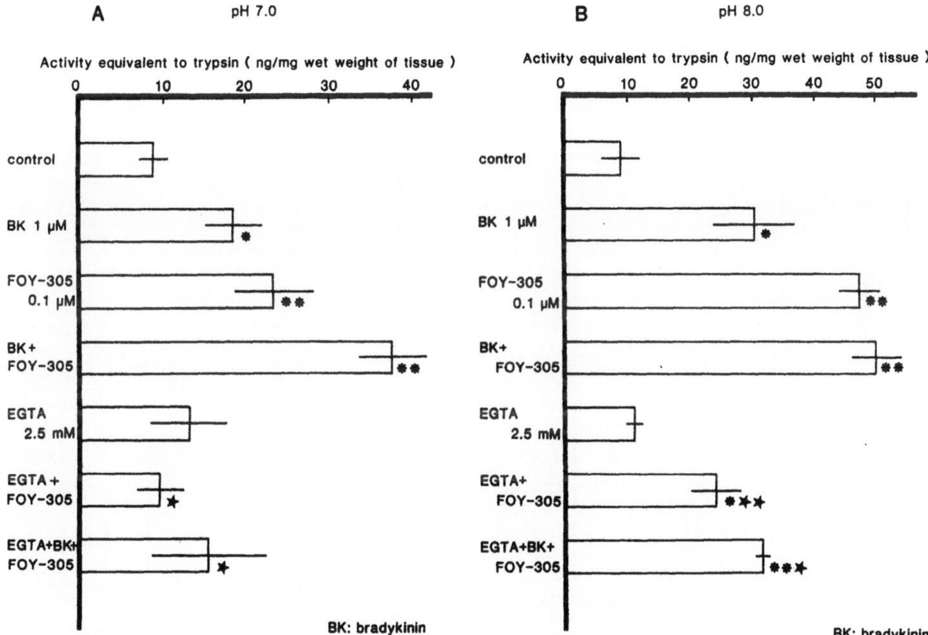

Fig. 2. Influences of FOY-305 and EGTA on BANA-degrading enzyme
activity in dental pulp. A: pH 7.0, B: pH 8.0. FOY-305
was added to the medium to be finally at 0.1 μM 3 min
before incubation of the pulp with BANA. EGTA was added
to the normal medium to be finally at 2.5 mM, prior to
preincubation of the pulp. Each value represents the
mean ± SEM. *p<0.05 and **p<0.01, in comparison with the
control. ★p<0.05 and ★★p<0.01, in comparison with corresponding control to show the EGTA-effect, respectively.

the rat using the same experimental system as that in the present study.

This difference appeared to show that there was a tissue-specificity of ME-like peptide processing between the dental pulp and the adrenal medulla of the rat. This suggestion seemed to be also supported by the facts that both cyclic AMP and GMP enhanced BANA-degrading enzyme activity in the pulp, while those nucleotides did not enhance the enzyme activity in adrenal medulla of the rat at pH 7.4(unpublished data). These results in the pulp suggested that a BANA-degrading enzyme activity of multi-enzyme system in the pulp might be interfered with serine proteinases, because BANA-degrading enzyme activity was markedly enhanced, unexpectedly, by FOY-305 itself in absence of BK. However, the enhanced activities by FOY-305 at both pH 7 and 8 were remarkably reduced after addition of EGTA(2.5 mM) to the normal incubation medium, suggesting that EGTA-sensitive enzymes might be involved in degradation of BANA in the pulp.

On the other hand, as shown in Fig. 2, it was found that at pH 7, combination of BK with FOY-305 significantly enhanced BANA-degrading enzyme activity, in comparison with the enhancement by BK alone or FOY-305 alone, but not at pH 8, and in addition, that at pH 7, EGTA completely inhibited the enhancement of the enzyme activity by FOY-305 or by combination of BK with FOY-305, while at pH 8, EGTA partially inhibited it. These results appeared to suggest that BANA-degrading enzymes at pH 7 were different from those at pH 8 in the pulp.

Secondly, the effect of calcium ion on the inhibition of BANA-degrading enzyme activity by EGTA was examined in the present study, in order to know a characteristic of EGTA-sensitive enzyme in the pulp. EGTA(2 mM) was added to Ca-free incubation medium at the time of preincubation.

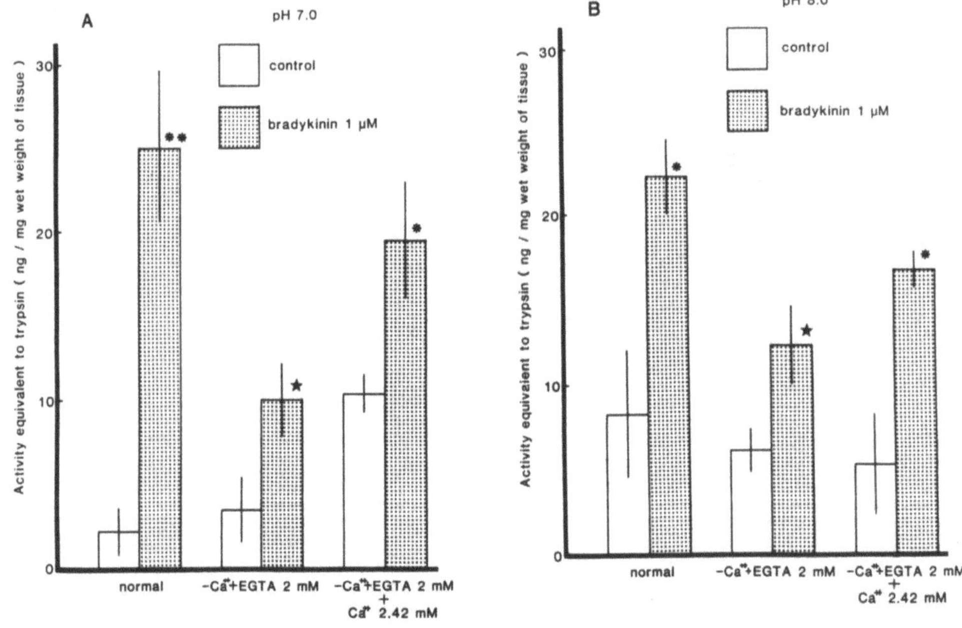

Fig. 3. Effects of EGTA and calcium ion on BANA-degrading enzyme activity in dental pulp. A: pH 7.0, B: pH 8.0. EGTA was added to Ca-free medium to be finally at 2 mM. CaCl$_2$ was added to EGTA-containing Ca-free medium to be finally at 2.42 mM. Each value represents the mean ± SEM. *p<0.05 and **p<0.01, in comparison with the corresponding control. ★p<0.05, in comparison with the BK-group(normal).

As shown in Fig. 3, addition of EGTA to the medium markedly inhibited
BK-induced enhancement of BANA-degrading enzyme activities in the pulp at
both pH 7 and 8. When calcium ion was added to the EGTA-containing medium
to be finally at 2.42 mM, the BK effects on the enzyme activities were significantly recovered from the inhibition by EGTA at both the pH. These
results suggested that calcium ion might play a role in BK-induced enhancement of BANA-degrading enzyme activities which were regarded as processing
enzyme activities of ME-like peptides in the pulp.

Further studies are necessary to elucidate the characteristics of the
enzymes involved in BANA-degradation which was increased by BK at both pH 7
and 8 in the pulp.

ACKNOWLEDGEMENTS

This work was supported partly by Grant-in Aid for Scientific Research
(No. 61570881) from the Ministry of Education, Science and Culture, Japan.

REFERENCES

1. T. Kudo, N. Yonehara, T. Hayashi, R. Inoki, T. Nishimoto and M. Akai,
    Opioid peptide in the dog canine pulp? in: Advances in Endogenous
    and Exogenous Opioids, H. Takagi and E.J. Simon, ed., p.173,
    Kodansha/Elsevier, Tokyo(1981).
2. T. Kudo, T. Nishimoto, R. Inoki, M. Akai and N. Yonehara, Met-enkepha-
    lin positive cells in the dog canine pulp, Acta Histochem. Cyto-
    chem., 15:449(1982).
3. T. Kudo, S. Maeda and R. Inoki, Opioid peptides in the tooth pulp,
    J. Osaka Univ. Dent. Soc., 28:167(1983).
4. T. Kudo, H.-L. Chang, S. Maeda, Y. Uchida, J. Nakamae and R. Inoki,
    Changes of the met-enkephalin-like peptide content induced by noxi-
    ous stimuli in the rat incisor pulp, Life Sci., 33(Sup. I):677
    (1983).
5. T. Kudo, H.-L. Chang, M. Kuroi, S. Wakisaka, M. Akai and R. Inoki,
    Influences of bradykinin and substance P on the met-enkephalin-like
    peptide content in the rat incisor pulp, Neuropeptides, 7:399
    (1986).
6. T. Kudo, M. Kuroi and R. Inoki, In vitro production and release of
    opioid peptides in the tooth pulp induced by bradykinin, Neuro-
    peptides, 7:391(1986).
7. R. Inoki and T. Kudo, Enkephalins and bradykinin in dental pulp,
    TIPS., 7:275(1986).
8. R. Evangelista, P. Ray and R.V. Lewis, A "trypsin-like" enzyme in
    adrenal chromaffin granules: a proenkephalin processing enzyme,
    Biochem. Biophys. Res. Commun., 106:895(1982).
9. V.Y.H. Hook, L.E. Eiden and M.J. Brownstein, A carboxypeptidase pro-
    cessing enzyme for enkephalin precursors, Nature, 295:341(1982).
10. M. Roth, Fluorimetric assay of trypsin, Clin. Chim. Acta, 8:574(1963).
11. Y. Tamura, M. Hirado, K. Okamura, Y. Minato and S. Fujii, Synthetic
    inhibitors of trypsin, plasmin, kallikrein, thrombin, $C_1\bar{r}$, and
    C_1 esterase, Biochim. Biophys. Acta, 484:417(1977).
12. E.-Q. Wei, T. Kudo and R. Inoki, Enhancement of proteinase activities
    by bradykinin in adrenal medulla of the rat, in this book(1987).

ENHANCEMENT OF PROTEINASE ACTIVITIES BY BRADYKININ

IN ADRENAL MEDULLA OF THE RAT

Er-Qin Wei, Teruo Kudo and Reizo Inoki

Department of Pharmacology
Osaka University Faculty of Dentistry
1-8, Yamadaoka, Suita, Osaka 565, Japan

SUMMARY

In the present study, a significant positive correlationship was found between the contents of bradykinin(BK)-like and met-enkephalin(ME)-like peptides in adrenal medulla of the rat with cavity-formed incisors in vivo, and the production of ME-like peptides was increased by BK in adrenal medulla of the rat in vitro. Influence of BK on the degradation of BANA, a synthetic substrate for trypsin, by the tissue enzymes was also studied. It was found that BK(0.1-10 μM) enhanced the enzyme activities in a dose-dependent manner, and the effect of BK(1 μM) was most effective at pH 6 and 8. The BK effect was inhibited by FOY-305, an inhibitor of serine proteinases, at pH 6, but not at pH 8. However, E-64, an inhibitor of cysteine proteinases, reduced the BK effects at both pH 6 and 8. These results suggested that 1) BK was an activator for BANA-degrading enzymes which were thought as processing proteinases of ME-like peptides in adrenal medulla of the rat, and 2) there may be, at least, two kinds of BANA-degrading enzymes activated by BK, one might be a serine proteinase with optimal pH at 6, and the others might be cysteine proteinases with optimal pH at both 6 and 8.

INTRODUCTION

It is believed, in general, that in adrenal medulla, ME-like peptides co-exist, and co-release with catecholamines by a variety of stimuli including noxious stimuli[1-4]. The peptides are produced from precursor protein by trypsin-like and carboxypeptidase B-like enzymes in adrenal medulla[5,6]. We have reported that ME-like peptide content of adrenal medulla was increased in adjuvant-induced arthritic rats, and there was a significant negative correlationship between the increase of the peptide content and pain threshold, suggesting that pain or pain producing substances may enhance the production of ME-like peptides in adrenal medulla[7-8]. On the other hand, we have also reported that formation of cavity on the rat incisors, a painful noxious stimulation, or BK, a pain producing substance, induced the increase of ME-like peptides in dental pulp of the rat in in vivo and in vitro experiments[9-11] . In the present study, we tried to examine a possible relationship between ME-like and BK-like peptides in adrenal medulla of the rat in vivo and in vitro.

MATERIALS AND METHODS

In vivo Experiments

Animals used were male rats(Sprague-Dawley strain) weighing 200-250 g.
The animals were anesthetized with urethane. Cavities were formed to expose
the pulp at necks of upper and lower incisors of the rat using a dental bar,
and then adrenal medullae were isolated 6, 24 and 72 hr after cavity formation, respectively. On the other hand, the adrenal medullae of anesthetized
rats without cavity were isolated as the control as mentioned above. The
adrenal medulla was homogenized in 0.1 N HCl. The homogenate was centrifuged at 100,000 x g for 20 min and the supernatant was lyophilized. The lyophilized materials were subjected to measure the contents of BK-like and ME-
like peptides by radioimmunoassays using antisera of ME and BK, respectively.
The values obtained were expressed as amounts equivalent to ME or BK(p mole/
g tissue).

In vitro Experiments

ME-like peptides in adrenal medulla. The adrenal medullae were isolated
from the anesthetized rat. After washing and weighing as mentioned above,
the tissue was preincubated in Hanks solution(pH 7.4) containing 20 μM of
bestatin and 1 μM of captopril at 37°C for 5 min and then incubated with BK
for 30 min. After the incubation, the tissue was immersed into ice-cold
0.1 N HCl to finish the reaction, while the medium was rapidly cooled on
ice. The adrenal medulla was homogenized in 0.1 N HCl and the homogenate
was treated to measure the content of ME-like peptides as mentioned above.
On the other hand, the incubation medium was desalted using SEP-PAK C18
cartridge and the ME-like peptides were collected from the resin with 50%
acetonitrile. The acetonitrile solution was lyophilized. The lyophilized
materials were subjected to measure the amount of release of the peptides
into the incubation by radioimmunoassay.

BANA-degradation in adrenal medulla. The adrenal medulla isolated as mentioned above, was preincubated in Hanks solution(pH 4-9) at 37°C for 5 min
and then incubated with BK for 30 min. Two μM of Nα-benzoyl-arginine-β-
naphthylamide(BANA), a synthetic substrate for trypsin-like enzyme, was
added to the incubation medium 2 min before incubation of the tissue with
BK. After the incubation, the reaction was finished by heating for 4 min at
90°C. The medium was rapidly cooled to 0°C on ice after removing the tissue. The cooled medium was subjected to measure BANA-degrading enzyme activity by fluorophotometry(ex. 338 nm, em. 410 nm)[12] using a spetrofluoropho-
tometer. Agents used were BK, FOY-305([N,N-dimethylcarbamoyl 4-(4-guani-
dinobenzoyloxy)-phenyl acetate]methanesulfonate)[13], E-64([L-3-trans-carbo-
xiran-2-carbonyl]-L-Leu-agmatin)[14]. TPCK(p-tosyl-L-phenylalanine chloromethyl ketone)-treated trypsin from bovine pancreas was used as a standard
enzyme in Hanks solution at pH 7.4. The values obtained were expressed as
activity equivalent to trypsin(μg/g tissue).

Statistical Analysis

Each value represents the mesn $\pm$SEM. The data obtained were analyzed
using Student's t-test or Mann-Whitney's U-test in order to examine the
significant difference.

RESULTS AND DISCUSSION

In the present study, influences of noxious stimulation on the contents
of ME-like and BK-like peptides in adrenal medulla of the rat was firstly
examined 6, 24 and 72 hr after cavity formation in the incisors. Both the

contents of ME-like and BK-like peptides in the tissue were significantly
increased 6 hr after cavity formation as compared with the control(p<0.05).
Twenty four hours after, BK-like peptide content was remarkably decreased
(p<0.05) and ME-like peptide content showed a tendency to decrease, while
72 hr after, both the contents were not changed(data not shown). A significant positive correlationship was found between the contents of BK-like
and ME-like peptides, as shown in Fig. 1, suggesting that BK was closely
related to production of ME-like peptides in adrenal medulla, as previously
found in dental pulp of the rat[9-11] .

Thus, we tried to examine whether BK could increase the content and
release of ME-like peptides in the adrenal medulla in vitro. The results
showed that the content of ME-like peptides was remarkably increased by BK
(1 µM) at pH 7.4, but not the release of the peptides, suggesting that BK
was an activator for processing enzymes of ME-like peptides in adrenal me-
dulla(Fig. 2A). In order to certify this suggestion, influence of BK on
degradation of BANA by the tissue enzyme was examined in vitro. As shown
in Fig. 2B, BANA-degrading enzyme activity in the adrenal medulla was remarkably enhanced by BK(0.1-10 µM) at pH 7.4, supporting the suggestion mentioned above.

Thirdly, influence of pH in the incubation medium on the enhancement
of BANA-degrading enzyme activity by BK was examined in order to know
characteristics of the enzymes in the tissue. The incubation media were
adjusted to pH 4, 5, 6, 7, 7.4, 8 and 9, respectively. The enhancing effect
of BK was found to be most effective at both pH 6 and 8(data not shown),
suggestng that there might be, at least, two kinds of BANA-degrading enzymes
activated by BK in the adrenal medulla. Thus, Further examinations on the
characteristics of the BANA-degrading enzymes activated by BK were performed
at both pH 6 and 8.

Since it was considered that one of the processing enzymes of ME-like
peptides might be a trypsin-like enzyme, the effect of FOY-305(0.1 µM), an

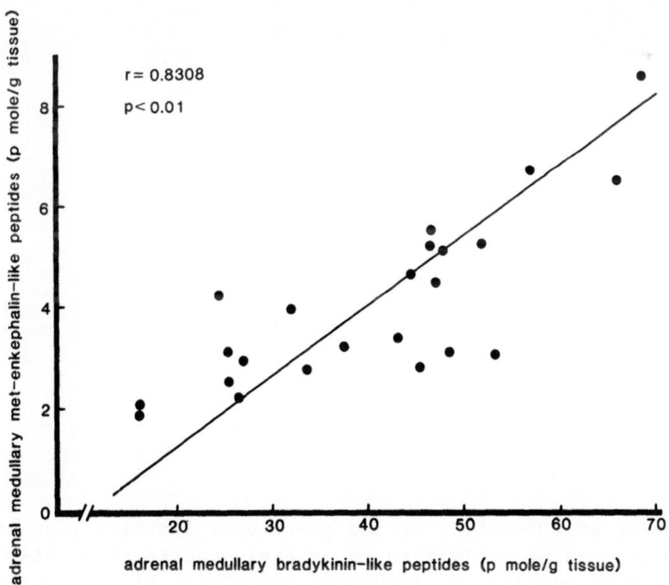

Fig. 1. Correlationship between the contents of BK-like and ME-like peptides
in adrenal medulla of the rat. Plots were obtained from the rats
with cavity-formed incisors 6, 24 and 72 hr after cavity formation
and from the corresponding control rats.

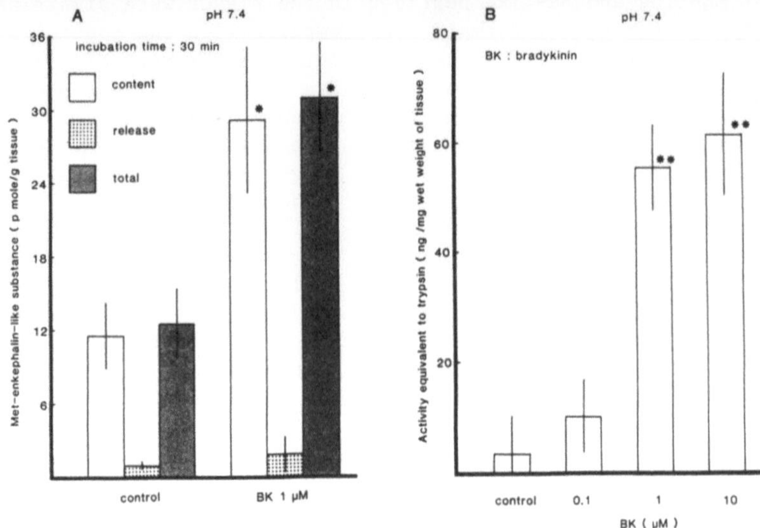

Fig. 2. Increase of ME-like peptide production by BK(1 μM)(A) and the effect
of BK on BANA-degrading enzyme activities(B) in adrenal medulla at
pH 7.4. After preincubation for 5 min, adrenal medulla was incubated with BK(1 μM) for 30 min, then both the tissue and medium were
subjected to radioimmunoassay for ME(A). Adrenal medullae were incubated with BANA(2 μM) for 2 min following to preincubation for 5 min
and then with BK(0.1-10 μM) for 30 min(B). *p<0.05 and **p<0.01, in
comparison with the controls.

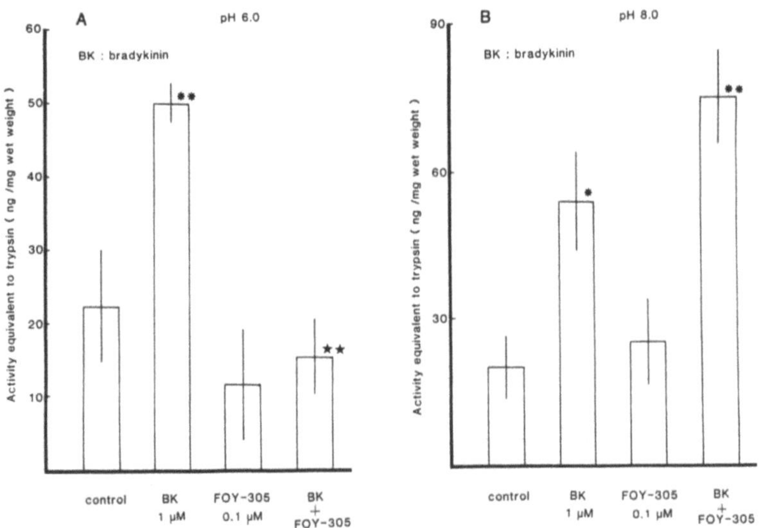

Fig. 3. Influence of FOY-305, a serine proteinase inhibitor, on BANA-
degrading enzyme activities in adrenal medulla at pH 6(A) and 8(B).
The adrenal medulla was incubated with BK(1 μM) for 30 min following to preincubation for 5 min. FOY-305 (0.1 μM) and BANA(2 μM)
were added to the medium 3 and 2 min before the incubation with BK,
respectively. *p<0.05 and **p<0.01, in comparison with controls.
★★p<0.01, in comparison with the BK-group.

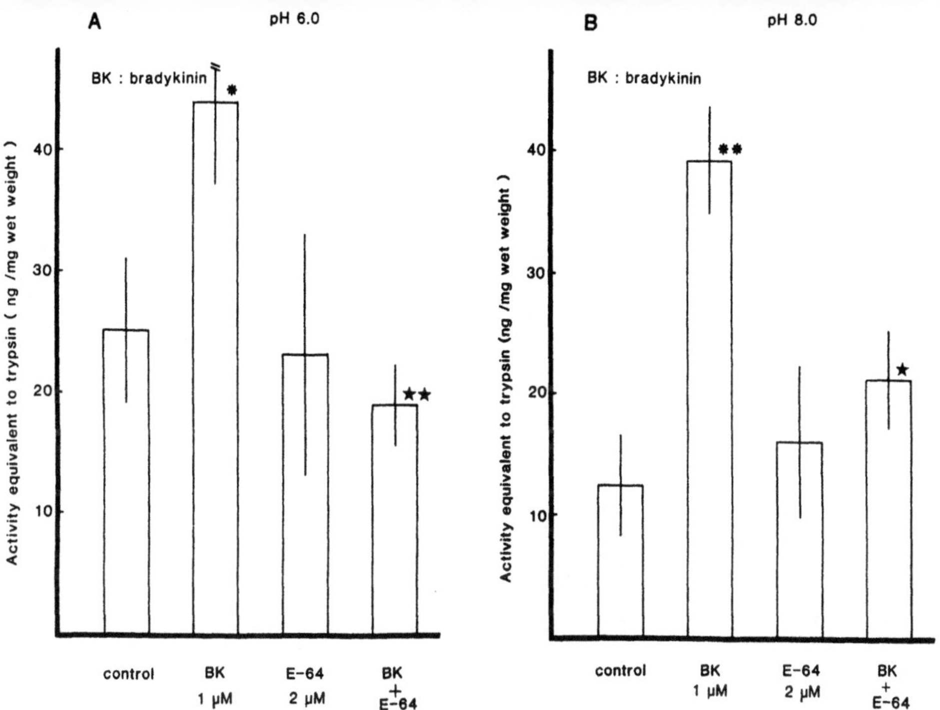

Fig. 4. Influence of E-64, a cysteine proteinase inhibitor, on BANA-degrading enzyme activities in adrenal medulla at pH 6(A) and 8(B). The adrenal medulla was incubated with BK(1 μM) for 30 min following to preincubation for 5 min. E-64(2 μM) and BANA(2 μM) were added to the medium, 3 and 2 min before the incubation with BK, respectively. *p<0.05 and **p<0.01, in comparison with the controls. ★p<0.05 and ★★p<0.01, in comparison with the BK-group.

inhibitor of serine proteinases, on BANA-degrading enzymes activated by BK was examined. As shown in Fig. 3, the results showed that the enhancing effect of BK on BANA-degrading enzyme activity at pH 6, but not at pH 8, was remarkably inhibited by FOY-305, suggesting that a serine proteinase was involved in BANA-degradation facilitated by BK at pH 6. This result seemed to show that there was a tissue-specificity of ME-like peptide processing between the adrenal medulla and the dental pulp in which, in contrast, FOY-305 enhanced BK-induced enhancement of the enzyme activity at pH 7[15].

In the next place, E-64, a specific cysteine proteinase inhibitor, was used to know whether cysteine proteinases were involved in BK-induced enhancement of BANA-degrading enzyme activities in the adrenal medulla. The results showed that the enhancing effect of BK was significantly inhibited by E-64(2 μM) at both pH 6 and 8(Fig. 4). From these results, it was suggested that there were, at least, two kinds of BANA-degrading enzymes activated by BK in the adrenal medulla, one of which was a serine proteinase with optimal pH at 6 and the others were cysteinases with optimal pH at 6 and 8. Mizuno et al[16,17] reported that there were a thiol-dependent protease, with optimal pH at 5.5 and a serine protease with optimal pH around 7.5-9.5 in bovine adrenal medulla which were related to conversion of pro-enkephalin to enkephalins. However, it was unclear, at present time whether BANA-degrading enzymes activated by BK at pH 6 and 8 were identical with the enzymes reported by Mizuno et al.

Further studies are necessary to elucidate the characteristics of the enzymes involved in BANA-degradation at pH 6 and 8 in adrenal medulla.

ACKNOWLEDGEMENTS

This work was supported partly by Grant-in Aid for Scientific Research (No. 61570881) from the Ministry of Education, Science and Culture, Japan.

REFERENCES

1. O. H. Viveros, E. J. Diliberto, Jr. E. Hazum and K.-J. Chang, Opiate-like materials in the adrenal medulla: evidence for storage and secretion with catecholamines. Mol. Pharmacol. 16:1101 (1979).

2. I. Hanbauer, S. Govani, E. A. Majane, H.-Y. T. Yang and E. Costa, In vivo regulation of the release of met-enkephalin-like peptides from dog adrenal medulla. in Regulatory Peptides: From Molecular Biology to Function, E. Costa and M. Trabucchi, eds., Raven Press, New York (1982), p209.

3. S. P. Wilson, K.-J. Chang and O. H. Viveros, Proportional secretion of opioid peptides and catecholamines from adrenal chromaffin cells in culture. J. Neurosci. 2:1150 (1982).

4. O. H. Viveros, E. J. Diliberto, Jr. E. Hazum and K.-J. Chang, Enkephalins as possible adrenomedullary hormones: storage, secretion, and regulation of synthesis. Adv. Biochem. Psychopharmacol. 22:191 (1980).

5. R. Evangelista, P. Ray and R. V. Lewis, A trypsin-like enzyme in adrenal chromaffin granules: a proenkephalin processing enzyme. Biochem. Biophys. Res. Commun. 106:895 (1982).

6. V. Y. H. Hook, L. E. Eiden and M. J. Bronstein, A carboxypeptidase processing enzyme for enkephalin procursors. Nature 295:341 (1982).

7. T. Kudo, E.-Q. Wei, R. Inoki, M. Terasawa and T. Nakao, Influence of Y-20003, an analgesic agent, on the endogenous opioid system in rats. in Progress in Opioid Research, J. W. Holaday, P.-Y. Law and A. Herz, eds., National Insititute on Drug Abuse, Rockville (1986), p236.

8. E.-Q. Wei, T. Kudo, R. Inoki, Terasawa and T. Nakao, Correlationships between pain threshold and met-enkephalin-like peptide levels in adrenal medulla and plasma of adjuvant-induced arthritic rats. Inflammation(Jap.) 7:355 (1987).

9. T. Kudo, H.-L. Chang, M. Kuroi, S. Wakisawa, M. Akai and R. Inoki, Influence of bradykinin and substance P on the met-enkephalin-like peptide content in the rat incisor pulp. Neuropeptides 7:399 (1986).

10. T. Kudo, M. Kuroi and R. Inoki, In vitro production and release of opioid peptides in the tooth pulp induced by bradykinin. Neuropeptides 7:391 (1986).

11. R. Inoki and T. Kudo, Enkephalins and bradykinin in the dental pulp. TIPS 7:275 (1986).

12. M. Roth, Fluorimetric assay of trypsin. Clin. Chim. Acta 8:574 (1963).

13. Y. Tamura, M. Hirado, K. Okamura, Y. Minato and S. Fujii, Synthetic inhibitors of trypsin, plasmin, kallikrein, thrombin, $Cl\bar{r}$, and Cl esterase. Biochim. Biophys. Acta 484:417 (1977).

14. H. Sugita, S. Ishiura, K. Suzuki and K. Imahori, Ca-activated neutral protease and its inhibitors: in vitro effect on intact myofibrils. Muscle Nerve 3:335 (1980).

15. T. Kudo, E.-Q. Wei and R. Inoki, Activation of calcium ion-dependent proteinases by bradykinin in dental pulp of the rat. in this book.

16. K. Mizuno, A. Miyata, K. Kangawa and H. Matsuo, A unique proenkephalin-coverting enzyme purified from bovine adrenal chromaffin granules. Biochem. Biophys. Res. Commun. 108:1235 (1982).

17. K. Mizuno, M. Kojima and H. Matsuo, A putative prohormone processing protease in bovine adrenal medulla specifically cleaving in between Lys-Arg sequences. Biochem. Biophys. Res. Commun. 128:884 (1985).

TRYPSINE-LIKE ESTEROPROTEASES, KININ AND KININASES IN SUBMAN-
DIBULAR GLAND, COLON AND PULMONARY LAVAGE FLUID OF MOUSE MODEL
FOR HUMAN CYSTIC FIBROSIS (CF)

O.L. Catanzaro, O.H. Pivetta,* G.N. Dodera Martinez
and S.B. Vila

Cátedra de Anatomía Comparada y Fisiología Animal
Facultad de Farmacia y Bioquimica, UBA
*Instituto Nacional de Genética Médica
Buenos Aires, Argentina

INTRODUCTION

Cystic fibrosis is a disease with a generalized disorder
primarily affecting exocrine glands and the pulmonary and gastrointestinal systems. We have demonstrated (1,2) in a mouse
model (Cribriform degeneration -cri/cri-) that significant decreasing of kallikrein enzyme is observed in different exocrine
glands. Several reports have postulated a defective transport
of chloride ions across epithelia (3), the defect could be
caused by an alteration in the number, characteristic or regulation of Cl^- channels in the plasma membrane of eptihelial
cells. Because the association of kallikrein with exocrine
glands and the regulation of transepithelial sodium and chloride
transport, the kallikrein and their products, kinin, and inhibitors are reasonable in vivo candidates to be involved in the
function of these tissues in CF.

In the present work we decided to study the kallikrein-
kinin system and inhibitors in a mouse model for human cystic
fibrosis (cri/cri mice).

MATERIAL AND METHODS

Males DBA/2J-cri inbred mice, genotypes cri/cri (affected
homozygotes) and +/? (representing the entire non affected
population) were used.

The animals were sacrificed by a blow on the head. Submax-
ilary glands, colon and pulmonary lavage fluid (PLF) were removed and chilled in PBS, homogenized at 4°C and centrifuged at
20,000 xg per 20 min at 4°C.

Caseinolytic activity was determined by the method of
Minato et al (4), esterolytic activity by the method of Takuma

Table 1. ESTEROPROTEASES AND KININASES IN SUBMANDIBULAR GLAND AND COLON

Submandibular gland	Esterases uM TAME/mg P/min	Kininases U/mg P/min
control male (10)	.320 ± .133	3.80 ± .89 P< .001
cri/cri male (10)	.192 ± .059 P .01	6.37 ± .71

Colon		
control male (10)	.137 ± .074	.95 ± .21 P<.001
cri/cri male (14)	.132 ± .055 N.S	4.12 ± .96

et al. (5). Kinin was determined incubating the PLF with rat kininogen, and with biological assays (6). Kininase was determined incubating the samples with bradykinin according to Kashimata et al. (7).

RESULTS

Table 1 shows the esterase activity in submandibular gland and colon from cri/cri mutant mice, respect to control (+/?). The enzyme activity was significantly reduced in submandibular gland but not in colon.

On the other hand kininase activity was significantly increased in the two organs of cri/cri mice.

The activity of kinin in PLF was significantly lower in cri/cri mice than control. In contrast kininase activity was higher in cri/cri mouse when compared with control (Table 2).

Table 2. KININ AND KININASE IN PULMONARY LUNG FLUID

PLF	Kinins ng BRD/mg P/min	
control male	1.810 ± .027	1.93 ± .37
cri/cri male	.290 ± .020	5.32 ± .90

DISCUSSION

The majority of studies related to disease states have
been focused on the plasma kallikrein-kinin system.

In spite of extensive investigations on CF, no comprehensive efforts have examined the levels of tissues kallikreins,
their modulators, substrates and products. There is not information about experimental data concerning tissues kallikreins,
specific tissues kallikrein inhibitors, kallikrein synthesis and
activation, kininases, kinins or kininogen, expecially in sites
rich in these components and affected by the disease (intestine,
pancreas, salivary glands, sweat glands, respiratory epithelia).
In this paper we used a DBA/2J-cri mouse mutation with many CF-
like alterations (cri/cri), including salivary gland electrolytic abnormalities, decreased pancreatic lipase, low submandibular and pancreatic kallikrein (8, 9, 10).

Our results clearly show a significantly lower esteroproteases in submandibular gland and colon.

Among other finding, it has been reported that a proteases
complex is missing in most CF patients, and that binding of tryp-
sine and other proteinases to α_2 Mproteases is decreased in plasma of CF patients respect to controls (11, 12). Also, a deficiency of arginine esterase activity has been reported in these
patients (13). In Human CF and heterozygotes a decrease of
"trypsine-like" or arginine esterase activity in plasma has been
described (13, 14). The decrease of submandibular esteroproteases
could be explained by an alteration in the duct cells of the
gland. The enzyme may be involved in water electrolyte regulation by the action on tubular epithelium or by a modification of
the local blood flow of the organ (15). The results observed in
colon and submandibular gland of cri/cri mice, show a marked
reduction of esteroproteases, with a significant increase of
kininase activity; on other hand PLF from the same animals show
a decreased activity of kinin with increased kininase activity.
It has been suggested that tissue kallikreins and their product
kinins are reasonable "in vivo" candidates for participation in
the regulation of transepithelia sodium and chloride transport.
The phenomen of decreased $Cl^=$ permeability, coupled with a enhanced Na^+ uptake, has been offered as an explanation of the
presumed dehydration of the respiratory mucus, with a impairment
of the function in colon absorption and lung infection seen
in CF patients. In colon, submandibular gland and PLF we see
an increased activity of kininases in cri/cri mice.

The last statement is very important, since the activation
of this inhibitor could account for the observed decreased activity of kinin and proteases. Further work is necessary to
clarify the main process of these findings.

ACKNOWLEDGEMENT

This work was supported by CONICET. República Argentina
Grants 1316/86.

REFERENCES

1. O.L. CATANZARO, M.I. VACCARO, S.B. VILA, A.L. MARTINEZ SEEBER and O.H. PIVETTA. Life Sc. 32, 825, 1983.
2. DODERA MARTINEZ G.N., S.B. VILA, O.L. CATANZARO, O.H. PIVETTA. Life Sc. (in Press)
3. P.M. QUINTON. Nature 301, 421, 1983.
4. A. MINATO, S. HIROSE, S. HAYASHI. Chem. Pharm. Bull. 15, 1356, 1967.
5. T. TAKUMA and M. KUMEGAWA. Bioch. Biophys Acta 584, 51, 1979.
6. A. POWERS and A. NASJLETTI. Endocrinology 112, 1194, 1983.
7. M. KASHIMATA, M. HIRAMATU, M. KUMEGAWA and M. MINAMI Enzyme 34, 22, 1985.
8. M.C. Green, r.l. SIDMAN and O.H. PIVETTA. Science 176, 800, 1973.
9. D. KAISER, O.H. PIVETTA, and O.M. RENNERT. Life Sci. 15, 803 1974.
10. O.H. PIVETTA and M.C. GREEN. Medicina 37, 379, 1977.
11. E. SHAPIRA, G. RAO, H.U. WESSEL and H.L. NADLER. Pediatr. Res. 10, 812, 1976.
12. G.B. WILSON and H.H. FUNDERBERG. Pediatr. Res. 10, 87, 1976.
13. G.J.S. RAO and H. NADLER. Ped. Res. 8, 684, 1974.
14. K.Y. CHAN, D.A. APPLEGARTH and A.G. DAVISON. Clin. Chim. Acta. 74, 71, 1977.
15. T.B. ORSTAVIK. Acta Physiol. Scand. 140, 431, 1978.

ROLE OF THE KALLIKRAIN-KININ SYSTEM IN HUMAN PANCREATITIS

Soichiro Uehara, Kyosuke Honjyo, Satoshi Furukawa,
Akio Hirayama and Wataru Sakamoto*

Dept. of Internal Medicine, Tonan Hospital, Sapporo 060, Japan
*Dept. of Biochemistry, School of Dentistry, Hokkaido University
Sapporo, 060, Japan

SUMMARY

Various factors in the kallikrein-kinin system were evaluated in acute and chronic pancreatitis.

It was noted in particular that plasma trypsin and glandular kallikrein increased markedly in acute phase of pancreatitis and its correlation with amylase was observed.

Plasma prekallikrein (PPK) decreased in acute pancreatitis, but increased in chronic pancreatitis. A negative correlation was noted between PPK and kallikrein like activity. Both HMW and LMW kininogen decreased in acute pancreatitis.

It was presumed from these findings that the increase in kinin and its activation at the acute phase of pancreatitis might be due to kallikrein or trypsin originating from the pancreas.

INTRODUCTION

Kallikrein, which is present not only in the plasma but also in organs such as the salivary gland, pancreas, and kidney, acts on circulating kininogens to release kinins which reduce blood pressure, increase vascular permiability, and cause pain.[1] Two kininogens are known to be present in humans. One is high-molecular-weight (HMW) kininogen, which is present as a complex with coagulation factor XII and prekallikrein in the plasma, and the other is low-molecular-weight (LMW) kininogen, which is activated by glandular (tissue) kallikrein.[2] Bradykinin is produced from the former, and kallidin the latter.[2],[3]

Since the author has been particularly concerned with the Kallikrein-Kinin (K-K) system in pancreatitis, the present study was initiated with the aim of further determining the various factors involved in the kallikrein system, and their relationships with respect to pancreatitis.

MATERIALS AND METHODS

The subjects of the study were 10 healthy adult subjects, 8 patients with acute pancreatitis and 25 patients with chronic pancreatitis.

Diagnosis of pancreatitis

Diagnosis of acute and chronic pancreatitis were made on the basis of measurements of pancreatic enzymes, clinical observations, and computerized tomography.

Measurement of pancreatic enzyme activity

Serum amylase was determined by the blue starch method (Seikagaku Ltd, Japan). Serum trypsin was determined by RIA (Hoechst, West Germany).

Measurement of the plasma kallikrein

Plasma levels of prekallikrein (PPK), Kallikrein like activity were determined by the method of Friberger[5] using chromogenic substrate S-2302 (Kabi, Vitrum AB., Sweden).

Measurement of glandular kallikrein

Radioimmunoactivity of plasma glandular kallikrein (GK) was determined by RIA (Green Cross Ltd., Japan).[6]

Measurement of plasma kininogens

To determine HMW and LMW-kininogens a bioassay employing the method of Uchida et. al.[7] was made. The content of isolated kinin was converted and determined using synthetic bradykinin (Peptide Institute Inc. Japan).

Measurement of the plasma proteinase inhibitors

Alpha$_1$-antitrypsin (α_1-AT), alpha$_2$-macroglobulin (α_2-M), antithrombin III (At-III), and C_1-inactivator (C_1-INA) were determined by the single rapid immunodiffusion method (Berhringwerke, West Germany) and alpha$_2$-plasmin inhibitor (α_2-PI) was determined by the same method (Mochida, Ltd. Japan). Protein was assayed by the method of Lowry et. al.[8] Blood samples were collected into plastic tubes containing 1/10 volume of 3.8% sodium citrate.

Statistical methods

The student's t-test comparing mean values for unpaired data was used and differences were considered statistically significant for $p < 0.05$.

RESULTS

The pancreatic enzymes in blood

During the acute phase of acute and chronic pancreatitis, the levels of amylase and trypsin were increased and these results were showed in Table 1.

A significant correlation was noted between trypsin and α_1-AT (r = 0.44, n = 56), trypsin and amylase (r = 0.36, n = 50) respectively.

Plasma Prekallikrein

Table 1. shows the results of measurements. PPK was significantly decreased in the patients with acute pancreatitis as compared to healthy subjects, whereas it showed an increase in the patients with chronic pancreatitis.

Table 1 Plasma levels of prekallikrein, glandular kallikrein, HMW and LMW kininogens and serum levels of amylase and trypsin in normal subjects and patients with pancreatitis

	normal subjects	acute pancreatitis	chronic pancreatitis
serum amylase (u/ml)	240.6 ± 64.2 (n = 22)	2944.5 ± 1127.5** (n = 12)	432.2 ± 177.7* (n = 45)
serum trypsin (ng/ml)	244.4 ± 71.0 (n = 15)	1028.0 ± 641.1** (n = 12)	365.1 ± 255.9 (n = 45)
plasma prekallikrein (%)	102.0 ± 5.6 (n = 10)	52.5 ± 24.0** (n = 12)	119.1 ± 41.5* (n = 45)
plasma glandular kallikrein (ng/ml)	50.8 ± 5.5 (n = 10)	89.3 ± 23.3** (n = 8)	63.3 ± 22.2* (n = 31)
plasma HMW-kininogen (μgBKeq./ml)	0.85 ± 0.06 (n = 10)	0.49 ± 0.22** (n = 8)	0.95 ± 0.30 (n = 11)
(ngBKeq./ml)	12.3 ± 1.2 (n = 10)	6.6 ± 2.6** (n = 8)	12.8 ± 4.1 (n = 11)
plasma LMW-kininogen (μgBKeq./ml)	2.87 ± 0.20 (n = 10)	1.81 ± 0.68** (n = 8)	2.20 ± 0.63* (n = 11)
(ngBKeq./ml)	41.4 ± 4.0 (n = 10)	24.6 ± 8.9** (n = 8)	30.3 ± 9.3* (n = 11)

$* \ p < 0.05, \quad ** \ p < 0.01$

The relationship between kallikrein like activity and PPK was examined. In this correlation a trend toward high levels of kallikrein like activity, with a decline in PPK in acute phase of acute and chronic pancreatitis is noted. (Fig. 1)

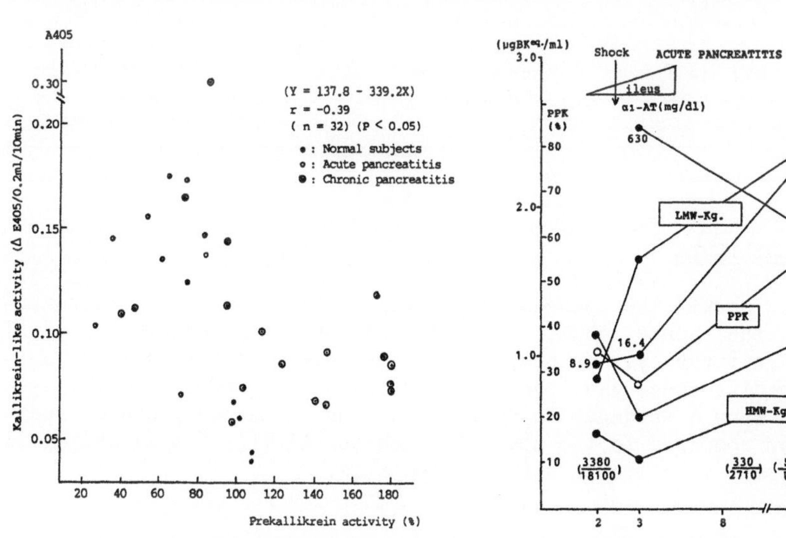

Fig. 1. Correlation between plasma Prekallikrein activity and plasma Kallikrein like activity in normal subjects, and patient with Pancreatitis.

Fig. 2. The behaviors of prekallikrein, HMW and LMW kininogen and proteinase inhibitors levels in plasma of patients with acute pancreatitis.

Glandular kallikrein

The level of plasma GK was significantly higher in acute and chronic pancreatitis than in healthy subjects. (Table 1)

Factors of kinin system

The level of HMW-kininogen in the acute pancreatitis significantly decreased, as compared to healthy subjects, while in chronic pancreatitis no difference was observed. The level of LMW-kininogen was significantly decreased in acute and chronic pancreatitis, as compared to healthy subjects. (Table 1)

Changes in the K-K system in acute pancreatitis

The patient (Fig. 2) presented with clinical signs (such as, abdominal pain, ileus and shock) together with an increase in pancreatic enzymes, and a decrease in HMW and LMW-kininogen, and PPK, which began to normalize following continued treatment.

Table 2 Plasma levels of α_1-AT, α_2-M, AT-III, C_1-INA and α_2-PI in normal subjects and patients with pancreatitis

		acute pancreatitis		chronic pancreatitis	
	normal subjects	acute phase	stabilized phase	acute phase	stabilized phase
α_1-AT (mg/dl)	253.4 ± 73.2 (n = 53)	439.5 ± 19.5** (n = 22)	235.0 ± 45.0 (n = 13)	298.3 ± 63.2** (n = 60)	216.4 ± 32.4 (n = 38)
α_2-M (mg/dl)	236.7 ± 65.1 (n = 53)	246.4 ± 63.8 (n = 22)	271.9 ± 68.8 (n = 13)	255.3 ± 68.3 (n = 60)	253.0 ± 83.5 (n = 38)
AT-III (mg/dl)	28.2 ± 2.7 (n = 14)	20.9 ± 5.5** (n = 16)		25.3 ± 2.5** (n = 20)	
C_1-INA (mg/dl)	29.9 ± 2.7 (n = 22)	23.8 ± 4.2** (n = 11)		32.5 ± 5.6 (n = 20)	
α_2-PI (g/ml)	60.0 ± 14.9 (n = 22)	41.4 ± 13.4** (n = 11)		47.1 ± 15.4* (n = 14)	

* $p < 0.05$, ** $p < 0.01$

Proteinase inhibitors

Table 2. shows the changes in proteinase inhibitors in pancreatitis. During the acute phase of acute and chronic pancreatitis, α_1-AT increased significantly, as compared to its levels in the healthy subjects, but no difference was found between these two groups in α_2-M. α_2-M did however, show a tendency to decrease during the acute phase of pancreatitis, as compared to the stabilized phase. AT-III, C_1-INA and α_2-pI showed a decrease in patients with pancreatitis.

DISCUSSION

In the cases of pancreatitis, the pancreas contains large amount of glandular kallikrein (GK) and trypsin which activate pancreatic kallikrein and plasma kallikrein.

Consequently, activation of the K-K system has been reported already
in pancreatitis, as one of its clinical symptoms.

This phenomenon was reported by Hollenberg et. al.[9] in their experiments on pancreatitis in dogs and was investigated further by
Thal,[10] Ryan,[11] Popieraitis[12] and Lasson et. al.[13],[14] who suggested that
activation of K-K system was caused by a mainly activated plasma kallikrein.

In this study, we measured plasma levels of various factors of K-K
system, and examined the relationship between the changes in these levels
and the pathology of pancreatitis.

Our measurement of various factors of the K-K system in acute pancreatitis patients showed decrease in PPK, HMW and LMW-kininogen, and
increase in plasma GK and trypsin. In chronic pancreatitis patients,
levels of the K-K system showed increase in PPK, plasma GK and trypsin
and decrease in LMW-kininogen.

However association of proteinase inhibitors such as the C_1-INA,
α_2-M, AT-III, α_1-AT and α_2-pI with this activation has also been shown.[15],[16]

Considering these findings, it was thought that the decrease in PPK
in acute pancreatitis was linked with the activation of kallikrein, and
that the increase in PPK in chronic pancreatitis showed, from its behabi-
viour in blood, a preparatory state (hypercoagulable state) to the activation of kallikrein.

In the course of acute pancreatitis it was further noted that,
simultaneously with the onset of shock, other symptoms and both
kininogens content showed a decrease in parallel with the decrease in
PPK, both of which were normalized in conjunction with the disappearance
of symptoms. These findings suggest that kinin production takes place in
the acute phase of acute pancreatitis. Due to these findings, the classification and measurement of HMW & LMW kininogens was carried out in order
to confirm the origin of kallikrein activity. These showed that a decrease in both kininogens occurred in acute pancreatitis. These results
might have been brought about by GK and trypsin of pancreas origin, and
these pancreatic enzymes might have activated plasma kallikrein.

In the case of chronic pancreatitis, on the other hand LMW-kininogen
alone showed a decrease. This is in explicable if only the theory of PPK
activation is considered. Therefore the action of pancreatic kallikrein
[17] or so called "non specific kininogenase" of leukocyte origin,[18] may
need to be investigated.

This kind of activation of plasma K-K system in the acute phase of
pancreatitis induced an acceleration of coagulation and fibrinolysis
through the activation of the XII factor, which was considered to bring
about the possibility of shock through the kinin system, together with
the onset of disseminated intravascular coagulation (DIC).

REFERENCES

1) E. Haberman: Kininogens, in: Handbook of Experimental Pharmacology,
   Suppl. 15, Ed. E.G. Erdoes. Springer-Verlag. Berlin, pp 250-288,
   1970.

2) D.M. Kerbiriou, B.N. Bouma, and J.H. Griffin: Immuno chemical studies
   of human high molecular weight kininogen and it complex with plasma
   prekallikrein or kallikrein. J. Biol. Chem. 255: 3952-3961, 1980.

3) H. Kato, S. Nagasawa, and S. Iwanaga: HMW and LMW kininogens. Methods
   Enzymol. 80: 117-119, 1981.

4) R.S. Telmer, and J.P. Felber: Radioimmunoassay of human plasma
   trypsin. Biochem. Boiphysi. Acta. 236: 78-85, 1971.

5) P. Friberger, E. Eriksson, S. Gustavsson, and G. Claeson: Determination of prekallikrein in plasma by means of a chromogenic tripeptide substrate for plasma kallikrein. in: Kinin-II, Ed, by S. Fujii, H. Moriya, and T. Suzuki, Pleum. New York. pp 67-82, 1979.

6) S. Morichi, E. Sako, Y. Iga, M. Nishida, and H. Moriya: Human urinary kallikrein (HUK): Large-scale purification and direct solid-phase radioimmunoassay (RIA). in: Kinin IV (Part B), Ed. L.M. Greenbaum, and H.S. Margolius, Pleum. New York, pp 549-555, 1986.

7) Y. Uchida, and M. Katori: Differential assay method for high molecular weight and low molecular weight kininogens, Thromb. Res. 15: 127-134, 1979.

8) O.M. Lowry, N.J. Rosebrough, A.L. Farr, and R.J. Randall: Protein measurement with the forins phenol reagent, J. Biol. Chem. 193: 265-275, 1951.

9) M. Hollenberg, E.E. Kobold, R. Pruett, and A.P. Thal: Occurrence of circulatory vaso active substances in human and experimental pancreatitis. Surg. Forum. 13: 302-311, 1962.

10) A.P. Thal, E.E. Kobold, and M.J. Hollengerg: The release of vasoactive substances in acute pancreatitis. Amer. J. Surg. 105: 708-713, 1963.

11) J. Ryan, W. Bethesda, J.G. Moffat, and A.G. Thompson: Role of bradykinin system in acute haemorrhagic pancreatitis. Arch. Surg. 91: 14-24, 1965.

12) A.S. Popieraitis, and A.B. Thompson: The site of bradykinin release in acute experimental pancreatitis. Arch. Surg. 98: 73-76, 1969.

13) A. Lasson, and K. Ohlsson: Changes in the kallikrein kinin system during acute pancreatitis in man. Thromb. Res. 35: 27-41, 1984.

14) A.O. Aasen, T.E. Ruud, R. Kaaresen and J.O. Stadaas: Evaluation of patients with acute pancreatitis by means of chromogenic peptide substrate assays and the proenzyme functional inhibition index. Scand. J. Gastroenterol. 21: Suppl. 126: 40-45, 1986.

15) S. Uehara, and A. Hirayama: Studies of antithrombin-III in pancreatitis (in Japanese). Acta. Haematol. Jap. 40: 248-254, 1977.

16) W. Sakamoto, O. Nishikaze, S. Uno, K. Yoshikawa, and S. Uehara: Relationship between salivary kallikrein, kininogen, and plasma proteinase inhibitors, in: Kinin III. Ed, by H. Fritz, G. Dietze, F. Fiedler, G.L. Haberland. Blinkhäusser. Basel, Boston Stuttgart, USA. pp 184-189, 1983.

17) Y. Uchida, and H. Katori: Independent consumption of high and low molecular weight kininogens in vivo. in: Kinin IV (Part A), Ed. L.M. Greenbaum, and H.S. Margolius, Pleum. New York, pp 113-117, 1986.

18) K.L. Melmon, and M.J. Cline: Interaction of plasma kinins and granulocytes, Nature, 213: 90-93, 1967.

STUDIES OF SWEAT KALLIKREIN IN NORMAL HUMAN SUBJECTS

Ronald K. Mayfield, Donald A. Sens, Ayad A. Jaffa and Harry
S. Margolius

Departments of Medicine, Pathology and Pharmacology, Medical
University of South Carolina and Veterans Administration
Medical Center, Charleston, SC

INTRODUCTION

Kinin-generating and kallikrein-like esterase activities have been
found in human sweat (1-6). Free kinins and kininase activity have also
been detected (4,6). These findings suggest that kallikrein and kinins may
have some role in sweat gland function. Since kinins are potent stimuli to
epithelial ion transport in other sites, the generation of kinins within
the sweat gland may be related to regulation of sweat ion concentration (7-
9). It has also been postulated that sweat gland kinin production may be
linked to the cutaneous vasodilation which occurs during sweating (1).

Despite measurements of kallikrein-like activity, no direct measurements of tissue kallikrein in sweat have been carried out, and sweat kallikrein levels have not been measured in relation to sweat gland function.
In the present study we measured both immunoreactive kallikrein and kininogenase activity in exercise-induced sweat collected from several body sites
of normal human subjects. Kallikrein levels were also measured in sweat
induced by heat or pilocarpine stimulation. Sweat kallikrein was assessed
in relation to sweat gland secretion of sodium and protein.

METHODS

During ad lib exercise, sweat was collected into clean glass vials
and pooled from several body sites by 9 male and 2 female normal subjects,
18-40 years old. Urine was collected over the 24-h period prior to exercise. Subsequently, sweat from six sites (forearm, abdomen, chest, back,
forehead and axilla) was individually collected by 4 male and 5 female
subjects during heat stimulation in a sauna. These samples were collected
with a Macroduct Sweat Collection System (Wescor Inc., Logan, UT). In
addition, forearm sweat was collected into a Macroduct coil following
pilocarpine iontophoresis (1.5 mA for 5 min). None of the subjects had any
chronic diseases and none were taking medications.

Sweat samples collected in vials were centrifuged and the aqueous
phase was separated from lipid or pelleted debris. Kallikrein was assayed
directly in this portion with a radioimmunoassay, using purified human
urinary kallikrein as standard (10). Kininogenase activity was measured
as previously described (11), using purified bovine low molecular weight
kininogen (10 µg/tube, Protein Research Institute, University of Osaka,

Osaka, Japan) or human low molecular weight kininogen substrate (15 µg/
tube), kindly provided by Dr. Kazuaki Shimamoto, Sapporo Medical College,
Sapporo, Japan. Sweat and urine sodium were measured by flame photometry
and sweat protein was measured by the method of Lowry et al. (12).

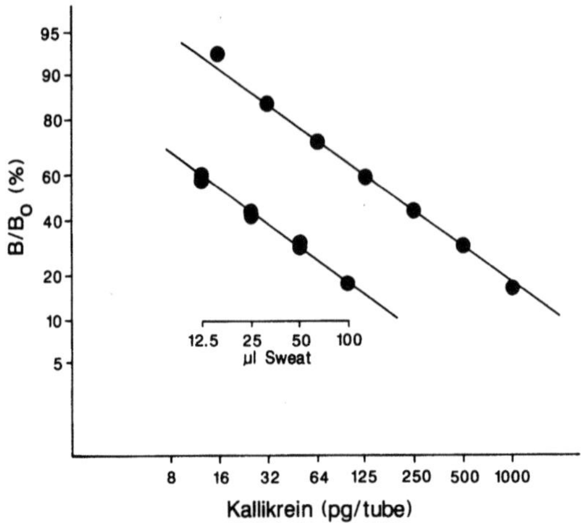

Figure 1. Sweat (lower line) and purified human urinary
kallikrein (upper line) in the kallikrein
radioimmunoassay.

RESULTS

As shown in Figure 1, pooled sweat in serial dilution produced a dis-
placement curve which was parallel to that of purified human urinary kallikrein in a kallikrein radioimmunoassay. Kallikrein concentration in sweat
pooled from several body sites showed a wide range (0.12 - 8.4 ng/ml sweat).
To determine whether this large variation was due to differences in the
protein content of sweat, kallikrein concentration was expressed relative to
total sweat protein. This relative concentration showed a similar wide
range (0.085 - 6.75 ng kallikrein/mg protein), suggesting that the variability in sweat kallikrein level was not simply due to differences in the
concentration of all sweat proteins. The absolute concentration (ng/ml)
and relative concentration (ng/mg protein) were highly correlated ($r = 1.0$,
$y = 1.3 x - 0.14$, $P < 0.001$).

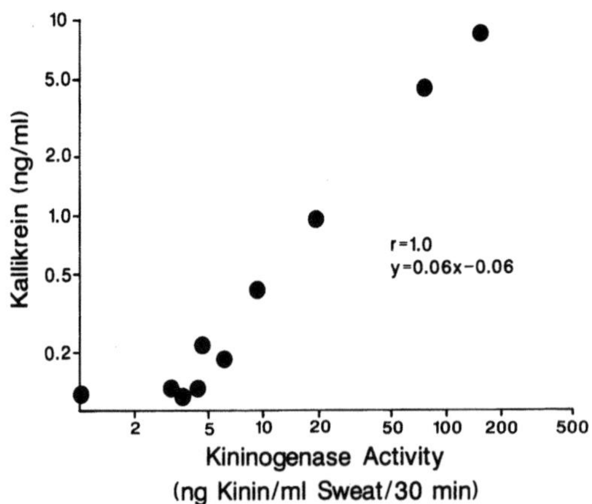

Figure 2. Correlation between sweat kallikrein content
(RIA) and kininogenase activity.

The pooled sweat collections showed kinin-generating activity when incubated with human or bovine low molecular weight kininogen. This activity also showed a broad range (< 2.0 - 152.5 ng kinin/ml sweat/30 min incubation, human kininogen). Kininogenase activity was directly correlated (P < 0.001) with the level of immunoreactive kallikrein (Figure 2). Using human kininogen the specific activity of sweat kininogenase activity averaged 0.6 ng kinin/min/ng kallikrein. Bovine low molecular weight kininogen was also cleaved during incubation with sweat, but this substrate was not as preferred as human kininogen. Incubation with similar amounts of bovine kininogen generated approximately 1% as much immunoreactive kinin as during incubation with the human substrate.

Figure 3 shows that the kallikrein concentration of sweat obtained from males during exercise (pooled from several body sites) was inversely correlated (P < 0.01) with the sweat sodium concentration. Furthermore, sweat sodium (meq/l) was directly and significantly correlated with urinary sodium excretion, measured during the 24-h period prior to the exercise-induced sweat collection (r = 0.67, y = 0.42 x + 59.4, P < 0.05).

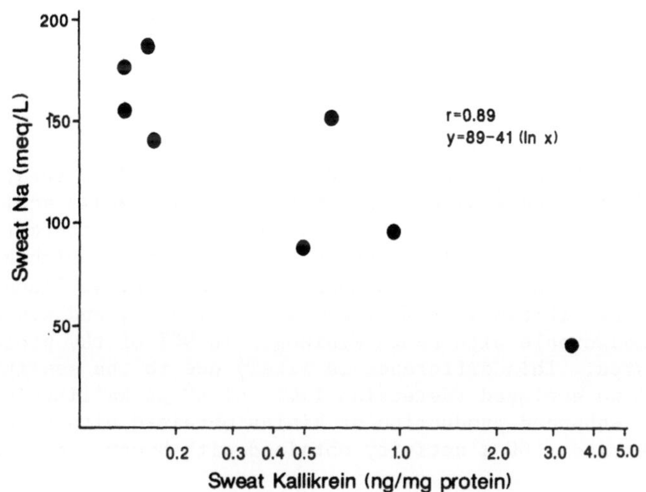

Figure 3.   Relation between sweat kallikrein level and
            sweat sodium concentration.

To further examine reasons for the broad range in sweat kallikrein level, immunoreactive kallikrein was measured in sweat collected into Macroduct coils, but not pooled, from six different anatomic sites (Figure 4). In the majority of collections from all sites, the kallikrein level was below 1 ng/ml. Samples with undetectable kallikrein were obtained from all but the axillary region. Except for the forearm and abdominal region, all sites also yielded samples with much higher concentrations (> 2 ng/ml), the highest level found in forehead sweat.

The kallikrein level of sweat was also compared in sweat collected from the forearm into Macroduct coils during heat or pilocarpine stimulation (Figure 5). There was no difference in the kallikrein level when sweating was stimulated by either of these agonists.

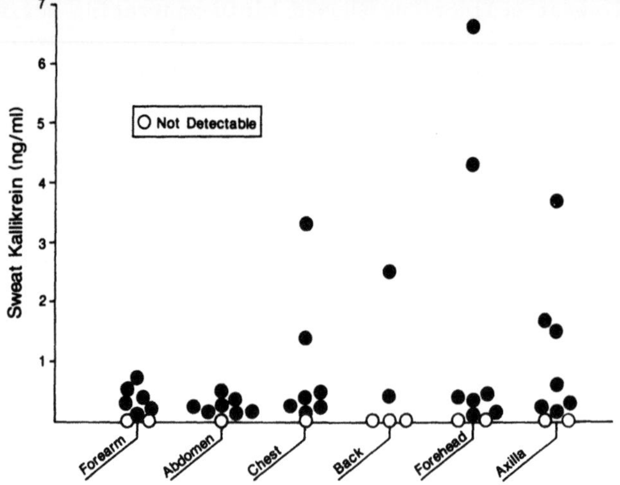

Figure 4.   Kallikrein level in sweat from various anatomic sites.

DISCUSSION

In this study we demonstrated that human sweat contains a tissue kallikrein which is immunologically similar to human urinary kallikrein and
cleaves low molecular weight kininogens to produce kinin.   Previous studies
have found that crude sweat or concentrated sweat fractions contain kallikrein-like esterase activity or kinin-generating activity (1-4), but immunoreactive kallikrein has not been directly measured in sweat.   Two of
the prior studies found a wide range in sweat kininogenase activity between
subjects (3,4).   Our study confirms that the kallikrein content of sweat
can range nearly 100-fold.   In contrast to one study in which kinin-generating activity was undetectable in most sweat samples, we found measurable
immunoreactive kallikrein in 80% of samples collected, and kinin-generating
activity was measurable with human kininogen in 90% of the pooled sweat
samples we tested.   This difference is likely due to the sensitivity of the
kallikrein RIA we employed (detection limit of 80 pg kallikrein/ml sweat)
as well as the enhanced production of kinins obtained with a homologous
kininogen substrate (100 x activity obtained with human compared to bovine
kininogen).

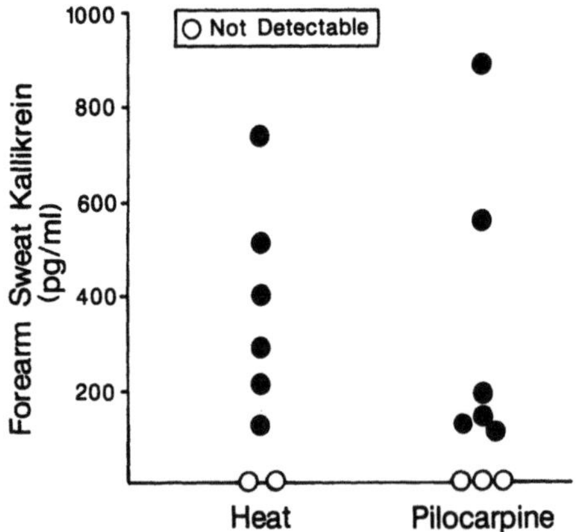

Figure 5.   Forearm sweat kallikrein levels following
heat or pilocarpine stimulation.

reasons for this wide range are uncertain. Evaporation during collection
of sweat may have occurred, as evidenced by the high level of sodium in
some collections. However, if variable evaporation was responsible for the
range in kallikrein level found, correction for protein content should have
reduced the range. This was not the case. Horie et al. (5) found that
sweat collected by simple scraping contains protease activity which may be
derived from the epidermis or deposited on the skin during previous sweating. This may account for some of the variability we found in sweat kallikrein levels in pooled collections. However, sweat collected with the
Macroduct coil also showed a wide range in kallikrein levels (Figure 4),
and this collection method has been shown to yield sweat with very little
contamination with epidermal protein (13).

Some anatomical sites yielded sweat with higher kallikrein concentration than others (Figure 4). This suggests regional differences in sweat
glands might account for differences in kallikrein production. The highest
levels were found in sweat from the trunk and forehead, sites where sebaceous glands are more prominent (14). Sebaceous glands secrete by a holo-
crine mechanism (disintegration of cells). If the kallikrein in sweat was
principally from sebaceous gland secretion we should have detected high
protein levels in sweat with high kallikrein, but did not. Apocrine sweat
glands, which are specialized sweat glands that produce a milky secretion
and are without cholinergic innervation, have regional differences in distribution and could contribute to the regional differences in sweat kallikrein (15). However, these glands are generally not found in some of the
sites which produced sweat with high kallikrein concentration (e.g. forehead). Furthermore, pilocarpine stimulation produced sweat containing kallikrein, suggesting that apocrine glands are not the source of kallikrein.

Eccrine sweat glands are an apparent source of the tissue kallikrein
in sweat. Differences in sweat flow rate from eccrine glands might account
for the wide range in kallikrein levels we found. Fox and Hilton reported
that kinin-generating activity of sweat increased as sweat flow rate accelerated (1). Some of the highest sweat kallikrein levels we measured (Figure
4) were in sweat from sites which demonstrate the highest flow rates during
heat stimulation (16).

Finally, our data show that sweat gland kallikrein excretion is related
to sweat gland sodium excretion. Sweat kallikrein and sodium concentrations
were inversely related in exercise-induced sweat from males. A similar inverse relation has been found between renal sodium and kallikrein excretion
in humans studied during high or low sodium diets (17). The influence of
dietary sodium intake on renal kallikrein is at least in part mediated by
mineralocorticoid and it is thought that kallikrein participates in sodium
handling by the kidney. The sweat gland regulates sodium excretion similar
to the kidney, in that increased dietary sodium increases sweat sodium concentration and mineralocorticoid administration reduces sweat sodium (18,
19). In our study sweat sodium and urinary sodium excretion were directly
correlated. From all of this, it is reasonable to suggest that tissue kallikrein in the sweat gland may participate in sweat gland sodium metabolism.
This notion is supported by the recent finding that kinins stimulate sodium
transport across cultured sweat duct epithelia (20). If kallikrein plays a
role in sweat duct sodium transport, it could explain our finding of high
kallikrein levels in sweat from sites with a high sweat flow rate.

It has been postulated that a tissue kallikrein abnormality may be involved in the disordered exocrine gland function and epithelial ion transport in cystic fibrosis. No substantial abnormalities of kallikrein have
been found in urine, saliva or plasma of cystic fibrosis patients, but sweat
kallikrein has not been examined (9,21,22). However, pancreatic and

salivary kallikrein are decreased in a mouse model which manifests some electrolyte abnormalities of cystic fibrosis (23). Our findings now make a case for studying sweat gland kallikrein and its regulation in cystic fibrosis.

ACKNOWLEDGEMENTS

We wish to thank Amy Frayser and Michael Bigelow for technical assistance and Barbara Whitlock for assistance in preparing the manuscript. This work was supported by grants from the National Institute of Diabetes, Digestive and Kidney Disease, DK 35977 and AM 11028, and the Veterans Administration.

REFERENCES

1. R. H. Fox and S. M. Hilton, Bradykinin formation in human skin as a factor in heat vasodilation, J. Physiol. 142:219 (1958).
2. J. E. Fraki, C. T. Jansen and V. K. Hopsu-Havu, Human sweat kallikrein. Biochemical demonstration and chromatographic separation from several other esteropeptidases in the sweat, Acta Dermatovener 50:321 (1970).
3. D. B. Frewin, D. J. McConnell and J. A. Downey, Is a kininogenase necessary for human sweating? Lancet II:744 (1973).
4. A. G. Scicli, G. Forbes, D. Goldberg and O. A. Carretero, Kininogenase activity and kinins in human sweat, Proceedings of Kinin '84, International Congress, Savannah, Georgia, p. 124, October (1984).
5. N. Horie, H. Yokozeki and K. Sato, Proteolytic enzymes in human eccrine sweat: a screening study, Am. J. Physiol. 250:R691 (1986).
6. T. Hibino, T. Takemura and K. Sato, Evidence that human eccrine sweat contains kallikrein and kininase, Clin. Res. 35:923A (1987).
7. A. W. Cuthbert and H. S. Margolius, Kinins stimulate net chloride secretion by the rat colon, Br. J. Pharmacol. 75:587 (1982).
8. A. W. Cuthbert, A. M. George and L. MacVinish, Kinin effects on electrogenic ion transport in primary cultures of pig renal papillary collecting tubule cells, Am. J. Physiol. 249:439 (1985).
9. A. W. Baird and H. S. Margolius, Bradykinin stimulates electrogenic bicarbonate secretion by guinea pig gall bladder, Br. J. Pharmacol. 91:369P (1987).
10. K. Shimamoto, J. Chao and H. S. Margolius, The radioimmunoassay of human urinary kallikrein and comparisons with kallikrein activity measurements, J. Clin. Endocrinol. Metab. 51:84 (1980).
11. M. Kondo, K. Shimamoto, N. Ura, T. Nishimiya, T. Mita, M. Nakagawa, T. Maeda, Y. Yamaguchi and O. Iimura, A simple and sensitive method for determination of human urinary kallikrein activity (kininogenase activity), using human low molecular weight kininogen, Endocrinol. Japon 31:635 (1984).
12. O. H. Lowry, N. J. Rosebrough, A. L. Farr and R. J. Randall, Protein measurement with the folin phenol reagent. J. Biol. Chem. 193:265 (1951).
13. D. A. Sens, M. A. Simmons and S. S. Spicer, The analysis of human sweat proteins by isoelectric focusing. I. Sweat collection utilizing the Macroduct system demonstrates the presence of previously unrecognized sex-related proteins, Pediatr. Res. 19:873 (1985).
14. S. Emanuel, Quantitative determination of the sebaceous glands' function, with particular mention of the method. Acta Dermato.-venereol. 17:444 (1936).
15. W. B. Shelly, Apocrine sweat, J. Invest. Dermat. 17:255 (1951).
16. K. Ikeuchi and Y. Kuno, On the regional differences of the perspiration of the human body, J. Orient. Med. 7:67 (1927).

17. H. S. Margolius, D. Horwitz, R. G. Geller, R. W. Alexander, J. R. Gill, Jr., J. J. Pisano and H. R. Keiser, Urinary kallikrein excretion in normal man: relationships to sodium intake and sodium retaining steroids, _Circ. Res._ 35:812 (1974).

18. J. W. Conn and M. W. Johnston, Salt economy of sweat glands under conditions of hard work in a tropical climate, _J. Clin. Invest._ 23:933 (1944).

19. R. J. Grand, P. A. di Sant'Agnese, R. C. Talamo and J. C. Pallavicini, The effects of exogenous aldosterone on sweat electrolytes, _J. Ped._ 70:346 (1967).

20. A. W. Cuthbert (personal communication).

21. J. Lieberman and G. D. Littenberg, Increased kallikrein content of saliva from patients with cystic fibrosis of the pancreas, _Pediatr. Res._ 3:571 (1969).

22. E. R. Hare and J. A. Verpoorte, Comparative studies on salivary kallikrein from cystic fibrosis patients and controls, _Pediatr. Res._ 19: 938 (1985).

23. O. L. Catanzaro, M. I. Vaccaro, S. B. Vila, A. L. Martinez Seeber and O. H. Pivetta, Kallikrein and amylase contents in tissues from a mutant mouse model for human cystic fibrosis, _Life Sci._ 32:825 (1983).

SIGNIFICANCE OF TISSUE KALLIKREIN IN CHRONIC ATROPHIC GASTRITIS

T. Sakai,* S. Otsuka,* K. Kizuki** and H. Moriya**

*1st Department of Internal Medicine, Toho University School
of Medicine, Omori-nishi 5-21-16, Ota-ku, Tokyo 143, Japan
and **Department of Biochemistry, Faculty of Pharmaceutical
Sciences, Science University of Tokyo, 12, Ichigaya-
funakawara-machi, Shinjuku-ku, Tokyo 162, Japan

SUMMARY

Seventy patients were diagnosed to have chronic atrophic gastritis,
because an atrophic border was distinguished by the endoscopic Congo red
method. The atrophic border was furthermore classified into the closed type
and the open type. Specimens of the gastric mucosa were obtained by biopsy
to measure tissue kallikrein as a marker of inflammation. The sandwich-type
ELISA showed that kallikrein significantly increased with the extension of
the atrophic area. Histopathological investigations also revealed that
kallikrein markedly increased with the appearance of intestinal metaplasia.
The peroxidase-antiperoxidase method located (1) a large amount of
kallikrein in the mucous granules which filled the goblet cells found in the
mucosa showing intestinal mataplasia and (2) a small amount discharged into
lumens. These findings suggested that atrophy of the gastric mucosa might
be an inflammatory change, and that the kallikrein-kinin system might be
associated with gastric inflammation regardless of the pathological stage.

INTRODUCTION

An atrophic change in the gastric mucosa is pathologically thought to
be an inflammatory change. However, many investigators insist that it is
basically an involutional change. The concept of chronic atrophic gastritis
still remains unclear. This study was designed to measure tissue kallikrein
as a marker for inflammation and find a key to the elucidation of this
disease from biochemical and histopathological aspects.

MATERIALS AND METHODS

Seventy patients were studied, who were diagnosed to have chronic
atrophic gastritis because an atrophic border was distinguished by the
endoscopic Congo red method (Okuda, 1977). The atrophic border was
furthermore classified into the closed type and the open type according to
the endoscopic atrophic patterns devised by Kimura and Takemoto (1969). As
a result, the atrophic border was proved to be of closed type in 20 patients
and of open type in 22 patients. Fundus glands were intact to a

considerable extent in the remaining 28 patients. Biopsy was performed
using a fiberscope under direct vision to take 5 specimens/patient (about 20
mg each) for kallikrein determination from the lesser curvature of the
corpus. The specimens were immediately kept at 4°C and their weight was
exactly measured. Thereafter, they were temporarily frozen until use for
test. One ml of Tris HCl buffer (pH 8.0) was added to the thawed specimens
at 4°C. After that, the specimens were homogenized using a teflon
homogenizer of Potter-Elvehjem at 340 r.p.m. for 1 minute. The homogenate
thus obtained were filtered using Millex HA microfilter (0.45 μm, Millipore
Japan Ltd.). The filtrate thus obtained was used to quantitatively
determine tissue kallikrein by the sandwich-type ELISA according to Suzuki
et al. (1986). Statistical analysis was performed using Student's t test to
compare the amount of tissue kallikrein in the atrophic area with that in
the intact fundus gland area.

The specimens obtained from 40 of the 70 patients were histo-
pathologically classified into the following 4 stages by modifying the
method of Ito et al. (1984): (I) almost normal, (II) decrease of gastric
glands and slight infiltration of inflammatory cells, (III) decrease of
gastric glands and marked infiltration of inflammatory cells, and (IV)
disappearance of gastric glands, moderate infiltration of inflammatory cells
and marked intestinal metaplasia. The relationship between this
histopathological classification and tissue kallikrein was also
investigated.

One spcimen was stained using the peroxidase-antiperoxidase (PAP)
method to locate tissue kallikrein in the microstructure of the gastric
mucosa.

Results

Mean tissue kallikrein in the atrophic area was significantly about 12
times higher than that in the fundus gland area, coming to 228.7 ng/g of
tissue. A further analysis revealed that mean tissue kallikrein levels in
the closed type and the open type were significantly about 4.8 times
($p < 0.05$) and about 19.3 times ($p < 0.001$) higher than that in the fundus
gland area, respectively. It should be noted that mean tissue kallikrein in
the open type was significantly about 4 times higher than that in the closed
type ($p < 0.01$) (Fig. 1).

Most specimens obtained from the fundus gland area were histo-
pathologically almost normal. On the other hand, intestinal metaplasia was
found in most specimens obtained from the atrophic area of the open type.
Tissue kallikrein was proved to become markedly high with the appearance of
intestinal metaplasia (Table 1).

The PAP method demonstrated that a large amount of tissue kallikrein
was present in the mucous granules (indicated by an arrow) which filled the
goblet cells found in the mucosa showing intestinal metaplasia, and that a
small amount of tissue kallikrein was discharged into lumens (Fig. 2).

Discussion

Otsuka et al. (1981) reported that tissue kallikrein appeared at the
early stage of water immersion-induced stress ulcer in rats, and suggested
that it might play an important role in the course of acute gastric
inflammation. In the present study, tissue kallikrein was also found in
patients with chronic atrophic gastritis. To our knowledge, this is the
first report that showed the presence of tissue kallikrein in the human
gastric mucosa obtained by biopsy.

In this study, atrophy was macroscopically demonstrated by the
endoscopic Congo red method. Tissue kallikrein was proved to increase with
the extension of atrophy. Furthermore, the largest amount of tissue

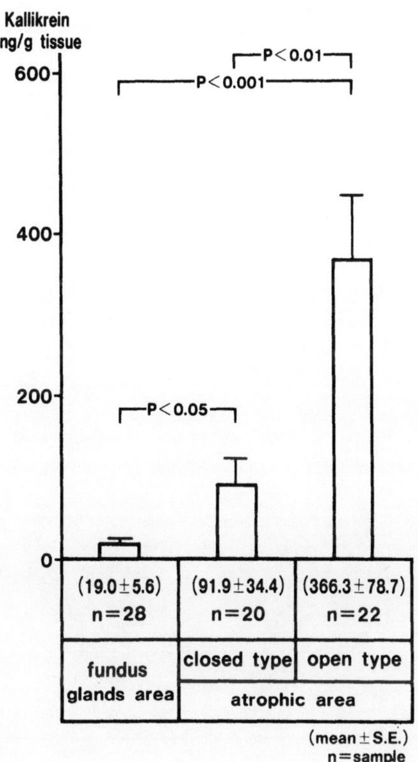

Fig. 1   Relationship between tissue kallikrein of gastric
mucosa and development of gastric mucosal atrophy

Table 1   Relationship between tissue kallikrein of gastric mucosa and development of intestinal metaplasia

	normal	inflammatory cell infiltration (slight)	inflammatory cell infiltration (marked)	intestinal metaplasia inflammatory cell infiltration
fundus glands	35.1 (n=9)	(n=0)	0.0 (n=2)	
closed type	23.5 (n=2)	48.7 (n=3)	(n=0)	173.2 (n=5)
open type	(n=0)	(n=0)	21.0 (n=4)	424.5 (n=15)

tissue kallikrein of gastric mucosa : ng/g tissue

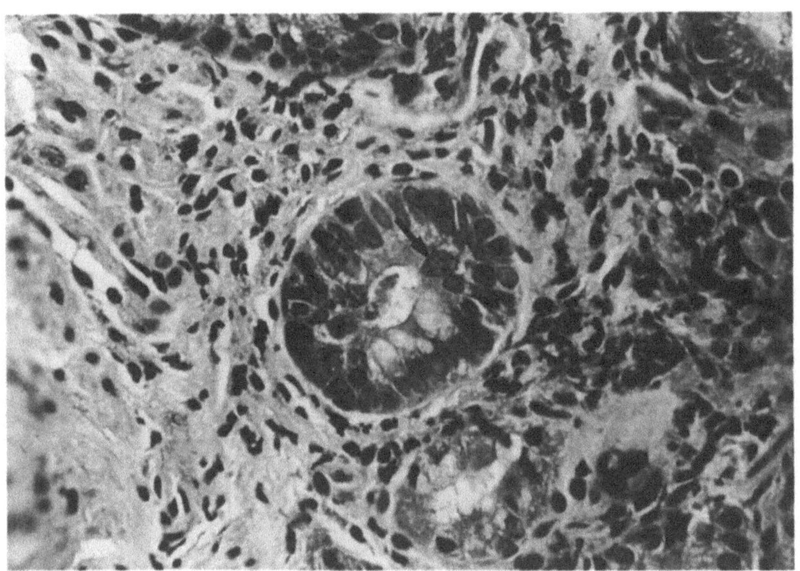

Fig. 2   Tissue kallikrein located in goblet cells by the PAP method

kallikrein was shown to be present when inflammation came to the final stage
with the appearance of intestinal metaplasia.

Since kinin is released by kallikrein into blood and makes blood
vessels hyperpermeable, the above findings suggest that atrophy in chronic
gastritis is an inflammatory change.

Uetsuji et al. (1981) demonstrated that the presence of tissue
kallikrein in the stomach obtained by resection from a patient with duodenal
ulcer. Although there is difference in pathology, animal species etc., the
findings so far obtained suggest that the kallikrein-kinin system may be
involved in the course of inflammation.

REFERENCES

Ito, M., Sato, N., and Kudo, M., 1984, The effects of vagotomy on the
    gastric mucosa activity, Japan Practical Surg. Soc., 45(1):1 (Jpn).
Kimura, K., and Takemoto, T., 1969, An endoscopic recognition of the
    atrophic border and its significance in chronic gastritis, Endoscopy,
    3:87.
Okuda, S., 1977, Measurement of gastric acid secretion by endoscopy, J.
    Adult Diseases, 7:49 (Jpn).
Otsuka, S., Suzuki, Y., Yoshida, M., Yoshida, R., and Igarashi, N., 1981,
    Correlation between glandular kallikrein and the course of
    experimental gastric ulcers in rats, Proceedings of the 3rd
    International Congress on Kinin, 384.
Suzuki, S., Ikekita, M., Kizuki, K., and Moriya, H., 1986, Measurement by
    EIA of tissue kallikrein present in human blood and its clinical
    application, Proceedings of the 26th Annual Meeting of Japan Society
    of Physical Chemistry (Jpn).
Uetsuji, S., Yamamura, M., Yamamoto, M., Uchida, K., Kushiro, H., Kodama,
    J., and Fujii, S., 1981, Human stomach kallikrein, Agent and Actions,
    (supl.) 137.

STUDIES ON THE INTESTINAL ABSORPTION OF TISSUE KALLIKREIN

Edwin Fink*, Xu–Chang Feng** and Elmar Richter**

Abteilung für Klinische Chemie und Klinische Biochemie in der
Chirurgischen Klinik Innenstadt* and Walther–Straub–Institut für
Pharmakologie and Toxikologie** der Universität München

INTRODUCTION

It has recently been reported that enteral administration of tissue
kallikrein (pig pancreatic kallikrein) can have an improving effect in
several pathologic disorders such as an increase in sperm output and sperm
motility in asthenozoospermia and oligozoospermia (1) and a decrease of
blood pressure in essential hypertension (2). These findings suggest that
tissue kallikrein can be absorbed intestinally in a biologically active
form. That this is indeed the case was recently shown by other groups and
by us (3,4,5). Here we present results on the intestinal absorption of
enzymatically active tissue kallikrein obtained with a new experimental
model.

METHODS

Perfusion of Intestinal Segments

Female Sprague–Dawley rats (270–310 g body weight) fasted for 18 h
were operated as described by Windmueller and Spaeth (6). Briefly, the rats
were anesthetized with urethane (0.8 g/kg, i.p.) and the mesenterial vein
draining a 8–10 cm segment of ileum as well as the jugular vein and the carotid artery were cannulated. Ligatures were secured around each end of the
selected segment. 0.2, 1.0 or 5.0 mg pig pancreatic kallikrein in 0.5 ml
saline was injected into the closed loop. In control experiments C-14 labeled polyethylene glycol 4000 (50 nCi) was administered together with 0.5
ml saline or 5 mg kallikrein. Blood was collected from the intestinal vein
for 60 min in 5 min fractions. The blood lost was replaced by infusion of
heparinized blood of donor rats into the jugular vein.

Analytical Procedures

Immunoreactive porcine pancreatic kallikrein was determined by a radioimmunoassay (7). Kininogenase activities were measured by assaying the
kinin released upon incubation of an aliquot of the respective sample with
partially purified kininogen (8).

Gel filtration experiments were performed using an Ultrogel AcA 44
column, 0.9 x 115 cm, eluted at a flow rate of 4.0 ml/h with 15 mM NaH_2PO4,

0.15 M NaCl, 0.01 M EDTA, 2 g NaN$_3$/l, pH 7.4. Fractions of 0.9 ml were
collected and analyzed for kininogenase activity and immunoreactive pig
pancreatic kallikrein.

RESULTS

Complex Formation of Pig Pancreatic Kallikrein (PPK) with Rat Plasma Components

Single plasma samples obtained during the absorption experiments were
subjected to gel filtration. Immunoreactive PPK was eluted in three peaks
(Fig. 1). The peak maxima at fractions 32, 40 and 54 correspond to molecular masses of $>$130, 82 and 32 kDa. Since PPK has a molecular mass around 32
kDa the two peaks corresponding to higher molecular masses obviously represent complexes of PPK with components of rat plasma.

The immunoreactivities of the three species of PPK were not identical:
when serial dilutions of single fractions of the three peaks were measured
by radioimmunoassay the slopes of dose-response curves of the two complexes
were not identical and they were also different from the slope of the standard curve.

The relative amounts of immunoreactive PPK eluted in the three peaks
varied when different plasma samples were subjected to gel filtration. It
seems that the complex formation depends on different concentrations of the
complex forming components of the individual rat plasmas or on not con-
trollable conditions during sample preparation.

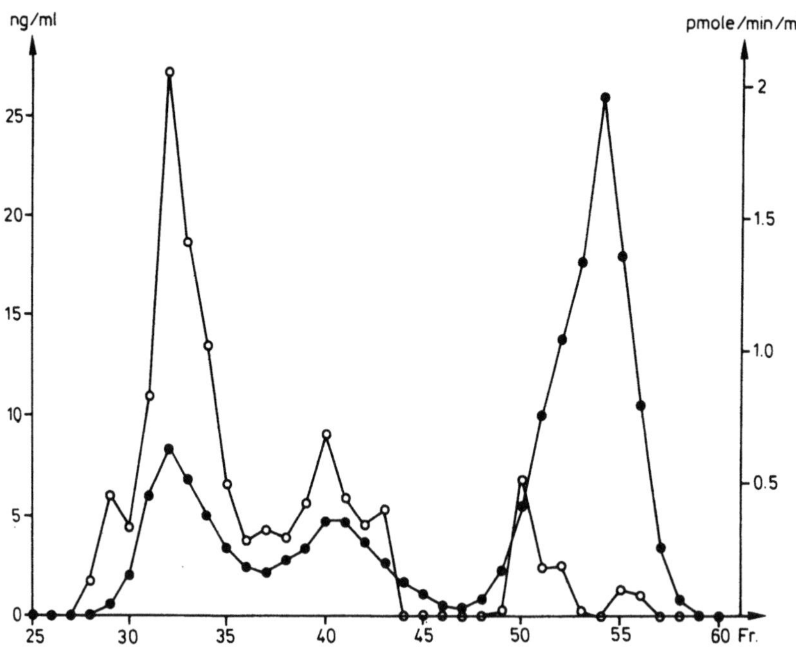

Fig. 1 Gel filtration of a sample of mesenteric venous plasma
        containing absorbed pig pancreatic kallikrein. The
        fractions were assayed for immunoreactive kallikrein
        (filled circles) and for kininogenase activity (open
        circles).

Kininogenase activity was also eluted in three peaks (Fig. 1), the highest activity was contained in the immunoreactivity peaks corresponding to the complexes, almost no activity was found in the peak of presumably free PPK (around fraction 54). The "free" PPK present in the sample obviously represents to a high degree an enzymatically inactive form, the active PPK is almost completely bound to plasma components. No kininogenase peaks were detectable when an identical gel filtration experiment was performed with a plasma sample which did not contain pig pancreatic kallikrein.

Radioimmunoassay of PPK in Rat Plasma

As a consequence of the complex formation the concentrations of PPK measured by radioimmunoassay are too low. This was shown by recovery experiments.

PPK was incubated with rat plasma in concentrations between 2 and 50 ng/ml and the PPK concentration determined by radioimmunoassay. The recoveries ranged between 25 and 8 percent. Thus, since the recoveries are dose dependent, a correction of the values is not possible.

Taken together, PPK and rat plasma components react under formation of complexes which have immunoreactivities different from and lower than free PPK. As a result, the value obtained as PPK concentration by radioimmunoassay varies with the dilution at which the sample is assayed and is significantly lower than the true PPK concentration in the sample. In addition, the ratio of the amounts of the three immunoreactive PPK species may vary from sample to sample, thus, even if the true concentrations of PPK in different plasma samples are identical the concentrations determined by radioimmunoassay may still be different.

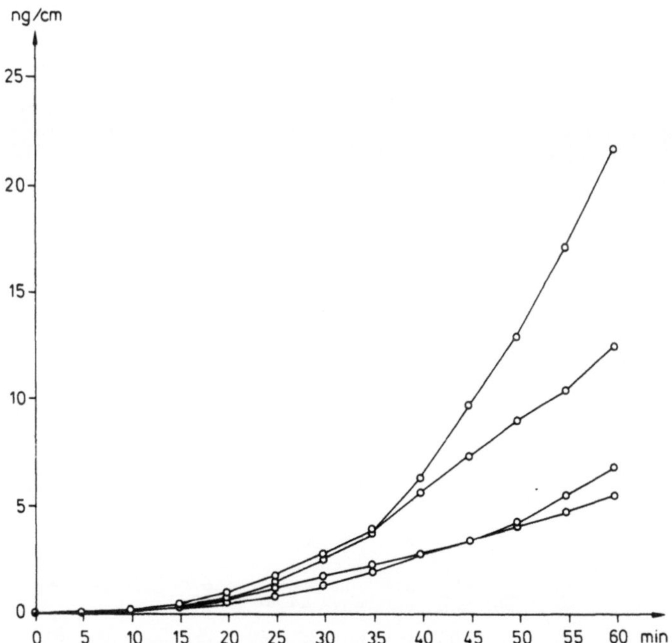

Fig. 2 Cumulative amount of pig pancreatic kallikrein in mesenterial venous blood of an intestinal segment after administration of 1.0 mg (four identically performed experiments, the amount of absorbed kallikrein is calculated per cm of the intestinal segment).

At present, these difficulties cannot be overcome and no other, more reliable method to determine low concentrations of PPK in rat plasma is at hand. Therefore, in spite of the problems just presented we used the radioimmunoassay procedure in our studies. However, one has to keep in mind that the concentrations determined represent "immunoreactivity equivalents" and not the true PPK concentrations. The true PPK concentrations will be significantly higher (certainly by a factor of ten) than the values presented here.

<u>Intestinal Absorption of Porcine Pancreatic Kallikrein</u>

Porcine pancreatic kallikrein was administered at dose levels of 0.2, 1.0 and 5.0 mg. When 0.2 mg were administered, only in one out of six experiments absorption of PPK was detectable whereas at doses 1.0 mg and 5.0 mg only one experiment out of eight and nine, respectively, was negative. The amount absorbed during one hour per 1 cm of ileum was 2.6 ng for dose 0.26 mg, up to 22 ng for dose 1.0 mg and up to 248 ng for dose 5.0 mg. Thus, in spite of the high variability of absorption a dose dependency is clearly recognizable. The time course of intestinal absorption for dose levels 1.0 and 5.0 mg is shown in Figs. 2 and 3.

The highest amount absorbed in one of the experiments was 0.05 % of the administered dose. However, one has to consider that this amount was absorbed by only 10 cm of ileum whereas the total length of rat small intestine is about 100 cm and that the shape of the curves clearly demonstrates that the absorption was still in progress at the end of the experiment. In addition, as discussed above, the PPK concentrations in the plasma samples are highly underestimated by the radioimmunoassay.

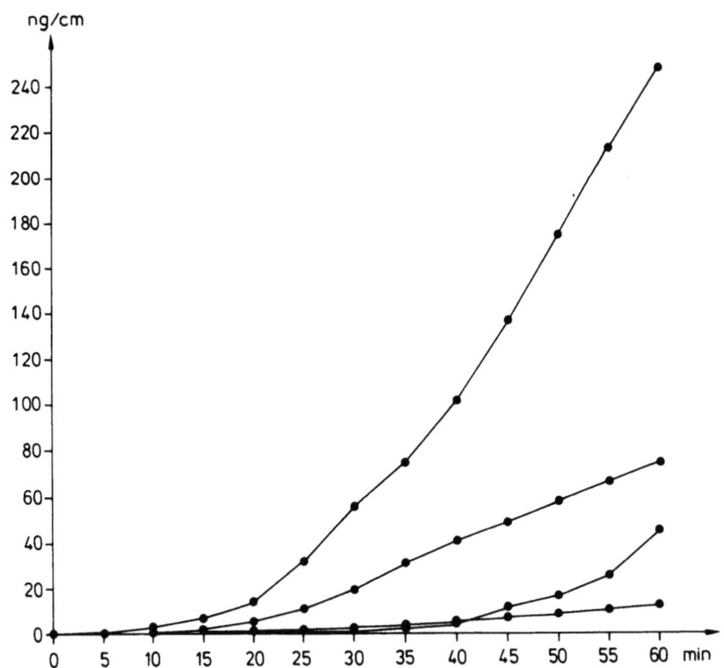

Fig. 3 Cumulative amount of pig pancreatic kallikrein in mesenterial venous blood of an intestinal segment after administration of 5.0 mg (four identically performed experiments, the amount of absorbed kallikrein is calculated per cm of the intestinal segment).

In a control experiment C-14 labelled PEG 4000 was administered together with 5 mg kallikrein. Only about 0.8 % of the radioactivity were
found in the blood which is in the same range as in the absence of kallikrein. Thus, neither the experimental procedure nor the presence of the
tissue kallikrein caused any significant unspecific permeability increase
of the intestinal wall for high molecular substances.

DISCUSSION

Earlier investigations (3-5) have shown that intestinal absorption of
tissue kallikrein is possible and some evidence has been presented suggesting that the absorbed kallikrein is to some degree still enzymatically
active.

The experimental model employed here will allow to study the intestinal absorption of tissue kallikrein on a fully quantitative basis as soon
as the problems of the radioimmunoassay can be overcome. The model is well
established for studies on the absorption of small molecules and seems to
be equally well suited for investigations on the tissue kallikrein absorption though further control experiments will be necessary to confirm that
the observed absorption is not an artefact of the experimental setup.

The present studies corroborate the earlier findings (3-4) and demonstrate clearly that tissue kallikrein can indeed be absorbed in an enzymatically active form. Virtually all of the active tissue kallikrein is bound
to plasma components, but these kallikrein complexes still display kininogenase activity. It is not clear whether this kininogenase activity is intrinsic or due to a partial dissociation of the complexes under the conditions of our assay.

At present, nothing is known on the nature and the physiological function of the complex forming proteins. One might speculate that they act
both as inhibitors and as carriers for tissue kallikreins preventing undesirable kinin release during the transport to the target site.

Compared to the administered dose the fraction of absorbed tissue kallikrein was quite low and it may be regarded as questionable whether such
small amounts can exert the pharmacological effects observed in human. However, for the treatment of asthenozoospermia and oligozoospermia as well as
of essential hypertension the tissue kallikrein is administered orally for
at least several weeks and under these conditions a pharmacologically active level may build up.

ACKNOWLEDGMENTS

This work was supported by the Deutsche Forschungsgemeinschaft, Sonderfor-
schungsbereich 207, B2. Pig pancreatic kallikrein was kindly provided by
Dr. P. Huber, Bayer AG, Wuppertal, FRG. We are very grateful to Mrs. G.
Godec and Mrs. C. Hirschauer for their excellent technical assistance.

REFERENCES

1. Schill, W.-B., Kinin-releasing pancreatic proteinase kallikrein. In:
   "Treatment of male infertility", J. Bain, W.-B. Schill and L. Schwarz-
   stein, eds., Springer-Verlag, Heidelberg, pp.125-142, (1982).

2. Overlack, A., K. O. Stumpe, R. Kolloch, C. Ressel, and F. Krueck, Anti-hypertensive effect of orally administered glandular kallikrein in essential hypertension. Results of a double blind study. Hypertension 3, Supp. 1:18-21, (1981).

3. Moriwaki, C., K. Yamaguchi, and H. Moriya, Studies on kallikreins. III. Intra-intestinal administration of hog pancreatic kallikrein and its appearance in the perfusate from the mesenteric vein. Chem. Pharm. Bull. 22:1975-1980, (1980).

4. Fink, E., R. Geiger, J. Witte, S. Biedermann, J. Seifert, and H. Fritz, Biochemical, pharmacological, and functional aspects of glandular kallikreins. In: "Enzymatic release of vasoactive peptides", F. Gross and G. Vogel, eds., Raven Press, New York, pp. 101-115, (1980).

5. Overlack, A., A. G. Scicli, and O. Carretero, Intestinal absorption of glandular kallikrein in the rat. Am. J. Physiol. 244:G689-G694, (1983).

6. Windmueller, H. G., and A. E. Spaeth, Vascular autoperfusion of rat small intestine in situ. Meth. Enzymol. 77:120-129, (1981).

7. Fink, E., and C. Güttel, Development of a radioimmunoassay for pig pancreatic kallikrein. J. Clin. Chem. Clin. Biochem. 16:381-385, (1979).

8. Fink, E., W.-B. Schill, F. Fiedler, F. Krassnigg, R. Geiger, and K. Shimamoto, Tissue kallikrein of human seminal plasma is secreted by the prostate gland. Biol. Chem. Hoppe-Seyler 366:917-924, (1985).

THE EFFECTS OF DIABETES AND INSULIN ON COLONIC TISSUE KALLIKREIN

Ayad A. Jaffa, Donald H. Miller, Harry S. Margolius, and
Ronald K. Mayfield

Departments of Medicine and Pharmacology, Medical University
of South Carolina and Veterans Administration Medical Center
Charleston, South Carolina, USA

INTRODUCTION

Gastrointestinal dysfunction is a frequent complication of diabetes
mellitus (1). Although disturbed gastrointestinal motility is thought to
be a major underlying cause of the diarrhea which frequently develops, recent studies show that impaired absorption of fluid and electrolytes occur
in the ileum and colon of streptozotocin-diabetic rats (2,3). Moreover,
insulin can stimulate ion transport in the colon, and receptors for insulin
have been identified in isolated normal rabbit colonic epithelia as well as
cultured human colonic tumor cells (4-6).

Tissue kallikrein and kinins are potent stimuli to ion transport across
several gastrointestinal epithelia, including the small intestine, colon and
gall bladder (7-9). We have recently discovered that the diabetic state
alters, and insulin regulates, the level and synthesis of kallikrein in the
kidney tubule, another site where kallikrein may function in water and
electrolyte transport (10). For these reasons, we investigated the effects
of diabetes and insulin on colonic kallikrein levels and synthesis rate.

METHODS

Male Sprague-Dawley rats (Charles River Laboratories, Inc., Wilmington,
MA) weighing 170-200 g were used in these studies. Rats were housed 4-
5/cage, and had free access to water and regular chow. Diabetes was induced
in 63 rats by a single intravenous injection of streptozotocin (STZ), 65
mg/kg body weight. Control rats (n=24) were not injected. After 24 h
diabetes was confirmed in STZ-treated rats by tail vein plasma glucose
levels. Plasma glucose was also measured in control rats at the same time.
Fourteen days after the injection of STZ, diabetic rats were divided into 3
groups. One group was not treated and the other two groups were treated
with insulin, 8 units regular, subcutaneously, and then killed 2.5 h or 5 h
after insulin treatment. The normal controls, diabetic and insulin-treated
diabetic rats were all injected with ^{35}S-methionine (1 µCi/g body weight,
i.p.), twenty minutes before being killed to measure kallikrein synthesis
rate.

The descending colon was removed, opened and rinsed free of luminal
content. The kidneys were removed and perfused via the renal hilus with
10 ml iced cold 0.9% saline. Both tissues were subsequently stored at

-20°C. The tissues were homogenized and extracted with deoxycholate as
previously described (10), for measurement of protein, kallikrein and kallikrein synthesis rate. Kallikrein was measured by radioimmunoassay incorporating a monoclonal antibody that recognizes only the active enzyme (11).
Prokallikrein was measured following its conversion to active enzyme by trypsin treatment, as previously described in detail (10). The in vivo kallikrein synthesis rate was measured by the method of Miller et al. (12).
Tissue protein was measured by the method of Lowry et al. (13).

Table 1. **Plasma glucose levels (mg/dl) in control, diabetic and insulin-
treated diabetic rats**

| | Day 1 | Day 14[a] | | |
		Pre-insulin	Post-insulin 2.5h	Post-insulin 5.0h
Control (n=24)	113 ± 2	118 ± 3		
Diabetic (n=24)	400 ± 20^b	476 ± 20^b		
Diabetic (n=16)	369 ± 25^b	471 ± 24^b	59 ± 9^c	
Diabetic (n=23)	363 ± 16^b	434 ± 19^b		258 ± 31^c

[a] Rats treated with insulin received 8.0 units regular insulin subcutaneously.
[b] $P < 0.001$ vs control
[c] $P < 0.001$ vs pre-insulin

RESULTS

Table 1 shows the plasma glucose levels in the control and diabetic
rats. One day after STZ injection (day 1) the diabetic rats showed hyper-
glycemia, which persisted over two weeks. On day 14, the diabetic rats
treated with 8 units of regular insulin and killed after 2.5 h showed a
marked reduction in plasma glucose level. Plasma glucose levels in diabetic
rats killed 5 h after insulin injection were also lowered, compared to pretreatment levels, but increased from levels at 2.5 h.

Colonic levels of prokallikrein and active kallikrein are shown in
Figure 1. In normal rats prokallikrein comprises more than 90% of the total
tissue kallikrein in the colon. After two weeks, diabetic rats showed a
44% reduction in colonic prokallikrein level, compared to control rats.
Active kallikrein was not significantly reduced. Following acute administration of insulin to diabetic rats, prokallikrein levels increased, and by
5 h prokallikrein in insulin-treated rats was significantly greater (38%)
than levels in untreated diabetic rats. In contrast, active kallikrein,
which was not significantly reduced by the diabetic state, fell markedly
2.5 h after insulin administration. At 2.5 h active kallikrein was only 50%
of the level in untreated diabetic rats and was 36% of the mean level in
normal rats. However, after 5 h, active kallikrein had risen and was not
significantly lower than the level in untreated diabetic rats, but remained

lower than control rat levels. This rise in active kallikrein occurred as
prokallikrein was also rising. All of these changes in kallikrein were observed in rats in which plasma glucose did not fall below normal.

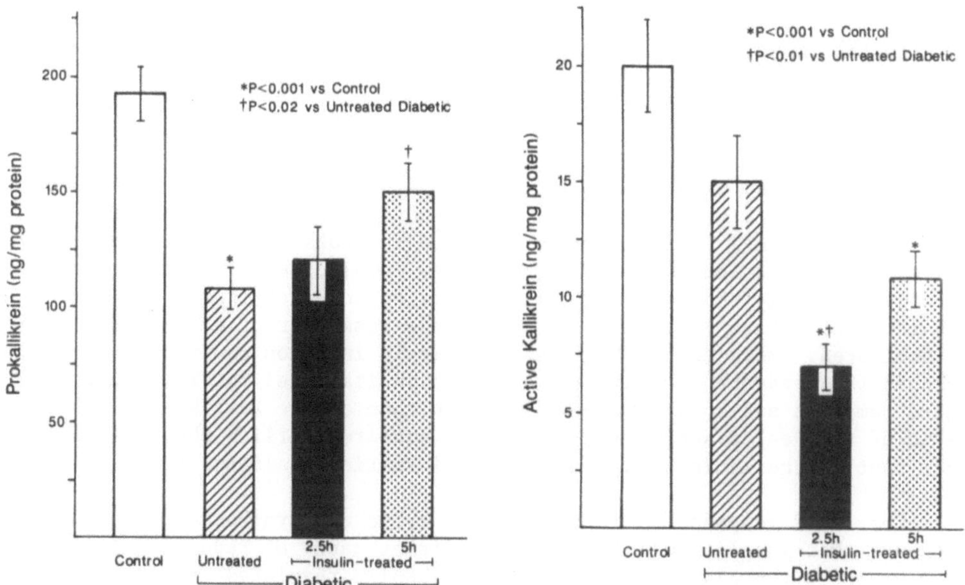

Figure 1.   Colonic prokallikrein and active kallikrein in control and
diabetic rats.

To examine the mechanism for these changes, the relative rate of prokallikrein synthesis in the colon was measured (Figure 2). Prokallikrein
synthesis showed a trend towards reduction in the diabetic rats, but this
was not statistically significant. However, 2.5 h after insulin treatment,
prokallikrein synthesis increased 50% over the rate in untreated diabetic
rats. By 5 h after insulin, synthesis had returned to a rate which was
nearly the same as in the untreated diabetic rats. This rapid increase in
prokallikrein synthesis preceded the rise in tissue prokallikrein level.

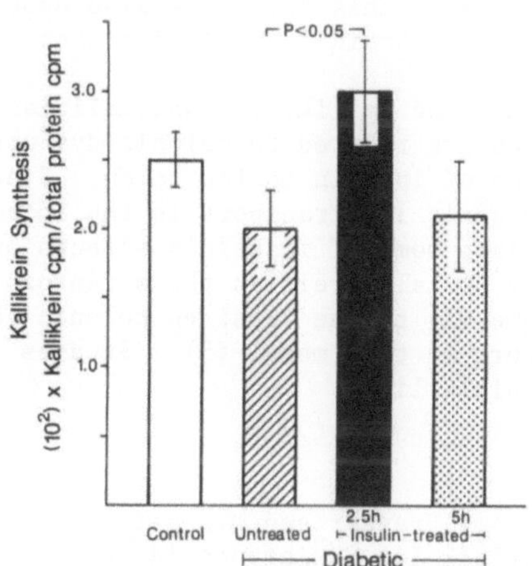

Figure 2.   Prokallikrein synthesis in the colon of control and diabetic rats.

We also examined the effect of acute insulin administration on active
and prokallikrein in the kidney, a tissue in which prokallikrein synthesis
and activation is impaired by the diabetic state (10). As previously observed, active renal kallikrein was reduced in diabetic rats compared to
normal controls (24.7 ± 2.1 vs. 54.7 ± 2.9 ng/mg protein, P < 0.001), and
prokallikrein was unchanged (24.3 ± 1.9 vs. 24.4 ± 3.1 ng/mg protein).
Over 5 h, neither active nor prokallikrein levels in the kidney were changed
by insulin treatment. Active renal kallikrein in diabetic rats, 5 h after
insulin treatment, was 30.0 ± 1.7 ng/mg protein, and prokallikrein was 23.3
± 2.7 ng/mg protein.

DISCUSSION

In this study we have shown that the diabetic state results in reduced
tissue prokallikrein in the distal colon and insulin rapidly restores the
level toward normal by inducing an increase in prokallikrein synthesis. Despite a 50% reduction in prokallikrein, the level of active kallikrein was
not significantly reduced. This may be due to the fact that, relative to
the level of active enzyme, there is a large reservoir of prokallikrein to
be activated. More than 90% of the kallikrein in colon is zymogen, and
even in the presence of a marked reduction in its level in diabetic rats
there remained six-fold more prokallikrein than active kallikrein. This
ratio of zymogen to active enzyme content confirms earlier observations
that most of the kinin-forming enzyme in intestine is latent (14).

The rapid response of prokallikrein levels and synthesis to insulin
suggests that insulin deficiency is the direct cause of reduced colonic
kallikrein in the diabetic rats and that insulin regulates colonic kallikrein. The 50% increase in prokallikrein synthesis in the colon following
insulin represents the largest and most rapid increase in kallikrein synthesis yet observed (10,12). We also reported that insulin replacement
increases prokallikrein synthesis in the diabetic kidney, but the effect
was seen over days (10). In the present study, the lack of an acute change
in renal kallikrein levels following insulin replacement is consistent with
those earlier findings.

The notion that insulin regulates colonic kallikrein is reasonable in
view of the action of insulin on renal kallikrein and the finding that colonic epithelia possess insulin receptors which physiologically respond like
insulin receptors in other target tissues (5). Furthermore, a human colonic
cancer cell line (HT29) also has insulin receptors, and both protein and RNA
synthesis are increased in these cells within two hours of exposure to insulin (15). A derivative of this cell line also appears to make considerable amounts of tissue kallikrein (unpublished observation).

It is uncertain how the kallikrein abnormalities and regulation we have
discovered in the colon are related to colonic dysfunction in diabetes or
the physiologic actions of insulin in the colon. Since kallikrein and kinins stimulate electrogenic ion transport in the intact colon, it is possible that they may mediate some of insulin's effects on colonic ion transport
(4,7). The deficiency of kallikrein in the streptozotocin-diabetic rat may
also be related in some way to the impaired colonic absorption of fluid and
electrolytes that occurs in this model (3). Studies in isolated cell models
may clarify these possible links.

ACKNOWLEDGEMENTS

We wish to thank Amy Frayser and Michael Bigelow for technical assistance and Barbara Whitlock for assistance in preparing the manuscript. This
work was supported by a grant from the National Institute of Diabetes,
Digestive and Kidney Disease, DK 35977, and the Veterans Administration.

REFERENCES

1. M. Feldman and L. R. Schiller, Disorders of gastrointestinal motility associated with diabetes mellitus, Ann. Intern. Med. 98:378 (1983).
2. R. N. Fedorak, M. Field and E. B. Chang, Treatment of diabetic diarrhea with clonidine, Ann. Intern. Med. 102:197 (1985).
3. E. B. Chang, R. M. Bergenstal and M. Field, Diarrhea in streptozotocin-treated rats. Loss of adrenergic regulation of intestinal fluid and electrolyte transport, J. Clin. Invest. 75:1666 (1985).
4. J. Crabbe, Insulin, glucagon and active transport: from man to amphibia and back, in: "Transport mechanisms in epithelia", H. H. Ussing and N. A. Thorn, ed., Academic Press, New York (1972).
5. D. J. Pillion, V. Garapathy and F. H. Leibach, Identification of insulin receptors on the mucosal surface of colon epithelial cells, J. Biol. Chem. 260:5244 (1985).
6. K. G. Mountjoy, I. M. Holdaway and G. J. Finlay, Insulin receptor regulation in cultured human tumor cells, Cancer Res. 43:4537 (1983).
7. A. W. Cuthbert and H. S. Margolius, Kinins stimulate net chloride secretion by the rat colon, Br. J. Pharmacol. 75:587 (1982).
8. A. W. Cuthbert, A. M. George and L. MacVinish, Kinin effects on electrogenic ion transport in primary cultures of pig renal papillary collecting tubule cells, Am. J. Physiol. 249:439 (1985).
9. A. W. Baird and H. S. Margolius, Bradykinin stimulates electrogenic bicarbonate secretion by guinea pig gall bladder, Br. J. Pharmacol. 91:369P (1987).
10. A. A. Jaffa, D. H. Miller, G. S. Bailey, J. Chao, H. S. Margolius and R. K. Mayfield, Abnormal regulation of renal kallikrein in experimental diabetes. Effects of insulin on prokallikrein synthesis and activation, J. Clin. Invest. 80:1651 (1987).
11. T. Ando, J. Chao, L. Chao and H. S. Margolius, An improved method for the measurement of rat tissue kallikrein using a monoclonal antibody which recognizes only active kallikrein, Adv. Exp. Biol. Med. 198B: 515 (1986).
12. D. H. Miller, J. Chao and H. S. Margolius, Tissue kallikrein synthesis and its modification by testosterone or low dietary sodium, Biochem. J. 218:37 (1984).
13. O. H. Lowry, N. J. Rosebrough, A. L. Farr and R. J. Randall, Protein measurement with the folin phenol reagent, J. Biol. Chem. 193:265 (1951).
14. I. J. Zeitlin, Pharmacological characterization of kinin-forming activity in rat intestinal tissue, Br. J. Pharmacol. 42:648 (1972).
15. J. Cezard, M. Forgue-Lafitte, M. Chamblier and G. Rosselin, Growth-promoting effect, biological activity, and binding of insulin in human intestinal cancer cells in culture, Cancer Res. 41:1148 (1981).

R. Tallman and L. K. Stahlar, Disorders of gastrointestinal motility associated with diabetes mellitus. Ann. Intern. Med. 98:378 (1983).

R. S. Fedoruk, H. Field and K. M. Chang, Treatment of diabetic diarrhea with clonidine. Ann. Intern. Med. 96:179 (1985).

L. D. Chang, K. M. Bergenthal and S. Blair, Diarrhea in streptozotocin treated rats, loss of adrenergic regulation of intestinal fluid and electrolyte transport. J. Clin. Invest.

THE EFFECTS OF HUMAN KALLIKREIN AND APROTININ ON NONMALIGNANT AND MALIGNANT

CELL GROWTH

M. Korbelik[1], J. Škrk[2], M. Poljak-Blaži[1], A. Suhar[3]
and M. Boranić[1]

[1]R. Bošković Institute, Zagreb; [2]The Institute of
Oncology Ljubljana; [3]J. Stefan Institute, Ljubljana
Yugoslavia

INTRODUCTION

Various exogenous proteinases, eg. trypsin, chymotrypsin and
thrombin, stimulate the growth of cells cultured in vitro (Scott 1987;
Chen and Buchanan 1975; Allen et al. 1981). The aim of this study was to
examine the effects of a urinary proteinase, kallikrein, and one of its
inhibitors, aprotinin, on the colony-forming ability of two cell li
nes: hamster fibroblasts (V79) and human laryngeal carcinoma cells (HEp),
and of human bone marrow cells in short-term culture. Effects on the activ
ity of intracellular proteinases (cysteine, serine and aspartic) of the
cells studied were also examined.

MATERIAL AND METHODS

Kallikrein from urine origin (Geiger et al., 1980) was kindly
provided by R.Geiger. Aprotinin is produced by Bayer Werk Inc.
The activities (concentrations) of agents tested in this work were chosen
from our experience gained in related studies (Korbelik et al., 1986;
Suhar et al., 1986).
Kallikrein and aprotinin were tested on the ability to affect clonal
growth of normal cells (Chinese hamster lung fibroblasts - V79, and human
bone marrow cells) and malignant cells (human carcinoma of the larynx -
HEp).

Monolayer cultures of Chinese hamster lung fibroblasts (V79),
representing non-malignant diploid cells, and malignant HEp cells (human
carcinoma of the larynx), were cultivated at 37°C in Eagle's Minimal
Essential Medium, supplemented with 10% foetal bovine serum (Gibco).
Synchronized populations of actively proliferating cells were obtained by
mitotic selection. Immediately after selection, mitotic cells were plated
for colony formation. Agents under study were added to the cell growth
medium for 1.5 hour intervals. With V79 cells the agents were applied
0-1.5 hours and 2.5-4 hours after the plating, and with HEp cells 0-1.5
hours and 8-9.5 hours after the plating, in order to coincide with M/G1 and
G1/S stage of the cell cycle or respective cells. After the termination of
1.5 hour incubation interval the treatment media were washed away and
replaced with fresh growth media. Samples were then incubated for 7 days
to allow for formation of macroscopic colonies. Non-proliferative (G0)
cells were maintained at contact inhibition of growth for 5 days before

the treatment with agents under study, which was 6 hours in this case. Cells were then harvested and either plated for colony formation, or used for the determination of specific activities of endogenous intracellular proteinases. In the latter case cells were concentrated by centrifugation, lysed in distilled water, sonicated and homogenized by Pierce homogenizer.

The activity of cysteine proteinases in the homogenate was determined using N-α-benzoyl-DL-arginine-1-naphtylamide (BANA) as substrate. Serine (neutral) proteinases activity was determined using 1% calf thymus histones as substrate at pH 7.5, while aspartic proteinases were followed using 2% bovine hemoglobin as substrate at pH 3.5.

Human bone marrow was obtained from healthy male donors. The short-term cultures in semisolid agar medium were prepared and grown for 10 days according to the original method described by Metcalf (1977) using enriched RPMI 1640 medium and placental growth factor. The aggregates consisting of more than 40 cells were scored as colonies, and smaller aggregates as clumps.

Aprotinin was added immediately before plating the cell suspension in complete growth medium and left in cultures throughout the growth of colonies. Kallikrein was added to the cells suspended in 0.3 ml of medium without serum and agar presented for one hour at 37°C. The medium was then completed with serum and agar in desired concentrations (final volume was 1.5 ml of medium per dish) and the cultures were further incubated for 10 days to obtain colonies.

The effect of kallikrein and aprotinin examined in this work were tested simultaneously on the same bone marrow specimen.

RESULTS AND CONCLUSION

The results of our study show that kallikrein (from human urine) stimulated colony-forming ability of human bone marrow cells, yielding in average 4.2 times more colonies compared to cultures without it (Fig.1a). In synchronized populations of V79 cells, stimulatory effect of kallikrein was most pronounced at the G1/S phase of the cell cycle (Fig.2a). Proteinase inhibitor interferred with colony-forming ability of human hemopoietic cells. Aprotinin, an inhibitor of kallikrein, was a weak inhib bitor of colony growth (Fig.1b). In synchronized populations of V79 cells, aprotinin was stimulatory (although less effective than kallikrein) (Fig.2a).

Effects of different concentrations of kallikrein and aprotinin on the colony-forming ability of V79 cells are seen in Fig.3.

In malignant HEp cell line, the effects of kallikrein and aprotinin were opposite to those in nonmalignant V79 cells. Kallikrein inhibited colony formation of HEp cells when added at the G1/S phase of the cell cycle (Fig.2b). Aprotinin inhibited colony formation of HEp cells at early G1, while with V79 cells at that phase it exerted stimulatory effect (Fig. 2b). Substances with such differential effects on normal and malignant cells may be of interest as potential chemotherapeutic agents.

Tested intracellular proteinase activities of V79 cells, incubated with kallikrein were decreased (Table I).

Thus the data show that kallikrein - although an extracellular proteinase by principal action, influences cellular proliferative activity. This supports the idea (Scott 1987) that extracellular or pericellular proteolysis is able to stimulate growth or division of cells, perhaps by means of a signal that crosses the cell membrane. Kallikrein seems to be able to modify the activity of membrane-bound or endogenous proteinase(s) of the cell. This might be coupled with activity of peptide growth factors and/or enzymes associated with them.

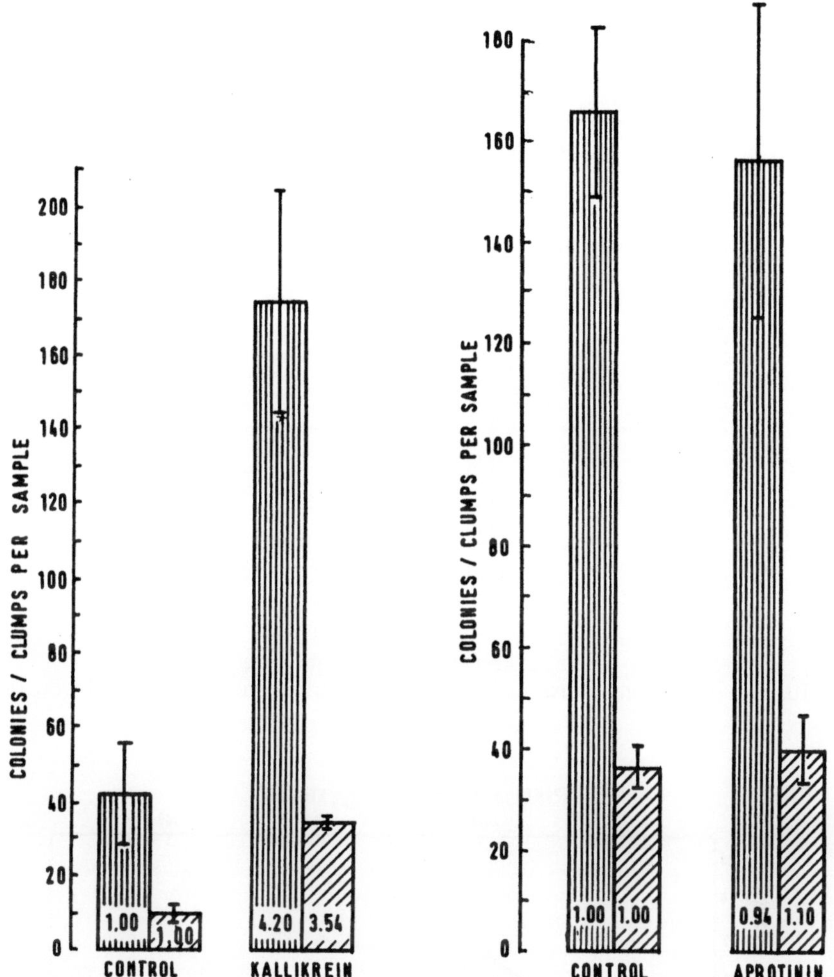

Fig.1. The effects of kallikrein (0.01 µg/ml - a) and kallikrein ihib
bitor aprotinin (10 KIU/ml - b) on colony formation of human bone
marrow cells. Proteinases were incubated with cells suspended in
serum-free medium for one hour at 37°C. Immediately serum and agar
solutions were added with rest of the medium, establishing growth
conditions for colony formation. 1.5×10^5 cells (a) and 2×10^5 cells
(b) in the final volume of 1.5 ml medium were seeded per dish. Each
of of twin columns represents number of colonies (left column) and
cell clumps (right column) scored after 10 days of culturing in
semi-solid medium. The numbers in columns are relative ratios of
colonies (clumps) in respective column/colonies (clumps) in control.
Each value is a mean of at least three identical samples (four
samples in control). Error bars represent standard deviations.

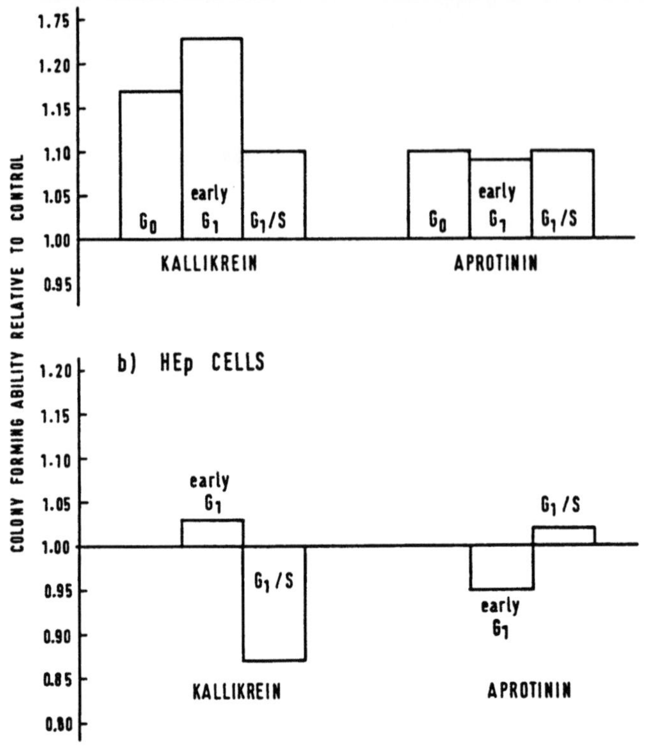

Fig.2. The effects of kallikrein (0.01 ug/ml) and aprotinin (10 KIU/ml) on colony forming ability of synchronized V79 and HEp cells.

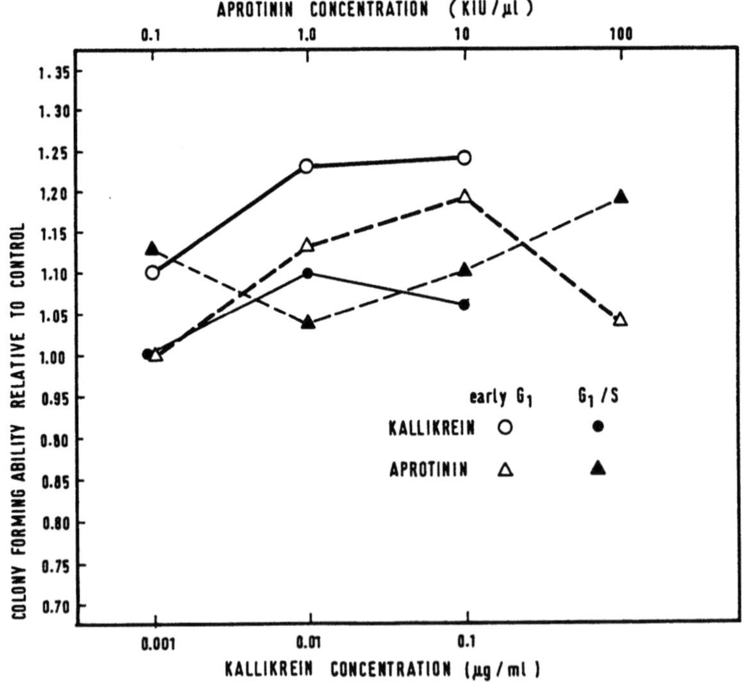

Fig.3. The effects of different concentrations of kallikrein and aprotinin on colony forming ability of V79 cells at specific points of the cell cycle.

Table I. The effects of proteinase and proteinase inhibitor added to the growth medium on endogenous proteinase activity in nonproliferating V79 cells.

AGENT	SPECIFIC ACTIVITY				
	Serine proteinases		Cysteine proteinases		Aspartic proteinases
	nmol Tyr/min mg protein	% control	nmol NA/min mg protein	% control	nmol Tyr/min mg protein
Control	0.72	1.00	2.55	1.00	0
Kallikrein (0.01 ug/ml)	0.31	0.43	2.17	0.85	0
Aprotinin (10 KIU/ml)	0.41	0.57	1.62	0.63	0.69

REFERENCES

Allen R.J., Rattray S., and Scott G.K., 1981, Preliminary evidence that
    thrombin may mimic a naturally occurring proteinase in cultured cells.
    Biosci.rep. 1: 881-884.
Chen L.B.,and Buchanan J.M., 1975, Mitogenic activity of blood components.
    I. Thrombin and prothrombin. Proc.nam.Acad.Sci.U.S.A. 72: 131-135.
Geiger R., Stuckstedte U., and Fritz H., 1980, Isolation and characterization
    of human urinary kallikrein. Hoppe-Seyler's Z.Physiol.Chem. 361: 10003-
    -1016..
Korbelik M., Škrk J., Suhar A., Schauer P., and Turk V., 1986, The role of
    intracellular proteinases in proliferative activities of mammalian cells
    in culture. Period.biol. 88: 142-144.
Metcalf H., 1977, Hemopoetic colonies (Recent Results in Cancer Research).
    Springer, Berlin.
Scott G.K., 1987, Proteinases and eukaryotic cell growth. Comp.Biochem.Physol.
    87B: 1-10.
Suhar A., Turk V., Korbelik M., Petrović D., Škrk J., and Schauer P., 1986,
    The role of cathepsins H and B, and inhibitors leupeptin and CPI in pro-
    liferative activities of non-malignant and malignant cells in culture.
    In: "Cysteine Proteinases and Their Inhibitors", V.Turk, ed., W. de
    Guyter, Berlin.

ACKNOWLEDGEMENT

    This work was supported by the research grant of the Research Council
of Slovenia.

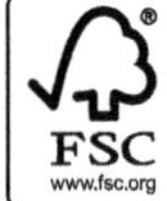

MIX
Papier aus verantwortungsvollen Quellen
Paper from responsible sources
FSC® C105338

If you have any concerns about our products,
you can contact us on
ProductSafety@springernature.com

In case Publisher is established outside the EU,
the EU authorized representative is:
Springer Nature Customer Service Center GmbH
Europaplatz 3, 69115 Heidelberg, Germany

Printed by Libri Plureos GmbH
in Hamburg, Germany